Occupation for Health
Volume 1

A Journey
From Self Health to Prescription

Ann A Wilcock

With a contribution from Clephane Hume

Foreword
HRH The Princess Royal

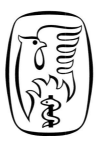

British Association and College of Occupational Therapy 2001

British Association and College of Occupational Therapists
106-114 Borough High Street
Southwark
London SE1 1LB
UNITED KINGDOM

Website www.cot.org.uk

ISBN number   0-9539375-1-8

British Library Cataloguing in Publication Data
A catalogue record for this book is available from the British Library

Editor: Clare Hocking, University of Technology, Auckland, New Zealand
Frontispieces: Therese Schmid, University of Newcastle, NSW, Australia and
Daniel Pitman, Tracey Greenway
Clerical Assistants: Kathleen Moran and Derek Wilcock

Indexed by Dr Laurence Errington in association with First Edition
Translations Ltd, Cambridge.
Printed by The Lavenham Press Limited. Suffolk

This history is dedicated to the memory of Nathalie Barr (née Smythe) MBE FCOT 1910-1993 whose generous legacy to the College of Occupational Therapists made it possible.

To
Patricia Fisher
Enjoy the Journey

[signature]
13ᵗʰ October 2001.

i

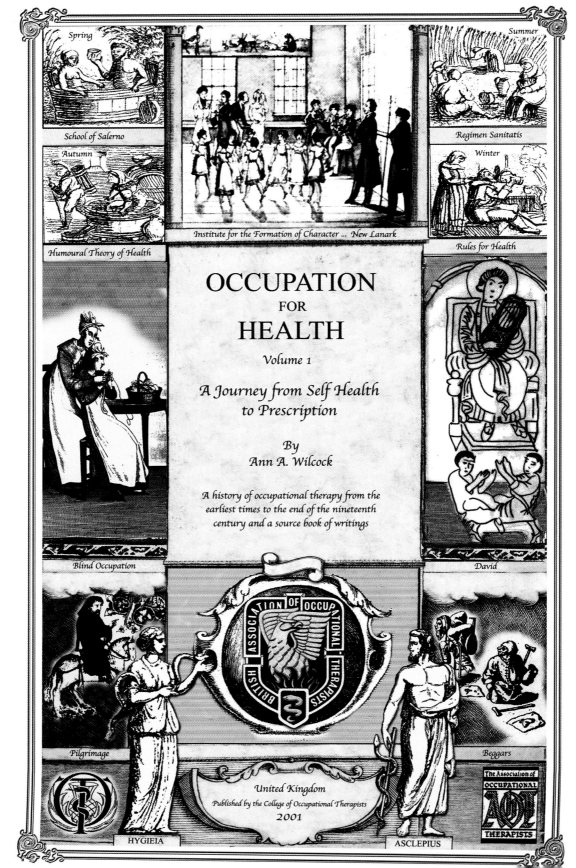

Spring

School of Salerno

Summer

Regimen Sanitatis

Autumn

Winter

Institute for the Formation of Character ... New Lanark

Humoural Theory of Health

Rules for Health

OCCUPATION
FOR
HEALTH

Volume 1

*A Journey from Self Health
to Prescription*

By
Ann A. Wilcock

A history of occupational therapy from the
earliest times to the end of the nineteenth
century and a source book of writings

Blind Occupation

David

Pilgrimage

Beggars

United Kingdom
Published by the College of Occupational Therapists
2001

HYGIEIA

ASCLEPIUS

The Association of OCCUPATIONAL THERAPISTS

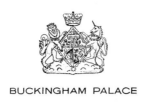

BUCKINGHAM PALACE

As Patron of the College of Occupational Therapists, I am delighted to commend this history to you.

I believe that it sets out, for the first time, the rich heritage of the occupational therapy profession, which came to be formally named in the early twentieth century but has its roots in the thinking and approaches to health of people from bygone times.

The story it tells of this long and exciting journey uncovers connections with some of the best known social and creative visionaries of past centuries. It also provides an opportunity for today's occupational therapists, students and support staff to revisit, with new insights, their approach to tackling the challenges of the modern day.

The history should be of interest not only to occupational therapists but also to people in all walks of life, enabling them to understand better the importance of occupation in health. We hope that it will contribute to a new understanding of this fundamental concept internationally so that it can be used to improve the lives of people across the world.

Anne

Contents

Volume one

Editor
Clare Hocking, University of Technology, Auckland, New Zealand

Frontispieces
Therese Schmid, University of Newcastle, NSW, Australia
Daniel Pitman
Tracey Greenway

Contributors
Clephane Hume

Clerical Assistants
Kathleen Moran
Derek Wilcock

Acknowledgements
My sincerest thanks go to:
- Natalie Barr, for her generous bequest which made the writing of this history a possibility.
- Beryl Steeden, Tracey Greenway, colleagues and associates at the College of Occupational Therapy who provided practical assistance, and encouraged me by making what proved to be an overwhelming task seem valuable and worthwhile.
- my family, friends and colleagues in Australia and the UK who provided invaluable support during what proved to be the most traumatic years of my life, and encouraged me to keep going with my occupational therapy - the history project. In particular I mention my late husband Derek, and companion dog, Polly, along with Cecilie Bearup, Ann Carnduff, Janet Crowe, Maeve Groome, Bruce Heyward, Clare Hocking, Peggy Jay, Anne and Peter Kendall, Coralie Law, Caroline Marshall, Jim May, the late Kathleen Moran, Catherine Paterson, Barry Pitman, Vee Pols, Hugh Stewart, Gail Whiteford, and Alison Wicks.
- Therese Schmid, and Daniel Pitman for hard work, and long days involved in the chapter frontispiece illustrations, and the University of Newcastle, NSW, Australia for providing financial support for Therese's contribution.
- Clare Hocking for her commitment, thoroughness, and long hours spent in editing this volume.
- To the friendly and efficient bespoke service provided by The Lavenham Press Limited, Terence Dalton, Elisabeth Whitehair and Trudy Wilcox.
- The Assistance provided by the Wellcome Library, the British Library, the Borthwick Institute, York, the Royal Star and Garter Homes, Richmond, the New Lanark Trust, The Octavia Hill Society, Wisbech, and the Bethlem Royal Hospital Archives and Museum.

Part 1

Primitive Times

Chapter 1

A History of Occupational Therapy

Contents

This text is the first volume of two devoted to a history of occupational therapy, centering on the United Kingdom. Such a history is important because it tells of the development of a relatively poorly understood approach to health, which differs from mainstream medicine yet, is complementary to it. That approach, which holds that engagement in meaningful and satisfying occupation is important to health, has a surprisingly long history in that this relationship has been recognised for many centuries by physicians and others for both its preventive and therapeutic potentialities. Tracing the origin of the profession up to the end of the nineteenth century is the focus of the first volume. The second tells the story of the profession's development in the United Kingdom during the twentieth century with its links to practice in other parts of the world.

In this short, introductory chapter, the need for and nature of the history will be discussed. The historical method used will be explained, along with a justification for making it a source book with major extracts of original material. The two aspects of its main title, occupation for health, will be considered briefly, and the story of the sub titles of the two volumes told. Next, what is included in definitions of occupational therapy in the twentieth century will be reviewed, because in many ways that provided the starting point for exploration and the boundaries to what is included. That last point is important to bear in mind, because what emerges from the historical exploration is not exactly the same as what has been central to practice in the twentieth century because the context and the needs of the times differed. That provides a rationale for including contextual material to make sense of the history, and to make analysis possible. A final point to consider concerns fascinating thoughts and facts about who were the occupational therapists before the profession was formally created.

The need for and nature of the history

The history of occupational therapy is a very young field of study. Authors of major occupational therapy texts have used potted histories to introduce readers to present approaches to the field[1]. A few books like Macdonald's history of the remedial services[2], Anderson and Bell's story of the profession in Australia[3], or Breines' perspective of the pragmatist origins of the profession in America[4], have specifically addressed the history of the profession from a national or particular point of view. The first of those has proved to be a very useful source of data in this history, and has been drawn upon extensively. Such histories have been augmented by chapters in books such as Paterson's historical perspective of work practice services in Work Practices: International Perspectives,[5] and papers in occupational therapy journals, like Peloquin's on Moral Treatment,[6] or MacDonald's tracing of the history of the British Association.[7] Internationally, possibly more is known about the history of the profession in America than the United Kingdom, because it was named and framed there. Despite that, many of the ideas that led to the establishment of the professional association in the United States early in the twentieth century originated in Europe and the United Kingdom. These ideas were of great social significance, worthy of teasing out and analysing in terms of present day practice.

Whilst histories of occupational therapy have, in the main, concentrated on developments in the twentieth century since people have been formally named and trained as occupational therapists, some have recognised its much earlier origin. Macdonald, for example linked it as part of:

> ... a common heritage of the experiments and discoveries to which the astrologers, artists, engineers, mathematicians, medicine-men, philosophers, physicians, priests and scientists contributed throughout the ages, and the common basic medical and scientific subjects which were ultimately evolved,[8]

suggesting that:

> Many of the particular elements which form the framework of each of the particular therapeutic services were distinguishable from an early date, and it would seem that some may have origins further back than history has recorded. Occupations were used to divert the tormented mind from disease or misery and to provide normal forms of exercise; massage was used even before anatomy was known; exercises were used for treatment and recreation; ... The techniques were not all fully assembled as bases for medical treatment however, until centuries later, and only in these last decades have the relevant parts been welded into the particular structures of the particular services.[9]

Occupational therapy historians have particularly noted Moral Treatment, a humane approach to mental illness in the late eighteenth and nineteenth century, as a precursor to the modern discipline.[10,11] Apart from this only a few references trace other origins in ancient forms of medical regimes. This may be because the mix of remedies in earlier times, and the overlap between modern day specialities, means that it is difficult to give examples of early forms of occupational regimes in a way that matches exactly 20th century professional interventions.

The apparent scarcity of information about the history of occupational therapy is partly due to its rather obscure place within medicine and to a lack of understanding of occupation as an entity in itself and of its relationship to health. Additionally, professional associations in the field are relatively recent and there are only small numbers of therapists in comparison to medicine. Because of this there has been little interest in the task from health historians or from overly busy occupational therapy practitioners, although in recent years interest, particularly from academics in the field, has increased. The history of medicine, despite it being written at all periods, usually by medical men in search of earlier observations on which to base their treatment claims, is itself a relatively new area of study. It has mostly been concentrated upon uncovering those past approaches to health most similar to the current discipline, such as pharmaceutical, surgical, dietary, and hygiene practices with regard to illness. There are, in medical histories, occasional references to exercise and occupations. However, like reference to the promotion of health or prevention of illness, they tend to be treated as peripheral by historians, and are often difficult to find because they not always catalogued in indexes in a relevant format. In putting this history together it has been necessary to seek out those occasional references, and to gather information from other sources about the kaleidoscope of concerns which form part of modern occupational therapy.

Another reason for the scarcity of information about the history of occupation work in health is that the social and economic role of occupation has meant that some initiatives were not viewed as contributing to health. This is particularly the case in terms of social and community health, until recent times when these have become specialist interests in public health and within occupational therapy. The latter interest is not surprising as occupation has provided much of the context for social and community interaction, and the use of occupational regimes towards health and well-being has to take into account their social and communal nature if a balanced lifestyle is to be attained.

Because occupation is so much a part of the fabric of everyday living,[12] healing by less ordinary means was more often seen as "health work" than a recommended regime of occupation. Additionally, whilst in most remedial health professions the services given direct attention towards the problems being overcome, the opposite has often been the case in occupational therapy; the therapist in many cases directing the recipient's attention away from the specific problems and towards occupational achievement.[13]

Writers tend to write about the unknown rather than the commonsense, the extraordinary rather than the ordinary, the explicit rather than the implicit. Because of this there are few historical texts dealing, in any depth, with the therapeutic effects of "doing" healthily, although many allude to it and address it as part of other health agendas. Even so, a substantial amount of information can be dredged from such sources as there are, providing a clear picture that occupational regimes for health have been ongoing throughout human history. This picture, and the various themes that form its substance, should provide insight into the important role of occupational therapy, and ground future developments in preventive, remedial, adaptive and health promoting directions.

It is of particular importance to trace earlier versions of the therapeutic use of occupations for health because people have tended to think of it as a recent phenomenon. Further, the therapeutic application of occupation is viewed as having relatively minor importance in the current health care climate, which values heroic, technological, expensive and life saving interventions over sensible and simple regimes aimed at prevention and/or well-being. Lack of awareness of a long and significant history has allowed many occupational therapists to base their practice on recent values or ideas, often founded upon those of other human service industries. For some in the profession, that tendency has resulted in a "rudderless ship without an anchor in an unchartered sea" syndrome, or the limiting of practice opportunities to those of a known "port" in which particular contributions are welcome. The discovery of a rich and surprisingly stable history of great antiquity, may help provide the courage to leave port, and supply a rudder and an anchor for the exciting journey ahead.

Because of the extent of twentieth century advances in all things medical and technological there is danger of condemning the past unheard, or treating it as interesting but largely irrelevant. Contemptuous tolerance and self contented application of modern standards to earlier practices, motives and conditions fails to appreciate the impact of context on service, or that change is possible. The many brilliant observations and vigorous search for factors important to health, well-being and happiness provide an invaluable resource on which to base future developments. Harnessing the brilliant ideas of great thinkers of the past can do more than display erudition about antiquarian points of view. It is only possible to understand policy if we know its history, and to understand the place and potential of occupational therapy if we know of initiatives and movements in the past. In that regard, a comment from the great medical historian Henry Sigerist is worth considering and rephrasing. He said, 'medical history is medicine also', which made valuable contributions 'by looking at medicine from the outside.'[14] This history of occupational therapy and its antecedents is also aimed at being therapeutic for the profession by providing a chance to consider itself afresh, according to assessment from outside its regular preoccupations that may then inform future directions.

The historical method

In trying to reconstruct the story of occupational therapy and its antecedents, source material has to be found for investigation. Because the evidence being searched out may be from hundreds or thousands of years ago the resources are scarce, and may not be recognisable at first glance. A historian often does not immediately understand the significance of some information until other glimpses from another perspective suddenly emerge and connections are made. That is more often than not because the world of the past is very different to the present. The closer the history comes to the present, the more numerous the sources and that is reflected in the following chapters. By the second volume the source material, in many ways, was at a point of overload, and arbitrary decisions about what or what not to include have had to be made. Those decisions will never satisfy all readers, but provide a place for more histories to be undertaken, and more insights to be experienced.

Because of the often hidden nature of occupational regimes and therapy, sources other than health texts need to be considered. For example, the ideas held by philosophers at various times provide an indication of the views held about important issues during their lifetimes. As these affect practical aspects of peoples lives such as how they deal with sickness, or spend their time, it is as important to use these as a source of contextual material as it is to record actual events, or the ideas held at any one time by physicians alone.

What this history will attempt to do is to uncover early forms of "occupation work" towards mental, physical, social and community health, including the evolution of adaptations to assist daily living, which is so much a part of modern practice. It will do so using a critical and analytical history of ideas approach because this sort of analysis enables the viewing of changing trends in theory and practice as part of societal and economic contexts and ideas. This will not only provide information about our past, it will help in the appreciation of the profession's present stance and possible future directions.

The selection of material that is gathered for any text, as well as the analysis, depends upon the point of view brought to the task. Like any history, the selection as well as the story told will reflect the interest and bias of the historian. This history is likely to reflect my long-term engagement in occupational therapy in both physical and psychological fields of practice and academia along with a current fascination in the relationship between occupation and health, and the need for occupational justice to ensure health and well-being for all people.

The task of selection in the first volume would be less unequivocal if there was a clear body of knowledge recorded within medical histories that dealt with, for example, prescribing occupation for remedial purposes or the independence of people with disability. As medical histories have not been directed to such ends, at first glance, many of them appear barren of relevant material and somewhat destitute of landmarks of specific interest to this history. Those factors, along with awareness of the wide-ranging interests of current day occupational therapists, required a searching out of material from a whole range of sources. Gradually the stories became entwined with the social history of economic change, government initiatives and policies, and causes of great significance deemed by social activists to be necessary for the well-being of individuals and communities. The long lasting effects of developments associated with the occupations followed in daily life at different periods had subsequent effects on health. It sometimes took many ages to effect changes to improve the health experiences of general populations, which in many cases were caused by occupational factors, and alleviated by better understanding of the "natural" occupational needs.

The movement of change was so gradual that it is only through comparison over considerable periods that it becomes apparent. For that reason the story is told in chapters which were picked according to predetermined periods of known change. Although many ideas arise, appear to flourish, only to fade out of the picture, few of them leave no trace, and many are rediscovered, time and time again. It has been startling to find that many of the practices or developments attributed to twentieth century occupational therapists had earlier but relatively unknown predecessors. That is true in the case of ideas and philosophies about occupation, health and happiness, as well as practicalities like the Nelson knife, the need for rails on steps and stairs, and the usefulness of rocking as a treatment technique.

Delving into primary sources, the texts of the time, has been necessary for much of both volumes. Particularly in relation to the first volume, it is important to know of such sources in their original form and context, so use will be made of substantial extracts. Because of this, the language included may not be that which is currently acceptable or politically or professionally correct. He, or man, for example is used almost to the exclusion of female nouns or pronouns unless addressing particular health concerns, or occupations of women. If the revisiting of the context of ideas, language and practices is not done in this way it is difficult for the author, and the reader, to appreciate approaches in terms of the values of the time in which they were written. Accordingly, the history could only be viewed from today's perspectives.

The use of extensive extracts from original sources will mean that this history can be used as a source book for other enquiries, which will be of benefit because some of the early texts are particularly difficult to uncover or are unusual to find in local or occupational therapy libraries. Seeing the words of the authors, in the style of the period, permits a greater understanding of their points of view and the context in which they wrote. It provides a different experience for readers than only being provided with the historian's interpretation of what was written. The source for much of this material has been the British Library and the Wellcome Library. Other specialist archives, such as the Imperial War Museum and the Bethlem and Maudesley Archives in London, the Borthwick Institute in York, the Lancaster Asylum Archives in Preston, and the Gartnaval Hospital Archives in Glasgow have also been accessed.

Many of the stories from the old, rich and stable history told in this volume were the unexpected rewards of an extensive and wide-ranging search of ancient texts. The exploration was wide ranging, because, in setting out to write about "early" history it was important to recognise the timeless intertwining of economics, politics, events and health carer roles. Such intertwining makes it impossible to trace a clear path of the development of the profession by studying, for example, only the history of medicine. Whilst it was valuable to view from a broad standpoint, it was also necessary to try to pick out and piece together that which appears relevant to current practice and thought. Again, so diverse is the modern profession, that disparate sources proved fruitful. Whilst few of the examples selected in the text appear to stand out as unequivocal antecedents of the twentieth century profession, the way in which they appear to inter-relate is remarkable, a fact which is hard to gauge from less extensive histories.

Also within the texts, there will be some original contributions by other authors, mainly in the second volume. They draw upon particular expertise within the community of occupational therapists, such as Clephane Hume in relation to the Bible, Catherine Patterson's extensive knowledge of Scottish occupational therapy history and the stories of specialist groups within the British Association and from schools of training.

The use of secondary sources, which are accounts 'reacting to the ideas of a primary author,' directed searches towards new or different sources of evidence as well as illuminating the original ideas. Tertiary sources, such as recent books and articles, were similarly useful especially because of the shortness of time available to gather the vast amount of data that there proved to be. In particular it is necessary to acknowledge the value found in the medical histories written by Roy Porter. These not only suggested lines of inquiry, but also presented cogent analyses and theories that were often relevant to this history and remarkably compelling. His work has been drawn on, extensively, to provide context as well as ideas, in part, again because of the shortness of time. Another particularly useful source has been Henry Sigerist, a medical practitioner and historian who provided substantial histories of medicine in the early middle period of the twentieth century which were enriched by some of his health philosophies that obviously emerged from his research. The story which emerges from this process, though, does not follow already well-trodden paths, or 'simply recreate another authors interpretation of the past', but opens up 'new avenues of investigation, criticism and reflection' from an occupational therapist's perspective of history.[15]

Immersion in the data was an important step in understanding and interpreting just what might be described as occupation for health (or occupational therapy) in each age. Whilst attempting to consider the context from the start of the exploration it was not until I was immersed in the data from a particular period that I began to experience some sense of what drove people's lives in terms of health. Of course this was a very limited experience, but I recall vividly the glow of understanding, when the breakthroughs occurred. Those were exciting times, like when I "knew" that spiritual health was the underlying and all-embracing belief system of the middle ages to the extent that health care encompassed only those physiological ideas which were compatible with the provider's faith. Their faith was the major force in what they believed about health and in what they did to restore or maintain it. So the occupations called upon in terms of maintaining or restoring health were those of a moral nature and spiritual purpose, as well as those considered useful according to humoural physiology.

In the early stages, prior to immersion in the data, and whilst my understanding was only intellectual, I continued to look for evidence of occupation being used as therapy in similar ways and for similar reasons as in modern times. It was only when I reached a deeper stage of understanding that it was possible to appreciate that the nature and philosophy of any "occupational therapy" of a given period would differ according to, not only the physiological explanation of health and illness, but also the dominant beliefs and social contexts. What was of fundamental importance in the process was becoming conscious of the context of people's lives, ideas and values, at any period, from their perspective.

Sigerist, recognised that context was of primary importance. In The Social History of Medicine, a paper read before a meeting of the California Academy of Medicine in San Francisco, on March 11, 1940, Sigerist drew his audience's attention to the degree to which context had been neglected in past histories. Rather, these histories, principally, told the stories of the great men of medicine's heritage rather than the social needs of their clients. In this history, an attempt has been made to address issues of both context and heritage in order to clarify why certain occupational initiatives towards physical, social, mental or spiritual health were paramount at any one time. That has meant that although the history is, in large part, dependent on the story of the great and of the books they wrote, and even of the "firsts" of what became more accepted practices, it was external circumstances which triggered the need for answers, in most cases. Sigerist added that he had found from his studies 'that many great discoveries were made simultaneously by various people', and in that belief, this history has supposed that the single stories told are representative of many similar ones.[16]

Sigerist shocked his medical audiences more than once by saying 'medicine is not so much a natural as a social science'. He suggested that the goal was not only to cure disease and restore an organism by applying methods of science, but to keep an individual 'adjusted to his environment as a useful member of society or to readjust him (or her) as the case may be'. Whilst many might say that those are often the last issues to be considered in much of modern medicine, with its interest in the scientific, the same cannot be said of occupational therapists, for whom it is central. Sigerist also reminded his audience of the two parties involved in the process of care, so that the history of medicine could not limit itself to:

> ... the history of the science, institutions, and characters of medicine, but must include the history of the patient in society, that of the physician, and the history of the relations between physician and patient. History thus becomes social history.[17]

Such is the case in occupational therapy, and so a broader range of texts has been consulted to provide some insights into what that might have been at any time. There is limited information on such relationships, however, so some inferences have to be made from the contextual information as a whole.

To further illustrate the importance of context a brief overview of spiritual health is useful. It can be suggested that that is a less central issue within modern occupational therapy in comparison to earlier times. Throughout history some people sought healing from religion not medicine. Religious medicine in ancient Greece and Rome drew upon the healing cult of Aesculapius, in whose temples miracle cures were performed. In the time of the early Christian church and in the Middle Ages prayer was a central aspect of treatment for all ailments. For those with mental disorder, incantations and exorcism were logical therapy, as they were believed to be possessed by evil spirits. Magic and witchcraft were once considered legitimate sciences and women could be persecuted as witches. Although, even in the present day, some Christian sects practice faith healing, those earlier therapeutic practices cannot be considered without understanding the culture and belief systems of the times.[18]

As times changed medicine excluded the transcendental, developing instead a rational, empirical base of observation and reason, followed by research and science. Treatment using occupation changed along side it and as part of it, and will continue to change. In the twentieth century most occupational therapists have been used to working for state-based health and social services which has resulted in them following certain types of practice. That context is beginning to change and it could be that future practice will be very different, just as the work of physicians differed over the centuries as medicine evolved.

Representative of the contextual nature of the history are the chapter frontispieces which provide a conceptual map of the material to be found in the chapter encased in pictorial material illustrative of the social fabric of the times. Often that material is based on sections of artwork of, or depicting the period.

The main frontispieces of each volume are based on the wonderful sepia Frontespiece of Robert Burton's 17th century Anatomy of Melancholy which is pictured in chapter 5 of this volume: The Renaissance, Humanism and Beyond: Occupational Regimes for Social and Mental Health. The collage in the Frontispiece for this volume is a collection of illustrations representing different periods in history, different aspects of occupation for health, linked with the current British Association badge, and the early badges of English and Scottish Occupational Therapy Associations. The classical gods represent Aesculapius, the god of medicine, and Hygiea, the goddess of health. Other representations include David playing the harp to sooth Saul with music; the occupations of the four seasons from early depictions of the Regimen Sanitatis, the six rules for health, which over the centuries maintained occupation, as action and rest as one of them; and Chaucer riding his horse on a pilgrimage. Also included are disabled beggars earning their livelihood with drawings and lute playing; children dancing as part the social health initiatives at the industrial community of New Lanark; and a blind child in the nineteenth century being enabled to learn knitting. See appendix for the source of these illustrations.

Explaining the title: Occupation, health, self health and prescription

Occupation for Health was the theme chosen by the College of Occupational Therapists for their 1998 annual conference, held that year in Belfast. As it was the year that research into this history commenced it seemed fitting to adopt that as the main title for the two volumes.

Occupational therapy is founded upon the notion that occupation can affect health in a positive way to such an extent that very complex therapeutic notions have developed over the twentieth century as part of a profession named and framed around it. As before then no such profession existed, it could be supposed that it arose according to the specific requirements of the time. That presupposes that the profession may only have a legitimate life whilst those conditions remain. If on the other hand, it had existed in various guises, and been carried on as part of other health or social service activities, then it can obviously be of continued use even when conditions change. That has proved to be the case, and so the title of occupation for health appears applicable to both volumes.

Occupation encompasses all the things that people do, is part of their being, and integral to their becoming whatever they have the potential to become. Occupation has a biological purpose in that it is the mechanism by which people, throughout time, have acquired all they require to survive and all they need to accomplish in order to be safe and feel good. Occupation is a natural mechanism for health in that it exercises mind and body, and has the potential to keep all parts of the human organism honed and working well. It is also the means of social interaction and spiritual well-being, all of which work together through the integrative functions of the central nervous system in a holistic way to create health. MacDonald named some of the occupations that she found had been used for health purposes throughout history. They included:

> ... *music, songs, violin playing and dancing; horse-riding, hunting, fishing, swimming, rowing and sailing; sawing and chopping wood, working with a hammer; digging and following the plow[19], ringing church bells; throwing stones and darts; boxing; walking or ambling; sweeping, sewing, weaving, pottery making; domestic activities and those of daily living; and, for those who could afford it, travelling.[20]*

Health has been described simply as the 'well working of the organism as a whole'[21] which clearly links it with occupation, the fundamental mechanism used to "work the organism". According the World Health Organisation it is more that the absence of illness but encompasses physical, social and mental well-being. In its Charter for Health Promotion it is suggested how that vision of health can be achieved. The Charter states that 'to reach a state of complete physical, mental and social well-being, an individual or group must be able to identify and to realise aspirations, to satisfy needs and to change or cope with the environment'.[22] As occupation is the fundamental mechanism by which people 'realise aspirations, satisfy needs and cope with the environment' the links between occupation and health are clear for all to see.[23]

In terms of the sub-titles, several different versions appeared to be appropriate at various stages of the exploration, but towards the end, the present ones, From self health to Prescription and From Prescription to self health, clearly emerged from analyses of the collected data, and were chosen. The "self health" ideology seemed to fit well with the profession's philosophies, and is becoming more and more central as therapists take an enabling approach to practice in the present day. In terms of prescription, it can be strongly argued that practice and development have been both facilitated and later proscribed by the medical profession's prescriptions.

Defining occupational therapy to set boundaries

Defining occupational therapy seems to be a surprisingly difficult task, and many occupational therapists confide that they hate being asked "what it is". Its difference from other health professions closer to the medical model is one of the perceived difficulties, yet that is also its strength.

The earliest formal definitions usually included aiding or hastening recovery following mental or physical disease or injury through the use of prescribed and guided activity. John Colson's 1945 definition in The Rehabilitation of the

Injured: Occupational Therapy is such a one. Colson was a member of the Chartered Society of Physiotherapy, and the Ling Physical Education Association, as well as of the Association of Occupational Therapists. In a series with a common main title, he chose to write about occupational therapy first, because of a dearth of books in the field, and requests for such a text. Those requests for 'a book which presents occupational therapy as a form of remedial exercise' came from 'many surgeons and medical men developing rehabilitation at home and in the Dominions.'[24] Colson's definition was:

> *… the use of any occupation which is prescribed and guided for the purpose of contributing to and hastening the rehabilitation of the unfit. It may be considered from both the physical and mental aspects, as it is employed in the rehabilitation of physical disabilities following trauma and disease, and in the treatment of mental disorders.*[25]

Definitions gradually became more complicated, adding notions of spiritual health, social dysfunction, prevention of disability, maintenance and promotion of health, enhancement of functional performance, facilitation of skills, adaptation to disability, environmental modification, independence, and quality of life.

On a quite different tangent around the idea of determining "what it is" is the notion of praxis. That notion, which is intimate to the idea of "doing" and well-being, has excited the interest of philosophers throughout time. It has been identified with the practice of occupational therapy by H. Tristram Englehart, a physician and philosopher who reflected that rather than a somatic, psychological, or even social work model of practice, occupational therapy followed a praxial model.[26] The word praxis, from the Greek for "of action", was adopted into Latin and the modern European languages. It is defined in the Oxford English Dictionary as 'doing, acting, action, practice', yet in another dictionary it is defined as "accepted practice or custom".[27] According to Lobkowicz it 'refers to almost any kind of activity which a free man is likely to perform; in particular, all kinds of business and political activity'.[28] In "praxiology" - the science of efficient action, the discipline deals 'with methods of doing anything in any way … from the point of view of its effectiveness'[29] Many writers, or translators of old texts replace the word praxis with the more common word "practical", although this is not its true meaning. It is, perhaps, the closest philosophical concept to how occupation is viewed by occupational therapists. To define occupational therapy as a praxial model of practice might be worth considering, if this definition was linked with mental, physical, social and spiritual health in order to make the difference clear. In a similar vein, Englehardt suggested, in line with the notion that "humans are occupational beings", that:

> *… in viewing humans as engaged in activities, realising themselves through their occupations … occupational therapy supports a view of the whole person in function and adaptation often absent in somatic medicine, the psychological health care professions, and social work as well. The virtue of occupation is engagement in the world.*[30]

MacDonald, in World-Wide Conquests of Disabilities: The History, Development and Present Functions of the Remedial Services, provided a combined practical definition of the work of the physiotherapists, remedial gymnasts, and occupational therapists which emphasised their similarities. She wrote that collectively they worked towards 'health and the ability of people to live as actively and as independently as possible in their social and economic conditions' by contributing to:

> ... the investigation and treatment of disease and injury, and to enable the patient to attain the highest level of his capacity, compatible with his life circumstances. This covers physical, psychological, social and economic considerations in the patients rehabilitation, although there may be more emphasis on one aspect or another according to the techniques used, and the particular needs of the individual patient.[31]

Of occupational therapy itself, she too claimed that it was 'the least easily definable treatment service, because it covers a wider range of forms of application and of cases to be treated'. Despite that, she provided the following description:

> Occupational therapy is the term applied to therapeutic work and to appropriate purposeful occupations which include recreations and certain forms of hobbies, and activities of daily living which include self-care, inter-relationships and travelling. It is prescribed for the distinct purpose of contributing to a patient's recovery from disease, injury or disability and to re-establishment in life. It was originally evolved from the sedative, pleasurable or pastime activities of early Egyptian and Greek days, which were used to divert, to heal, and to fit men for war. It should be emphasised that occupational therapy has as its aim assessment, contributions to diagnosis, and treatment; it is not wholly aimed at production or money making, nor actual vocational training, but patients can be prepared for the latter, and can be passed on to special training centres when they have been improved in their treatment. In some cases it is necessary for diversions to be offered.
>
> Physical occupational therapy includes assessing and contributing to the patients' abilities in their activities of daily living, and the planning of their resettlement. This calls for equipment adaptation as it involves the muscle re-education, training in coordination, mobilisation of joints, building up of strength, dexterity and work tolerance, re-education in work habits, retraining in specific movements and skills, and preparation for resettlement through special units, when applicable.
>
> Psychological occupational therapy includes re-socialisation of the patients who have psycho-social dysfunctions, and it contributes to encouragement in re-adaptation for normal living, helps in overcoming anxiety, and in satisfying basic needs ... Some patients need to be persuaded to take an interest in other people in their community, to relate more easily to them, and to recognise the interests and responsibilities which they can adopt to develop a satisfactory degree of competence and acceptance.
>
> Occupational therapy for children is applied to those with physical

disabilities, including the cerebral palsied, and to those with psychological problems. It calls for an understanding and secure relationship between the therapist and the child-patient. The purpose is mainly to help these children to live their lives as normally as possible, and to give them the appropriate security and interests.[32]

There have also been definitions particularly associated with one or other aspect of the work. In mental health definitions in the 1950s, experts in the field explained their ideas further. Stafford Clark, for example, in Psychiatry Today, described occupational therapy as an active method of treatment with a profound psychological justification,[33] and Fleming in Social Psychology of Education that occupational therapy for patients with psychosocial dysfunction helps to satisfy basic needs for security, adventure, recognition and response.[34]

In the Directory of Private Practitioners 2000, the British College of Occupational Therapists defines it as:
… the treatment of people with physical and psychiatric illness or disability through specific selected occupation for the purpose of enabling individuals to reach their maximum level of function and independence in all aspects of life. The occupational therapist assesses the physical, psychological and social functions of the individual, identifies areas of dysfunction and involves the individual in a structured programme of activity to overcome disability. The activities selected will relate to the consumer's personal, social, cultural and economic needs and will reflect the environmental factors which govern his/her life.[35]

The definitions, although very general, provide some indication of the scope of the history and the range of ideas to be researched. The words occupation (specific, selected) and activity (prescribed, guided, structured) are, of course, paramount, but others are of obvious importance. Those range through mental or physical disease, disability, injury or fitness; hastening recovery, rehabilitation, enabling individuals, function and independence; and personal, social, cultural and economic needs. Also important are environmental factors; all aspects of life; active method of treatment with a profound psychological justification; basic needs for security, adventure, recognition and response; re-socialisation, resettlement, work tolerance, re-education and skills; recreations, activities of daily living, self-care, inter-relationships, diversion, healing, and fitting men for war. Others have emerged as the history progressed and include important concepts such as spiritual health, social health and activism; environmental and economic factors; health promotion and illness prevention; and communal, philosophical and political activity.

In some respects, data will be looked for which address any of those aspects. In the main, the ongoing health-care task of occupational therapists is bounded within five major headings, namely the application of an occupational approach to:

- Adaptation following disability and handicap
- Rehabilitation and habilitation
- Restoration of health
- Prevention of illness, or the
- Promotion of health.

Pride in a holistic perspective to the work suggests that within all those broad areas of practice occupational therapists are interested in mental, physical, social, and spiritual health for individuals or communities of any age group, or social strata.

In order to position and analyse the past, occupational therapy historians, in a way similar to medical historians, must ascertain what the health and occupational conditions were in any given society and period. They must ask what the environmental, economic and ideological conditions were that influenced those conditions in order to appreciate the occupational measures taken to promote or improve health, to prevent or reduce illness. That means that public and occupational health histories, social and educational histories, social activist or philosophy histories, are as important to consider as remedial service histories. Inclusion of such material will make clear some of the restrictions or possibilities open to those endeavouring to use an occupational approach to health care at any time, including the explanations for the nature of health problems and for the intervention. They are not judged as good or bad in comparison with modern day approaches, but with an eye to similarities and differences. As Sigerist, so aptly, wrote 'Nothing could be more foolish in comparing ancient theories with ours than to call progressive what corresponds to our views, and primitive what is different'.[36]

Proto-occupational therapists

An important question for this text to address is "who were the occupational therapists before the modern profession?" Just as for other current day professions, initially they were ordinary individuals living their lives the best way they could within their family and kinship groups and extended communities. They followed practices which instinctively made them feel good, and which did not appear to cause discomfort or death, just as they would have applied their own methods of justice to create an effective working community to meet the needs of survival, and as animals living naturally do today.

Therapy probably also included some altruistic action towards others in their social group, and particularly for those with kinship ties. This will be discussed further in the next chapter, but points to the first occupational therapists being individuals acting altruistically towards themselves and towards kin. This trend is still apparent in the common sayings of today like 'I am doing this as therapy' or 'what you need to do to feel better is …,' and was a fact of life for the vast majority of the population up to the arrival of "modern medicine" and some notion of "welfare states". Based on evidence of the period, and despite the existence of physicians and surgeons, people, other than the well-to-do, acted as their own health providers even as late as the eighteenth and nineteenth centuries.

Indeed Sigerist asked,

> … who was a physician and who not? … The great majority of all cases of illness, moreover, even today, are never seen by a physician. They are treated by the patient himself or by his relatives. And this self treatment may be according to principles of the scientific medicine of the time.[37]

Apart from self-medicine and kin-medicine, anyone could, and many did, call themselves physicians, until legislation to counter that practice in the 19th century. Yet the history of medicine is timeless, and includes the stories of practitioners long before specific university training began.

In similar vein, as there is no evidence of particular people whose job it was to provide health care through occupation as their sole role until possibly the nineteenth century, it is important to recognise other people who included it as part of their life roles. In this way it is possible to identify medicine men, shaman and priests along with other religious personnel such as monks and nuns, and people appointed by socio-political institutions to encourage healthy and strong regimes based on how the population engaged in occupation, as in some of the Greek States of the classical period. Also recognised are philosophers and social activists such as those who will be discussed in the Chapters dealing with industrial times; philanthropists, physicians, surgeons and nurses; as well as people employed for various duties relating to the occupation of the poor, prisoners, and patients or inmates in hospitals, institutions and asylums.

As well as socio-political structures to maintain occupation as a central agency in people's lives, there were some people who evaluated people's functional capacities with a socio-political purpose. In that regard, some other legal and political figures, as part of their duties, played theoretical or practical parts in enacting earlier versions of some of occupational therapists' current work. For example, at least from the middle ages onwards, legal systems in England, such as The Court of Wards and the Chancellery, assessed the competence of those thought to have some mental incapacity by using tests devised according to the practical skills people required in their day to day life and occupations.[38]

The history of occupational therapists should not try to prove that their tasks and the results they achieved have always been the same, they will not be and can not be, just as in the future, they will differ again. Any similarities can be noted, and the differences celebrated and learnt from.

In summary, the chapter has introduced this history of occupational therapy, which will tell the story of how engagement in meaningful and satisfying occupation has been used for health and well-being throughout the existence of humankind. It has a surprisingly long history. Whilst the second volume tells the story of the profession's development in the United Kingdom during the twentieth century with its links to practice in other parts of the world, the chapter also introduced the focus of the first volume which traces the origins of occupational therapy up to the end of the nineteenth century. Both the need for and nature of the history were discussed and the historical method and boundaries to what is included explained. That latter point is critical, as what emerges from the historical exploration is not identical to practice in the twentieth century because of differences in context and the needs of particular periods. As Sigerist explained in the mid twentieth century:

> *The scope of medicine broadened from century to century. The society in which we live is different from that of our ancestors. The physician is no longer a medicine man nor a craftsman nor a priest. He has new tasks, new functions, and new weapons. A new medical science serving a new type of society necessarily requires new forms of medical service. … I think that the sociological approach to the history of medicine not only gives us a better understanding of the past but can also help us in planning for the future.*[39]

That can be re-stated in terms of occupation for health:

> *Occupation for health changed from century to century. The society in which we live is different from that of our ancestors. The practitioner is no longer a shaman, nor a nun, nor a craftsman nor a physician. She or he has new tasks, new functions, and new weapons. An emerging occupational science underpinning practice that serves a new type of society necessarily requires new forms of occupational therapy service. I think that a socio-cultural contextual approach to the history of occupational therapy not only gives us a better understanding of the past but can also help us in planning for the future.*

---

[1]See for example: Haworth NH, MacDonald EM. *Theory of Occupational Therapy.* London: Bailliere, Tindall & Cox, 1940 & 1944; Hopkins HL, Smith HD, eds. *Willard and Spackman's Occupational Therapy.* 7th ed. Philadelphia: J.B. Lippincott Co., 1988.

[2]Macdonald EM. *World-Wide Conquests of Disabilities: The History, Development and Present Functions of the Remedial Services.* London: Bailliere Tindall, 1981.

[3]Anderson B, Bell J. *Occupational Therapy: Its Place in Australia's History.* Sydney: NSW Association of Occupational Therapists, 1988.

[4]Breines E. *Origins and Adaptations: A Philosophy of Practice.* Lebanon, NJ: Geri-Rehab, Inc., 1986.

[5]Paterson C. An historical perspective of work practice services. In Pratt J, Jacobs K, eds. *Work Practices: International Perspectives.* Oxford: Butterworth-Heinemann, 1997; 25-38.

[6]Peloquin SM. Moral treatment: Contexts reconsidered. *American Journal of Occupational Therapy* 1989; 43(8): 537-544.

[7]Macdonald EM. History of the Association. *Occupational Therapy* June 1957; 30-33.

[8]Macdonald. *World-Wide Conquests of Disabilities…*; 1.

[9]Macdonald. *World-Wide Conquests of Disabilities…*; 13.

[10]Peloquin. Moral treatment: Contexts reconsidered…; See also: Peloquin SM. Moral treatment: How a caring practice lost its rationale. *American Journal of Occupational Therapy* 1993; 47(2): 167-173.

[11]See, for example: Paterson CF. Rationales for the use of occupation in 19th century asylums. *British Journal of Occupational Therapy* 1997; 60 (4): 179-183; Paterson CF. A short history of occupational therapy in mental health. In: Creek J, ed. *Occupational Therapy in Mental Health*. Edinburgh: Churchill Livingstone, 1996; 3-14.

[12]Wilcock AA. *An Occupational Perspective of Health*. Thorofare, NJ: Slack Inc., 1998.

[13]Macdonald. *World-Wide Conquests of Disabilities…*; 3.

[14]Sigerist HE. *A History of Medicine, Volume I: Primitive and Archaic Medicine*. New York: Oxford University Press, 1955; 6.

[15]Hamilton DB. The idea of history and the history of ideas. *Image: Journal of Nursing Scholarship* 1993: 25(1); 47.

[16]Sigerist HE. The social history of medicine. In: Marti-Ibañez F, ed. *Henry E. Sigerist on the History of Medicine*. New York: MD Publications, Inc.; 1960: 25.

[17]Sigerist. The social history of medicine…; 26.

[18]Sigerist. The social history of medicine.

[19]Mitchell RJ, Lays MDR. *A History of the English People*. London: 1950; 280. (the prescription for Anthony A Wood, of Oxford)

[20]Macdonald. *World-Wide Conquests of Disabilities …*; 13.

[21]Kass LR. Regarding the end of medicine and the pursuit of health. In: Caplan AR, Engelhart HT, McCartney JJ, eds. *Concepts of Health and Disease: Interdisciplinary Perspectives*. Massachusetts: Addison Wesley Publishing Co., 1981.

[22]World Health Organisation, Health and Welfare Canada, Canadian Public Health Association. *The Ottawa Charter for Health Promotion*. Ottawa, Canada: 1986.

[23]Wilcock AA. Biological and sociocultural aspects of occupation, health and health promotion. *British Journal of Occupational Therapy* 1993; 56(6): 200-203.

[24]Colson JHC. *The Rehabiltation of the Injured: Occupational Therapy*. London: Cassell and Company, Ltd., 1945.

[25]Colson. *The Rehabilitation of the Injured…*; 1.

[26]Englehart HT. Defining occupational therapy: The meaning of therapy and the virtues of occupation. *American Journal of Occupational Therapy* 1977; 31(10): 666-672.

[27]*The Oxford English Dictionary*, 2nd ed., Vol XII. Oxford: Clarendon Press, 1989: 130, 633; *The Standard English Desk Dictionary*. Sydney: Bay Books, 1976; 663.

[28]Lobkowicz N. *Theory and Practice: History of Concepts from Aristotle to Marx*. Notre Dame, Ill. and London: University of Notre Dame Press, 1967; 9.

[29]Kotarbinski T. The goal of an act and the task of the agent. In: Gasparski W, Pszczolowski T, eds. *Praxiological Studies: Polish Contributions to the Science of Efficient Action*. Dordrecht, Holland: D Reidel Publishing Company, 1983; 22.

[30]Englehart. Defining occupational therapy…; 672.

[31]Macdonald. *World-Wide Conquests of Disabilities…*; 1-2.

[32]Macdonald EM *Occupational Therapy in Rehabilitation*. London: Bailliere Tindall, 1976.

[33]Stafford Clark D. *Psychiatry Today.* London: Pelican, 1952.

[34]Fleming CM. *Social Psychology of Education.* London: 1959; ch. iv.

[35]Occupational therapists in private practice. *Directory of Private Practitioners 2000.* London: College of Occupational Therapists, 2000; 5.

[36]Sigerist. *A History of Medicine, Volume I…*; 10.

[37]Sigerist. *A History of Medicine, Volume I…*; 7.

[38]Porter R. *Mind-Forg'd Manacles.* London: The Athlone Press, 1987; 112.

[39]Sigerist. The social history of medicine…; 28-33.

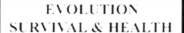

EVOLUTION
SURVIVAL & HEALTH

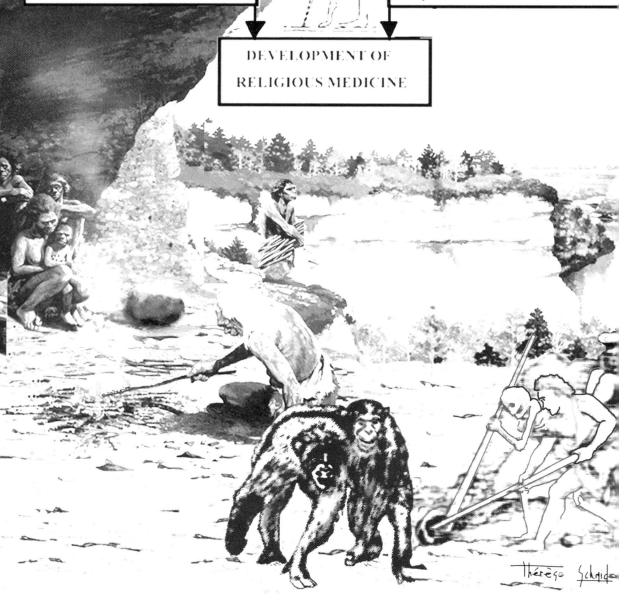

SCIENTIFIC EXPLANATION

Animal species
Natural lifestyle/safety
Instinctive behaviour
Self-health - kin-health
  occupations/exercise, rest
  diet - remedies
Communal health
Spiritual explanations

CHRISTIAN EXPLANATION

God's creation
Fall of humankind
Work for survival and health
Natural lifestyle
Self-health - kin-health
  occupation/exercise, rest
  diet - remedies
Spiritual & social rules

DEVELOPMENT OF

RELIGIOUS MEDICINE

Chapter 2

Nature's Regimen in Primitive and Spiritual Times: Evolution, Survival and Health

Contents

In this chapter some of humankind's journey throughout their early existence is considered from the perspective of the relationship between health and occupation. It is an appropriate place to start the journey of exploration about the history of occupational therapy because what people did, how they engaged, through their occupations, with the outside world was, and still is, an essential aspect of their survival, health and well-being. Whilst health care is traditionally regarded as healing, curing and, in some cases, preventing disease, the characteristic features of any health profession are determined to a large extent by the structure of a society within time; by its general conception of the world, by its attitude towards the human body, and by its valuation of health and disease. In some places, at particular times, the principle focus has been towards health promoting regimens at a societal level, at other times, the saving of individual lives, at any cost, has been deemed the most important part of care.

With the view that occupation is a major physiological mechanism for health, it follows that some aspects of its use for health maintenance and as a means of therapy may be visible across the spectrum of human time. There are, however, different views about how humankind's health journey started, according to the tales told by the ancients, by evolutionary scientists, by Bible chroniclers, and by medical historians. All will be explored briefly.

Early stories tell of gods and mythological creatures and places at the very birth of existence with special powers and attributes that seem essential to the life of humankind on earth. Two such creatures, the phoenix and the snake, were chosen by the English and Scottish Associations of Occupational Therapists as their symbols, the stories of which are told in the second volume of the history.

Because the modern world has largely embraced the scientific stories of evolution that have unfolded in the last century, the place of occupation for health will be traced in those terms. As well, the Bible provides another version of the origins of humankind and also stories about occupation for health in biblical times. As Christianity is the most followed religion in the Western World, it is appropriate that those views are put forward as part of the total picture. The final section will draw on particular tales about the origins of health care told by medical historians that are important to understand as they to, in some places, tell of occupation for health.

Stories told by the ancients

Many modern civilisations organise their lives through faith in the future, believing that humankind will overcome the problems of ill-health and injustices with beneficent politics, technology and scientific knowledge. That belief in a golden age in the future is opposite to stories told by the ancients of a golden age in the remote past which was free from toil and grief. Yet both, somehow, imply that perfect health and happiness are possible–sometime. That illusion has been manifest in many different forms throughout history.

Legends of primitive religions and folklores of most ancient peoples are wont to place this idyllic state in the past, their stories of better times telling of strong and healthy longevity. According to their legends, the ancient Greeks believed such people existed somewhere, and were perhaps people from the Isles of the Blest at the edge of the Western Sea, the Hyperboreans and the Scythians in the north, or the Ethiopians in the south. All of them were supposed to be happy, vigorous and virtuous, free from labour, warfare, disease and old age, feasting 'gaily, undarkened by sufferings', in fact either living in everlasting bliss, or dying, 'as if falling asleep'.[1] In China in the Yellow Emperor's *Classic of Internal Medicine* published in the fourth century BC, it is said that in the distant past 'people lived to a hundred years, and yet remained active and did not become decrepit in their activities'.[2] A reason given was that 'the ancients followed Tao and the laws of the seasons under the guidance of their sages who were credited with the realisation of the value of education in the prevention of disease'.[3] Lao-tzu in *Tao Te Ching* (The Way)[4] and Chuang-tzu also tell how 'the ancient men lived in a world of primitive simplicity' which 'was a time when the yin and the yang worked harmoniously, ... all creation was unharmed, and the people did not die young'.[5] At a later date, Pao Ching-yen asserted that 'man in the morning went forth to his labour on his own accord and rested in the evening. People were free and uninhibited and at peace ... Contagious diseases did not spread, and long life was followed by natural death.'[6]

Such tales and legends are reflected in more recent rationales, which are also based on the notion that perfect health and happiness are possible. Those ideas are apparent in the stories about Utopias, and in the recurrent thought that a return to nature and to naturally healthy ways of living will provide the answers. In the twentieth-century Western people still try to re-establish contact with their forgotten natural past in their choice of food, in natural remedies, country cottages and "get away from it all" holidays.

The occupation for health journey told by evolutionary scientists

There is some truth behind those behaviours and ideas about natural ways of life. Physiological change is very a slow process and humans are little different, in biological terms, from thousands of years ago when they lived a simpler life, much more dependent on the fluctuations of nature to survive and to remain healthy. Because of the biological relationship between occupation and health, when people lived naturally, in a way similar to other species in the wild, nature itself imposed an occupational regimen that maintained health. That is, in order to survive, occupations that provided food, shelter, safety and superiority over predators were a daily requirement. Darwin's theory of evolution implies that any individual with defects that prevented them being effective actors on the environment would usually fail to survive to reproduce.

Life, then, was an adventure in an unpredictable and poorly understood world where dangers must be overcome, and mere existence was a response to challenges between individuals and their environments, often resulting in injury or disease.[7] People's occupations were the way in which they dealt with the dangers and challenges of their environment. Furthermore, these occupations were often of an active nature, demanding a range of physical exercise and mental cunning, as well as being dependent on the social collective of the community in which they lived. Occupations, coupled with times of rest according to diurnal variation and the seasons, and adventure, stimulation and novel experiences through the challenges of a nomadic way of life, kept physical, mental and social capacities honed and healthy. This way of life also supported hygiene because there was little build up of debris to support parasites and bacteria.[8]

Apart from this, in a state of nature people would, in many instances, have determined what occupations made them feel better when they were sick and whether their health improved with restful or energetic activity. Perhaps they adapted occupations or tools so that they were able to carry out their activities of daily life despite dysfunction. Relatives, or other members of a close knit tribe may have recommended particular occupations or adaptations as a result of their own experience. In addition, and in a way similar to the experience of most people with regard to physicians until fairly recently, they would probably not have called upon outside experts to advise on such matters. The caring for self in all matters of health, including the application or use of everyday occupations for therapeutic purposes, is what the title of this history is calling "self health". Finding out about self and kin as self health occupational therapists is important because such activity points to the essential basis of the profession.

In a similar vein, the nurturing, protective and enabling roles of parents and other people within a related or social group lasted until the young were ready, albeit at an early age, to take responsibility for themselves and share in the protection of self and others. Such altruistic caring behaviour is important to bear in mind because it is the basic requirement for people entering the health professions to work with people who are in some ways disadvantaged. To claim that self health and kin-health care was apparent amongst early humankind is an essential part of the history of occupation based therapeutics.

Lack of written records from the times makes substantiating such claims about occupation for health difficult. Use has been made, instead, of accounts provided by evolutionary scientists, historians, anthropologists and ethologists who have drawn conclusions informed by archaeological fragments and by inference from twentieth century cultures which appear similar to those of early humans.

De Waal, a zoologist and ethologist who specialises in primate behaviour, supports the self health hypothesis when he suggests that 'it is hard to take care of others without taking care of oneself first', and that paradoxically 'altruism starts with an obligation to oneself'. He goes on to argue that:

> The form of altruism closest to egoism is care of the immediate family. In species after species, we see signs of kin selection: altruism is disproportionally directed at relatives. Humans are no exception. A father returning with a loaf of bread will ignore the plight of whomever he meets on his path; his first obligation is to his family ... If his family were well fed and everyone else were starving, it would be a different matter - but if his family is as hungry as the rest, the man has no choice. [9]

Altruism, he says, is dependent on what can be afforded, with the potential recipients of morality extending only if 'the health and survival of the innermost circles are secure', and benevolence decreasing 'with increasing distance between people'. When survival appears secure people take care of kin and 'the circle of altruism and moral obligation widens to extended family, clan, and group, up to and including tribe and nation'. People 'build exchange networks with fellow human beings both inside and outside the group' and in comparison with other primates are 'remarkably giving'. Whilst moral inclusion does not imply that everyone is valued equally it is possible that it could embrace all of humanity, and even other species 'depending on what society can afford'.[10]

Providing an even stronger claim that altruism and moral behaviour was apparent in early humans is the knowledge that it can be observed in other primates. Table 1.2.1 from De Waal's *Good Natured: The Origins of Right and Wrong in Humans and Other Animals*, summarises his findings from years of study and observation, which he illustrates with stories. One of interest is about Mozu, a Japanese monkey that roamed the Shiga Heights of the Japanese Alps despite having no hands or feet, a congenital malformation attributed to pesticides. When her story was told, Mozu was eighteen years old and had successfully raised five infants. This is all the more remarkable when it is realised that she was unable to travel through the trees as her peers did, and in the winter had to carry her offspring through shoulder high snow. She was well accepted by her group mates, which at least infers a relatively tolerant attitude toward the handicapped, even though she might not have been able to contribute effectively to her group in accepted ways. Similarly, that is, perhaps, all that can be inferred from fossil remains of adult Neanderthals and early humans known as Shanidar 1, Romito 2, the Windover Boy, and the Old Man of La Chapelle-Aux-Saints, who had physical impairments. In their cases, however, claims were made that their survival was evidence of compassion and moral decency.[11]

Table 1.2.1: Animal behaviour that suggests morality[12]

It is hard to imagine human morality without the following tendencies and capacities found also in other species.

Sympathy-Related Traits
Attachment, succorance, and emotional contagion
Learned adjustment to and special treatment of the disabled and injured
Ability to trade places mentally with others: cognitive empathy*

Norm-Related Characteristics
Prescriptive social rules
Internalisation of rules and anticipation of punishment*

Reciprocity
A concept of giving, trading and revenge
Moralistic aggression against violators of reciprocity rules

Getting Along
Peacemaking and avoiding of conflict
Community concern and maintenance of good relationships*
Accommodation of conflicting interests through negotiation

It is particularly in these areas - empathy, internalisation of rules and sense of justice, and community concern - that humans seem to have gone considerably further than most animals.

Zoologists and ethologists have made interesting observations, which appear to make sense of some of human's occupational behaviour. Ethologists study animal and human behaviour. Central to their approaches is the notion that behaviour demonstrates the interactions between the inborn, natural aspects of behaviour and those determined by experience and learning, and is subject to both evolution through natural selection and development in cultural history. In part, they seek to discover the survival function of the behaviour under study. One highly regarded ethologist (and zoologist) was Konrad Lorenz (1903-89) who explained it as examining:

> *... animal and human behaviour as the function of a system owing its existence, as well as its special form, to a development process that has taken place in the history of the species, in the development of the individual and, in man, in cultural history.*[13]

He maintained that species evolve in 'unforeseeable ways' that are not 'predetermined and directed toward some purpose'.[14] This is in line with standard evolutionary thought that the origin of humankind was a consequence of 'a long series of events, each depending on the other, and each unpredictable and unique'.[15] Ethologists and other evolutionary scientists pose the question - What has this (or that) behaviour, or biological characteristic to do with survival? Rephrasing that fundamental question to be relevant to this history, which suggests that occupation was used in the earliest days of humankind as part of the practice of self health and kin-health, it becomes–What has occupation for health to do with survival?

In the exploration underlying an earlier text *An Occupational Perspective of Health* it was proposed that the brain has "healthy survival" as its primary role, which continually draws upon human's occupational nature. In turn, human's occupational nature results from evolution/phylogeny, genetics, ontogeny, socio-cultural and ecological environments, and opportunity. The human brain is both an occupational and a healing brain, and engagement in occupation forms a three-way link with health and survival as depicted in figure 1.2.1.

Figure 1.2.1: Three-way link between occupation, health and survival[16]

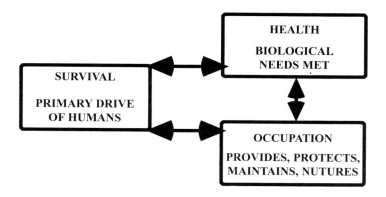

Survival is the primary drive of humans and depends on occupations that provide for essential needs of the organism. The extent and quality of survival depends on individual's physical, mental and social well being. Health is the outcome of each organism having all essential sustenance and safety needs met; on the provision of safety and education for the next generation; and on having physical, mental and social capacities maintained, exercised and in balance. This is achieved through occupation, which depends on a level of health and well-being sufficient to provide the energy, drive and functional attributes necessary for engagement in occupation.

The range of capacities available to people permits the pursuit of many options which, although not obviously related to survival or health, enable people to hone their skills, capacities and flexibility. In this way, people become competent to deal with new situations as and when they happen, as well as providing exercise to maintain the 'well working of the organism as a whole' which is the way Kass defines health.[17] A mix of physical characteristics, such as bipedalism and an opposable thumb, highly developed cognitive capacities, and consciousness endow unprecedented flexibility to human occupation, enabling people to meet the challenge of different environments by freeing them from functional and instinctive constraints. They result in people being able to engage in obligatory occupations to meet socio-cultural expectations and, mostly, to welcome new or adventurous ones. Zoologists Desmond Morris[18] and Lyall Watson[19] argue, along those lines, that people actively pursue the new and different and can, therefore be described as neophilic, whilst psychologist, Bruner, suggests that, perhaps, particular learning experiences are necessary for people to brave exploration of the unknown.[20] Those issues are of interest to the supposition that people acted as self health therapists using occupation, because without such capacities they would not have been able to do so.

Stephenson, in *The Ecological Development of Man*, suggested that the "animal" ability of primitive humans developed into a commonsense approach to health and illness.[21] So, it is both possible and probable that people acted as their own therapists, adjusting what they did according to their health status. This may have included seeking out and preparing food substances which seemed to be either what they had observed as useful in other cases and times or which they craved when feeling unwell.[22] As Sigerist, put it:

> *Empirically, guided by his instinct, man learned to distinguish what was good from what was harmful. The taste of different herbs indicated their effect to a certain extent, and so we must admit that a certain amount of hygienic* (health) *knowledge was acquired empirically at a very early period.*[23]

Indeed, it is recognised that 'with his omnivorous feeding habits and experimental frame of mind, primitive men established the curative values of a wide range of plant products, many of which are still in medicinal use'.[24] Such behaviours, it can be supposed, led, eventually, to medical science and physicians' concentration on both nutrition and remedies that were taken orally.

If that was the case, then self health occupational intervention preceded and led to the development of medical science.

An important aspect of self health occupational intervention was the development of tools. These extended the possibilities of improving safety, shelter and comfort through, for example, the building of thatched-roof shelters on stilts and fashioning needles out of bones and containers from hollowed out stone, wood, or leather. The range of food available was extended through the invention of fish-hooks and harpoons and the transportation of goods and people with boats and rafts made from hollowed-out trunks or tree branches and, eventually, through the invention of the wheel. (Some tools were later adapted for use in surgery, such as trephination, which involved the cutting of a hole in the skull to allow the removal of the evil spirit responsible for the disease state.) Such inventions not only, on the whole, improved living conditions for primitive humans but also maintained their beings through providing exercise in the use of their capacities.[25]

The next issue to be considered concerns the type of health problems faced by early humankind. It has been supposed that the natural demands of the lifestyle were health maintaining and enhancing for the majority as long as they were living in an environment which could support their survival needs adequately. Because of the very small human population on earth that would have been the most usual experience, subject to seasonal variations, and natural disasters. However, despite those supposed advantages, a high level of mortality at all ages is believed to have been the common experience. Those who survived and procreated were those most able to provide the requirements of life, and could be designated, in hindsight, as having 'a tolerable state of health ... such as exists among wild primates of the forest today'. Similar to other species living a natural lifestyle in supportive environments, Coon observed that 'natural selection is not thwarted, and in their breeding populations they do not build up increasing loads of disabling genes'.[26]

As well as occupational accidents, aggression and infanticide, the cause of most mortality and morbidity was from ecological forces acting on the population. Obvious examples were availability of food and water, as well as climatic factors like 'older people suffer(ing) gradual loss of the ability to buffer temperature extremes'.[27] Additionally 'parasites with high transmission rates and little or no induced immunity' such as worms, lice and ticks, and pathogens such as salmonella and trypanosoma (sleeping sickness) were, probably a fact of life.[28] That was because, as McNeill explains, like other animals, early humankind were 'caught in a precarious equilibrium' of a self balancing and regulating ecological system, preying on other forms of life, as they were preyed upon by micro-organisms, parasites, and large bodied predators. Despite the fact that in a natural state some microparasites provoke acute and deadly disease, others achieve a stable relationship with the host who experiences low-level disease. Yet others set up immune reactions, or are carried to become, perhaps, the cause of disease in others. Within the natural world, any change to one living creature is compensated for by genetic or behavioural change in co-organisms.[29]

Whilst to many modern individuals such demographic and epidemiologic factors appear too awful to contemplate, in fact, they do not contradict the claims that primitive hunter-gatherer peoples experienced general well-being. Rather, they sustained ill health and accidents much as modern people do, although the illness was sometimes of a different nature. The early deaths of many of the population can be laid at the door of lack of specialist knowledge. Because of their occupational nature and potential, humans were able to work at decreasing the experience of ill health to improve mortality odds. Survival pressures, in fact, provided meaning, motivation and opportunity for individual and communal occupations that addressed the obvious health risks of the day. Those deductions support the notion that occupation, survival and health are inextricably linked, especially if it is understood in terms of the World Health Organisation's belief that health includes the ability 'to identify and to realise aspirations, to satisfy needs and to change or cope with the environment'.[30]

When humans began to develop culturally, and to change different habitats through their occupations, they also changed the balance of nature and patterns of disease. For example, populations increased as people began to dominate the food chain, and many parasites and disease organisms were left behind following mastery of the use of clothing, shelter and fire which allowed expansion into colder environs. In new environments populations escalated and occupations proliferated,[31] but because of little resistance to unfamiliar infections which resulted in an increase of those diseases, the experience of morbidity was still high and low life expectancy remained the common experience.[32]

It has been noted that there are "many records" of peoples living natural, primitive life-styles exhibiting remarkable healing capacity after injury. Additionally it is well known that 'the knowledge of homeopathic medicine held by the women was considerable'. That coexisted with the use of shamans at times of ill health, but without the expectation that "good health" was 'an inalienable right of life'.[33,34]

It appears that it must have been early in history that people gave some form of spiritual or magical significance to the experience of illness. Special people within a community were often chosen, because of apparently unique circumstances, particular events at the time of birth, or family reasons, to become the medicine man, shaman, witch doctor or healing practitioner. In some cultures such positions were hereditary. Usually they had some form of training and were initiated at an elaborate ritual ceremony. Some of those were more than medicine men. Expected to make contact with divinity during trances as part of ecstatic rituals, their role was to ward off evil, bring rain, foretell the future, and practise black magic towards personal enemies as well as to heal sickness.[35] Sometimes they lived separately from the other members of their tribe, whilst in others their healing role was practiced only occasionally.[36]

Sigerist, who believed religious medicine to be timeless,[37] explained to the New York Academy of Medicine in 1933 how, in some instances, primitive health care was probably quite complex. While minor disorders would be subject to self health regimens, he said, those of a more serious nature needed explanation, often of a magical or religious nature, which pointed the way to a cure. Other people, the gods or demons may take possession, punish, or cause harm.[38] 'As civilisation reached a higher stage, magical beliefs that at the time had been generally accepted came to be regarded as mere superstitions; religion attained a higher plane'. However the ancient view that 'the sick man is branded with the odium of sinfulness' has 'survived the centuries and millennia'.[39]

Macdonald agreed that disease was attributed to the influence of magic, or to malignant spirits that were thought to take possession of those affected, and that it was through magical procedures that people tried to counteract the effects. Those took the form of incantations, the wearing of specially made amulets which acted preventively as well as remedially, and musical rituals in the form of chants and dances, in which the practitioners frequently wore masks and adorned mantles. Such treatments were mixed with 'the use of herbs, bathing, diets, bleeding, limb immersion in hot oil, the baking of painful joints by heat, the soaking of fevered persons in icy water and, in some cases, applying massage'. Those kinds of treatment continued as primitive medicine gradually lost some of its hold.[40]

Stories of occupation for health told in the Bible

As well as being a spiritual guide telling the story of God and Christ, the Bible is, without doubt, the most read history book of the Western World. In the words of the ancients, even if written, in many cases, after the events, details of how people lived in biblical times, their occupations, what they believed in, and matters of health are recorded. They have been subject to numerous interpretations, but the story that has been referred to more often than any other in the search of medical histories is the story of "the fall of humankind" in *Genesis*. Readers will probably recall those Bible verses that refer to the fact that from the time of eating the forbidden fruit, people were condemned to work for their survival and health:

Unto the woman he said, I will greatly multiply thy sorrow and thy conception; in sorrow thou shalt bring forth children; and thy desire shall be to thy husband, and shall rule over thee.

And unto Adam he said, Because thou hast hearkened unto the voice of thy wife, and hast eaten of the tree, of which I commanded thee saying, Thou shalt not eat of it: cursed is the ground for thy sake; in sorrow shalt thou eat of it all the days of thy life;

Thorns also, and thistles shall it bring forth to thee; and thou shalt eat the herb of the field;

In the sweat of thy face shalt thou eat bread, till thou return unto the ground; for out of it wast thou taken: for dust thou art, and unto dust shall thou return …

Therefore the Lord God sent him forth from the Garden of Eden, to till the ground from whence he was taken.

So he drove out the man; and he placed at the east of the garden of Eden Cherubims, and a flaming sword which turned every way, to keep the way of the tree of life.[41] (See figure 1.2.2)

Figure 1.2.2: The fall: Expelled from Eden, Adam and Eve raise a family and set to work. Engraving by Scotin, c 1765
(The Wellcome Library)

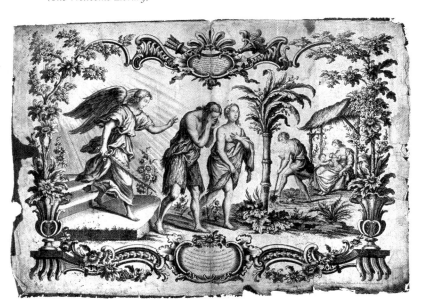

Projecting forward, during the Medieval period that story was to become of extreme importance in all matters of the rationale attributed to illness and to the provision of health care. Siraisi explains that in the most general terms, 'sickness was conceived as a consequence of the Fall of Man, and hence as a consequence of sin'. On that point, she refers to St. Augustine's writings: 'This very life, if life it can be called, pregnant with so many dire evils, bears witness that from its very beginning all the progeny of mankind was damned.' Augustine (354-430) developed the notion that 'Christ himself was the true physician, that is, the physician primarily of souls but also of bodies'. The question can be asked whether Jesus attributed disease and injury to the 'Fall'. He certainly, on two occasions, did not subscribe to the notion that it was due to the sinfulness of the sufferer. For example in Luke chapter 13 verses 4-5 he said:

Or these eighteen, upon whom the tower in Siloam fell, and slew them, think ye that they were sinners above all men that dwelt in Jerusalem?

I tell you, Nay: but, except ye repent, you shall all likewise perish.[42]

In all cases, though, for Christian theologians and writers it was an accepted principle that cure of the soul took precedence over cure of the body, and that some illness might have been sent or allowed by God as a spiritual test and ought to be accepted and suffered. Occupation, as labour, was central to that creed. Early Christianity also accepted natural causation of disease and attempted to restore spiritual and bodily health.[43]

Because of the historical importance of the Bible the following section of the chapter was solicited from Clephane Hume, a minister of the church as well an occupational therapist, which tells of examples from within it about occupation and health.

Health and occupation: Biblical examples
by Clephane Hume

The Bible tells of a long era in the world's history from creation to the early church, and encompasses the world of the Old Testament, the lifetime of Jesus told in the *Gospels*, and the early Christian era told in the *Acts* and *Epistles*. In its entirety the Bible also provides an example of multicultural living, both in harmony and dissent. Other great religions have a parallel history.

The social context and social health

In relation to health and occupation it is necessary to consider the lifestyle of the people who, broadly, included city dwellers; village dwellers living a mainly agricultural existence; and nomads who travelled from place to place, taking their tents with them. City dwellers ranged from rulers with great wealth to slaves, who, as neighbouring nations competed with one another, might have been hostages of war or prisoners. Slavery could perhaps be regarded as a non-healthy occupation although there are stories in the *Epistles* of former slaves being well treated. The educational side of life was not neglected - there are, for example, many references to writers and recorders, just as in relation to commerce there are stories of stewards and tax collectors. Similar to later periods of history, there are also instances of sexual needs being met, as illustrated by reference to Old Testament prostitutes and the brothels of Ephesus, and early use of aromatherapy could perhaps be deduced from the use of precious ointments and oils.

In the villages, many people lived a subsistence-focused life, working in the fields and pursuing domestic tasks. The writers of the gospels reveal an understanding of farming,[44] and in *Deuteronomy* accounts of people cultivating and harvesting grain, olives and grapes includes attention to the different occupations which contributed to the entirety of the process. The advice given in the passage below also gives an indication of steps that were a part of everyday life which provided for the sustenance needs of the disadvantaged and needy as part of social and community health practices. Acting in a preventive way, such procedures would reduce the incidence of diseases of poverty in a way that did not seem to make the recipients beholden.

When thou cuttest down thy harvest in the field, and hast forgot a sheath in the field, thou shalt not go again to fetch it: it shall be for the stranger, for the fatherless, and for the widow: that the LORD thy God may bless thee in all the work of thine hands.

When thou beatest thine olive trees, thou shalt not go over the boughs again: it shall be for the stranger, for the fatherless, and for the widow.

When thou gatherest the grapes of thy vineyard, thou shalt not glean it afterward: it shall be for the stranger, for the fatherless, and for the widow.[45]

"Give to the needy" was a recognised duty encompassing health, and beggars would congregate at the gates of the houses of the wealthy in the hope of receiving food and care as in the story of Lazarus told in Luke 16: 19-31. The story of Jesus, in Matthew 15: 32, feeding the multitude because he was worried that they might collapse from hunger, illustrates similar compassion and practical care for others. He said: 'I have compassion for these people; they have already been with me three days and have nothing to eat. I do not want to send them away hungry, or they may collapse on the way.'

There are, of course, because of the extensive time it covers, variations in social health between Biblical periods which, in more than a few instances, was concerned with issues resulting from foreign occupation of Palestine, such as those of sovereignty or slavery. In Old Testament times for example, the Greeks and Persians occupied Palestine. This gave rise to confrontation and resistance to the ruling powers, and the necessity of defending their kingdoms that required that kings maintain armies, soldiers, weapons, chariots and horses.[46] All the social ill-health problems associated with war must have been paramount. In the period between the Old and New Testaments, Roman occupation was an example of the continued domination of one people over another and this, including references to slavery, continued into early Christian time.

Not surprisingly, the insecurity of rulers persisted, with the most well known example being that of King Herod, who in his feelings of anxiety, killed all the young boys in Bethlehem, lest they become a threat to his sovereignty.[47] A more positive example in the face of similar feelings is that of Moses in the bulrushes. Moses, who would otherwise have been slain together with all male children, by a jealous and insecure pharaoh, was placed in a basket and put among the bulrushes. Secretly watched over by his sister, he was seen by the pharaoh's daughter who rescued him. The little girl fetched her mother as a possible nurse and thus Moses was brought up by his mother, in the court of the king, later becoming a great leader.[48]

A major down side of social health for approximately 50% of the population was that, throughout the Biblical era, there was a patriarchal society in which women were devalued or, even, regarded as outcasts. That was more so if they came from one of the tribes not regarded as socially acceptable. *Luke* 19: 1-5 provides an example of an unjust judge penalising a widow, but also how in the end the judge is worn down by her persistence. Counter to that dominant social more, Jesus demonstrated the importance of valuing all people. Development of that sense of equality, or at least need to care for others, is described in the *Acts of the Apostles*. Co-operative living is suggested by the reference to guilds of tradesmen in *Acts* 19: 25, and in the early church, many needs were clearly met within a community style of living where people shared and looked after those in need such as widows who, because of the discrimination against women had few rights.[49]

Ruth, in her widowhood and poverty gleaned the stubble for enough corn to meet her needs and those of her mother-in-law, Naomi. She attracted the eye of the owner of the field and there is a happy ending when he marries her. He shows understanding of her situation at both physical and emotional levels:

> *Ruth the Moabitess said to Naomi "let me go to the fields and pick up the leftover grain behind anyone in whose eyes I find favour". Naomi said to her "go ahead my daughter", so she went out and began to glean in the fields behind the harvesters. As it turned out, she found herself working in a field belonging to Boaz, who was from the clan of Elimilech. At mealtime, Boaz said to her, "Come over here. Have some bread and dip it in the wine vinegar". When she sat down with the harvesters, he offered her some roasted grain. She ate all she wanted and had some left over. As she got up to glean, Boaz gave orders to his men, "Even if she gathers among the sheaves, don't embarrass her. Rather, pull out some stalks for her from the bundles and leave them for her to pick up, and don't rebuke her." So Ruth gleaned in the field until evening. Then she threshed the barley she had gathered and it amounted to about an ephah. She carried it back to town and her mother-in-law saw how much she had gathered. Ruth also brought out and gave her what she had left over after she had eaten enough.*[50]

Occupation for physical health

In order to sustain health, people were required to give attention to basic subsistence needs - clean water, food, clothing and shelter. Thus, for many, occupation for health centred around self maintenance and self health activities following a pattern consistent with Maslow's hierarchy of needs. As well as the calling and lifestyle of the disciples as fishermen of Galilee, mentioned in *Matthew* 4, which also supposes the activity of boat builders, there were grinders and bread makers, shepherds, spinners, weavers and embroiderers, builders and tent makers. Building included tradesmen such as brick makers as mentioned in *Exodus* 5: 6-18, stonemasons, architects and carpenters. Joseph, the father of Jesus, was a carpenter and Mark described Jesus' possible apprenticeship to the trade.[51] Oil from the production of olives lit the lamps, and wine from the grape harvest was used for daily life as well as celebratory events such as the wedding at Cana, described in *John* 2.

In terms of professional help in cases of illness, *Leviticus* chapters 13 to 15 suggest there was a temple based form of care. That source details various examples such as the requirement for lepers to go to the priest, which was echoed in Jesus' words in *Luke* 15: 14 to those he healed, 'Go show yourselves to the priest'.

It appears that remedial bathing, which has been suggested as the origin of rehabilitation,[52] was deemed therapeutic even in those early times. The pool of Siloam and the pool of Bethesda were recognised as places of healing and people would enter the water, sometimes with the assistance of others. See figure 1.2.3, which depicts Jesus visit to the therapeutic pool of Bethesda. Christ's interest in assisting in the healing process was carried on by his followers. However an element of caution in the use of healing is shown when Paul advises Timothy to 'not be hasty in the laying on of hands'.

Figure 1.2.3:   **Christ cures the paralytic at the therapeutic pool of Bethesda. Engraving by Ravenet and Picot 1772 after Hogarth**
(The Wellcome Library)

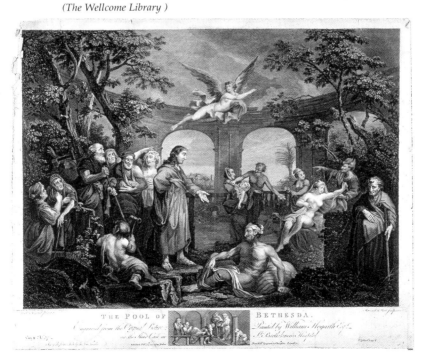

Mental health

Early Christians seem to have valued direct contact in relationships, as *John 2* suggests: 'I have much to write to you, but I do not want to use paper and ink. Instead I hope to visit you and talk with you face to face, so that our joy may be complete.' Talking to others and discussing issues would have had some benefits as people shared problems and feelings. That perhaps illustrates a spirit of communal self health. An appreciation of personal self health with regards to balancing mental and spiritual needs within a busy lifestyle was indicated by the story told in *Mark* 1: 35 of how Jesus took time to withdraw into a quiet place to meditate and pray. However, he not only recognised his own needs, but also those of the stigmatised and marginalised. On one occasion, he requested water from a Samaritan woman, which was a contentious thing to do since she was an outcast. This obviously not only slaked his thirst, but raised her self esteem:

> *Jesus, tired as he was from the journey, sat down by the well. When a Samaritan woman came to draw water, Jesus said to her "Will you give me a drink?" The Samaritan woman said to him "you are a Jew and I am a Samaritan woman. How can you ask me for a drink?", (For Jews do not associate with Samaritans). Jesus answered her "If you knew the gift of God and who it is that asks you for a drink, you would have asked him and he would have given you living water". "Sir" the woman said, " you have nothing to draw with and the well is deep".[53]*

Various instances of stress are recorded, though not necessarily met. There are, for example, the instances of Mary the mother of Jesus worried about the events in the temple; of Jesus at Gethsemane, where his friends failed to stay awake to support him; and of Mary and Martha in a conflict situation until Jesus reasoned with them, pointing out the advantages of listening versus doing.[54] The latter story provides an example of passive but positive occupational behaviour.

In the Old Testament, emotion was freely expressed in poetry and music through the psalms, such as in *Psalm 137*: 'by the waters of Babylon we sat down and wept'. These were written down and familiar to those who heard them in the temple in later times. In terms of treatment, the use of music soothed Saul who had said:

> *Find someone who plays well and bring him to me. Whenever the spirit from God came upon Saul, David would take his harp and play. Then relief would come to Saul; he would feel better and the evil spirit would leave him.[55]*

David is featured playing the harp on the Frontispiece of Volume 1, and in figure 1.2.4.

Public health, and occupation

In *Leviticus* chapters 13-14, the Old Testament records Moses' words to the Israelites in what is essentially a series of lectures in public health, presumably

Figure 1.2.4: **An aging David strums his harp, reciting psalms. Engraving by van Pandere c. 1620 after Arpinas**

(The Wellcome Library)

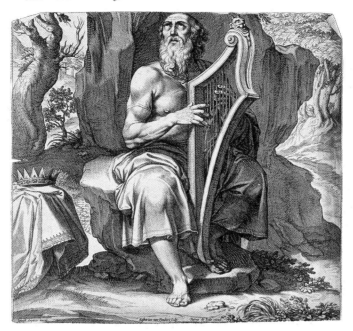

targeted at preventing the spread of disease such as leprosy. Detailed regulations about rashes and infectious skin diseases, require the individual to show the lesion to the priest and to present himself for re-examination 7 days later, and so on, until pronounced clean. Chapter 13 also includes advice on baldness, boils and mildew. The next chapter records equally detailed regulations for cleansing from infectious skin diseases, with attention to the economic status of the individual. Other chapters address diet, childbirth, menstruation and ejaculation.

NB. Sigerist notes:

> *… cleanliness was meant to imply spiritual cleanliness. But it was necessary that this spiritual cleanliness should have an outward expression. The priest was robed in spotless garments. He avoided touching unclean things, and so the man who came to the temple in order to worship his god had to be clean also. Although the cleanliness was taken in a spiritual sense, it had great hygienic consequences.*

All ancient cults, he said, demand similar cleanliness:

> *… but these precepts are probably most distinctly defined in Leviticus, where we find a great many regulations concerning the daily life of the Jew. These laws were not based upon hygienic reasoning, and yet they served to improve hygienic conditions vastly. Thus it was postulated that only clean animals should be set apart to be eaten, that such animals should be slaughtered alive with an unnotched knife, and that only animals were to be slaughtered that had no disease or injury.*

In this way only sound cattle were slaughtered and the method of slaughtering ensured free bleeding, so that the meat was better preserved. It was much the same with the other laws. The man who becomes unclean must be purified before he steps into the temple, and the ritual of purification required that the clothes of the impure man be washed and that he himself had to bathe. Uncleanliness is contagious. Whoever touches an unclean man becomes impure himself. The menstruating woman was considered unclean for seven days. The woman in labour was unclean from the moment her pains began and remained unclean for forty days after delivery if her child were a boy and eighty days if it were a girl.[56]

There were regulations governing behaviour and some of these applied particularly to priests or members of certain groups. In the story of the Good Samaritan, told in *Luke* 10: 30-37, the priest and the Levite, traditionally held up as examples of uncaring behaviour, would have become ritually unclean had they touched a dead person.

Clean water was essential to public health, and a striking and practical Old Testament example of meeting that requirement is that of King Hezekiah. He organised the building of a tunnel to carry water to the city of Jerusalem, a job that must have entailed hard labour for many but with beneficial results. 'It was Hezekiah who blocked the upper outlet of the Gihon spring and channelled the water down to the west side of the City of David.'[57] The tunnel can still be seen today. Perhaps reflecting an understanding of the potential dangers of unclean water, was the suggestion made to Timothy to 'stop drinking only water, and use a little wine because of your stomach and your frequent illnesses'.[58] That is an interesting remedy in terms of modern day thoughts about the pros and cons of taking wine.

Spiritual needs and spiritual health

Spiritual needs and spiritual health were important throughout the long Biblical period. Priests, leaders of worship, temple officials and workers all had health focussed occupational roles, which included time to fulfil rituals and to pray as an integral part of daily life, as it was for many others. They were also incorporated into the re-enactment of narratives from history such as the Passover meal which recalled the saving of the people of Israel and helped to bond the later generations as told in 2 *Chronicles* 35 and *Matthew* 26: 17-39. In that spiritual sense, psychosocial life requires a sense of individual "place" and belonging in the scheme of things. Hence there was careful recording of the history of the Exodus: the escape from Egypt.

In the New Testament a focus on spiritual rather than material matters is central. The notion of doing, being, and becoming, for example, takes on a strong spiritual dimension. Paul wrote, in *Ephesians* 3: 16, 'I pray that out of his glorious riches he (the Father) may strengthen you with power through his Spirit in your inner being'. For Christian believers, indeed, the ultimate sense of "becoming" is in the theological message of the gospels: that we might have eternal life - 'God sent his one and only son into the world that we might live through him … an atoning sacrifice for our sins'.[59] Other, more practical examples include statements such as: "Life is more than food" in *Luke* 12: 2; or, when in *Matthew* 19: 21, a rich young man is told, to his consternation, 'If you want to be perfect, go, sell your possessions and give to the poor, and you will have treasure in heaven'; or, in *Matthew* 6: 19-21: 'Do not store up for yourselves treasures on earth where moth and rust destroy, and where thieves break in and steal. But store up for yourselves treasures in heaven. … For where your treasure is, there your heart will be also.'

An important part of spiritual health was the notion of loving and caring which later in history took on the notion of "moral" health. In the New Testament, there is great emphasis, through the healing miracles of Jesus, on healing from illness, with health including the commandment to care for others: Love your neighbour as yourself.[60] That command to love was central and was expressed in various ways as a form of spiritually healthy behaviour within the early church: 'Dear friends, let us love one another, for love comes from God. Everyone who loves has been born of God and knows God'. (1 *John* 4: 7) Several passages exhort people "do not love the world" but to focus their ultimate love on God who loved them first.[61] Many examples in the New Testament record the concept of grace through Christ. Grace was a word used to indicate the love shown by God to human beings (sinners) in making their forgiveness and salvation possible. Thus early Christians greeted each other with the words "grace and peace to you", recorded, for example, in the *Epistles of Paul* and used in liturgy today - 'Grace and peace to you from God our Father and the Lord Jesus Christ'.[62]

In contrast, the God of the Old Testament is recorded in different ways, often chastising his people for their wayward behaviour but always loving them as demonstrated by his behaviour. During the exodus, food was provided in the desert, manna and quails miraculously appeared to sustain the people. Noah was warned of the flood, enabling him to build the ark and thus save creatures and people.[63]

Philosophical beliefs and values in relation to occupation for health

In very general terms the focus varies between the old and new testaments. In the Old Testament, health is related to worshipping God and obeying his commandments. The Ten Commandments, listed in *Exodus* 20, encompass principles for healthy living in terms of avoiding conflict with others, by not coveting, for example, or not committing adultery.

In the New Testament, the healing miracles of Jesus demonstrate clearly how a disadvantaged or previously handicapped individual can become a productive member of society and is thus made whole in the broadest sense, like the lepers[64] or the man with the palsy to whom Jesus said 'Get up and take your mat and go home. And the man got up and went home.'[65] Likewise stories tell of those who made a dramatic change in lifestyle and were able to find a sense of self-fulfilment like Zacchaeus' story told in *Luke* 19: 1-9. In other accounts of healing miracles there are several instances of people being made whole through exorcism of demons. There was obviously a belief in possession by evil spirits, in ways that would not nowadays be acceptable. Fevers were rebuked and demons cast out. Mark described a boy with epilepsy:

> *Teacher I brought you my son, who is possessed by a spirit that has robbed him of speech. Whenever it seizes him it throws him to the ground. He foams at the mouth gnashes his teeth and becomes rigid … It has often thrown him into fire or water to kill him …*
>
> *Jesus heals the boy and explains to the disciples that "This kind can come out only by prayer".*[66]

Macdonald reported that the medical approaches taken by the people of Israel were influenced by the Egyptians and other successful practices of nearby countries.[67] To gain an appreciation of what they may have been, the last section of the chapter goes on to discuss what happened in Babylonia, Egypt and neighbouring states.

Stories of occupation for health told by medical historians

Many of the famous physicians and surgeons throughout history have reflected on past practises in order to inform their own observations, approaches and prescriptions. Paré, for example, in the early 17th century, set forth his views on the origins of medicine:

> *Most men derive the original of phisicke from heaven … Neither could mans capacity ever have attained to the knowledge of those things [herbes and plants] without the guidance of the Divine Power. For God the great creator and fashioner of the world, when first he inspired Adam by the breathe of his mouth into a living and breathing man, he taught him the nature, proper operations, faculties and vertues of all things contained in the circuit of this Univers … this knowledge was not buried in oblivion with Adam: but by the same guift of God was given to those whom he had chosen and ordained for physicke, to put their helping hands to others that stood in need therof. … we find it recorded in ancient histories, before the invention of Physicke, that the Babilonians and Assyrians had a custome amongst them, to lay their sicke and diseased persons in the porches and entries of their houses, or to carry them into the streets and market places, that such as passed by and saw them, might givee them counsell to take*

those things to cure their diseases, which they had formerly found profitable in themselves or any other in the like affects, neither might any passe by a sicke man in silence.[68]

Those notions support the suggestion of occupations as part of self health initiatives being the foundation of medicine. Sigerist, that early twentieth century medical historian, appears to agree, as well as holding the premise that it is closely linked with the occupations of daily life to provide the requirements of the human organism. In 1936 in the *Wesley M. Carpenter Lecture*, he said:

> *It is the destiny of man that he has to work to maintain his life. He has to produce and gather the food that his organism requires and has to produce goods to protect himself against the climate and to make his life easier and more enjoyable. The greatest advance in the history of human civilisation was the step from the Paleolithic to the Neolithic Age, from the food-gathering to the food-producing stage, when man had learned to cultivate plants, to domesticate animals, to perfect his tools. Man struggled with nature, and he is conquering it gradually through his intelligence, inventiveness, and skill. The productive forces, animate and inanimate, active and passive, man and his raw material, the labourer and his tool, were the decisive factors in history.*
>
> *Man has to work in order to live - and this is good. Work gives significance to our life. It ennobles it. It allows us to create material and spiritual values without which life would not be worth living. If society progressed, it was due to the cooperative efforts of all its members. Man has a duty to work, but he should also have a right to work. Work balances our life and is therefore an essential factor of health.*[69]

In a later history he put forward a further opinion which supports the self health hypothesis. Humans are mammals, he said, and "like other animals" are equipped with instincts which drive them to 'commit actions tending to preserve the individual, to propagate his kind', and that 'when illness has taken hold of the animal organism, instincts manifest themselves in a special way. The body craves what it needs to overcome the lesion and restore health.' Instinct led similarly to many methods of treatment apart from diet and oral remedies, such as rubbing or massage, heat and cold, and bathing. Whilst 'instinctive self-help came first' he suggested that 'mutual aid can be assumed at an early stage, since it is common amongst animals.' There were differences in the treatment of the sick, the aged, the weak, and the disabled which could still be observed in primitive peoples remaining in the twentieth century. 'Some accept the burden, treat them kindly, feed them, attend to them, honour the aged, and are prepared to bring any sacrifice to have the sick treated … Others, however get rid of the handicapped.' It was the more primitive groups of hunter-gatherers who adopted the first scenario in the main, and those with more developed agricultural and pastoral tribes who have more complex social organisations and property relations who ignored or repudiated the disadvantaged. There are still a few primitive tribes of higher civilisation within which a person suffering from serious disease is abandoned, dead socially before physically. The sick person is considered the victim of evil forces - 'Witchcraft, the action of evil spirits, or the wrath of a deity may be responsible for his illness'.[70] Despite such theoretical rationales, and in some cases it was out of 'respect and compassion' to relieve them of their 'suffering and misery', economy undoubtably plays a major part in the elimination of the sick and infirm.[71]

Of the early civilisations, Babylonia and Egypt stand apart for their sophisticated social structures. Both had medical writings, which provide a surprising amount of accurate observations, and of accumulated empirical knowledge. Babylonia, which came into being round about 5500 BC, was an ancient state in the fertile region watered by the Tigris and Euprates rivers. It was subdivided into Akkad, Sumer and Chaldaea, all of which, at various times, were used as the name for the whole State.[72]

In Babylonia, which was of an entirely religious character, theology encompassed all of the sciences, and as was to be the case for much of history, it was the priests who were the physicians. The physician-priest, as well as carefully noting and giving a meaning to the symptoms of disease, watched for and interpreted omens telling the intentions of the gods. From watching the stars or the flickering of a flame, or analysing the organs of sacrificed animals, or what happened to a drop of oil poured into water he was able to tell the fate of a patient and what would be appropriate treatment. That might be to placate the gods as well as keeping them benevolent. Treatment often consisted of incantations given with the physician-priest dressed in a red cloak, and holding a raven in one hand, and a falcon in the other. [73]

The first regulations to be picked up subsequently and similarly elsewhere detailing a collection of laws and code of conduct for physicians, are to be found in the Code of King Hammurabi which were inscribed on stone columns in 2000 BC. Known as The Judgement of Righteousness, the rules included, what is thought may be, the first reference to industrial conditions. Surgeons were declared liable for their interventions, and if a fatality occurred after an operation his right hand was cut off. In the same rules a fee structure was prescribed which varied according to the social standing of patients. Later regulations stipulated that surgeons were not allowed to practice before they had performed three successful operations on infidels.[74][75]

As Paré recorded, the sick were indeed carried to the market place so that they might receive advice from those with knowledge or who had similar diseases or disabilities, which perhaps provides an example of an early form of support group. One of the earliest forms of modern physical treatment techniques was hydrotherapy. 'Even in 2000 BC in Babylonia the words *A Su* connected water with healing.'[76] Another institution of occupation for health significance started in Babylon, namely–a weekly day of rest from labour. In Babylonia, because the seventh, fourteenth, twenty-first, and twenty-eighth days of the month were considered unlucky, no work was done. This practice was adopted into Judaism, and thence into Christianity and Islam giving it a moral significance by making it the day of the Lord dedicated to worship as well as rest.[77]

Between 626-539 BC, a strong Chaldaean dynasty ruled an independent Babylon.[78] Halle, in the 1789 French *Encyclopedie Methodique*, published a treatise on hygiene which included a history of preventive and health promotive methods. He wrote:

> *The Chaldeans, and above all the Egyptians, who were in the habit of uniting all the useful sciences and all public institutions to their religious mysteries, were the first, as far as our knowledge extends, who joined these two departments of medicine and of legislation. We ought not, at least, to ascribe this honour to the inhabitants of India, to whom some philosophers have allowed a priority of claim over the natives of Egypt and of Chaldea. It will be universally admitted, that the Hebrews and the Greeks borrowed the greatest part of their customs from the Egyptians.*[79]

Assyria was an ancient state in Mesopotamia, bounded on the south by Babylonia. It was at the zenith of its power in the 7th century BC, although of greater antiquity.[80] It seems that physicians and surgeons there specialised in particular physical and mental illnesses, as well as 'surgeons– "knife doctors", physicians– "herb doctors", and psychiatrists– "spell doctors"'. The nature of diseases appear to have included abscesses, arteriosclerosis and arthritis; a variety of ear, eye and heart troubles; gastro-intestinal and genito-urinary disorders; mental illnesses and physical injuries. Illnesses and disabilities were treated by drugs, massage, manipulations, heat, baths, exercises, and music. "Splints" were made of clay and wood. Arad-Nana, the physician of King Esarhaddon, prescribed baths for his royal patient's fever and, for his arthritis and gout, vigorous massage and exorcism from a magician.[81]

Sigerist, who held that 'at all times and everywhere work is one of the chief determining factors of health and disease'[82] discussed how people had been in ancient times, and still were, exposed to all kinds of hazards in the pursuit of their work to the extent of them being life-threatening. Stone Age people gathering food and hunting animals were subject to accidents, but subsequent economic developments created new and different hazards. He deplored the value heaped on civilisations such as that of ancient Egypt for its treasures, without concurrent horror at the working conditions of the labourers. Its pyramids and temples of great art and beauty 'were built with the blood and tears of thousands of human beings' engaged in slave labour, as they are depicted on wall paintings and reliefs. Other workers hardly fared better, as a few scraps of preserved ancient Egyptian literature from the Middle Kingdom told in, what must be, some of the earliest occupational health literature:

> *I have never seen a blacksmith acting as ambassador or a foundry worker sent on a mission, but what I have seen is the metal worker at his work: he is grilled at the mouth of the furnace. The mason, exposed to all weathers and all risks, builds without clothing. His arms are worn out with work, his food is mixed up with dirt and rubbish: he bites his nails, for he has no other food. The barber breaks his arm to fill his stomach. The weaver engaged in home work is worse off in the house than the women: doubled up with his knees drawn up to his stomach, he cannot breathe. The laundryman on the quays is the neighbour of crocodiles. The dyeworker stinks of fish spawn: his eyes are tired, his hand works unceasingly and as he spends his time in cutting up rags he has a horror of clothing.*[83]

The work-rest cycle is an important aspect of occupation for health, as is the need to balance physical, mental and social occupations as well as obligatory and self-chosen ones. As Sigerist stated:

> *Rest and recreation are important factors in health, and sleep and food are not enough to restore a human being, because man is endowed with a mind and he experiences hopes and fears, joys and sorrows, love and hatred. Man must have emotional outlets; and hope and joy are as necessary for his well-being as sunshine is to the life of the plant.*[84]

He asked how the ancient Egyptians fared in that respect. The wealthy, as would be supposed, fared best. They followed what were to become the age old pastimes of the rich, hunting and fishing from their country homes, entertaining with dancing girls, musicians, juggling or ball games. They also played board games like senet or hounds and jackals. See figure 1.2.5. The workers had little opportunity for recreation except of the most basic physiological nature or religious festivals, which were days of rest dedicated to the worship of the gods.[85]

Whilst later in the history it will be deplored that prisoners have no occupations, the other extreme seemed to be the case in ancient Egypt where 'condemned prisoners, prisoners of war and others … sometimes alone, sometimes with their entire families' were sent to the gold mines:

> *… these workers can take no care of their bodies and have not even a garment to hide their nakedness, there is no one, seeing these luckless people would not pity them because of the excess of their misery, for there is no forgiveness or relaxation at all for the sick, or the maimed, or the old, or for women's weakness, but all with blows, are compelled to stick to their labour until worn out they die with servitude.*[86]

Physicians received their training in schools connected with the chancelleries, the courts, or the temples. Egyptian temples the most famous of which were in On, Memphis, Thebes, and Sais, were the repository of civil records, as well as medical schools which provided training according to the patron gods they were built to honour. Individual gods were thought to be

Figure 1.2.5: Sketch of a XIX-XXth Dynasty wall painting depicting a board game

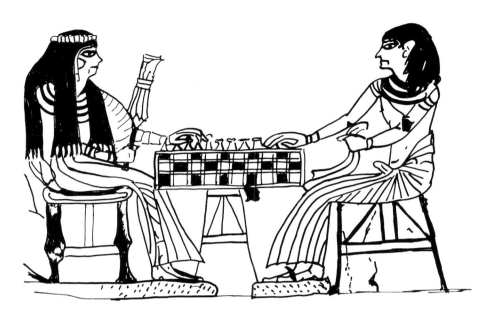

responsible for certain parts of the human body. Each temple had its scribes, and although physicians belonged to their class, they were sometimes priests, just as priests might also be magicians and doctors, or might act as statesmen or poets. Medical training was conducted in schools connected with the temples or courts. An empirical approach to treatment was sometimes used which might include massage, baths, bloodletting and spells as well as drugs amongst their remedies. Women priestesses or health practitioners, who were said to be given less status than the men, attended childbirths and "less-serious" conditions using massage and herbs in their treatments.[87 '88]

Thoth was both a sun god and the god of medicine who had revealed writing and other skilled crafts to humankind. In his temple gymnastics, music, dancing, painting, sculpture, mathematics and astronomy were encouraged. Possibly, in reference to his temples, and with regard to the mentally ill, Phillipe Pinel, at the end of the 18th century explained how he viewed the Egyptian system of treatment:

An intimate acquaintance with human nature, and with the character in general of melancholics, must always point out the urgent necessity of forcibly agitating the system; of interrupting the chain of their gloomy ideas, and engaging their interest by powerful and continuous impressions on their external senses. Wise regulations of this nature, are considered as having constituted in part the celebrity and utility of the priesthood of ancient Egypt. Efforts of industry and of art; scenes of magnificence and grandeur; the varied pleasures of sense; and the imposing influences of a pompous and mysterious superstition, were, perhaps, never devoted to a more laudable purpose. At both extremities of ancient Egypt, a country which was at that time exceedingly populous and flourishing, were temples dedicated to Saturn, whither melancholics resorted in crowds in quest of relief. The priests, taking advantage of their credulous confidence, ascribed to miraculous powers the effects of natural means exclusively. Games and recreations of all kinds, were instituted in these temples. Voluptuous paintings and images were every where exposed to public view. The most enchanting songs, and sounds of the most melodious, "took prisoner, the captive sense". Flowery gardens and groves, disposed with taste and art, invited them to refreshing and salubrious exercise. Gaily decorated boats sometimes transported them to breathe, amidst rural concerts, the purer breezes of the Nile. Sometimes they were conveyed to its verdant isles, where, under the symbols of some guardian deity, new and ingeniously contrived entertainments were prepared for their reception. Every moment was devoted to some pleasurable occupation, or rather to a system of diversified amusements, enhanced and sanctioned by superstition. An appropriate and scrupulously observed regimen; repeated excursions to the holy places; preconcerted fêtes at different stages to excite and keep up their interest on the road, with every other advantage of a similar nature, that the experienced priesthood could invent or command, were, in no small degree, calculated to suspend the influence of pain, to calm the inquietudes of a morbid mind, and to operate salutary changes in the various functions of the system. Those ancient establishments, so worthy of admiration, but so opposite to the institutions of modern times, point out the objects to be aimed at in every asylum, public or private, for the reception of melancholics.[89]

It was not only in the use of occupation for the cure of mental illness that Egypt provides examples of being in the forefront of ancient regimes for health, in ways similar to occupational therapists of the modern age. The other aspect is their use of splints. The splinting of fractures with palm fibre splints was practised as early as the 5th Dynasty (2750-2625 BC).[90]

They also used mouldy bread on wounds. The Edwin Smith papyrus, which contains the remains of a surgical treatise of the seventeenth century BC, systematically and logically describes 48 histories of surgical cases, mainly wounds and injuries to the head, chest and spine.[91] The Ebers papyrus, which is dated about a century later, is encyclopaedic with regard to detailed descriptions of diseases. Osteoarthritis, "hardening of the limbs", appears to have been a common complaint of later years.[92] By the fifth century, over specialisation and religious restrictions appear to have resulted in a gradual demise of its prominence. But it did not die completely, and in the third century BC, Herophilus of Chalceon following his Greek medical training went to Alexandria. Apparently a notable practitioner, writer, and pioneer of anatomy, his contribution included the combining of anatomical knowledge with diet and exercise aimed at maintaining and restoring health.[93] Erasistratus, described by Celsus as the "father of physiology," followed on with Herophilus's work on the nervous system providing a more accurate description of the brain including a differentiation of cerebellum and cerebrum, and came close to Harvey's discovery of the circulation of blood. Because of ethical concerns about the dissection of human bodies, such work was not continued as would have been expected as part of Classical medicine.[94]

In ancient Persia too, where they worshipped the Sun God, Mithras, dissection was not permitted because of religious beliefs, but they accepted help from Egyptian physicians, and appear to have been influenced by other neighbours. Thrita, one of their own physicians was famous for following the themes of Aesculapius, and like the Mesopotamians, they had "knife-doctors", "herb-doctors", and "word-doctors" rather than "spell doctors".[95] The ancient Persians also made great use of gymnasia during the time of Cyrus (c. 600-529).[96]

In summary, two different scenarios of evolution have been provided in this chapter. The first is an evolutionary account of the use of occupation for health as the scientific world understands it at present, and the second is a biblical account of the same story. Both are told because occupational therapists in the twentieth century have been largely tied to the scientific world through their association with modern medicine. Despite that, the profession has never quite fitted because of its interest in the spiritual as well as the physical, mental and social aspects of illness. Few medical professions aim for holism to quite the same extent as occupational therapy, and so, it may not be surprising that it appears that quite a number of its practitioners embrace the second of the two explanations. For those who are comfortable with the scientific account, the creationist version offers a historical glimpse at one of the rare ancient accounts of life before the Classical period. Both the evolutionary and biblical accounts support the idea of a self health scenario, which grew from the occupational nature of humankind, and from their instinctive drives. They observed, deduced, and practiced in an exploratory way, which eventually led to medical science, and ultimately to occupational therapy.

[1]Hesiod. *Works and Days.* c. 8th Century BC.

[2]Ilza Veith. Huang Ti Nei Ching Su Wen. *The Yellow Emperor's Classic of Internal Medicine.* Baltimore: Williams and Wilkins, 1949; 253.

[3]Dubos R. *Mirage of Health: Utopias, Progress and Biological Change.* New York: Harper & Row, 1959; 131.

[4]Lao-tzu. *Tao Te Ching* (The Way). Circa 500BC.

[5]Chuang-tzu. In: Dubos R. *Mirage of Health…; 10.*

[6]Pao Ching-yen. In: Needham J. *Science and Civilisation in China, Vol 2, History of Scientific Thought.* Cambridge: Cambridge University Press, 1956.

[7]Dubos. *Mirage of Health…; 1.*

[8]Wilcock AA. *An Occupational Perspective of Health*. Thorofare, NJ: Slack Inc., 1998.

[9]De Waal F. *Good Natured: The Origins of Right and Wrong in Humans and Other Animals*. Cambridge, Mass. & London, England: Harvard University Press, 1996; 212.

[10]De Waal. *Good Natured…*; 212-214.

[11]De Waal. *Good Natured…*; 6-7.

[12]De Waal. *Good Natured…*; 211.

[13]Lorenz K. *Civilized Man's Eight Deadly Sins*. Translated by Latzke M. London: Methuen & Co Ltd., 1974; 1.

[14]Lorenz K. *The Waning of Humaneness*. Munich: R Piper & Co Verlag, 1983. Translated USA: Little Brown and Company, 1987; 5.

[15]Pilbeam D. What makes us human. In: Jones S, Martin R, Pilbeam D. *The Cambridge Encyclopedia of Human Evolution*. Cambridge: Cambridge University Press, 1992; 1.

[16]Wilcock. *An Occupational Perspective of Health…*; 36.

[17]Kass LR. Regarding the end of medicine and the pursuit of health. In: Caplan AL, Englehardt HT, McCartney JJ, eds. Concepts of Health and Disease: Interdisciplinary Perspectives. Massachusetts: Addison Wesley Publishing Co., 1981.

[18]Morris D. The Human Zoo. London: Jonathan Cape, 1969.

[19]Watson L. Neophilia: The Tradition of the New. Great Britain: Hodder and Stoughton Ltd, 1989.

[20]Bruner JS. Nature and uses of immaturity. American Psychologist 1972; August: 687-708.

[21]Stephenson W. The Ecological Development of Man. Sydney: Angus and Robertson, 1972; 136.

[22]Stephenson. The Ecological Development of Man…; 136.

[23]Marti-Ibañez F, ed. Henry E. Sigerist on the History of Medicine. New York: MD Publications, Inc., 1960; 17-18.

[24]Stephenson. The Ecological Development of Man…; 136.

[25]Macdonald EM. World-Wide Conquests of Disabilities: The History, Development and Present Functions of the Remedial Services. London: Bailliere Tindall, 1981.

[26]Coon CS. The Hunting Peoples. London: Jonathan Cape Ltd., 1972; 390.

[27]Dobson A. People and disease. In: The Cambridge Encyclopedia of Human Evolution…; 411-412.

[28]Meindel RS. Human populations before agriculture. In: The Cambridge Encyclopedia of Human Evolution…; 410.

[29]McNeill WH. Plagues and People. London: Penguin Books, 1979; 13, 25. (first published by Doubleday, USA, 1976).

[30]World Health Organisation, Health and Welfare Canada, Canadian Public Health Association. The Ottawa Charter for Health Promotion. Ottawa, Canada: 1986.

[31]McNeill. Plagues and People.

[32]Hetzel BS, McMichael T. L S Factor: Lifestyle and Health. Ringwood, Victoria: Penguin, 1987.

[33]King-Boyes MJE. Patterns of Aboriginal Culture: Then and Now. Sydney: McGraw-Hill Book Company, 1977; 154-155.

[34]Wilcock. An Occupational Perspective of Health.

[35]Girling DA. New Age Encyclopaedia. 7th ed. Sydney & London: Bay Books. 1983; vol 26: 75; vol 30: 157.

[36]Sigerist HE. A History of Medicine, Volume I: Primitive and Archaic Medicine. New York: Oxford University Press, 1955; 4.

[37]Sigerist HE. A History of Medicine, Volume II: Early Greek, Hindu, and Persian Medicine. New York: Oxford University Press, 1961; 44.

[38]Sigerist. Paper to The New York Academy of Medicine, October 18, 1933. In: A History of Medicine, Volume I; 4.

[39]Marti-Ibañez. Henry E. Sigerist on the History of Medicine…; 26.

[40]Macdonald. World-Wide Conquests of Disabilities…; 15-17.

[41]The Holy Bible. The Oxford Pictorial Edition. London: Oxford University Press; Genesis 3: 16-19, 23-24.

[42]The Holy Bible. The Oxford Pictorial Edition…; Luke 13: 4-5.

[43]Siraisi NG. Medieval and Early Renaissance Medicine: An Introduction to Knowledge and Practice. Chicago and London: University of Chicago Press; 8-9.

[44]The Holy Bible. New International Version. Hodder and Stoughton, 1988; Matthew 13: 24-30.

[45]The Holy Bible. The Oxford Pictorial Edition…; Deuteronomy 24: 19-21.

[46]The Holy Bible. New International Version…; I Kings 10: 28; II Kings 7: 6.

[47]The Holy Bible. New International Version…; Luke 2: 16.

[48]The Holy Bible. New International Version…; Exodus 2: 1-10.

[49]The Holy Bible. New International Version…; Acts 2: 44-46.

[50]The Holy Bible. New International Version…; Ruth 2: 2-3, 14-18.

[51]The Holy Bible. New International Version…; Mark 6: 3.

[52]Kersley GD, Glyn G. A Concise International History of Rheumatology and Rehabilitation: Friends and Foes. London: Royal Society of Medicine Services Limited, 1991; 1.

[53]The Holy Bible. New International Version…; John 4: 6-9.

[54]The Holy Bible. New International Version…; Luke 10: 38-42.

[55]The Holy Bible. New International Version…; 1 Samuel 16: 14-23.

[56]Marti-Ibañez. Henry E. Sigerist on the History of Medicine…; 18.

[57]The Holy Bible. New International Version…; 2 Kings 20: 20; 2 Chronicles 32: 30.

[58]The Holy Bible. New International Version…; 1 Tim 5: 23.

[59]The Holy Bible. New International Version…; 1 John 4: 9-10.

[60]The Holy Bible. New International Version…; Matthew 22: 34-40.

[61]The Holy Bible. New International Version…; 1 John 2: 15.

[62]The Holy Bible. New International Version…; 2 Corinthians 1: 2.

[63]The Holy Bible. New International Version…; Genesis 8: 8-12.

[64]The Holy Bible. New International Version…; Matthew 9: 1-8.

[65]The Holy Bible. New International Version…; Luke 5: 24 -26.

[66]The Holy Bible. New International Version…; Mark 9: 14-29.

[67]Macdonald. World-Wide Conquests of Disabilities…;23.

[68]Johnson T. The Workes of that Famous Chirurgion Anbrose Parey Translated out of Latin and Compared with the French. London: Printed by Th Cotesand R Young, 1634; A2-A3.

[69]Sigerist HE. The Wesley M. Carpenter Lecture: Historical background of industrial and occupational diseases. October 19, 1936. In: Marti-Ibañez. Henry E. Sigerist on the History of Medicine…; 46.

[70]Marti-Ibañez. Henry E. Sigerist on the History of Medicine…; 26.

[71]Sigerist. A History of Medicine, Volume I…; 114-117, 154-156.

[72]Girling. New Age Encyclopaedia…; Vol. 3: 38.

[73]Sigerist HE. Paper to The New York Academy of Medicine, October 18, 1933. In: Source Book of Medical History: Compiled with Notes by Logan Clendenning, Toronto,

Canada: General Publishing Company, Ltd., London, UK: Constable and Company, Ltd. 1942; 4.

[74]Sigerist. Paper to The New York Academy…; 5.

[75]Macdonald. World-Wide Conquests of Disabilities…; 19.

[76]Kersley & Glyn. A Concise International History of Rheumatology…; 1.

[77]Marti-Ibañez. Henry E. Sigerist on the History of Medicine…; 19.

[78]Girling. *New Age Encyclopaedia*…; Vol 6: 154.

[79]Halle R. Treatise: Hygiene. In: Encyclopedie Methodique, Medicine. Tome 7, part 1. Livraison 65. Translated in: Sinclair J. The Code of Health and Longevity Vol III. Edinburgh, Printed for Arch Constable and Co.; and T Cadell and W Davies, and J Murray, London, 1806; 260-475.

[80]Girling. New Age Encyclopaedia…; vol 2: 235-236.

[81]Macdonald. World-Wide Conquests of Disabilities…; 17-18.

[82]Sigerist. A History of Medicine, Volume I…; 254.

[83]Papyrus Sallier, 2, 4, 6. Cited in: Marti-Ibañez. Henry E. Sigerist on the History of Medicine…; 46-47.

[84]Sigerist. A History of Medicine, Volume I…; 261.

[85]Sigerist. A History of Medicine, Volume I…; 261-262.

[86]Diodorus, III, 12ff. Translated by G. Booth. London, 1814. In: Sigerist. A History of Medicine, Volume 1…; 260.

[87]Sigerist. A History of Medicine, Volume I.

[88]Macdonald. World-Wide Conquests of Disabilities.

[89]Pinel P. A Treatise on Insanity. Trans from French by D. D. Davis. Sheffield: Strand, London. Printed by W Todd, for Messrs. Cadell and Davies, 1806; 180-182.

[90]Smith GE. The most ancient splints. British Medical Journal 1908; 1: 732-737.

[91]Breasted JH. The Edwin Smith Surgical Papyrus. Chicago: 1930.

92Ebbell B. The Papyrus Ebers. The Greatest Egyptian Medical Document. Copenhagen: 1937.

[93]Jackson R. Doctors and Diseases in the Roman Empire. London: British Museum Press, 1988; 14-15, 27.

[94]Jackson. Doctors and Diseases in the Roman Empire…; 28.

[95]Macdonald. World-Wide Conquests of Disabilities…; 23.

[96]Halle. Treatise…; 291.

Part 2

Classical Times

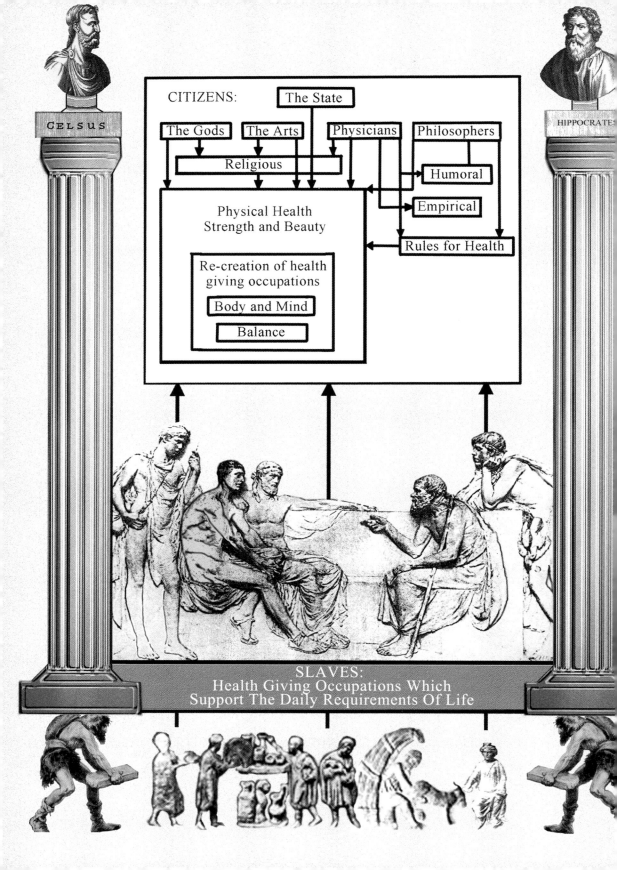

CITIZENS:

The State

The Gods   The Arts   Physicians   Philosophers

Religious

Humoral

Empirical

Physical Health
Strength and Beauty

Rules for Health

Re-creation of health
giving occupations

Body and Mind

Balance

CELSUS

HIPPOCRATES

SLAVES:
Health Giving Occupations Which
Support The Daily Requirements Of Life

Chapter 3

Occupation for Health in Classical Times

Contents

Ancient Greek and Roman culture are described as "Classical" and upheld as examples of civilised and sophisticated life. The period is recognised as the time when early scientific medicine emerged, it being particularly associated with Hippocrates who many regard as its founder. In view of the association of occupational therapy with medicine in the twentieth century, it seems to be particularly important to look for clues about a possible association between them at the time of medicine's dawning. This chapter will consider how some occupations that formed part of the cultural expression of Greco-Roman civilisations were recognised as contributing to the health of both individuals and nations as a whole. In order to do this, literature which describes particular aspects of life in that period, as well as the history of classical medicine have been consulted, along with translations of work by celebrated medical authorities, particularly those which provide evidence of the use of occupation for health. It is worthwhile to bear in mind some of the cultural differences in order to understand better the occupation for health information, which emerges in this chapter.

Ancient Greece was a collection of city-states established by conquest during the third and second millennia BC. At this time the citizens managed, largely, to rid themselves of the need to labour, leaving this to slaves, free peasants, artisans and craftsmen who were usually the indigenous people of the acquired lands.[1] Labour was seen as 'brutalising the mind, making man unfit for thinking of truth or for practising virtue; it was a necessary evil which the visionary elite should avoid'.[2] There was 'a conscious abstention from all activities connected with merely being alive'.[3] Indeed, a great distinction was made between labour of that sort and other occupations, which were the domain of the citizens and particularly of the upper social strata. Those occupations included literature, the arts, architecture and building, philosophy, mathematics, politics, sport and other expressions of bodily prowess, such as the age-old manly activities of fighting and making war. Indeed, these are the occupations that, in the present time, are applauded as representative of the Greco-Roman cultures.[4]

Women were also, generally, excluded from citizenship because it was associated with the bearing of arms. In principle women were excluded from most public life, spending their time in the "gynaeceum" - the women's quarters in the home. However many of them, apart from slaves, had much more freedom than that. Women of high status who were over sixty acted as messengers for their younger counterparts, and performed public ceremonial duties. Poor women were occupied in trades, such as retail and catering, and crafts, like vase painting and working in wool. Those who were foreign born, including women traders, were also entertainers and sex workers. Additionally there was a group who appeared to have independent status as philosophers, such as Hipparchia, wife of Crates, and Themista known as the lawgiver, wife of Leon. Others were mathematicians, physicians, poets, poet-musicians, and similar, outside the usual traditions. Some were wives, most were not, and some were foreign born. They were often referred to as "hetairae"–courtesans and the like–although they do not appear to have sold sexual favours, and their numbers were not inconsiderable. There were 76 women hailed as significant poets around the time of Sappho (c. 612 BC). Medicine was a forbidden occupation to them in Athens during the time of Pericles, whose companion Aspasia was a "hetairae" and the acknowledged teacher of Socrates.[5]

Despite the ancient Greeks' lack of understanding about the potential value of everyday occupation, it was, perhaps, associated cultural beliefs and attitudes that contributed most to a time of exceptional progress in health care. In particular, it was their attitude toward the human body that created a new system of personal health. Their ideal was a world of the healthy and sound, the harmonious, the beautiful and the balanced. Perfect balance was of both body and mind, and education was aimed at developing individuals to meet that cultural ideal through physical occupations in the main, along with intellectual stimulation provided within schools of philosophy situated at the gymnasia.[6]

Physicians adhered to a similar ideal, following rather than leading it, and not generating an overwhelming interest in, or slavish following of, medical ideas. In a way similar to gymnastic advisers, fourth century doctor Diocles of Karystosof recommended that in order to achieve health people should get up before sunrise, engage in physical training twice a day at the gymnasium, take only two simple meals a day, and maintain a high level of personal hygiene. Such regimes, though, were recommended mainly for 'the upper social strata. The great mass of the common people, the slaves, farmers, and labourers, had no part in it.'[7]

Because 'health was considered one of the highest goods, and disease a great curse because it removed man from the condition of perfection', the position of people who were sick or disabled was problematic. They were considered inferior. The physician, whose duty it was to maintain and restore health, was unlikely to have anything to offer:

> To attend a hopeless case was regarded as unethical since the end in view, the complete restoration of the patient, was unattainable. Weaklings and crippled children were destroyed. The sick man was an inferior being, and this too made his position particularly hard to bear.[8]

The custom of killing infants with disability is difficult for people of modern civilisations to understand, but it does appear to have been the case. Halle reported that this was a state decision rather than a personal one:

> It was an established custom at Sparta, as among the most ancient states of Greece, as well as at a later period among the Romans, to decide upon the fate of every infant at its birth; and according to its strength, and the indications which it gave of a sound constitution, to receive it into the number of the living, or to exclude it from this privilege, when its condition authorised the presumption that, in its future life, it would only become a feeble being, destitute of ability to serve its country.[9]

That being the case it is unlikely that historical research will uncover occupational regimes for the remediation of, or adaptation to, long term disability. Instead it is more likely to find that the use of occupation for health within the Classical cultures would be aimed at maintaining harmonious and balanced lifestyles, at developing the body beautiful and, probably, an inquiring mind, and, also, possibly, at preventing disease. Too, it might be used in a communal way to keep the State itself healthy and strong, and, indeed, in some instances it was the State itself that imposed an occupational regime for the well-being of its population.

Some recommendations for the use of occupation come from the stories of the gods, from literature, or from the wise utterances of long respected philosophers, and still others from physicians. Each of these will be considered separately.

Occupation for health: Recommendations of the state

Classical Greek culture upheld a code of personal hygiene which was to be the model for centuries,[10] hygiene being used, in that case, to imply more than clean, sterile and germ-free, but "health" itself or, more probably, "healthy living". It also upheld a particular kind of public health, which had more to do with the promotion of a healthy and fit race than the prevention of diseases, although it aimed at both. Halle, in the 18th century, pointed to an important distinction made in early societies between public and private health which was not obvious in his time. As he saw it, public health in societies such as that of ancient Greece constituted a part of the governance, in order to prepare future generations to be healthy and vigorous. The inference being that they would also be well able to defend their country:

> *In studying the legislation of ancient nations, we must never forget that their chief aim was to furnish the state with hardy citizens and able defenders. Every citizen was a soldier; and every private consideration was invariably sacrificed to the interests of the republic. It is in this order of things that we must sometimes seek for the origin of customs, which in our own times appear barbarous and inhuman.*[11]

Those specific public health needs, Halle also implied, were integrated with their more holistic view for 'without doubt, the ancients were more convinced than the moderns of the mutual dependence between the physical and moral virtues'. In Greece, and especially in Sparta, in order to prepare a race of healthy 'heroes each child's education became the most important concern of the state'.[12]

Across much of Greece, the education of children of both sexes was carried on at public expense in gymnasia, where the officials were responsible for the development and maintenance of their pupils' health, exercise and morals. With some of those officials it is difficult to clearly identify their role in modern terms. Herodicus (470-440 BC), for example, who is said to have cured himself from hypochondria by exercise, has been described as a physician, a teacher, or a wrestling master. This suggests that much less differentiation was made between those roles in classical times, that overlap between them was an accepted occurrence, and that their holistic view of health recognised that there is an interaction between mental and bodily occupation, education, and health status.

It appears difficult to equate closely the education system of ancient Greece with those in current use as what occurred seems to have been less structured in a classroom sense, with training of the body apparently taking precedence over focussed training of the mind. Indeed, the system of education appears to have been more aimed at the promotion of health and inherent strengths than the economic futures of the pupils. Because of that personal growth and remedial focus, the subject of education and gymnasia is relevant to this history. That is, places of education were also the places where health promotion and remediation took place.

In line with the health direction and the objective of healthy, strong, sound, beautiful and balanced citizens, the leaders of Ancient Greece deemed physical training to be of the utmost importance in education. As it was the custom to strip or at least to remove the greater part of clothing according to the demands of specific exercises, from *"gymnos"*, the word for naked, came the descriptor *gymnasium* for the place in which that occurred. This term was used not only for the venue for physical exercise but for educational complexes as a whole. Apart from academic instruction, the State-built and operated gymnasia were almost an ancient equivalent of the modern-day "health and leisure centre" with gymnasts providing instruction. (In addition to gymnasts there was a class of physicians called *Iatroleiptic* from their making use of massage and advice for the purpose of curing.[13]) The physical occupations practised in them were diverse, but mainly consisted of racing, leaping, hurling, and quoits as well as wrestling and boxing. They also included diverse types of dancing, rhythmical and harmonious movement, riding, driving chariots, swinging, climbing ropes, and swimming.

The gymnasia were large complexes, with separate buildings for different uses. These included as a stadium, baths, palaestra (which term was applied to either a private school of exercise or to places especially set aside for boxing and wrestling), and an outer portico where philosophers and teachers made known their ideas on philosophy and the arts and discoursed with students.

Women were educated as carefully as the men, in the belief that 'with the feebleness of the mother begins the feebleness of the man'.[14] In Ionia, Teos, Chios, and Sparta the early education of boys and girls was shared, whilst in other city states they were educated separately, the girls sometimes at home.[15] It is said that Lycurgus, the traditional legislator of Sparta, (many scholars suspect that he is a legendary figure[16]);

> *... turned his attention to the great object of preparing vigorous stamina, and sought, in the education of the Spartan women, the ingredient of that strength of body, which, combined with energy of soul, was to form the heroes whom he wished to give to his country.*[17]

To accomplish that, until the time of marriage when they had to cease frequenting the gymnasium so as to concentrate on wifely and motherly duties, Spartan women trained with men in the same exercises. During pregnancy they were constantly exposed to images which combined strength and beauty because of a belief that external impressions could affect developing embryos.

Sparta provides a definitive illustration of a State's use of occupation to enhance the health of populations. It was even the elders who decided solemnly upon the life or death of the babies, in the name of the republic. Until the age of seven Spartan infants were entrusted to the care of their parents, and during that time were permitted great liberty so that their physical, mental and moral faculties unfolded "unshackled" by "straitening bonds" or harshness. At seven they became the children of the state and began 'to inure themselves to fatigues proportionate to their age', performing their sport and exercise in public to harden their bodies gradually and improve their physical skill and movement. At twelve, living frugally and temperately, they spent almost the whole day in the gymnasium engaged in violent exercises. Less accustomed to the use of baths than the other states of Greece, the Spartans were habituated to bathing in rivers and streams. By the age of eighteen they had been taught to despise and resist pain, and to funnel their passions towards the love of their country.

Sensuality was discouraged, and the arts were encouraged only so far as they inspired noble and manly sentiments, and daring and courageous occupations.[18]

The Athenians instituted three *gymnasia* near to their city, despite, it was said, making less use of them, except for the education of the young, than in other parts of Greece. One of them was known as the Academy. This was where Plato instructed his followers in Socratian philosophy. Another, the Lyceum, was where Aristotle held forth to his students.[19][20][21] Thucydides, the Greek historian who lived about 455-401 BC, described some aspects of life in Athens, in his *History of the Peloponnessian War*. His descriptions are probably worth considering as he is credited with attempting to faithfully represent the past so that it might serve the future, seeking accuracy as well as making profound observations of people and events.[22] He explained that in Athens:

> Our constitution does not copy the laws of neighbouring states; but we are rather a pattern to others than imitators ourselves. Its administration favours the many instead of the few; this is why it is called a democracy. If we look to the laws, they afford equal justice to all in their private differences; if to social standing, advancement in public life falls to reputation for capacity, class considerations not being allowed to interfere with merit; while as to poverty, if a man is able to serve the state, he is not hindered by the obscurity of his condition.

He went on to explain how those democratic principles extended into the daily lives and occupations of the residents:

> The freedom which we enjoy in our government extends also to our ordinary life … we do not feel called upon to be angry with our neighbour for doing what he like …
>
> Further, we provide plenty of means for the mind to refresh itself from business. At stated periods of the year we celebrate games and sacrifices; beside which the elegance of our private establishments forms a daily source of pleasure and helps to banish the spleen; …
>
> … while in education where our rivals from their very cradles by a painful discipline seek after manliness, at Athens we live exactly as we please, and yet are just as ready to meet every legitimate danger …
>
> Cultivating refinement without extravagance and knowledge without effeminacy, we employ our wealth more for use than show, and place the real disgrace of poverty not in owning to the fact but in declining to struggle against it …
>
> These take as your model and judging happiness to be the fruit of freedom and freedom of valour, never decline the dangers of war.[23]

The different attitude of Athenians towards gymnasia is also apparent in the pamphlet written by Xenophon (c. 430-354 BC) and known as *Old Oligarch*, which told that:

> Citizens devoting their time to gymnastics and the cultivation of music are not to be found in Athens; the sovereign people has disestablished them, not from any disbelief in the beauty and honour of such training, but recognising the fact that these are things the cultivation of which is beyond its powers.[24]

The cult of gymnasia, notwithstanding, continued for several hundred years more, apparently also in Athens. Indeed, both Plato and Aristotle considered that the gymnasia based system of education was indispensable in "every well-ordered commonwealth," and hypothesised it necessary for the harmonious and simultaneous development of mind and body. The latter belief is close to occupational therapy's fundamental philosophy so, perhaps, it comes as no surprise that such systems were employed not only for development of mind and body, but were also applied to the cure of chronic diseases.[25,26]

On a different "occupational" tack, Pericles (490-429 BC), an Athenian statesman of unimpeachable honour, dignified bearing and eloquence, and leader of the Democratic party, advanced public health and well-being using the economic skills and abilities of the populace. He spent the time between 440-432 beautifying Athens with public buildings, to the extent that it was under his leadership that Athens attained 'the zenith of her artistic glory, her imperial greatness and her commercial prosperity'.[27]

The Periclean building program was in the first place 'a means of providing employment for the population of Athens'.[28] However, it offered much more in terms of community health, in that it provided not only financial benefits but purposeful occupation which was valued, demanding a range of skills and talents as well as ongoing physical and mental exercise. Plutarch described how:

With the variety of workmanship and of occasions for service, which summon all arts and trades and require all hands to be employed about them, they do actually put the whole city, in a manner, into state-pay; while at the same time she is both beautiful and maintained by herself.[29]

In supporting many types of occupational capacity and talent, the scheme must have promoted a sense of occupational justice amongst the artisans and workers, as it gave opportunity to most to make their living engaged in economically valued work, rather than only to those engaged in warfare and defence. This was so:

... that the undisciplined mechanic multitude that stayed at home should not go without their share of public salaries, and yet should not have them given them for sitting still and doing nothing ...

and so that they may:

... no less than those that were at sea or in garrisons or on expeditions, have a fair and just occasion of receiving the benefit and having their share of the public moneys ...

Thus, to say all in a word, the occasions and services of these public works distributed plenty through every age and condition.[30]

The Romans, who imitated many aspects of Greek culture, also established gymnasia, but usually on an even grander scale, suggesting that gymnastic occupations were valued in their society as they had been in Greece. They did remain a venue for the education of the young[31] but many argue that they existed, principally, for military training. Marcus Terentius Varro (116-27 BC) recognised the need for gymnasia when the nature of the physical occupations of the populous changed. He commented that, whilst Romans had engaged in agriculture they had derived the strength and vigour which preserve health and purity of morals from the labours of the field, but they had 'remained ignorant of the gymnastic art'. That kind of exercise became necessary 'when they quitted their fields, to surrender themselves to the tedious sloth of their cities and to fatal inactivity'.[32] From then on to the fall of the empire, physicians carefully encouraged its practice for the preservation of health and the cure of disease.[33]

Notwithstanding the probable military focus of gymnasia and thermae, Sigerist suggested that 'it was the merit of the Romans to develop public health. An effective public health organisation is possible only where there is a strong and steady government.' It had not been possible in Greece because of its division into small states that perpetually fought each other. In Rome, however, the organising power tended to be centralised, which made possible engineering feats such as the great aqueducts. Public health was enhanced, and the occupations of daily life changed when water was brought to the city on eleven aqueducts, and through eighteen conduits. Sigerist noted in 1961 that 'four are sufficient today to make Rome the city having the best water supply in Italy'. From 11 BC no tax was paid for the water.[34]

Some of the Roman gymnasia were called *"thermae"* (from which the word thermal derives) because hot and cold baths formed an essential element in their regimes after physical exercise.[35] Rome in the fourth century AD housed 11 great thermae, 856 baths, 1,352 water basins and fountains, and almost every house had its own water cistern.[36] It is from that tradition that spa treatments grew.[37] "Baths" were centres for the treatment of joints and urinary tract, to aid relaxation, and as beauty therapy as well as for cultural pursuits and sometimes debauchery, as at Ephesus where a brothel was incorporated.[38]

Story claims that baths were the forerunners of physical medicine and rheumatology,[39] and as occupational therapy in Britain was strongly connected to those branches of medicine in the middle part of the twentieth century, it becomes part of this history. Indeed, the holistic health education through physical and intellectual occupations that was followed in the gymnasia and thermae suggests that there are valid reasons for the profession to claim an early connection with public health, even if hesitant to claim debauchery. At Bath, in Roman England, baths established in 45 AD, as *Aquae Sulis*, were also a place for debates and teaching. These were on the site of hot springs, which had been valued for occult and religious purposes before the advent of the Roman occupation.[40]

The decline of many sports, including gymnastics followed the closure of the ancient Olympic Games in AD 393. They had become increasingly professional and then corrupt. But the final factor in their demise was a reduction of interest

Figure 1.3.1: **Woman bathing at the Roman Bath in the Strand, London by F. Matania**

(The Wellcome Library.)

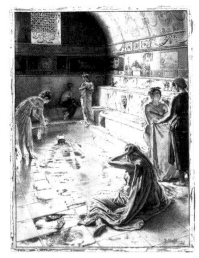

in any occupation that celebrated or increased the strength of the body. That major shift away from interest in the "body" followed the spread of Christianity across the Roman Empire and the concurrent and rigorously held belief that it housed Satan.[41] This factor punctuated an extraordinary change in beliefs about health, and about its care and remediation, from one which had used physical occupations to maintain and promote a healthy mind, body and State, to one in which the health of the soul was paramount, and occupations were centred on its salvation.

Occupation for health: Recommendations of the gods

In Classical times spiritual and religious needs were met by the gods, the lives of whom were not necessarily eternal, although they were regarded as immortal, omnipotent, and omniscient. Their powers were great: they had extraordinary strength and wisdom; carried out their actions with speed; were just but judgmental; and, on the whole loved and cared for humankind, rewarding those who were "good" with the fruits of the after-world, where sinners, who had escaped retribution, were duly punished.[42]

Belief in those deities influenced the occupations that were part and parcel of the daily lives of the masses. There were gods who looked after the farmer and his crops or livestock or the sailor's, fisher's or trader's safety on the waters. Some assisted the craftsman, artisan or artist to develop skills, new ideas or inspiration. Others upheld the natural world of sun, moon, mountains and rivers, or who cared for the health of individuals.[43]

Sigerist observed about "religious medicine" that:
> ... *we come upon it in the initial stages and throughout the course of every*

civilisation, no matter what other forms of medicine may have been developed. It is always present because it satisfies an ever-existing need. In all civilisations, at all times, there have been religious individuals who in case of illness sought help from the priest rather than the physician. Temples and churches, furthermore, were the last resort of those patients who had been given up by their physicians and were hoping for a miracle. And finally, there was also an economic factor which must not be overlooked. Religious therapy was, as a rule, cheaper than diets, drugs, and operations. The god was satisfied with a small sacrifice while physicians had to be paid in hard cash. We have records of many rich people who sought healing in temples and presented them with opulent gifts, but we also know that many more poor people, who could not afford a doctor, went to the temple praying for health.

Greece was no exception to the rule.[44]

In gymnasia and elsewhere, exercises aimed at developing the human body were practised to honour the gods and so physical training took on almost a religious fervour and character. It is therefore appropriate that the original Greek god of healing was Apollo, usually depicted as a youth of dazzling appearance. The son of Zeus and Leto, and twin brother of Artemis, he was born on the island of Delos, but was entrusted to the care of Themis (whose name signifies justice). Apollo was fed on nectar and ambrosia, so that within a few hours of his birth he had grown to manhood. His role was conceived in a number of ways: as a god of the Sun, throwing light on 'the dark ways of the future', as a god of music and song that can only be heard when 'light and security reign', and as a god of grazing herds who feed on the grass warmed by the sun. Apollo was also understood to be the god of earthly blessings and the personification of youth and beauty, as well as the god of medicine who 'provided for the growth of healing plants' and protected the young in athletic contests and war.[45] His godly responsibilities encompassed a holistic concept of health that included notions of the inter-relatedness of the sun and earth, of plants and animals, of renewal and regrowth, and of physical and creative occupations. With such responsibilities he seems to personify or deify many of the characteristics central to occupational therapy. Indeed, Macdonald, in her history of the remedial professions, records that Apollo displayed:

… sensitivity and moderation to medicine, art, law, music and poetry, and to the health and gaiety of youth, involving these factors in his religious and prophetic approach to life. He also showed great interest in astronomy, mathematics, medicine, philosophy and science, and used music and poetry therapeutically to relieve depression and pain …[46]

Apollo shared his knowledge of medicine with Chiron, the Centaur, who was said to be wise, kindly, and just, to understand philosophy, and to be skilled in arts like music, hunting, and astronomy, as well as the healing arts including chiropractics and surgery. Chiron had many well-known pupils such as Achilles, Hercules and Jason to whom he is said to have taught the art of healing. The most famous of his pupils has to have been Aesculapius, the son of Apollo and Koronis, a Thessalian princess. The story has several versions. In one, at Aesculapius' birth, his mother was killed by Artemis's arrows, though some say that it was by Apollo's arrows. In another Apollo saved his son from his paramour's womb when she was to burn at the stake for adultery. The stories, however, agree that the boy was saved by his father and given, by him, into the care of his trusted friend Chiron.[47][48][49]

Figure 1.3.2:   Aesculapius[9]

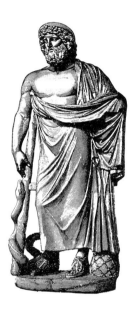

Aesculapius grew to be an outstanding physician and surgeon, and even, it is said, resuscitated some people who were already dead, for which presumption Zeus killed him with his thunderbolt. However, despite the cause and nature of his death, he was regarded as a god afterwards, and his cult dominated the "medical scene" and set a pattern for the cults of other healing deities.[50] Dubos' assessment of that tale, in *Mirage of Health*, maintains that:

> *To ward off disease or recover health, men as a rule find it easier to depend on healers than to attempt the more difficult task of living wisely. Asclepius, (Aesculapius) the first physician according to Greek legend, achieved fame not by teaching wisdom but by mastering the use of the knife and the knowledge of the curative virtues of plants. In contrast to Hygeia, the name Asclepius is of very ancient origin. Apparently Asclepius lived as a physician around the twelfth century BC. He was already known as a hero during Homeric times and was created a god in Epidaurus around the fifth or sixth century BC. His popularity spread far and wide, even beyond the boundaries of Greece ... In most of the ancient iconography from the third century on, as well as in all subsequent representations, Asclepius appears as a handsome, self assured young god, accompanied by two maidens: on his right Hygeia and on his left Panakeia.*[51]

His story as man and deity provides an illustration that the medicine of the Greek gods is inseparable from the cultural context and the development of classical medicine. His priests, known as Aesculapiads, were probably physicians, and his temples appear to have been 'sanatoria, centers of research and training, where medical experience accumulated and was passed on to younger generations'[52] His earthly contribution to this history will be discussed in the section relating to physicians.

Hygeia, who in many of the mythical tales is described as Aesculapius's daughter, sister or wife, or was 'relegated to the role of a member of his retinue' is also said, in early legends, to be the goddess who watched over the health of Athens.[53] In all of the versions, her role was the preservation of good health subservient to and distinct from restoration following illness. That role was attributed to Jaso or Panikeia, and in Rome to Meditrina. Dubos argued that 'Panakeia became omnipotent as a healing goddess through knowledge of drugs either from plants or from the earth. Her cult is alive today in the universal search for a panacea'[54]

Figure 1.3.3: **Hygeia Feeding the symbolic serpent of health**

(The Wellcome Library)

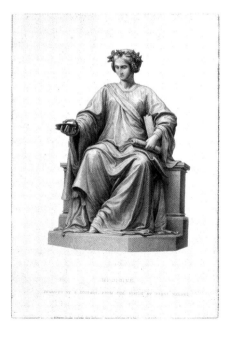

The way Dubos told of the myth of Hygeia provides insight into a different understanding of how health can be viewed, apart from the glories of heroic medicine. His notion of Hygeia's role appears to have much in common with many, but not all, of the aspirations of occupational therapists. Initially, by analysis of her name and what it has come to signify he alludes to the repression of joyful, health-giving occupations in the pursuit of the sanitary:

The word "hygiene" now conjures up smells of chlorine and phenol, pasteurised foodstuffs and beverages in cellophane wrappers, a way of life in which the search for pleasurable sensations must yield to practices that are assumed to be sanitary. Its etymology, however, bears no relation to this pedestrian concept. Hygiene is the modern ersatz for the cult of Hygeia, the lovely goddess who once watched over the health of Athens. Hygeia was probably an emanation, a personification of Athena, the goddess of reason. Although identified with health, she was not involved in the treatment of the sick. Rather, she was the guardian of health and symbolised the belief that men could remain well if they lived according to reason .... Throughout the classical world Hygeia continued to symbolise the virtues of a sane life in a pleasant environment, the ideal of mens sana in corpore sano.[55]

As he puts it, Dubos provides a cautionary and insightful vision of how health professions following in the footsteps of Hygeia are almost doomed to being overlooked in favour of the apparently miraculous effects of invasive techniques. Occupational therapists, who help ordinary people to overcome difficulties they experience in going about their everyday lives and to realise their potential, have experienced the frustrations such lack of recognition inevitably causes and will continue to cause, despite the value of what they do.

In Greece she eventually came to be more closely identified with mental health and in Rome she was known as Salus, a divinity of well-being in general. But in reality Hygeia was not an earthbound goddess of ancient origin. Her name derives from an abstract word meaning health. For the Greeks she was a concept rather than a historical person remembered from the myths of their past. She was not a compelling Jeanne d'Arc but only an allegorical goddess Liberty and she never truly touched the hearts of the people. From the fifth century BC on, her cult progressively gave way to that of the healing god, Asclepius ...

... The myths of Hygeia and Asclepius symbolise the never-ending oscillation between two different points of view in medicine. For the worshipers of Hygeia, health is the natural order of things, a positive attribute to which men are entitled if they govern their lives wisely. According to them, the most important function of medicine is to discover and teach the natural laws which will ensure to man a healthy mind in a healthy body. More sceptical or wiser in the ways of the world, the followers of Asclepius believe that the chief role of the physician is to treat disease, to restore health by correcting any imperfection caused by the accidents of birth or of life.[56]

From other tales of the gods come notions linked to that of occupation's relationship to health. The lives of Orpheus and Musaeus, for example, illustrate how music and poetry can exert a powerful effect on the soul and through it, in holistic terms, influence a healthy or sick body. Orpheus, an inspired bard and seer, was said to have bewitched people, animals, and plants, moved rocks, and halted rivers by the power of his words, sung to the strains of his lyre as he wandered throughout Greece. He was a purification priest and founder of a religious sect whose followers, the Orphics, were pledged to lead pure lives.[57] He was also a physician who used incantations and magic formulas to cleanse patients of impurities and appease the wrath of the gods. Musaeus was possibly a friend or disciple of Orpheus, and like him was a bard, seer, and physician.[58,59]

Occupation for health as described in literature

The early Greek writers were mainly poets. Probably the best and earliest known of the literary masters is Homer, who was born, it is thought, sometime between 1050 and 850 BC, somewhere on the west coast of Asia Minor. He is typically depicted, at least in his old age, as blind and poor, so, for that period, appears to have been a rare specimen of disability and disadvantage. Whilst parts of the Homeric epic probably embody an earlier oral tradition which goes back far into the past, he is generally accepted as the author of the classic poems the *Iliad* and the *Odyssey*. The *Iliad* tells the story of Agamemnon, Helen, Achilles and the Trojan War, and the *Odyssey*, the story of Odysseus's wanderings on the journey home from Troy.[60] In the *Odyssey*, Homer provides some idea of the place of physicians in society when he classes them with prophets, shipwrights and minstrels as "workers for the public good", and the respect still accorded to Egypt as a medical authority.[61]

Sigerist, in his discussion of "Homeric medicine", explained that Homer's heroes fitted the cultural ideal of being healthy and fit:

> *Their meals were frugal, as a rule, although large banquets were held on festive occasions. They drank wine, but it was mixed with water; drunkenness was frowned upon. They exercised in a variety of games and sports, and measured their strength and skill in various contests. They were clean, had bathrooms at home, and also bathed when at war.*[62]

In the Iliad, for example, after battle, Odysseus and Diomedes bathed first in the sea, and then in a regular bath before being anointed with oil. Games and sport constituted a part of the gymnastic art, which was used as natural exercise for soldiers. Homer, again in the Iliad, described military gymnastics. The interest excited amongst spectators and competitors resulted in them becoming adopted generally, through the efforts of people such as Hercules, Pelops, and Iphitus, king of Elis, who established the Olympic games. Philosophers and physicians, perceiving the value of exercise to health and strength in states of health, illness or convalescence, to the preservation of function, and the reduction of illness, communicated their observations to others. The practice of gymnastic exercise was extended, and buildings were constructed to allow it to be combined with other institutions that composed the education of youth.[63]

The gods played a large role in Homer's sagas, and it was they who inflicted disease, just as was the case in other ancient civilisations. As health was so highly desirable, it is not surprising that Homer also depicted disease as a great evil, and death the worst fate that could befall mankind. For example, in Hades, Achilles' soul told Odysseus that rather than being a king in the realm of the dead he would prefer to be still living on earth as a starving labourer on a farm.

Macdonald, in her history of the remedial professions, centred on Homer's interest in the use of occupations for health, whilst noting that he also recognised 'the value of music, sunshine, fresh air and appropriate diets and baths'. She described how Homer wrote of 'the diversionary and prophylactic value of crafts, gymnastics, games and exercises', and went on to discuss how in the *Iliad*:

> … *he tells of the noble craftsman-god, Hephaetus, who was lame, and having been disowned by his mother on this account he was saved by being given, by Thetis and Eurynome, opportunity and equipment for producing "much cunning handiwork"… It is interesting to note that at this time it was customary to encourage blind men to become minstrels and lame men to become smiths, the latter in imitation of their artisan-god, Hephaetus.*[64]

The legend of Hephaetos, in fact has several versions. The son of Zeus and Hera, he was either thrown from Olympus by his father, or by his mother, or on separate occasions by each parent, and with whom he later established a more friendly relationship. On his return to Olympus he set up a workshop in his palace with an anvil and "twenty pairs of bellows", becoming the god of those occupations dependent upon fire, such as pottery and blacksmithing. He made gifts for many of the gods but for himself fashioned what must have been considered the ultimate in mobility aids, 'two wonderful handmaidens of gold, who, like living beings, would move about and assist him as he walked'.[65,66] Maybe an enterprising robotic mobility aid manufacturer of the future will design something similar.

Another early poet was Hesiod, who wrote during the eighth century BC and, like Homer, believed that it was the gods who inflicted disease. His poems have particular interest for he was not born into the affluent classes, but was of peasant-farmer stock, from Boeotia, where he worked as a herdsman for his father. This means that from his writing it is possible to glean a common sense and plebeian way of regarding both health and occupation. He turned to literature and wrote what is described as "didactic verse", after his brother Perses inherited the family farm.[67]

One of three famous poems is known as *Works and Days*, and this, Sigerist analysed from the perspective of medicine. He suggested that Hesiod was obviously a firm believer in the gods, as the poem discussed "the days which come from Zeus", the countless plagues and diseases that sprang "soundless" from Pandora's box, and famine and plague as a punishment for sins and presumptuous deeds. The poem includes elements of primitive medicine such as views on religious medicine, old peasant taboos, and common-sense health care. Being written at a time when the division between rich and poor was increasing, it extols industry, justice, and moral behavior proclaiming that wealth is created by labour, and that the gods prefer work to idleness which itself is a disgrace. That mixture of common sense, religion, medicine and magic provided rules about urination and hygiene; and advice about husbandry, rising early, drinking wine mixed with water, not postponing for tomorrow what could be done today, when to marry, and the advantages of sons. From the mix of concepts in the poem comes the thought that, with the belief that health comes from the gods and that work was viewed positively by them, then it followed that ill health was likely seen as a potential outcome of idleness. Similarly, health and longevity, the ultimate good, could be seen as the outcome of engagement in well-chosen occupation.[68]

Sigerist also points to later poets, Martial, Juvenal, and Lucretius, who wrote during the 1st century BC, as sources to learn about aspects of occupational health. Their works, he said, reflect the layman's views about the dangers of certain occupations, 'of the diseases of sulphur workers[69] and blacksmiths[70] of the varicose veins of the augurs[71] and the hard fate of the gold miners'.[72]

Occupation for health as described by philosophers

Medicine and philosophy were closely linked and grew alongside each other, which explains why early in its history Greek medicine developed a theoretical framework.[73] Celsus explained:

At first the science of healing was held to be part of philosophy, so that the treatment of disease and contemplation of the nature of things began through the same authorities ... Hence we find that many who professed philosophy became expert in medicine ...[74]

Philosophy was not regarded at that time as an academic exercise with little or no practical day by day benefit, perhaps because 'most Greek philosophers took an active part in the political life of their country or at least showed great interest in problems of state and statesmanship'. They also taught the very young. To them philosophy was very practical, providing guides to action, and teaching people 'how to understand the world and how to act in it intelligently'.[75]

Thales (6-7thC BC) was a case in point. A wealthy and practical man, he was a mathematician, poet, physician, scientist and statesman as well as a philosopher, made contributions to astrology, geometry and navigation, and displaced 'many mythical notions by reason'.[76] He was a leader in the earliest Greek philosophy which originated in the Ionic colonies of Asia Minor, led principally by physicists and cosmologists such as himself, Anaximenes of Miletus (6thC BC), Heracleitus of Ephesus (5-6thC BC), Pythagorus of Samos (5-6thC BC), and Empedocles of Sicily (5thC BC). They mainly 'sought to reduce the universe to a first principal or single element'.[77] Thales, for example, believed water to be the first principle of the universe, 'claiming that it was the basis of all substances and that life depended on it'.[78] Apart from their central preoccupation, most of that early group also tended to have wide-ranging interests including medicine.[79] In fact it was from them that humoural theories of physiology and pathology are said to have originated, evolving naturally from their philosophical interest in the nature and structure of the universe.[80]

Of these it was Pythagoras (6thC BC), whose wife Theano, was 'devoted to medicine, hygiene, the arts of ethical living' and a commentator of healing arts, amongst other accomplishments,[81] who probably exerted the deepest influence upon medicine. Indeed, Edelstein's study appears to make it clear that the Hippocratic Oath was a Pythagorean document.[82] Pythagoras is also believed, with others such as Anaxagorus and Empedocles, to be responsible for 'the theory of the four humors, which were thought to constitute the substratum of life and disease'.[83] Provoked by the religious fervour that swept through Greece in the second half of the sixth century, amongst people no longer satisfied with the primitive worship of the Homeric gods, Pythagoras is said to have travelled widely. He finally emigrated to Croton in Italy, with a group of followers around 530 BC. There, he organised them into a well-disciplined school with somewhat the character of a religious order. It is worth noting here that such mobility was possible because 'schools of learning were free associations of masters and disciples, not burdened by buildings, endowments, or other earthly goods which tie a school to a certain locality'.[84]

Despite an interest in science, the Pythagoreans' chief concern was the progress of the soul and its redemption. To that end they led an ascetic and pure life, trying to maintain perfect physical and mental balance. They used meditation and mnemotechnics such as not rising in the morning before recalling in detail the previous day's happenings. Their interest in science centred on mathematics, which appeared to them as "the first principle", in that they believed it could be applied and make sense of everything, even such a creative thing as music. For example, 'tradition relates that Pythagoras while plucking a string discovered that the tone given was determined by the length of the string and that harmony was a mathematical proportion'.[85]

As harmony, perfect equilibrium and perfect balance were the goal of the Pythagorean's life and numerical interest, they believed that investigating numbers could also provide 'a key to the riddle of the universe and an instrument for the purification of the soul' as well as being the key and instrument to health.[86] Apparently the number four was considered particularly important, as logically two pairs of forces with opposite qualities would constitute an ideal balance. That idea was complementary to the Pythagorean doctrine of opposites which was to have a profound influence on medical theory as well as explaining the harmony of the world. 'Aristotle tells that some Pythagoreans spoke of ten such pairs, namely, limited-unlimited, odd-even, one-many, right-left, male-female, rest-motion, straight-curved, light-darkness, good-bad, square-oblong, a theory that may be of Babylonian origin.'[87'88] Some of those opposites might be worthwhile subjects for occupational therapists seeking to understand the notion of occupational balance.

With the view that health is a condition of perfect equilibrium, the way of life followed by the disciples of Pythagoras was meant to preserve that equilibrium. They practiced moderation and maintaining equanimity at all times and in all situations. However, if in spite of careful living a person's equilibrium became upset it was restored using "medicine" to regain physical balance and music to regain mental balance.[89] Music was, apparently, the occupation chosen as most health giving by Pythagorus, perhaps because of the mathematical connection with harmony. Macdonald reported that 'like Orpheus, he advised the use of music as a treatment for depression, and added that he also favoured gymnastics for promoting good health'.[90]

Empedocles (c. 490-430 BC) proposed the doctrine of elements, philosophising that fire was the essence of life, and water, earth and air formed the basis of other matter.[91] As well as Pythagorus and Alcmaeon of Croton (c. 450 BC) he was influential in the development of humoural theory.[92] Those four elements were closely associated with the primal qualities of warm, cold, dry and moist, and with four body fluids, blood, phlegm, yellow and black bile. The fluids, known as the humours, were present throughout the body, forming the foundation of humoural theories of physiology and pathology. The correct balance and mix of these was thought crucial to health, and so a lexicon of terms developed which was used to explain the range of possibilities. These included *crasis* for "the proportional mix of humours", *eucrasia* for the right balance and *dyscrasia* for the wrong balance. The latter was believed responsible for systemic disorders. *Abundatia* was the term given to over supply of any of the humours, *corruptio* to deterioration, *coagulatio* to curdling, and *putrefactio* to decomposition.[93] Empedocles also developed biological theories about perception and thought.[94]

Without doubt the best known of the Ancient Greek philosophers were Socrates (469-399 BC), Plato (427-347 BC) and Aristotle (384-322 BC). The first two, who were master and pupil, influenced thought in relation to the individual; to the origin of languages; and to the community, ethics and politics. Following a brief interest in the physical sciences of the earliest Greek philosophers, Socrates was influenced by Pythagorean teaching. However his particular focus came to be in individuals knowing themselves, their life, their personality, and what their thoughts should be, so his contribution was, in many ways, that of a precursor to psychology. He postulated a spiritual view of knowledge and conduct, substituting scientific notions with beliefs of mind and soul, and the value of truth, virtue, knowledge and appropriate action and conduct. Socrates attended the gymnasia for study and exercise as well as to teach. He trained his followers *"skepsis en logois"*, that is systematic examination of fundamental assumptions from which conduct and morality arose, and in that can be regarded as the founder of formal logic. With a high public profile, he was found guilty of corrupting Athenian youth, by encouraging them to criticise the existing order, and condemned to death. He committed suicide by taking hemlock.[95'96]

Plato had been born in Athens but, after Socrates death, he travelled extensively through Greece, Italy and Egypt before returning to his hometown and establishing himself at the Academy, where he taught for the remainder of his life.[97] Despite holding the opinion that women were inferior to men in every branch of industry, he taught both men and women believing that they should have the same educational opportunities. A prolific and eloquent writer, he was the author of numerous publications which covered topics such as art, education, ethics, gymnastics, literature, logic, mathematics, music, politics, "psychology", religion and science.[98] Although not a physician, he both respected Hippocrates and held particular "humourally based" medical theories and beliefs himself:[99]

> *The origin of diseases should be obvious. The body is composed of four elements - earth, fire, air and water; and disorders and diseases are caused by an unnatural excess or deficiency of any of them, by their shifting from their proper place to another, by any part of the body taking in an unsuitable variety either of fire or other element ... and by similar disturbances ... The only way in which good health can be maintained is for replacement and waste to be uniform, similar and on the same scale.*[100]

There was also a worse kind of disease due to 'an unhealthy way of life' leading to 'deterioration caused by a reversal in the process of their (marrow, bone, flesh, sinew, blood) formation'.

> *When flesh decomposes and the result of the decomposition is discharged back into the veins, the blood in the veins is extensively mixed with air and takes on a variety of colours and bitternesses, as well as acid and salty qualities, and develops bile, serum and phlegm of all sorts.*[101]

These destroyed the blood, which could no longer supply nourishment to the body as it circulated, and conflicted with each other, attacking parts of the body and spreading destruction and decay.

A third type of diseases was caused by changes or imbalance in breath, phlegm and bile, and a fourth were diseases of soul and mind. Of the latter, he cites as cause, 'acid and saline phlegm and bitter bilious humours' trapped in one of the three places where he believed the soul was housed, which caused irritability and depression, rashness and timidity, or forgetfulness and dullness.

He also argued that any condition which brought on madness or stupidity 'must be called a disease'. Because of that he ranked excessive 'pleasure and pain among the worst diseases of the mind,' but excused over-indulgence on both genetic and socially determined grounds.

> *And indeed it is generally true that it is unjust to blame over-indulgence in pleasure as if wrong doing were voluntary; no one wishes to be bad, but a bad man is bad because of some flaw in his physical make-up and failure in his education, neither of which he likes and chooses.*[102]

When people lived in "bad" communities, he said, and when there were no courses of study available to correct their faults, the blame for mental illness rested with parents and educators.[103] That theory implies an occupational cause and remedy to prevent mental illness from occurring at all. Indeed he went on to say about fitness of the mind 'that any of these forms (three distinct forms of soul mentioned above) that lives in idleness and fails to exercise its own proper motions is bound to become very feeble, while by that exercise they will become very strong '.[104]

In tune with his times, Plato expressed strong views about gymnastics and baths, the first medicinal use of which he credited to Herodicus of Selymbria and, sometimes, those opinions were at variance with each other:

> *Among movements, the best is that we produce ourselves - for it is most nearly akin to the movement of thought and of the universe; next is movement produced in us by another; worst of all is movement caused by outside agents in parts of the body while the body itself remains passive and inert. So the best way of perging and toning up the body is by exercise; next is the motion of a ship or any vehicle that does not cause fatigue; last, and for use in extreme necessity, though not otherwise if we have any sense, is purging by medicine and drugs.*[105]

In the third book of *Republic* he asserts that in his "ideal world" people would be trained in gymnastics from infancy throughout life. He said 'what music is to the inner man, gymnastics is to the frame-work that encloses his mind and spirit,' meaning that gymnastics provided for the harmonious and proportional development of the intellect, spirit and body.[106] Indeed, he is said to have recommended all kinds of exercises for limbs and sense organs. At other times Plato stated that gymnastics and bathing might have detrimental effects on people.[107]

Also in tune with the national notions about proportion and balance in health, Plato espoused balance of mind and body by avoiding 'exercising either body or mind without the other, and thus preserv(ing) an equal and healthy balance between them'. Following the example of his mentor, he advocated that those engaged in "strenuous intellectual pursuit" must also exercise the body, and those interested in physical fitness should develop "cultural and intellectual interests". In a similar way, engagement in occupations must be "properly proportioned" so that the exercise of individual human capacities was balanced, harmonious and health giving, and 'rightly called a fully developed personality'.[108,109]

Macdonald reported that Plato expressed opinions about issues which relate occupation to health, such as the health giving value of work, and the need for patients not being unnecessarily isolated by treatment so that they were still able to engage in usual occupation. He said, 'all kinds of diseases … should, so far as leisure permits, be controlled by proper regimes of life'.[110] Attributing thought and feeling to the brain, Plato advocated involving the patients' minds in their therapy, without dwelling over-much on their problems. He stressed that 'the cure of a part should not be attempted without the treatment of the whole'.[111] In a way similar to more modern ideas about "people as occupational beings", Plato recognised that all people have a unique collection of physical, mental and spiritual capacities which enables each to make a distinct contribution to their community.[112]

Those ideas were compatible with Plato's occupational ideology for which he used the term, praxis, from earlier reference in Greek mythology. That interest was picked up by a student of his, Aristotle, who was destined to become as famous as he was. Aristotle sometimes used praxis to describe every human activity although he mainly regarded it as one of three activities with *theoria* and *poiesis*. The difference between them can be distinguished by their goal: for theoria this was truth, for poiesis the production of something, and for praxis, action itself. Aristotle divided praxis into economic, ethical and political activity. Sometimes he restricted praxis to the sphere of ethics and politics, and on other occasions he identified praxis with eupraxia (good praxis) as opposed to dyspraxia (bad praxis or misfortune), and on still others he combined praxis and poiesis.[113] Aristotle's school followed the latter trend dividing all human activity between the theoretical and the practical. This dichotomy was accepted in medieval scholastic philosophy, and was integral to the philosophies espoused by Bacon, Kant, Hegel and Marx. It remains part of modern thinking.[114]

Figure 1.3.4: **A sketch of Plato and Aristotle from the Raphael fresco in the Vatican**

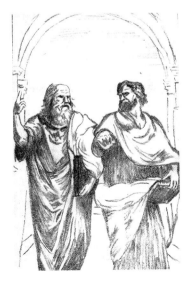

Aristotle was born in Chalcidice, the son of Nicomachus, who had been a court physician to Amyntas II of Macedonia. He left there when he was 17, journeying to Athens and becoming a pupil at the Academy, where he so distinguished himself that Plato nicknamed him "the mind of the school". In his thirties, in 347 BC, he opened a "Platonic" School in Assos with some colleagues, but five years later accepted an invitation from Philip of Macedonia to tutor his son Alexander, destined to become Alexander the Great.[115]

Aristotle, as could be anticipated, provided Alexander with a broad ranging curriculum. As well as the mandatory reading, writing and physical skills of the gymnasia, Alexander learnt rhetoric, astronomy, mathematics, and to make music. When he was ill he was 'encouraged to play with dice as a diversion', and when wounded by an arrow 'to undertake horse-riding to improve his bodily and mental conditions'. As King, Alexander founded Alexandria, in Egypt, which became an important centre of Greek learning and of world trade. An interest in biology and medicine, apparently gleaned from Aristotle, meant that the new City had both a famous gymnasium and a medical school.[116]

On Alexander's succession, Aristotle had returned to Athens and opened his school, the Lyceum. He was said to be a good organiser and an energetic teacher who encouraged reasoning and logic and the collection of encyclopaedic data.[117] During his 14 years at the Lyceum, until he retired to Chalcis when his life became endangered following his former pupil's death, Aristotle wrote many of his famous works. These traversed his wide ranging interests including topics such as metaphysics, "psychology", biology, logic, ethics, politics and literary criticism.[118]

Aristotle's exploration of medical issues was philosophical rather than practical, although he did engage in animal and fish dissections as part of his biological research. A founder of comparative anatomy, he described the major organs but, erroneously, considered that the heart was the seat of intelligence rather than the brain. He recognised Hippocrates' humoural theory, recommending walking and exercise for the maintenance of health, and writing about such things as balance, leverage and the use of pulleys in *Mechanica.* He also addressed the underlying effects of the soul, and introduced the term "Katharsis", but specifically in relation to experiencing emotions when attending theatrical tragedies.[119]

Somewhat anticipating Jeremy Bentham's Utilitarianism, Aristotle supposed that the supreme end for human endeavour is happiness, that the function of "man" is reasoning, and that happiness for "man" is the good performance of reasoning.[120] In concurrence with the cultural norms of his day, Aristotle did not argue for the greatest happiness for the greatest number of people, because he excluded a major group from his suppositions. Slaves who laboured or worked were viewed as less than human because their occupations were degrading, and that the true human condition was demonstrated by the leisure pursuits of Athenian gentlemen.[121] He recognised that without labour it is not possible to provide all the necessities of life, but that to master slaves was the human way to master necessity and thus was not against nature.[122,123]

Occupation and health as recommended by physicians

In the early days of Greek civilisation magic and religion were part and parcel of a physician's stock-in-trade. Treatment was often based on superstition, and depended on prayers, offerings to the gods, incantations, and the use of charms. It was a time when the present day medical symbol of the serpent was adopted as a sign of renewal, although the legends behind that adoption are a good deal earlier. Because serpents cast off their slough, they were thought to represent the elimination of disease and the retention of good health. Although some religious and superstitious beliefs continued, many were gradually ignored, and observation, philosophy and science began to emerge as the basis for diagnosis and treatment.

Because of the sparsity of written records, it may not be possible to find much information about prescriptions and recommendations of an occupational nature from the majority of physicians who worked during the Classical age. It is however possible to uncover the basis of modern medicine and to consider the central figures and the ideas they advanced, which support the basic premise of occupational therapy. In view of the previous sections of this chapter, it is already possible to predict that they will value physical activity for the health of both mind and body, balance between occupation and rest, and harmony within the range of occupations pursued. It is also probable that they would emphasise health rather than sickness, and be far from forthcoming about disability.

The first of the influential physicians to be discussed is Aesculapius who, as part god, learned his art from Chiron, the physician-centaur, and from his father, Apollo. He was revered during his lifetime because he was said to have cured vast numbers of people of their ills, to have successfully treated many war wounded, with surgery if required, and was one of the first physicians to visit patients in their homes and at their bedside. Machaon and Podaleirius, his two sons, followed him as physicians serving the wounded and sick in the armed forces.[124]

Aesculapius founded a number of treatment centres, which were described as temples, at Cos, Cnidus, Epidaurus, Pergamus, and Rhodes, amongst others. They were built near healing springs amidst attractive gardens, and became popular health resorts in which free treatment was offered to the poorer sick whilst wealthier patients were asked to contribute to temple funds. The centres appear similar to the gymnasia in that they were equipped with spas to bath in, an athletic centre, and a theatre. Hostels were provided for the sick, and patients with both spiritual and medical problems were treated with massage, medicinal herbs, special diets, rest, and exercises, such as horseback riding and activities wearing armour, as well as with magic and religious interventions: prayers, sacrifices, incantations and the "lick" of sacred snakes. Additionally, songs, mimes, drama and music were prescribed for patients with mental illnesses.[125]

His priests, the Aesculapiads, have sometimes been described as the first doctors of Greece. This, however, has been challenged, because what they provided was, in the main, religious medicine which bore little resemblance to later practice which some say originated with the pre-Socratic philosophers who have already been discussed. It was the latter which found its highest expression in the school of Hippocrates. It becomes confusing, though, because Hippocratic physicians also called themselves Aesculapiads because Aesculapius was the patron of their group or "guild".[126]

Early Greek physicians were craftsmen who trained as apprentices with other physicians, the art of medicine being 'transmitted by oral and practical instruction from father to son, from master to apprentice'.[127] They were not numerous as only the larger cities employed their own doctor, contracting more in times of special need, like war or epidemics. Social philosophers came to believe that a need for many doctors or hospitals earmarked a bad city. Indeed, Plato asked, 'to stand in need of the medical art through sloth and intemperate diet … obliging the skilful sons of Asclepius (ie. Aesculapius) to invent new names of diseases, such as dropsies and catarrhs - do you not think this abominable?' The same was obviously true in Rome where Tiberius argued that people who consulted a doctor after the age of thirty were fools for not having learned to regulate their lives properly without outside help.[128]

Figure 1.3.5: A sketch of patients with walking aids attend the *iatreion*, a doctor's place of business. From a vase painting, c. 470 B.C.

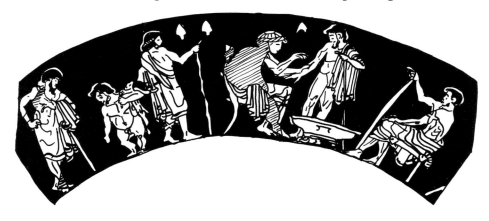

The doctor's place of business, known as the *iatreion*, offered scant privacy as it was open to everybody and 'medical questions were discussed publicly in the market place'. Other physicians practiced their art as wandering craftsmen, *'demiourgoi,* "men who work for the people"; as such they first appear in the *Odyssey* and such they still were in the days of Hippocrates'.[129] Hippocrates referred to their travelling status, when discussing the fact that they needed to be well aware of what and how particular geographical and physical environments affect health:

> For if a physician know these things well, … he will not, on arrival at a town
> with which he is unfamiliar, be ignorant of the local diseases, or of the nature of
> those that commonly prevail; so that he will not be at a loss in the treatment of
> diseases, or make blunders …[130]

As well as taking those external factors into account, itinerant doctors had to spend time and effort attracting potential clients' attention, by extravagant dress, perfume, and display of "showy instruments", along with impressive, fast, and correct prognostications, particularly if they had competition from others. Their social position was not high, but most were esteemed on account of the cultural attitude towards the human body.[131]

There were four main schools of medical thought: the Empirics, the Dogmatists, the Pneumatists, and the Methodists. The first of those, the Empirics based treatment on observation, providing remedies that had been found effective to treat observable symptoms. They rejected research and dissection, unlike the Dogmatics who advocated for them because they believed in understanding disease processes as the core to practice. They were, however, theoretical rather than practical. The Pneumatists were a splinter group of the Dogmatics who concentrated on the pneuma as the basis of all life, believing that disturbance of that caused illness. All three were exponents of humoural theory. The Methodists, however, were not. They stressed that there were a few general conditions common to all diseases and they developed "methods" to treat those conditions. They stressed the basic importance of "regimen".[132]

During the period of Pericles' political leadership, Hippocrates (c. 460 - c. 375 BC), the son of Heracleides, was born in Cos. This at least, is the most favoured of his biographies. His father was a physician, expert in the treatment of eyes, who belonged to the guild of Asclepides, a follower of the deified Aesculapius. Hippocrates was apprenticed to his father, becoming renowned as a medical teacher, and of such eventual skill that he is still known as the "father of medicine". With him, it was said, 'medicine stepped out of the temples and emancipated itself from religious bonds'.[133] This was because he encouraged the separation of magical and religious methods from those of empirical observation and deduction and the division of medicine from philosophy despite his interest in both.[134]

Figure 1.3.6: **Hippocrates Line engraving by P Pontius, 1638 after P.P.Rubens.**
(The Wellcome Library)

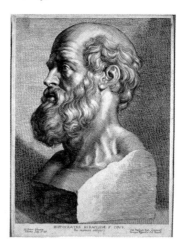

Hippocrates argued that medical decisions should be based on judgement, experience and ethics, as well as consideration of anatomy, although the study of that was rudimentary at the time. Diagnoses and prognoses took note of the personal, environmental and physical nature of the patients, stressing their individual predisposition and the inter-connectedness of body and mind. He taught that people would have a good chance of escaping illness if they lived reasonably. Somewhat surprisingly at that time, and maybe influenced by Athenian democracy, he claimed that everyone was entitled to the same degree of care and treatment.[135]

One of the views that Hippocrates held which anticipates later neurological and psychological thought, as well as the modern practice of neurological and psycho-social occupational therapy, was that it is the brain which integrates external and internal stimuli, and is the seat of action, emotion and experience:

Men ought to know that the brain, and from the brain only, arise our pleasures, joys, and laughter and jests, as well as our sorrows, pains, grief and tears. Through it, in particular, we think, see, hear, and distinguish the ugly from the beautiful, the bad from the good, the pleasant from the unpleasant, in some cases using custom as the test, in others perceiving them from their utility. It is the same thing which makes us mad or delirious, inspires us with dread and fear, whether by night or by day, brings sleeplessness, inopportune mistakes, aimless anxieties, absent-mindedness, and acts that are contrary to habit.[136]

Whilst he appears to attribute more to the effect of the "air" on the brain than is common at present in medical spheres, the importance of aerobic exercise to maximise brain function has received much attention in recent years within the broader health arena:

> *... I hold that the brain is the most powerful organ of the human body, for when it is healthy it is an interpreter to us of the phenomena caused by the air, as it is the air that gives it intelligence. Eyes, ears, tongue, hands and feet act in accordance with the discernment of the brain; in fact the whole body participates in intelligence in proportion to its participation in air.*[137]

Obviously Hippocratic medicine had its antecedents but little is known of it because, in Greece, the writing of medical books was a new phenomenon of the fifth century. The craftsman-physician training followed an oral tradition, which was sourced as medical authorities began to write down what probably had been done for a long time. Perhaps the best known of those, the *Corpus Hippocraticum,* is a collection of medical works often attributed to Hippocrates, but it is more commonly believed to be by different authors, most of them written in the fifth or fourth centuries BC, with possibly some from earlier times. This is probable because, as well as Hippocrates and his followers keeping careful case histories, it is believed that he also collected together the works of others. Paré provides evidence for that claim in his reflections on the origins of medicine. He wrote of ways in which early physicians and their patients recorded and stored information about successful treatments, and that Hippocrates accessed those records:

> *Strabo (c. 63 BC - c. AD 22, a Greek geographer and historian) writes that it was the custom in Greece that those which were sicke should report to Aesculapius at his temple in Epidaurum, that there as they slept, by their dreames they might be admonished by the God what meanes they should use to be cured; and when they were freed from their diseases, they writ the manner of their infirmities and the means by which they were cured, in tables & fastned them to the pillars of the temple, not only for the glory of God, but also for the profit of such, as should afterwards be affected with the like maladies. All which tables (as same reports) Hippocrates transcribed, & so from those drew the arte of physicke.*[138]

The collection in the Corpus Hippocraticum conveys a wealth of medical knowledge. It includes observations and evaluations of diseases, symptoms and their course; therapeutic regimes using dietetics, pharmaceutics and surgery; and theory about the nature of the health of humankind and the mechanisms of illness according to a humoural view of physiology.[139] "Dietetics" was used to encompass physical regimes of exercise, rest and bathing as well as food and drink.

Although the humoural theory is believed to have originated at an earlier date around Pythagorus' and Empedocles' time, it is at Hippocrates' door that its promulgation began. Halle, in 1789, suggested that Hippocrates was the first to illustrate the nature of *hygiene* or of health giving regimens. According to Halle, the art of medicine originates from that, since, Hippocrates said, its 'object had been, by changing the regimen which produced both his sufferings and his diseases, to secure, the support, the health, and the preservation of man'.[140]

Those rules and regimens were based on 'the choice, the preparation, and the admixture of aliments' which were 'the offspring of observation'. Similarly, observation led to the understanding that the selection needed to differ accorded to temperaments and state of health, and that other factors were important in the maintenance and restoration of health. The other factors included:

> ... the measure and proportion of exercise and of rest, as well as of sleep and of watchfulness, and the second step of the art has been the introduction of gymnastics, to which the use of baths must be added, which, especially in hot climates, have become one of the daily necessaries of man, as well as an object of pleasure and of luxury.[141]

The humoural explanation was to remain the ascendant physiological theory until the eighteenth or early nineteenth century, and so will be revisited several times in this history.

The approach was based on the state and effects of four humours, blood, phlegm, yellow bile and black bile, of which the body was thought to be mainly composed and which were related to the four basic elements of nature: fire, air, water and earth as Empedocles and Pythagoras had argued earlier. It was thought that maintaining the harmony of and equilibrium between the elements and humours would ensure health; that deviation from that balanced state would result in illness; and that careful diagnosis could detect imbalance and rectify it, by mainly natural means. Treatment was therefore holistic rather than particular to a body part, and consisted of adjustments to lifestyle, diet and physick, and attention to the elimination of waste matter through bloodletting as well as natural processes such as urination, menstruation, sweating, crying, vomiting, or sneezing. On the whole, treatment adopted opposition of the humoural or elemental imbalance, so if the disorder was thought to be the result of too much warmth and dryness or yellow bile, treatment would apply cold and moist remedies.[142]

Hippocrates discussed many of the problems and regimens to prevent or remedy disease in *On Regimen* and in his famous *Aphorisms*. His regimens contain much to interest occupational therapists with a broad perspective of health. Included in Book I are propositions as to diet and knowledge of the powers of food, drink, labour, the heavens and climates; a comparison of some of the actions and affections of human beings, whether derived from nature or art confirming and illustrating the doctrine of birth and of growth;[143] and the idea that medicine, along with other arts, is but an imitation of nature. Digressions commented about issues in occupational health for workers in iron, medical gymnastics, fulling, shoemaking, carpentry, architecture, cookery, tanning, sculpture, music, goldsmiths, potters, writing, public schools, merchants, and actors.[144] In Book II Hippocrates included: anointing, sweat, vomition, sleep, labour, rest, eating - and all such things that in any way are admitted to the body; exercise, both general and particular;[145] baths, and venery;

sleep and waking. Inactivity and repose; gymnastics. Exercise natural and ill timed. The exercise of sight, hearing, thought and voice, in talking, reading and so on; and walking at different periods such as before or after eating. Running, riding, racing, leaping, wrestling, and frictions (massage); playing at ball, holding the breathe; fatigue from want of exercise or from unaccustomed or excessive exercise, and its effects explained as arising from ideas of circulation and so on.[146] Book III included: observations on the impossibility of prescribing exercise and diet suitable for everyone; general rules for regimen of labouring people in the four different seasons of the year; the regimen for people in easy circumstances; observations on the need for individual regimens; and finally, the effects and symptoms of excess in walking and gymnastic exercise.[147]

Within the breadth of those topics is his acknowledgment that what people do and how they do it affects their health status, and that occupations of various kinds can be used for remedial purposes. That suggestion is confirmed in Jones' 1939 translation of Hippocrates' *Airs, Waters and Places*:

Whoever wishes to pursue properly the science of medicine must proceed thus …

He must consider with greatest care …

The mode of life also of the inhabitants that is pleasing to them, whether they are heavy drinkers, taking lunch, and inactive, industrious, eating much and drinking little.[148]

Not only did he consider occupations that were part of people's daily life as a factor in their own right, he linked them with food and drink. He made a differentiation between those who were inactive, gluttonous and imbibers, against the active participants in occupation who ate well but were abstemious. Making those sorts of links clearer through appropriate research might be one aspect of occupational therapy to be pursued in the future.

In *Aphorisms*, Hippocrates made particular recommendations and gave advice about dietetics and exercise. In the latter case, Hippocrates claimed for himself the credit of systematising exercises: and observed that 'exercise gives strength and firmness to the body and vigour to the mind'. Examples of his aphorisms include the following:

APHORISM XLVIII: In every Exercise of the Body, when it begins to be wearied, Rest presently mitigates the Weariness.

EXPLANATION: Rest is the Cure for Weariness. So likewise Diseases that happen after too much Rest, and from too lazy a Life, are cured by Exercise. For Weariness is too great a Tensity of the Fibres; but Rest relaxes the too tense Fibres again; and therefore cures Weariness.

Dubos noted, especially in relation to classical medicine, that helping patients to rest was part of any early physicians' knowledge base, notwithstanding the apparent simplicity of the concept.[149]

APHORISM XLIX: Those who are accustomed to daily hard Labour, tho' they are weak or old Men, more easily endure it, than those who are not accustomed to it, tho' they be strong and young.
EXPLANATION: Custom makes every Thing more easy and agreeable.

APHORISM L: Things we have been long accustomed to tho' worke, are wont to be less troublesom, than those we are not accustomed too. And therefore a change is not made to Things we are accustomed to.
EXPLANATION: This is more fully explained by the following Aphorism.

APHORISM LI: It is dangerous much and suddenly either to empty, fill, heat, or cool, or by any other Means to move or stir the Body. For whatever is beyond measure is an Enemy to Nature. But that which is safe which is done little by little, and especially when a Change is to be made from one Thing to another.[150]

Hippocrates' use of the word exercise was broad. It included activities which would most often be called so in the present day like using a punch-ball or hanging balls, and doing arm exercises or military forms of drill, as well as occupations of daily life such as labour and recreational pursuits. It also included those that he described as natural (as opposed to "violent") exercise, which embraced intellectual activities such as thought, and bodily functions such as sight, hearing, walking and speech. However, he did not see any particular exercise as useful or curative in all circumstances. For example, despite including walking as a natural exercise, and recommending the taking of many walks in the early morning and short walks in the sun after dinner, he deemed it to have some violent tendencies, so disapproved of it for remedial purpose when illness was acute. Similarly there were times when he recommended running, and other situations when it would not be prescribed because of 'the power to heat, concoct and dissolve the flesh'.[151]

Like modern day occupational therapists he recommended particular occupations for particular purposes, although, perhaps the choice of some occupations was different, such as prescribing horse riding, pugilistic movements and wrestling to develop the muscular parts of the body. In conjunction with that, or maybe as a singular treatment he advocated rubbing the body with oil and water to soften it and prevent overheating. He prescribed work or labour particularly for muscular skeletal purposes. 'By labour is meant strong exercise or exercise turned into business.'[152] In this period riding began to be mentioned as an occupation of choice for many remedial purposes, which was to continue for, at least, a further 2000 years. Such was its popularity at that time that it was used in the treatment of gout, head pains, sciatica, epilepsy, deafness, hiccoughs, dropsy and possibly other disorders.[153]

Many of Hippocrates ideas appear to have been incorporated into later physicians' work. Asclepiades (125-56 BC), a Bithynian physician provides an illustration through his work in Rome. He used many physical methods of treatment which Hippocrates and his school had advocated, introducing them as "mechano-therapy". As well as gymnastics, labour, massage, baths, and "open air", he became well known for his use of hanging, rocking and swinging beds, which might remind recent therapists of sensory integrative therapy. Such "moving" occupations were in accord with his physical theory of the human organism that viewed the body as a composite of atoms in constant motion. The occupations were applied as part of five dietetic principles, two of which were "walking" and various kinds of "carriage rides",[154] with both of those occupations being adopted in medieval to industrial health regimes. He prescribed hanging and rocking for children because they provided passive rather than "over-active" exercise, and also for those with mental illness. For the latter he also suggested 'many different kinds of baths; (and) he prescribed music and harmony and pleasant company and occupation'.[155] He went on to found a medical school in Rome, and probably to influence Celsus (who also prescribed rocking), the first of the renowned Latin medical writers.[156]

There is doubt that Aurelius Cornelius Celsus (25 BC - 50 AD) was a physician, but an intelligent layperson with an interest in medicine along with many other topics. His best known work was a treatise in eight books, *De Medicina* which was originally part of an encyclopaedia addressing philosophy, jurisprudence, agriculture, martial arts, and rhetoric.[157] Printed in 1478, it was one of the first medical books to use the new form of publication. The prescriptions given in his texts differed between people according to different builds and ages, rather than simply because of their medical condition, which fitted well with one of his principle messages which was to "let nature take its course".[158]

Figure 1.3.7: **Aurelius Cornelius Celsus. Lithograph by PR Vigneron (1789- 1872)**
(The Wellcome Library)

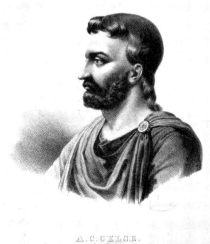

Celsus described how following Hippocrates, Greco-Roman medicine could be divided into dietetics, pharmacology and surgery. This did not mean that he ignored occupation, for it must be recalled that the word "dietetics" was used in a much broader way at that time and included exercise and rest.[159] Indeed, like earlier Greek authorities, Celsus advised "occupational" exercise to maintain health and as treatment for particular illness or condition, including walking, swimming, sailing, hunting, handling of arms, ball games, and reading aloud. The latter was recommended for weak stomachs, digestive organs and lungs. Some of the other disorders and diseases for which active and passive exercise was prescribed were 'functional disorders of the heart, liver, spleen, and digestive tube, palsy, neuralgic affections, (and) epilepsy'.[160] For losing weight, bathing in 'warm salt water, running, walking and violent exercise were advocated, and for putting on weight, warm baths, moderate exercise and relaxation'.[161] Celsus believed "rocking" was useful for people recovering from chronic illness and fevers, and advocated being on board a ship, being carried on a litter, carriage and horse-riding, the latter, a more energetic form of rocking, for convalescents and those with diarrhoea.[162]

With an essentially pragmatic approach which followed his belief that most people could regulate and maintain their own health through dietetics, and should seldom need recourse to a physician, Celsus thought it more difficult for urbanites, scholars and the weak. He articulated an idea, which was obviously becoming more general, that demanding schedules in gymnasia were not conducive to good health. 'Bodies thus fed up', he said, 'age very quickly and become infirm.'[163] Instead Celsus applied regimes of healthy living to everyday occupations. It is obvious, however, that he addressed his advice mainly to the wealthy when he prescribed moderation and variety, people spending more time in the country, but some in the town, sailing, hunting, and taking exercise, such as marching, running or playing hand-ball, and then resting:[164]

> *He who has been engaged in the day, whether in domestic or on public affairs, ought to keep some portion of the day for the care of the body. The primary care in this respect is exercise, which should always preced the taking of food … and … ought to come to an end with sweating, or at any rate, lassitude.*[165]

Celsus also wrote aphorisms which Sprengell, in 1708, published in a collection with those of Hippocrates. Some that pertain to occupation read as follows:

APHORISM II: Idleness and Luxury first corrupted Mens Bodies in Greece, and afterwards afflicted them here.
EXPLANATION: The Romans received most of their Discipline and Learning from the Greeks; to which beget Pride and Ambition, and hence, Luxury and Idleness, the Parents of most Diseases.[166]

APHORISM XVIII: A Sound, healthy, and active Man, (if he is at his own liberty) ought not to confine himself to any Rules, neither has he any need of the

Physician or the Quack. He ought to lead a various Course of Life, be sometimes in the Country, sometimes in Town, but yet oftener in the Country: He ought to sail, hunt, sometimes rest, but oftener be in Exercise; since Laziness slackens and dulls the Body, but Labour strengthens and makes it firm; the former hastens Old Age, the other prolongs Youth.[167]

APHORISM XXV: He ought to set apart some share of his Time for the Care of his Body, that has in the Day-time been employed either in domestic or civil Affairs. The first thing he is to take care of is, that he should always use a little Exercise before Meat, which should be continued so long till he finds himself in a Sweat or weary, but not too much fatigued.[168]

APHORISM XXXV: Too lazy a Life should be avoided, for there may happen a necessity to work.[169]

APHORISM XXXVII: Even the very Change of Labour will ease Weariness; and he that is fatigued by an unusual sort of Work, is refresh'd again by that which he has accustom'd himself to.[170]

Celsus also discussed mental illness. In the third book of *De Medicina* he referred to 'several kinds of madness and their cures', and suggested massage, exercise, and the use of occupations 'suitable to the temper of each'. He recommended that: 'The sorrowful thoughts of others must be dispelled, for which purpose concerts of music and symbals and noise are useful … Sometimes also the attention of the person must be strongly engaged'.[171]

The treatment he described varied between kindness and harshness despite advising 'yet these patients must be oftener humoured than contradicted'.[172] Pinel, the famous French physician, whose views of moral treatment revolutionised the treatment of the mentally ill towards the end of the eighteenth century said of that trait:

> *In the writings of the ancients, and especially of Celsus, a sort of intermediate and conditional mode of treatment is recommended, founded, in the first instance, upon a system of lenity and forbearance; and when that method failed, upon corporal and physical punishments, such as confinement, chains, flogging, spare diet, &c. Public and private mad-houses, in more modern times, have been conducted on similar principles.*[173]

In Rome, the first physicians were slaves with limited medical knowledge, but, from the fourth century BC on, these had gradually, and largely, been superseded by Greek physicians, as frequent wars necessitated well trained doctors. Despite initial reluctance to employ foreigners, the immigrants' superior knowledge was recognised to the extent that, in 46 BC, Julius Caesar presented all free-born Greek physicians on Roman soil with the right of Roman citizenship. Physicians had many privileges accorded them, such as freedom from taxation and military service, so to avoid abuse of the privileges some restrictions were introduced. Roman cities, according to their size, could employ only five to ten "city" doctors (*valde docti*) who had to prove their medical knowledge. Many families also had family physicians employed on an annual basis.[174]

A world-renowned Greek physician who worked in Rome was Claudius Galen (c. 131-201 AD). He was an architect's son, born in Pergamos in Asia Minor, studying medicine in his hometown and at Corinth and Alexandria, before going to Rome where he became the physician to five successive emperors. Galen was a prolific writer, producing about 130 medical books, as well as about 125 others on philosophy, law, mathematics, and grammar. He remained a medical authority of current note for 15 centuries.[175] From the point of view of this history, it is his versions of the humoural theory that were the basis of medieval medicine, the *Regimen Sanitatis* and later rules for health, which included occupations as part of mainstream medical recommendations.

Figure 1.3.8: **Galen. Line engraving by G.P. Busch.**

(The Wellcome Library)

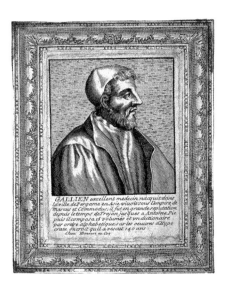

Galen both accepted and adopted the humoural system of medicine proposed by earlier master-physicians and philosophers, to the extent that his name is more closely linked with it than any of the others. He based his doctrine upon nine possible combinations of the four primal qualities:
1. The correct blend of warm, cold, dry and moist,
2.- 5. Prevalence of warm, or cold, or dry, or moist,
6. Combination of cold and dry associated with the earth and black bile,
7. Combination of warm and dry associated with fire and yellow bile,
8. Combination of cold and moist associated with water and phlegm, and
9. Combination of warm and moist associated with air and blood.

Those combinations and associations had affiliations with the temperaments, the life cycle, the seasons and the cardinal points.

Galen's theory was that the humours were formed as food underwent a series of digestive processes through the stomach and intestines to the spleen or liver, then to the blood vessels, body and heart, the tissues and organs, until finally the residue escaped as sweat. In this way three separate systems were serviced. The first was the respiratory system with the heart as its major organ, which he called the "vital spirit". The second was the digestive system with the liver as principal organ known as the "natural spirit". The third, the sensory system with the brain as principal organ known as the "animal spirit".[176]

The theory was that the humours underlay the *"complexio,"* the name given to a person's constitution and predisposition towards one or other type of disorder according to the probable dominance of one of the four humours, which were evident in the temperaments. These, the melancholy, the phegmatic, the choleric, and the sanguine were thought to determine both body and mental health characteristics. The temperaments along with the humours were two of seven physiological components that made up the *naturals*. The others were the elements, primal qualities, body parts, faculties, and spirits. There were three *contra-naturals:* diseases, their causes, and their signs, and six *non-naturals* which were lifestyle factors, air, food and drink, motion and rest, sleep and waking, evacuation and repletion, and the passions of the mind.[177] See figure 1.3.9.

Figure 1.3.9
The four elements, four qualities, four humours, blood, phlegm, black vile, yellow vile,four seasons, spring, winter, autumn, summer and four ages of man, childhood, decrepitude, old age, manhood. By Lois Hague, 1991
(The Wellcome Library)

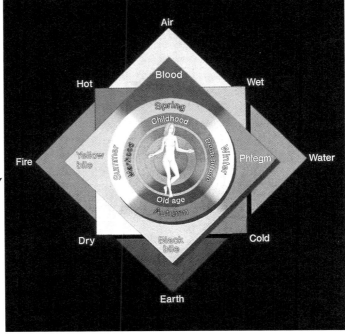

Galen was at one point in his career in charge of a gymnasium and his interest in physical methods of treatment as an essential part of therapeutics was evident. In the humoural theory those methods were considered within the non-naturals - "motion and rest". He approved highly of baths, 'warm, with sweet waters, cold, and of spring waters', prescribing them as treatment for many conditions and after exercise.[178] He paid great attention to massage, and different kinds of movement, both active and passive, recommending systems of exercise combining body and mind which, like many of his earlier counterparts, he considered to be interdependent.[179] Fuller saw his similarity to Hippocrates:

> As for Galen, he follows Hippocrates in this, as close as in other things, and declares his opinion of the benefit of exercises in several places; ... he has wrote a little tract, "de Parva Pila", wherein he recommends an exercise, by which the body and mind are both at the same time affected.[180]

Galen, argued Fuller many centuries later, pondered the interesting question of whether medicine or gymnastics were the most advantageous in promoting and maintaining health. Burton, just a little earlier, in his 17th century Anatomy of Melancholy, went so far as to suggest that 'Galen prefers Exercise before all Physick, Rectification of diet, or any Regiment in what kinde soever; 'tis Natures Physician' and then commented, particularly, on a type of ball game which featured in his recommendations:

> Amongst bodily exercises, Galen commends ludum parvae pilae, to play at ball, be it with hand or rackey, in Tennis courts or otherwise, it exerciseth each part of the body, and doth much good, so that they sweat not too much. It was in great request of old amongst the Greeks, Romanes, Barbarians, mentioned by Homer, Heroditus, and Plinius.[181]

So valued were Galen's systems that physician-gymnasts detailed prescriptions according to individual requirements, whilst assistants were also employed to dispense (or perhaps physically administer) the gymnast's prescription.[182] That implied that the physician-gymnasts and their assistants needed to know how to avoid fatigue caused by over-exercise, tension, and anxiety, as well as the kinematics of the occupations they used for exercise. Those could differ according to the methods and, in some cases, materials employed.[183]

The occupations for maintenance of health and strengthening of cognition, intellect and body, which Galen recommended, were, firstly, those of a sporting nature such as earlier experts had prescribed like ball-throwing, boxing, dancing, hunting, jumping, riding, rope-pulling, rowing, sailing, swimming, walking, wrestling, and swinging on ropes. "Work" occupations that he considered a source of good health and well-being were country pursuits like wood splitting, digging, ploughing, pruning, reaping, threshing, and the bearing of burdens. In general though he differentiated between labour and exercise, perhaps in line with the general belief that labour was principally an animal function, beneath the interests of the affluent, and because labour was compulsory. In order to prescribe or contra-indicate particular occupations,

Galen studied them in a way similar to the activity analyses of the 20th century. He detailed the body movements demanded by the occupations; of spine, loins, arms, legs, hands and fingers, the intrinsic actions of the muscles, tendons, sinews, bones, veins, flesh and ligaments, and took into account the effects on heart, arteries, pulse and respiration. As well he considered their singular qualities; their rhythm, slowness, lightness, speed and vigour, for example, and, 'in some cases their passive application'. Horse riding was again selected out for special mention, for Galen noted, as others who followed did, that the motion of the horse largely caused the motion of the rider. It was long valued for that "extrinsic" factor. Such careful analysis led naturally to his belief that occupations must be well chosen and carefully graded to meet the needs of the person for whom they were prescribed. He also recommended to people alternative ways of making a living such as handcrafts, mechanics, bronze work, house or shipbuilding, and plough and arms making.[184]

Galen's interest in mental health encompassed the condition of the mind in all forms of illness and even for those receiving physically focussed treatments he stressed the importance of mental attitude. He studied problems caused by emotional pressures, lack of temperance, insomnia and epilepsy, using drugs and "shock" treatments as well as recreation and occupation, and was said 'to have been emphatic about the importance of the element of volition in remedial exercises and occupations'.[185]

Apart from the principle directions taken by those eminent physicians a beginning interest in "occupational health" emerged. Galen, for example, at the start of his career, was a physician and surgeon to a school of gladiators. Classical physicians, and others of a scientific bent, noticed the influence of particular forms of employment on the health of the workers. Hippocrates correctly described a case of lead poisoning,[186] and Pliny (23-7 AD), a wealthy and learned Roman encyclopaedic writer, spoke of the noxious effects of lead, mercury, and sulphur on those who handled them,[187] and recommended protective masks of "bladder skin" to overcome toxicity.[188] Vitruvius, a Roman architect warned of "mighty currents of air" when digging wells which could choke and kill. He recommended the digging of additional air vents and anticipated the Davey lamp by recommending the lowering of a lighted lamp before descending the shaft and that if it remained alight it was safe.[189]

However, physicians were not much concerned with the health of manual workers, devoting most of their attention to the higher social strata. In the Hippocratic treatise *Peri Diaites,* for example, the author provided special dietary rules for the upper classes who, because of business interests, were unable to devote all their time and attention to their health.[190] 'It would never have occurred to him to prescribe any definite hygiene to craftsmen or workers', although medical care was provided to gladiators, the popular entertainers of the day. For them, and for the elite whom recreational occupations in the gymnasia provided the hazards, orthopaedic surgery was available, which probably reflects the frequency of injuries such as dislocations and fractures.[191]

Great value was placed on the culture 'shared by only a small upper class, and endless human lives had to be sacrificed and a great deal of suffering had to be endured to allow this culture to flourish'. In fact, as the workers were often slaves, prisoners of war, defeated original inhabitants, or convicts, no steps were taken to protect them other than those they instigated themselves. Pliny described how:

> ... persons employed in the manufactories in preparing minium protect the face with masks of loose bladder-skin, in order to avoid inhaling the dust, which is highly pernicious; the covering being at the same time sufficiently transparent to admit of being seen through.[192]

They were lucky to some extent, in that, because technology was mostly small-scale the labourers frequently worked in the open air, reducing the hazards occurring in later centuries.[193]

Because of the actions taken to reduce the number of handicapped people at birth, and the cultural attitude towards chronic illness and disability, little attention would have been given to helping them to establish or re-establish independent patterns of life. Neither would they have felt encouraged to take part in community activities. This being the case, there is little evidence during the Classical period of aids and adaptations or of mobility devices except for litters, walking aids, and lower limb prostheses.

A litter, which was basically a plank wide enough for someone to recline upon with handles at both ends, was a common form of device for moving people from place to place during the time before streets were sufficiently smooth to allow for vehicles like chairs with wheels. In Ancient Greek and Roman times litters were in common use, especially to transport injured soldiers. Some designs included seats or chairs and some were protected with a shade or covering.[194] It is likely that these were used for the elderly and infirm, as well as some of high social strata.

Amputation was probably fairly common when gangrene followed injury. Many lower limb amputees would have coped with a stick, crutch or a wooden peg. For those able to afford it, prostheses could be made out of sheet bronze over a wooden core. It is unlikely though, that they had moveable parts. One such as that was excavated in a tomb at Capua probably dated about 300 BC. Possible also for upper limb amputations, at least one, an iron hand was made for Marcus Sergius Silus, who lost his hand in the second Punic War (218-201 BC).[195]

In summary, during the Classical period, when modern medicine is said to have had its genesis, the use of occupation as part of health regimes was commonplace. It formed part of the daily lives of everyone to the extent that it is reflected in the myths of the gods and religious medicine, in the tales and poetry of master story-tellers, in philosopher's views of health and medicine as they sought answers to the essence of all things, and in the recommendations of legendary physicians who are immortalised in subsequent practice and in today's culture. Fuller, in the 18th century, was still admonishing the public in terms of the use of occupations as advocated by Herodicus, Hippocrates, Mercurialis and Galen. The use of occupation for health was seen as important enough to warrant state intervention to ensure that it did, in fact, form part of the population's daily life. Although the promotion of health and subsequent prevention of illness was important, early Italic medicine was chiefly interested in the treatment of symptoms because all else was deemed to be in the hands of the gods. When, in 295 BC, Romans suffered an epidemic of the plague, help was sought from the god Aesculapius rather than Greek physicians.[196]

Because of the time and place, and the cultural attitudes held, some occupations were more valued than others were, although most were recognised as health giving to some extent by one or other group of experts. For the citizens, the idea of youth, strength and physical beauty emerged as central, which is hardly surprising in a world in which wars and conquest were commonplace. That occupational reality, together with lack of technological medical know-how, led to other occupational directives in the provision of health programs. Not dissimilar to today, when youth and physical beauty are once more ascendant, gymnasia and physical exercise reigned supreme as providers of healthful occupation. Interestingly, in recent years occupational therapists have neglected specialisation in physical occupations to maintain health per se, although it is an important component of occupation for health and therapy. Perhaps this is because of the professional boundaries fostered by the relationship between occupational therapy, physiotherapy and the earlier discipline of remedial gymnasts. However, during at least the first thirty or forty years of occupational therapists' training, physical exercise, occupation and dance, and sometimes, beauty therapy as well, were taught as therapeutic media for both mental and physical conditions.

Apart from the glorification of physical strength and beauty at a time when martial arts were paramount, gymnasia served another health giving purpose. Because of the demotion of everyday physiologically based occupation into the hands of slaves and conquered peoples, it was necessary, though probably unconscious, to invent occupations to take their place. Occupation is a necessity for more than supplying the obvious basic requirements of life. It is also the means of giving life purpose, as well as satisfying the clamour of faculties, which need to be used or lost. Gymnasia met those needs especially because they were all embracing, supplying physical, mental and social occupations in combination.

The idea of wisdom was also linked with gymnasia, and intellectual exercise proceeded alongside its physical and social counterparts. This was, in part, because there was a strong belief in mind and body interaction, an idea which is central to modern day occupational therapy, and if that was a new thought, then the Classical period was important to the profession in that regard.

It was also important because it was the time when the notion of balance was first articulated, the idea being central to the Greek view of health, just as it is in present day occupational therapy. The Greeks came to believe that illness resulted from imbalance of the four humours and that a physician's job was to advise on due proportion, to 'restore a healthy balance' in order to aid 'the natural healing powers believed to exist in every human being'.[197][198][199] Current occupational therapists, whilst not adherents of the humoural theory, espouse a doctrine that balance between engagement in different types of occupations, and the capacities that they use, should be a central concern of healthful living.

Two aspects, particularly, jarred the goodness of fit of classical health regimes with those most highly regarded by occupational therapists. One is the difference made between the health needs of slaves and citizens, which was founded on a totally unacceptable notion that the mundane activities of daily life concerned with people's physiological requirements were inhuman, unhealthy, and brutalising. The second is the practice of infanticide for those regarded as less than perfect children.

[1]Neff WS. Work and Human Behaviour. 3rd ed. New York: Aldine Publishing Co., 1985; 33.
[2]Parker S. Leisure and Work. London: George Allen and Unwin, 1983; 14.
[3]Parker. Leisure and Work…; 17.
[4]Wilcock AA. An Occupational Perspective of Health. Thorofare, NJ: Slack Inc., 1998; 80.
[5]Boulding E. The Underside of History; A View of Women Through Time. Volume 1. Newbury Park: Sage Publications, 1992; 221, 227-229.
[6]Sigerist HE. A History of Medicine, Volume II: Early Greek, Hindu, and Persian Medicine, New York: Oxford University Press, 1961.
[7]Sigerist. A History of Medicine, Volume II…; 20.
[8]Marti-Ibañez F, ed. Henry E. Sigerist on the History of Medicine. New York: MD Publications, Inc., 1960; 27.
[9]Halle R. Hygiene. (Originally in: French Encyclopaedia Methodique, 7, 3. 1789). In: Sinclair Sir J. Code of Health and Longevity. Edinburgh, Arch Constable and Co., 1806; 276.
[10]Sigerist. A History of Medicine, Volume II…; 20.
[11]Halle. Hygiene…; 275.
[12]Halle. Hygiene…; 266.
[13]Georgii A, ed. Ling's Educational and Curative Exercises. London: Renshaw, 1875; 11.
[14]Georgii. Ling's Educational and Curative Exercises…; 8.
[15]Boulding. The Underside of History…; 221.
[16]Girling DA. New Age Encyclopaedia, 7th edition. Sydney, London: Bay Books, 1983; vol 18: 108.

[17]Halle. Hygiene…; 276.

[18]Halle. Hygiene…; 276-281.

[19]Plato. Republic (Third Book). In: Georgii. Ling's Educational and Curative Exercises…; 8-9.

[20]Georgii. Ling's Educational and Curative Exercises.

[21]Girling. New Age Encyclopaedia…; vol 13: 216.

[22]Girling. New Age Encyclopaedia…; vol 28: 147.

[23]Crawley R. The History of the Peloponnesian War by Thucydides. London: Longman's Green and Co, 1874; 121-127.

[24]Attributed to Xenophon but probably earlier. In: Dakyns HG. The Works of Xenophon. London and New York: Macmillan and Co., 1892; vol ii: 280.

[25]Georgii. Ling's Educational and Curative Exercises…; 10-11.

[26]Sigerist. A History of Medicine, Volume II.

[27]Girling. New Age Encyclopaedia…; vol 22: 200-201.

[28]Alexander PJ, ed. The Ancient World: To 300 AD. New York: The Macmillan Co., 1966; 88.

[29]Clough AH. Plutarch's Lives. Boston: Little, Brown and Company, 1905; vol 1: 337.

[30]Clough. Plutarch's Lives…; Vol 1: 337.

[31]Halle. Hygiene…; 268.

[32]Varro MT. De Re Rustica. Lib. ii, Proem (Goetz G, 1922).

[33]Halle. Hygiene…; 292.

[34]Marti-Ibañez. Henry E. Sigerist on the History of Medicine…; 20.

[35]Georgii. Ling's Educational and Curative Exercises…; 10.

[36]Marti-Ibañez. Henry E. Sigerist on the History of Medicine…; 20.

[37]Marti-Ibañez. Henry E. Sigerist on the History of Medicine…; 20.

[38]Kersler GD, Glyn G. A Concise International History of Rheumatology and Rehabilitation: Friends and Foes. London: Royal Society of Medicine Services Limited, 1991; 1.

[39]Story GO. A History of Physical Medicine: The Story of the British Association of Rheumatology and Rehabilitation. London: Royal Society of Medical Services Ltd., 1992; 1.

[40]Kersler & Glyn. A Concise International History of Rheumatology…; 1.

[41]Goodbody J. The Illustrated History of Gymnastics. London: Stanley Paul, 1982; 11.

[42]Murray AS. Who's Who in Mythology: Classic Guide to the Ancient World. London: Bracken Books, 1994.

[43]Murray. Who's Who in Mythology.

[44]Sigerist. A History of Medicine, Volume II…; 44.

[45]Murray. Who's Who in Mythology.

[46]Macdonald EM. World-Wide Conquests of Disabilities: The History, Development and Present Functions of the Remedial Services. London: Bailliere Tindall, 1981; 23-24.

[47]Van der Meulen JC. Man and his hand. The Hand, 8(1): 1976; 1.

[48]Murray. Who's Who in Mythology.

[49]Macdonald. World-Wide Conquests of Disabilities.

[50]Sigerist. A History of Medicine, Volume II.

[51]Dubos R. Mirage of Health: Utopias, Progress and Biological Change. New York: Harper and Row Publishers, 1959; 130.

[52]Sigerist. A History of Medicine, Volume II.

[53]Hygeia. 1995 Grolier Multimedia Encyclopedia. CD Rom. Grolier Electronic Publishing, Inc., 1995; Dubos. Mirage of Health…; 129.

[54]Dubos. Mirage of Health…; 131.

[55]Dubos. Mirage of Health…; 129.

[56]Dubos. Mirage of Health…; 130-131.

[57]See: Rohde. Psyche, vol. II; 109ff.

[58]Aristophanes. Frogs, 1033; Plato. De Republic, 2, 364E.

[59] Sigerist. A History of Medicine, Volume II…; 49.

[60]Girling. New Age Encyclopaedia…; vol 14: 136, 180; Georgii. Ling's Educational and Curative Exercises…; 10-11.

[61]Homer. Odyssey IVII, 382-4 & Odyssey IV, 219-34. In: Jackson R. Doctors and Diseases in the Roman Empire. London: British Museum Press, 1988; 12.

[62]Sigerist. A History of Medicine, Volume II…; 20.

[63]Halle. Treatise…; 290.

[64]Macdonald. World-Wide Conquests of Disabilities…; 26-27.

[65]Murray. Who's Who in Mythology…; 80.

[66]Girling. New Age Encyclopaedia…; vol 14: 65.

[67]Girling. New Age Encyclopaedia…; vol 14: 100.

[68]Hesiod. Works and Days, c. 8th Century BC. 102-5, 240-45, 308-11. In: Sigerist. A History of Medicine, Volume II…; 86-87.

[69]Martial. Epigrams XII, 57,14. In: Sigerist. A History of Medicine, Volume II.

[70]Juvenal. Satires X, 130. In: Sigerist. A History of Medicine, Volume II.

[71]Juvenal. Satires VI, 397. In: Sigerist. A History of Medicine, Volume II.

[72]Lucretius, VI, 811. In: Sigerist. A History of Medicine, Volume II.

[73]Jackson R. Doctors and Diseases in the Roman Empire…; 17.

[74]Celsus. De Medicina. Prooemium, 6-8. In: Jackson. Doctors and Diseases in the Roman Empire…; 19.

[75]Sigerist. A History of Medicine, Volume II…; 98.

[76]Macdonald. World-Wide Conquests of Disabilities…; 30.

[77]Girling. New Age Encyclopaedia…; vol 13: 137.

[78]Macdonald. World-Wide Conquests of Disabilities…; 30.

[79]Sigerist. A History of Medicine, Volume II.

[80]Berger M. Hildegard of Bingen: On Natural Philosophy and Medicine: Selections from Cause and Cure. Cambridge: D.S. Brewer, 1999; Beard MR. Women as a Force in History; A Study in Traditions and Realities. New York: Macmillan, 1946.

[81]Beard MR. Women as a Force in History; A Study in Traditions and Realities. New York: Macmillan, 1946; 326.

[82]Edelstein L. The Hippocratic Oath. Text, Translation and Interpretation (Bull. Hist. Med., Suppl. 1), Baltimore, 1943.

[83]Sigerist. A History of Medicine, Volume II.

[84]Sigerist. A History of Medicine, Volume II…; 94-95.

[85]Sigerist. A History of Medicine, Volume II…; 96-97.

[86]Cited in: Sigerist. A History of Medicine, Volume II…; 97.

[87]See Gomperz T. Griechische Denker, 4th ed. Berlin and Leipzig, 1922; 90.

[88]Sigerist. A History of Medicine, Volume II…; 97.

[89]Sigerist. A History of Medicine, Volume II.

[90]Macdonald. World-Wide Conquests of Disabilities…; 30.

[91]Diels H. ed and transcriber. Die Fragmente der Vorsokratiker. Hamburg: Rowohlt, 1957; Fragm. 17 and 21: 60f. In: Berger M. Hildegard of Bingen…; 15.

[92]Jackson. Doctors and Diseases in the Roman Empire…; 17.

[93]Berger. Hildegard of Bingen…; 15-16, 18.

[94]Girling. New Age Encyclopaedia…; vol 10: 150.

[95]Macdonald. World-Wide Conquests of Disabilities…; 33-36.

[96]Girling. New Age Encyclopaedia…; vol 26: 243-244.

[97]Girling. New Age Encyclopaedia…; vol 23: 68-69.

[98]Plato. De Republic. Translated by Jowett B. Oxford: 1938.

[99]Macdonald. World-Wide Conquests of Disabilities…; 34-35.

[100]Plato. Timaeus. Translated with an introduction by Lee HDP. Penguin Classics, 1965; 110.

[101]Plato. Timaeus…; 109-110.

[102]Plato. Timaeus…; 118-119.

[103]Plato. Timaeus…; 115-116.

[104]Plato. Timaeus…; 118-119.

[105]Plato. Timaeus…; 115-116.

[106]Georgii. Ling's Educational and Curative Exercises…; 9.

[107]Macdonald. World-Wide Conquests of Disabilities.

[108]Plato. Timaeus…; 117-118.

[109]Wilcock. An Occupational Perspective of Health…; 137.

[110]Plato. Timaeus…; 118.

[111]Plato. De Republic. Translated by Jowett B. Oxford, 1938. In: Macdonald. World-Wide Conquests of Disabilities…; 34.

[112]Macdonald. World-Wide Conquests of Disabilities.

[113]Petrovic G. Praxis. In: Bottomore T, ed. A Dictionary of Marxist thought. 2nd ed. Oxford UK; Blackwell Publishers, 1983; 435-440.

[114]Petrovic. Praxis…; 435-440.

[115]Girling. New Age Encyclopaedia…; vol 2: 155.

[116]Macdonald. World-Wide Conquests of Disabilities…; 36.

[117]Macdonald. World-Wide Conquests of Disabilities.

[118]Girling. New Age Encyclopaedia…; vol 2: 155.

[119]Macdonald. World-Wide Conquests of Disabilities…; 35-36.

[120]Aristotle. Nicomachean Ethics. In: Barnes J, ed. The Complete Works of Aristotle. Revised Oxford translation. UK: Princeton University Press, 1984.

[121]Arendt H. The Human Condition. Chicago, Ill: University of Chicago Press, 1958. Arendt recognised the lack of modern day theory about animal laborans (the labour of the body) and homo faber (the work of our hands) which she found surprising because of the present day glorification of labour and work as 'the source of all values' (83-85).

[122]Aristotle. Politics. In: Barnes. The Complete Works of Aristotle.

[123]Wilcock. An Occupational Perspective of Health.

[124]Macdonald. World-Wide Conquests of Disabilities.

[125]Macdonald. World-Wide Conquests of Disabilities…; 2-25.

[126]Sigerist HE. A History of Medicine, Volume I: Primitive and Archaic Medicine. New York: Oxford University Press, 1955; 5.

[127]Sigerist. A History of Medicine, Volume II…; 85.

[128]Dubos. Mirage of Health…; 143.

[129]Sigerist. A History of Medicine, Volume II…; 85.

[130]Jones WHS, trans. Hippocrates: Airs, Waters and Places, Vol. I. Cambridge, Mass: Harvard University Press; London: William Heinemann Ltd., 1939; 71-73.

[131]Sigerist. A History of Medicine, Volume II…; 6.

[132]Jackson. Doctors and Diseases in the Roman Empire…; 30.

[133]Sigerist. A History of Medicine, Volume II…; 45.

[134]Macdonald. World-Wide Conquests of Disabilities.

[135]Macdonald. World-Wide Conquests of Disabilities.

[136]Jones WHS, Trans. Hippocrates: The Sacred Disease, Vol II. London: William Heinemann Ltd., 1923; 179-183.

[137]Jones. Hippocrates: The Sacred Disease…; 179-183.

[138]Johnson T. The Workes of that Famous Chirurgion Anbrose Parey Translated out of Latin

and Compared with the French. London: Printed by Th Cotes and R Young, 1634; A2-A3.

[139]Sigerist. A History of Medicine, Volume II…; 85-86.

[140]Halle. Hygiene…; 264-265.

[141]Halle. Hygiene…; 265.

[142]Berger. Hildegard of Bingen…; 15-16,18.

[143]Haller: Hippocrates. On Regimen, Book I. chaps ii & viii.

[144]Gardeil: Hippocrates. On Regimen, Book I. sections ii & viii.

[145]Haller: Hippocrates. On Regimen, Book II. chaps x & xi.

[146]Gardeil. Hippocrates. On Regimen, Book II. sections ix-cxxi, cxxi, cxxii, cxxv-cxlv, cxlvi.

[147]Gardeil. Hippocrates. On Regimen, Book III. sections i, ii, vii, ix, xxii.

[148]Jones. Hippocrates: Airs, Waters and Places, Vol. I…; 71-73.

[149]Dubos. Mirage of Health…; 141.

[150]Sprengell CJ. The Aphorisms of Hippocrates and the Sentences of Celsus; with Explanations and References to the Most Considerable Writers in Physick and Philosophy, both Ancient and Modern. To which are added, Aphorisms upon the Small-pox, Measles, and other Distempers, not so well known to former more Temperate Ages. London: Printed for R Bonwick, W Freeman, Tim Goodwin, John Watho, Matt. Cotton, John Nicholson, Samuel Manship, Richard Parker, Benj Tooke and Ralph Smith, 1708; 41-42.

[151]Hippocrates. On regimen, On diet and hygiene, Aphorisms. Cited in: Macdonald. World-Wide Conquests of Disabilities…; 32.

[152]Hippocrates. On epidemics, book 6. Cited in: Stother E. An Essay on Sickness and Health. London, 1725; 341.

[153]Macdonald. World-Wide Conquests of Disabilities…; 31-32.

[154]Rackham H, Jones WHS, Eicholz DE, trans. Pliny Natural History. 10 vols. London: Loeb Classical Library, 1942-63; XXVI, 13.

[155]Macrae AKM. The historical development of modern psychiatric practice. Scottish Journal of Occupational Therapy June 1955: 21; 17-24.

[156]Macdonald. World-Wide Conquests of Disabilities…; 38-39.

[157]Jackson. Doctors and Diseases in the Roman Empire…; 9.

[158]Girling. New Age Encyclopaedia…; vol 6: 120.

[159]Jackson. Doctors and Diseases in the Roman Empire…; 32.

[160]Georgii. Ling's Educational and Curative Exercises…; 12.

[161]Macdonald. World-Wide Conquests of Disabilities…; 40.

[162]Jackson. Doctors and Diseases in the Roman Empire…; 34.

[163]Jackson. Doctors and Diseases in the Roman Empire…; 33.

[164]Spencer WG, trans. Celsus De Medicina. 3 vols. London: Loeb Classical Library, 1935-8; I, I, I.

[165]Spencer. Celsus De Medicina…; I, 2, 5-7.

[166]Sprengell. The Aphorisms of Hippocrates and the Sentences of Celsus…; 230.

[167]Sprengell. The Aphorisms of Hippocrates and the Sentences of Celsus…; 239.

[168]Sprengell. The Aphorisms of Hippocrates and the Sentences of Celsus…; 244.

[169]Sprengell. The Aphorisms of Hippocrates and the Sentences of Celsus…; 248.

[170]Sprengell. The Aphorisms of Hippocrates and the Sentences of Celsus…; 249.

[171]Celsus AAC. Of Medicine (c100 AD.) Book III, Translated by Grieve. London: 1837; 128-131.

[172]Macdonald. World-Wide Conquests of Disabilities…; 39-40.

[173]Pinel P. A Treatise on Insanity. Trans from French by D. D. Davis. Sheffield: Strand, London. Printed by W Todd, for Messrs. Cadell and Davies, 1806; 64.

[174]Sigerist. A History of Medicine, Volume 1…; 7.

[175]Girling. New Age Encyclopaedia…; vol 12: 101.

[176]Berger. Hildegard of Bingen…; 16-17.

[177]Berger. Hildegard of Bingen…; 16-17.

[178]Macdonald. World-Wide Conquests of Disabilities.

[179]Georgii. Ling's Educational and Curative Exercises…; 11.

[180]Fuller F. Medicina Gymnastica: Or, A Treatise Concerning the Power of Exercise with Respect to the Animal Oeconomy; and the Great Necessity of it in the Cure of Several Distempers. London: Printed by John Matthews for Robert Knaplock, at the Angel and Crown in St Paul's Church-yard, (MDCCV) 1705; 228-233.

[181]Burton R. The Anatomy of Melancholy. Oxford: Printed for Henry Cripps, 1651; 267.

[182]Georgii. Ling's Educational and Curative Exercises…; 11.

[183]Macdonald. World-Wide Conquests of Disabilities…; 44.

[184]Macdonald. World-Wide Conquests of Disabilities…; 43-44.

[185]Macdonald. World-Wide Conquests of Disabilities…; 45.

[186]Hippocrates. Epidemics VI, 25; ed. Littré V; 164-166.

[187]Rackham, Jones & Eicholz. Pliny Natural History…; XXXIV, 50; XXXIII, 40.

[188]Rackham, Jones & Eicholz. Pliny Natural History…; XXVI, viii; 14.

[189]Grainger F, ed & trans. Vitruvius on Architecture. 2 vols. London: Loeb Classical Library, 1970; VIII, VI; 12-13.

[190]Hippocrates. Peri Diaites III, 68; ed. Littré VI, 594.

[191]Marti-Ibañez. Henry E. Sigerist on the History of Medicine…; 47-48.

[192]Pliny GPS. Historia Naturalis XXXIII, 40.

[193]Sigerist. A History of Medicine, Volume II…; 47-48.

[194]Covey HC. Social Perceptions of People with Disabilities in History. Springfield, Illinois: Charles C. Thomas, 1998; 47, 50-51.

[195]Rackham, Jones & Eicholz. Pliny Natural History…; VI, xxviii, 105.

[196]Jackson. Doctors and Diseases in the Roman Empire…; 1988; 11.

[197]Risse GB. History of Western medicine from Hippocrates to germ theory. In: Kiple KF, ed. The Cambridge World History of Human Disease. Cambridge: Cambridge University Press, 1993; 11.

[198]Hippocrates. Regimen. In: Hippocratic Writings: On Ancient Medicine. William Benton, Publisher, Great Books of the Western World, Encyclopaedia Britannica, Inc., 1952.

[199]Wilcock. An Occupational Perspective of Health.

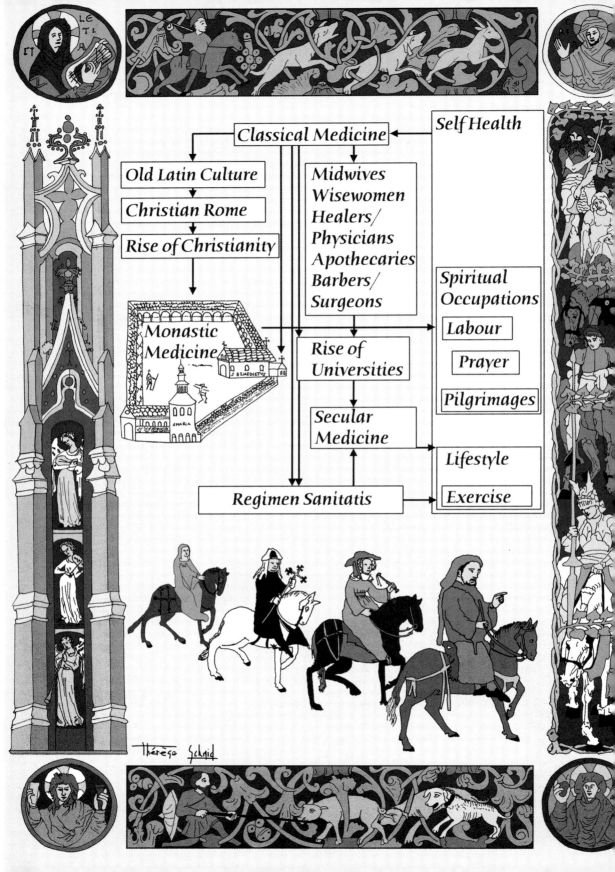

Classical Medicine ← Self Health

Old Latin Culture

Christian Rome

Rise of Christianity

Midwives
Wisewomen
Healers/
Physicians
Apothecaries
Barbers/
Surgeons

Monastic Medicine

Rise of Universities

Secular Medicine

Regimen Sanitatis

Spiritual Occupations

Labour

Prayer

Pilgrimages

Lifestyle

Exercise

Thérèse Schnid

Chapter 4

Spiritual Health Ascendant: Occupational Regimes in Medieval Times

Contents

From the fall of the Western Roman Empire in the fifth century until the Renaissance of Classicism in the fourteenth came a period variously described as medieval, the Middle Ages, and the Dark Ages. In this period, Europe experienced a time of invasions, power struggles, and the growth of a feudal society.[1] In the same period Christianity unfolded from a vulnerable, little known, religion to become dominant in medieval culture. The position of the sick in society was radically changed by Christianity, which was a healing religion appealing to the sick, the weak, and the crippled, in sharp comparison with the old religions, which were essentially for the sound. It promised healing both spiritually and physically. In previous eras, disease was considered the work of the demons, a punishment for sin, or a sign of inferiority. In the Christian world, disease offered purification and grace. In this chapter an attempt is made to understand what happened during that time in terms of health care, and whether occupation was understood to have a place within it. To do that it is necessary to appreciate, in some measure, how people lived, the changing role of church and secular organisations, and the physiological suppositions upon which health care was based. What emerges from that exploration, apart from some indications of occupation used with a similar rationale to the present, are three different views of occupation for health. First, that labour was an essential component of spiritual wellness, second a view that good or moral occupation leads to good health and the opposite to illness and, third, that occupation as physical exercise was one of six important principles to maintain and promote health based on Galen's understanding of that process.

To come to an understanding of how people lived, a brief overview of the times is essential. Along with the rest of Europe, England remained primarily rural, so that by the eleventh and twelfth centuries, about one tenth of the population lived in very small urban settlements whilst maintaining an agriculturally based lifestyle. They cultivated the land that surrounded their villages as part of an open field system in which strips of earth allocated throughout the fields were the responsibility and livelihood of families. The land was usually owned by the church, which was paid a tithe of goods and labour or, in the later Middle Ages, by feudal lords who were then owed homage and military service. Although few towns or cities, except London, were as large as their counterparts on the continent, places described as boroughs were usually quite sizeable, and Lincoln, Norwich, York and Winchester, for example, had populations of about ten thousand. Boroughs and towns were often walled, had their own markets and customs, and some were granted privileges and protection from the Crown. Real government though was a local affair. In twelfth century boroughs, merchants (or burgesses) who made their living from trade were generally well housed in private residences with gardens. They had a say in town governance with other significant members of the population such as those of its dominant industry which more and more was likely to be weaving. Some of the centres of industry became so wealthy that they began to assume importance in the political and economic life of the Country.

Despite that, the period is depicted, by many, as a time of depression because of an apparent decline in scientific thought and endeavour. Medical practice was seen as stagnating because of its adherence to translated accounts of previous authorities, and also because, in many cases, it became subordinate to the dogma of religious zeal and monastic creeds. Unlike older religions, which were essentially for the sound, beautiful, strong and pure, Christianity was one of healing, Jesus having performed miracles which enabled the ill, weak, and crippled to recover and to take their place in the world once more. That changed, to some degree, their place in society and that of physicians. Sigerist argued that:

> Christianity gave the sick man a position in society that he had never had before, a preferential position. The new religion addressed itself to the poor, the oppressed, the sinners, and the sick. It addressed itself to suffering humanity and promised healing and redemption.[2]

However, epidemics and other natural catastrophes were frequently considered punishments inflicted by God whilst 'mental diseases were the result of a disordinate life', and venereal diseases were 'punishment for sexual promiscuity'.[3] Indeed, "Patristic" literature, that is the writings of influential fathers of the first few centuries of the Christian Church, considered anatomy, physiology and pathology as being little different from other secular learning. In the latter regard, differentiation was made between Plato's theories, which were acceptable and Aristotle's, which were not. Likewise classical medicine was given modified acceptance and interest, contingent on Christian explanation and beliefs. However, notwithstanding such limitations, monasteries did provide new centres for medical learning, often according to what was available of classical medicine, alongside the practices of physical and spiritual healing that were followed by their order.[4]

The advent of Christianity and the subsequent establishment of monasteries in Ireland, too, led to the sick and destitute coming under their care. This replaced a long tradition in which, under Brehon law, there had been an obligation for territorial rulers to provide "hospitaller facilities for the sick and the homeless" (*briugu*). The "hospitals," apart from beds for patients and a physician in attendance, had "four doors and a stream of water running through". In fact Ireland boasts one of the earliest known hospitals, the "house of sorrow" (*Broin Berg)*, founded by Princess Macha about 300 BC near Armagh. It formed part of Ulster's royal residence until it was destroyed in 332 AD. It was, reputedly, the Druids who practised healing and a primitive type of surgery, who originally established a "hospital" on that site.[5]

Classical medicine had been kept alive by its adoption by Arabic men of letters and physicians. Arabic scholarship had been gradually advancing from the time when Ptolemy set up a museum in Alexandria in the fourth century BC, which, it is thought became the first centre of study at university level. A medical school was started there at about the same date.[6] Later, following the demise of Greco-Roman dominance, the Arab speaking world gradually increased its influence, establishing centres of learning at Basra, Baghdad, Cairo and Cordova, which ultimately became universities.[7]

The Arabic understanding of classical medicine was, in part, the result of translations carried out by the Nestorians, an early Christian sect. Founded by Nestorius, a fifth century bishop of Constantinople who was deposed because of his extreme views about the Virgin Mary, the sect prospered under Muslim rule, and continued its work in Mesopotamia with great and far reaching missionary zeal. Members of the sect translated many of Hippocrates' and Galen's works into Syriac, and later into Arabic. These ultimately became available to scholars of the west when Latin translations were also made.[8,9] It is possible to recognise an evolution in medieval medicine according to the timing of importation and translation of classical works, often via the Arabic versions of the texts. Of particular note are works from Ravenna from the fifth to seventh centuries, Monte Casino and Salerno in the tenth and eleventh, and Toledo in the twelfth, led by Gerard of Cremona.[10,11] The re-adoption of classical doctrines into Europe through the Arabic connection, particularly those of Hippocrates and Galen, led to rules (regimens) of health (sanitatis) being formulated. These provided the basis of medicine for centuries to come.

There was also a spreading of ideas by particular practitioners such as Aetius of Amida, a Christian physician of the sixth century and an imperial medical adviser. Educated in Alexandria, he wrote sixteen medical books, which referred to classical medicine and to the treatment of patients of all ages. On the rehabilitation front, he included breathing exercises for vocal paralysis, and recommended massage and active, passive and resisted exercises for physical disorders, along with the use of amulets and incantations.[12]

Paulus Aegineta (625-690), a Greek physician, provides another example. Born in Aegina, he practised at the medical school of Alexandria, and was considered by Muslim physicians to be one of the most eminent of Greek medical authorities. That was borne out by his production of seven important and descriptive volumes on the medicine and surgery of the Middle Ages. He specialised in the treatment of children, gynaecology, obstetrics, surgery of the reproductive systems, ophthalmology, and the treatment for apoplexy and epilepsy, and also supported the theories of general exercise. A particular occupation that he favoured in that connection was mountain climbing.[13]

Macdonald reports that Arabic physicians based much of their practice on keen observation, so it is interesting to observe that they evinced some appreciation of the need for occupation. For example, at "El Nasiti", a hospital in Cairo, 'convalescent patients were entertained by singers and musicians', and in another, St Basil's in Caesarea, programmes similar to 'rehabilitation schemes were provided, so that the patients might be able to return to their work on discharge'.[14] Dr James Walsh, a respected medical historian of the early 20th century described the latter hospital this way:

> St Basil's magnificent foundation at Caesaria in Cappadocia, called the Basilias, which took on the dimensions of a city (termed Newtown) with regular streets, buildings for different classes of patients, dwellings for physicians and nurses and for the convalescent, and apparently even workshops and industrial schools for the care and instruction of foundlings and of children that had been under the care of the monastery, as well as for what we would now call reconstructive work, shows how far hospital organisation, even in the latter part of the fourth century, had developed[15]

The Church as health and social welfare provider

As the Romans had withdrawn from England following the fall of their empire, some able physicians, surgeons, oculists and other health specialists continued, particularly in well established Roman towns like Colchester, Gloucester, Lincoln and York, many of which had medicinal bath-houses. Whilst the remaining Anglo-Saxon population also believed in the therapeutic application of water, they had reintroduced elements of primitive and magical medical theories, in which charms, spells and herbal treatments were used.[16] These elements lingered even after the gradual establishment of religious houses and medical assistance compatible with the Christian creed, which held a different attitude towards the human body. Medical historian, Sigerist explained that:

The Christian conception was strictly dualistic; mind and body are in opposition, and what matters is the soul. Why, then, care for the body, ie, the earthly, sinful part of man? It is obvious that such an attitude was not favourable for the development of hygiene. The great hygienic achievement of antiquity vanished not merely because the first centuries of the Middle Ages were hard times, troubled by wars; it vanished chiefly because of that different attitude. And yet in the Middle Ages, too, people wanted to lead a healthy and joyful life. It is true that the body is the perishable part of man, but it is the abode of the soul and is therefore to be preserved and to be cared for too, whence the church reconciled itself with medical science and attempts were made to improve sanitary conditions.[17]

The Roman Empire had established Christianity as its official religion in the 4th century. This resulted in the spread of Christian ideas throughout Europe, blended with a modified version of ancient Latin culture, which combination influenced the relationship between religious and secular healing and attitudes towards medical knowledge. The churches' beliefs were unequivocal: 'the divine was above the temporal … the body was to be subordinated to the soul, and healing, like any other temporal activity had to be under ecclesiastical regulation'.[18] Bearing that in mind, though, essentially medicine was learned from those classical texts that were available. For example, in the 6th century Cassiodorus had his monks refer to works by Hippocrates, Dioscrides and Galen. In the early 7th century, the bishop of Seville, Isodore, compiled both an encyclopaedia, *Etymologiae*, and a thesis *On the Nature of Things (De Natura Rerum)* which contained Hippocratic and Galenian medical lore. In the 9th century, Hrabanus Maurus the archbishop of Mainz, reorganised much of the former work in *De Universo*. As could be expected, and typical of the time, such texts combined secular with religious interpretations.

The monastic establishments, which were developed as Christianity spread, provided the first extensive health and social welfare services for mass populations. In that regard, rather than being considered a time of depression because of the apparent decline in scientific thought, the churches' adherence to religious zeal and monastic creeds set up a different way forward. Rather than being based on the revolutionary findings of a few forward thinkers, it was founded on an appreciation of human need, even if that was largely with a spiritual objective. Taking in the sick was considered a duty that benefited the soul of those doing the good deed. But this differed from medicine, for Jesus had healed without "potions" or "physic".[19]

From the medical point of view the Benedictine Order, the oldest in the Latin west, was the most active of all. Christian monasticism had begun in 4th century Egypt when men chose to occupy themselves with prayer and physical labour whilst living as hermits in the desert.[20] Similarly, St Benedict of Nursia (c. 480-547), pictured in figure 1.4.1, lived for over forty years as a religious recluse in a cave near Subiaco in Southern Italy. Such was his reputation that he was accepted as an unofficial leader of about twelve communities of anchorites who gathered near him. In 529 he founded a monastery at Monte Casino near Naples. After his time, all was not peaceful for the brethren. Between late in the 6th and the 9th centuries the monastery at Monte Casino was sacked twice, so that the monks had to flee, in both cases only returning to carry on their work many years later. It remained a monastery until 1866 when it was preserved by the intervention of English well wishers, resident in Italy, and classed as a national monument with monks retained as its custodians.[21]

Figure 1.4.1: **Saint Benedict.**
Abbot of
Monte Casino. F.
L. Schmitner
(1703-1761)
(The Wellcome Library)

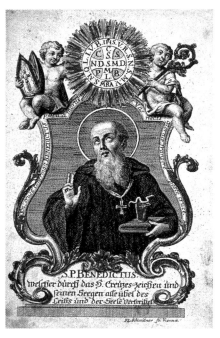

At Monte Cassino, St Benedict wrote his "Rule", which was organised around alternating periods of prayer, labour and rest. His prescription for monastic life, which appears occupationally well balanced between "doing and being", 'became normative for western monasteries and dominated the structure of religious communities from the sixth to the thirteenth century'.[22] Benedict deemed that labour (occupation) was essential for spiritual health and well-being as one of his Rules attests. This ordained that 'idleness is the enemy of the soul and therefore, at fixed times, the brothers ought to be occupied in manual labour, and again at fixed times, in sacred reading'.[23] That Rule gives some indication of the church's perspective of health, when prayer received more emphasis than what would now be called medical care. It was a time when the spiritual was considered more important than the physical, as distinct to the opposite in the modern world, because disease was often attributed to sin. In an age when medicine had no sophisticated tools to aid recovery Benedictine's view was particularly useful, especially when it is borne in mind that spirit, mind and body are closely connected and influence each other. Because of this, spiritual health was considered the key to ensuring physical and mental health, as far as was possible then.

In the early days of monastic settlements monks of any denominations were forced, usually by their isolation, to perform all subsistence occupations. Later, as monasteries grew rich, it was often the lay workers and villagers owing tithes who carried out many of those tasks. Bitel describes how hagiographers in Ireland 'described whole families of tonsured monks labouring with an almost Benedictine zeal for the work of the hands'. Whilst some neglected labour for the more obvious spiritual duties, most regarded 'manual labour not as essential to survival but as a spiritual option'. They did this even though many of the spiritual elite 'lacked the skills with which to support themselves and their communities'.[24] Bitel adds that:

> Almost from the arrival of Christianity in Ireland, monks took on the duties of doctors of body and soul … and because of the medieval notion that external illness reflected inner decay, the monks were able to use their curative powers to reinforce the links between disease and disorder and between health and social equilibrium[25]

De infirmis fratribus, which is Chapter 36 of Benedict's Rule, states that:

> Care of the sick must rank above and before all else, so that they may truly be served as Christ, for he said: "I was sick and you visited me" (Matt. 25: 36) and "What you did for one of these least brothers you did for me" (Matt. 25: 40). Let the sick on their part bear in mind that they are served out of honor for God, and let them not by their excessive demands distress their brothers who serve them.[26]

The Rule also charged the "infirmarian" with being "thoroughly reliable" as well as being pious, diligent and solicitous towards those in his charge.

As one of the chief duties of the Order was to care for the sick, it is not surprising that Monte Casino was referred to as a hospital at a very early date. Despite St Benedict having forbidden the monks to act as teachers, it was also known as a medical school by, at least, the 9th century.[27] Within its health care system, forerunners of psychotherapy, physiotherapy, and hydrotherapy were used,[28] however, most of the cures wrought were said to be of a miraculous nature. In this regard it is important to understand that it was for illnesses thought to have a moral basis that most 'patients sought cures and monks healed'. Hagiographers in Ireland, where monastic settlements were established early, recorded that "saintly cures" were routine for 'paralysis, blindness, deafness, and muteness'.[29]

Gasquet, in his 19th century history of Henry VIII and the English Monasteries, quotes an early source as saying that monastic establishments:

> … made such provision daily for the people that stood in need thereof, as sick,

sore, lame, or otherwise impotent, that none or few lacked relief in one place or another. Yea, many of them, whose revenues were sufficient thereto, made hospitals and lodgings within their own houses, wherein they kept a number of impotent persons with all necessaries for them with persons to attend upon them[30]

There was a need for facilities as well as people to carry out such duties. Chapter 66 of Benedict's Rule laid down that everything that was necessary should be contained within the monastic enclosures, all of which had a common lay out of buildings for particular functions. A drawing of part of an enclosure is included in the frontispiece to this chapter. From about 820 the health care buildings, with the infirmary and physicians' house, were located in the north east corner with the novitiate house, the bloodletting house, the medicinal herb garden, and the monks' cemetery. The physician shared his house, which contained his pharmacy, with the critically ill.[31]

The Cistercians, who had many establishments in Ireland, followed St Benedict's Rule, and offered shelter and care to anyone arriving at one of their monasteries. 'Let a thoughtful care be had for the reception of the poor and strangers from afar; for in these do we must truly welcome Christ.' If poor, they were not only received with kindness but given food, drink and clothing. All had infirmaries and many had leper houses.[32] The Augustinians too deemed that it was the role of monasteries to care for the sick and elderly. The original record of the Augustine priory, or hospital, of St John the Evangelist in Kilkenny clearly decrees that the religious house be to honour God and St John by providing support of the sick and indigent.[33]

It is worth noting that in the early part of this era physicians were usually ordained priests, and that later, many Northern university-trained physicians took priestly orders.[34][35] However it is probably true that 'monks did not compete with physicians, but encouraged and even employed them'.[36] In a similar vein, from the thirteenth century those in major monastic orders, such as the Benedictines, were forbidden by the fourth Lateran Council of 1215 to carry out surgery that shed blood.[37] This regulation, which was initially intended 'to detach clergy from a manual and bloody craft' and from "gain",[38] was to deepen the later distinction made between physicians and surgeons.

There was general agreement between religious healers and secular physicians that their functions differed, an agreement that was well understood by prospective patients.

Secular physicians attended cases in which the injury and its cure were singular phenomena, and in which the patient either became completely well or died soon after the trauma. Religious healers, on the other hand, ministered to chronic and degenerative afflictions.[39]

It appears from this that the type of illness treated within religious organisations had much more in common with the type of patients traditionally helped by modern day occupational therapists, than those for whom secular physicians cared.

Bearing in mind the particular type of patients seeking help from medieval monasteries, it follows that, from an early date, most maintained a hospice which provided medical care as well as food and shelter.[40] Some also provided 'study centres for adults and children, hospitality for travellers, care for the sick, isolation for lepers, general welfare centres, and work-shops'.[41]

In the general population any "defect" was feared, in part, because defects were still viewed as an indication of sin or spiritual flaws. Only "holy men and women" who could deal with those problems and to whom re-socialising the victims of isolation presented no problems, 'could cure that fear'. Additionally many societies, like that in early Ireland 'found little use for disabled people in their pastoral and agriculturally based subsistence economy', especially as disabilities 'kept people from performing ordinary jobs and from attending social gatherings'. Indeed, Bitel proposes that throughout Europe most disabled people were considered not only a burden but also 'a shame to families of fighters and farmers'. She adds that 'the diseased, the disabled, the sterile, and the mad', although 'rejected by the healthy community', were not only in a 'position to gain spiritually from their physical distress', but also to profit 'socially in the long run'. 'By seeking a cure, the afflicted entered into a series of exchanges with the religious elite' which ultimately benefited and supported them as they were 'transformed from disabled, immoral outcasts into virtuous, sociable Christians'.[42]

However, because it was believed that 'illness spread outward from the soul, patients had to achieve the proper spiritual condition before the saints or their representatives would consider attempting to cure them'. The patient had to make the first approach, usually in a holy place, and in their explanation of the nature of the illness, humbly acknowledge the spiritual weakness to which it could be attributed. 'The entire process was ineffective if the patient failed to achieve a state of inner awareness.'[43] If the result of the consultation were negative, the acceptance of a potentially faulty spiritual condition on the patient's part meant that the religious healer had only successes to report.

Women shared the development of monasticism. For example, St Scholastica, Benedict's sister, also founded a Benedictine establishment. Most were less well endowed than their male counterparts. However, particularly in Germany, some convents were wealthy and restricted entry to noble women, especially those who were deemed unmarriageable, or for whom a dowry could not be found.[44] Macdonald suggests that the:

> *Christian influence on the care of the sick encouraged the development of medical and nursing roles for women, based on the newly developed monastic*

hospitals. The women doctors were highly respected and popular, but some were said to indulge in quackery![45]

It is worth noting that one of the most famous medical authorities of monastic life was a woman, Saint Hildegard (1098-1179), a Benedictine Abbess pictured in figure 1.4.2, who founded a new convent at Bingen on the Rhine. When writing about health she followed the prevailing view about it being the result of balance, that is, 'the right order and the correct measure', between the four humours. The humours, she said, 'temper one another, just as the world consists of four elements that are harmoniously combined'.[46] Touching on the relationship between what people do and the four elements, fire, air, water and earth, of which, it was believed as in classical times, the world consisted, Hildegard argued that:

> *The elements, in fact, are subject to humans, and as they are touched by the humans' deeds so they perform their tasks. … This derives from God's primal ordinance because God established that the elements should work according to human's deeds. … When human beings are on the right path, doing good and evil within measure, then the elements perform their tasks according to the humans' needs*[47]

She went further than that, maintaining that just as the elements 'hold the world together so they are also the fastening of the human body', and related their function to health and illness. 'When the elements operate in an orderly manner in human beings they maintain them and make them healthy; when they are at variance they make them ill and kill them.'[48] Only some selected people such as Samson, Solomon, or Jeremiah, or even a pagan, like Plato, 'whom God's grace has imbued' with special gifts, were thought able to be healthy despite an excess of one or other humour. As part of that, they were thought to have the potential to engage in exceptional occupation.[49] It is contrary to present day occupational therapy thought that particular human potential is restricted to the few. Now it is understood that all people are different and have different and particular occupational potential[50]

Figure 1.4.2: Hildegard von Bingen. W. Marshall
(The Wellcome Library)

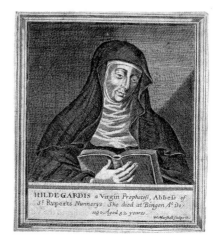

Apart from that, the central tenet of her overall argument, based as it was upon both a spiritual and secular medieval understanding of human physiology, supplies a very different way of considering the relationship between occupation and health to the present day. It advances, very strongly, the idea that human deeds should be considered in terms of right or wrong according to the Christian creed, that health results from doing mainly good, and that ill health results from engaging in immoral actions. This idea, which is a further development of Benedict's Rule concerning labour being necessary for the soul, remained part of the general and medical patterns of thought until the advent of humanism and the scientific revolution of the Renaissance. It accounts, in some measure for the difference between the provision and types of health care which were offered then, as compared to later. It also suggests that it was those with religious affiliations who were best qualified to be the "occupational therapists" of the time, advising, sanctioning and enabling the masses, as well as sick or "impotent" individuals, to engage in moral occupations for their spiritual, and hence, physical and mental health and well-being.

In addition to this moral view of human occupation and health, the exercise potential of physical doing was also considered important, although not so carefully thought out in terms of individual needs or detail as nutritional health care. Hildegard recommended:

If a male who is physically healthy walks for a long time or is on his feet for a long time, he will not harm himself by keeping his body in motion, provided he does not walk or stand excessively. Those who are weak should sit; for if they walked or stood too much they might harm themselves. But because woman is weaker than man and has a different cranium, she should walk and stand with moderation. To avoid causing harm to herself she should sit rather than run. It will however not hurt anybody to ride a horse, though it may make one very tired because one moves around in the air and wind. One should take care of one's feet and legs and exercise them, now and then, by bending and stretching.[51]

In considering the occupations that were used by spiritually based practitioners as agents for health, the first has got to be "labour". In terms of those times, labour would mostly have been of a physical nature–working in the fields and in husbandry (figure 1.4.3.), or in the production and manufacture of buildings or items needed for daily life. The second would have been those obviously to do with the well-being of the soul. These included prayer, visiting and helping with the sick and elderly, and special occupations such as making pilgrimages to the resting place of saints or their relics, or taking part in a crusade to rescue holy places. Whilst both labour and spiritual occupations were aimed at the soul's health, they would by their nature have assisted the body and mind at the same time, and thus vindicate the foundation beliefs. The third type of occupation, which according to St Hildegard was prescribed, was exercise mainly through walking or riding. All three were done, at least in the case of those taking part in monastic life, according to a prescribed balance of physical, mental, spiritual, social and rest occupations, however pilgrimages, being somewhat outside that prescription, deserve special mention.

Figure 1.4.3: **Labour such as ploughing would have been used for spiritual health (monastic occupational therapy) as well as subsistence.** *(British Library)*

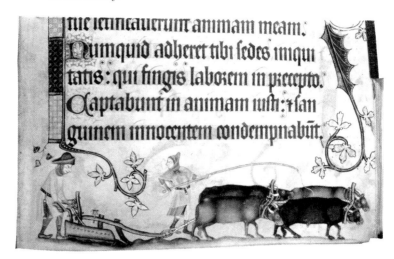

It is thought that pilgrimages to Jerusalem, Bethlehem and other places of Christian significance had started in the fourth century and remained popular throughout the Middle Ages. Many people visited shrines in their own countries, the most visited in England being the tombs of St Thomas Becket, St Alban, St Edward the Confessor, and St Cuthbert, although relics kept in other holy places were also thought to have healing powers. St Thomas's blood, for example, was believed to cure blindness, insanity, leprosy, and deafness.[52] 'Few large churches were without some important relic, and even the poorest people could therefore make at least one pilgrimage in a lifetime.'[53] It is supposed that so intense was the popular piety of medieval Christendom that little encouragement was required from members of the church to augment the belief that visiting, touching or even looking at a saint's relics was sufficient to heal the diseased and calm the troubled.

Pilgrimages have some aspects in common with much later medical recommendations, when physicians prescribed that people take a holiday from their day to day life to refresh themselves in body and mind and recover their health. In these later times there was often acknowledgment that a change of air might be helpful, or that "taking the waters" at a spa or seaside place might be effective. During the Middle Ages pilgrimages offered even more than that. As well as an ultimate goal or purpose, which is clearly understood by modern day occupational therapists as of vital importance in the health outcomes of the therapy they prescribe, there was adventure, the mobility demands of getting there, and the stimulation of meeting different people on the way and sharing the journey. Chaucer's *Canterbury Tales* provides a truly magic account of the latter.

Figure 1.4.4: **Pilgrimage**
(British Library)

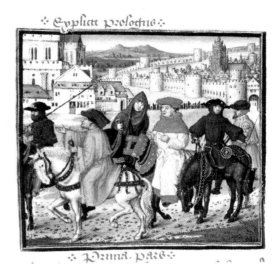

With regard to mental health in the Middle Ages, four main categories of disorder: frenzy, mania, melancholy, and fatuity, were recognised by medical authorities according to Galen's view that such illness occurred as a result of humoural imbalance. Other authorities held different views, such as that it was caused by the moon, lovesickness, sorcery or possession by the devil, so it is not surprising that treatment varied. The latter belief led to the insane being linked to witchcraft, and the torture and execution of thousands of people, mainly women, in an attempt to get rid of Satan's menace.[54]

Walsh maintains that despite there being no large asylums or poorhouses at that time, treatment was less subject to abuse than in the early 20th century. This was because each community looked after their own often, early in the disorder, in small local hospitals, which he says were numerous, or in monastic establishments if there was a link between patient and monastery. In the convalescent stages, kin usually gave care. The more well-to-do, he says, also found refuge in monasteries or convents, which sometimes had separate facilities for the purpose, such as small houses set apart but within the enclosure.[55] One can imagine that in both monastery and home, the sufferers were encouraged to take part in, at least some aspects, of everyday life.

Walsh's, and more recently, Porter's descriptions of medieval care of the insane illustrate how different facilities existed in different parts of Europe, not only originating in monasteries. In Spain, as a result of Moorish influence,

Granada had an apparently well-managed asylum for the insane by 1365. This was the first of others established at Valencia, Zaragoza, Seville, Barcelona, and Toledo in the following century. In Germany, as well as monasteries, there were madmen's towers known as narrenturme, and at Geel, in Flanders, a community-care system for the mentally handicapped. The latter came about as a result of such children being brought to the shrine of St Dympna, an Irish girl martyr, whose intercession was believed to have particular value for them. Often children were left near the shrine, supposedly to benefit from long term exposure to the Saint's influence. Surrounding villagers, proud of their patron saint, cared for the children, gave them various simple occupations to perform, and protected them from being abused or taken advantage of. As adults, many became attached to monasteries where they engaged in humble tasks in a protected environment. Other villages, especially in the Low Countries and France, followed the Geel example and took up similar work. Other shrines apart from that of St Dympna were believed to hold the power to cure madness such as St Mathurin and St Acairius in northern France.[56][57]

Hospitals established during this period usually had church affiliations. St Maria Nuova in Florence, said to be the "first hospital among Christians", was initially a small establishment which was gradually medicalised and enlarged.[58] St Jerome recorded that at least two were founded in Rome early in the fifth century and, later in the same century, Pope Symmachus built three more in the Papal City connected to St Peter's, St Paul's, and St Lawrence's Churches. As Christianity spread, other hospitals were established in Germany, where they were particularly associated with Pope Innocent III or the Teutonic Knights of the Crusades; in France, where the Paris Hotel Dieu had physicians in attendance from 1231; and also Britain.[59] In the latter, St Alban's Hospital was set up in 794; St Bartholomew's, London, in 1123; Holy Cross, Winchester in 1132; St Paul's, London, in 1137; St Mary's, London, in 1197; St Thomas', London, in 1215, and St Leonard's, York, in 1287 which had 225 beds for the sick and poor.[60][61]

Some medieval hospitals were, undoubtedly, poor by modern day standards, but not all. For example, Tonnerre in France, which was built for Marguerite de Bourgogne, the sister of St Lois, in 1293, allowed each patient plenty of space and privacy, effective ventilation and subdued lighting, as well as being a place of architectural beauty. The Hospital of St Jean of Bruges, dating from the next century, was also light and airy, and had pleasant gardens suitable for convalescents. Walsh reported in 1920 that the original building was still used as a storeroom in the current hospital, and its advantages were obvious including, he said, 'occupation of the patients' minds with details of the construction'.[62] This suggests yet other aspects of occupation for health used at that time, and probably neglected or deemed less important in the present day, that of involving curiosity and thought in speculation when there is an inability to engage in more physically demanding occupation, and doing so in an environment that refreshes the spirit.

One of the most serious health problems of the time was leprosy. The 'spread of that disease by pilgrims and crusaders returning from the East' led to the setting up of numerous "leper hospitals" throughout Europe and England.[63] There were possibly 19,000 in Europe, altogether, and in England about 130. In Bury St Edmunds alone, for example, six such establishments were set up between 1150 and 1260. These also had a brief to cater for pilgrims, the infirm and the aged, though leprosy was highly stigmatised and those people with leprosy were targets of strict social exclusion according to ancient Levitical decrees reiterated by the 12th century Lateran Council. That enforced segregation of people with leprosy from the general population, whilst inhumanly horrendous for its victims, resulted in the disease being in decline by the 1350s, and its gradual dying out. Leprosariums, or lazarettos as they were called, became useful for other purposes, like housing others with infectious diseases, or the mentally disordered, indigent syphilitics, or the poor.[64,65]

Secular experts and the development of university education

Apart from the "healing" services provided by religious institutions, there was no great change from previous periods of history in the intellectual assumptions about the nature and expectations of health, secular practice, and delivery of health care. In medieval society, as earlier, those differed according to the cultural milieu of which they were a part. For most people, health care still, largely, depended upon self, family, and neighbours, especially in the case of ordinary maladies like headache or urinary infection, or even for disorders like gout or dropsy. The first recourse was often a prayer, sometimes to a saint believed to have special curative powers for the particular ailment, along with ministrations provided by kin in their own home or the home of others. 'With or without medical guidance, patients practised self-help in the form of self medication, visits to medicinal baths, pilgrimages, or prayer; and religious shrines offering alternative forms of healing were omnipresent.'[66] As dwellings, on the whole, were tiny and crowded, sufferers would not have been able to avoid being involved in the day to day life of those around them, which might have been therapeutic in some cases, or made the situation worse in others. When all else failed a health worker of some kind, perhaps a self styled or "trained" physician might be called. In most cases, like monastic healers, their practices were compatible with church teachings because Christian values were ingrained amongst doctors and patients alike. In modern terms all physicians were untrained, as there were no formal requirements, licensing or university education, although there is some indication, that even then, in many instances, some held higher than normal social status.[67]

There were people in country areas who were known as healers, but they, in the main, practised medicine as only one of several occupations. In some places there were wise women or others who were known as "empirics" (craftsmen). In urban locations, although doctoring by the family was also the norm, there were bloodletters and "healers" in addition to midwives. As well, there were guilds of apothecaries (or pigmentaries) responsible for the preparation and dispensing of medicines; practically trained surgeons (or chiurgeons) who, like the modern day orthopaedic surgeon, were expert in the treatment of fractures and dislocations. In addition there were barber-surgeons whose members were available, for a fee, to provide advice, nostrums, bleedings, and more.[68] For the more affluent, midwives and nurses were available to visit people in their homes, or, sometimes to look after them in the practitioner's own residence when suitable care was not possible elsewhere.

In terms of public health, any of the experienced health practitioners could be given the task of advising magistrates about illicit practice, and help guard the towns and boroughs from lepers and plague carriers. In return they were often granted a monopoly on aspects of the medical trade, and access to imported spices and drugs. Little indication has been found in the literature that occupation was used as a particular remedy except as "exercise," of which it appears horse riding was the most favoured. The exercise remedies were prescribed, as in the rules of health handed down from Galen according to the humoural theory, probably in a way similar to Hildegard, and discussed later as part of the *Regimen Sanitatis*. Health experts who encouraged physical exercise included Amand de Tournay, Petrus of Apono, and a woman, Francesca Barbaro, who particularly encouraged girls and young women to exercise.

Here and there, in pockets of time and place, aspects of more sophisticated medical practice existed. There were, indeed, even a few physicians, such as Oribasius and Caelius Aurelanius, who embraced some almost familiar notions about rehabilitation. Oribasius (325-403) was an outstanding Byzantine physician from Pergamun, where Galen was born, and physician to the Emperor Julian. He compiled, in *Medicinalia Collecta,* a collection of seventy medical works, largely from Galen and other earlier authorities, which might otherwise have been lost. The subjects his manuscripts addressed were wide and included children's illnesses, dieting, childbirth, brain diseases, the causes of strabismus and the treatment of accidents. His apparent interest in "rehabilitative media" encompassed vocal exercises, graded massage and active therapy. In the latter he recommended the use of an inflated leather ball for exercise and the punching of hanging flourbags or sandbags to encourage arm action. He recommended the use of swimming, prescribing warm baths and sea bathing for strengthening the body and for reducing swelling (he mentioned, in particular, those suffering from elephantiasis). Contrary to modern views, but apparently in line with several contemporaries, such as Actuarius (1250-1300) who recommended avoiding excessive exercise,[69] he advised against extensive walking or running.[70,71]

Caelius Aurelanius, a Roman physician born at Sicca in Africa late in the fourth century wrote a couple of practical medical texts on chronic and acute diseases that included the translated works of Soranus of Ephesus. Apparently particularly interested in neurological disorders, he described motor and sensory paralysis, encephalitis, epilepsy and speech defects.[72] Caelius advised bathing in warm spring baths, and sun bathing for chronic infections and, like Oribasius, swimming in the sea, but he suggested it should be with the assistance of inflated supports to prevent accidents and the over-use of energy. He prescribed exercises for eye disorders, and for problems relating to the tongue, including patients experimenting with speech exercises such as word forming, counting, voice production, and chewing nuts. For paralysed fingers, hands, arms, and legs he recommended massage, the use of wax baths, and graded exercises using passive assistance or resistance, assistance with pulleys, and using dumb-bells and inflated leather balls. Caelius also gave attention to mobility aids. He recommended the use of a chair with arms to assist with rising, and the support of one or two people, crutches, or the use of a type of hand controlled mobile support, to encourage walking. When supports were no longer required he prescribed a graded programme to improve mobility which included walking in specially designed ditches, up and down graded steps, or over hurdles, possibly with weighted footwear.[73] As well as this portent of things to come, the late Middle Ages saw the development of at least another couple of "aids to daily living". The glass workers of Venice introduced the use of eyeglasses,[74] and descriptions of trusses survive from the thirteenth century on.[75]

As well as different initiatives occurring around Europe, some medieval physicians evinced particular interest in the mentally ill. Caelius Aurelianus in the 4th–5th century is a case in point. He is said to have taken a well-balanced psychological approach to insane patients, recommending sensible and humane treatment.[76] Paulus Aegineta, the eminent 7th century Greek physician connected with the medical school of Alexandria mentioned earlier, as well as his many other interests, advised on the care of people suffering mania or melancholia. There can be little doubt that Aegineta referred to specially chosen occupations with therapy as the intent when he recommended "exhilaration of the mind". He wrote his prescription thus:

> Those who are subject to melancholy from a primary affection of the brain are to be treated with frequent baths and a wholesome and humid diet, together with suitable exhilaration of mind, and without any other remedy unless, when from its long continuance, the offending humour is difficult to evacuate, in which case we must have recourse to more powerful and complicated plans of treatment.[77]

Whilst it is possible to assume that this message, which appears to recognise the importance of occupation as therapy for mental illness, was from a lone voice, it is also conceivable that Aeginata's view was more widely held. In particular, it is echoed by Bartholomaeus Anglicus (the Englishman) in the thirteenth century, towards the end of the Middle Ages. Bartholomaeus was not a physician but a learned clergyman and teacher, so it is possible that he chose to discuss treatments he observed rather than carried out. His encyclopaedia is said to have been very widely read, probably in early manuscript form and prior to its being printed some 200 years later. In it Bartholomaeus prescribed, as well as prevention of self harm, the treatment of insanity as quiet and peaceful retirement, diversion from disturbed thought processes, and music and occupation to restore health and mental well-being by gladdening the mind. He expressed it this way: 'And namely such shall be refreshed, and comforted, and withdrawn from cause and matter of dread and busy thoughts. And they must be gladded with instruments of music and some deal be occupied'.[78]

Another of great renown in the 13th century was Gilbertus Anglicus, an English physician, who was apparently well liked, being commonly known as "the loveliest of doctors." He wrote *Compendium Medicinae* which its full title explains is "useful not only to physicians, but to clergymen for the treatment of all and every disease".[79] Gilbertus was particularly interested in mental disorders, and clearly discriminated between 'the symptoms of anxieties, hallucinations, mania and melancholia, and for the latter condition recommended music, sweet smelling herbs and wine'.[80]

Porter reports in *Mind-Forg'd Manacles* that in England, protection started in medieval times for those with mental handicap and from families of different social orders (but where property was at stake). Handled, sympathetically, by the Court of Wards, the judiciary 'provided a facility of trusteeship for idiots or lunatics in legal matters —property, contracts, estates, heirships, and inheritance'.[81]

The eighth to thirteenth centuries saw a number of universities established throughout Europe. They evolved initially when groups of students gathered to study under famous experts, many of whom were clerics. For example, at Salerno and Montpellier centres of learning were set up in which medical study was central. Universities started to flourish in Italy, Spain, France and England at about the same time as the great age of hospital building.[82] New universities were opened by scholars from others, such as Oxford in 1167 by students who came from Paris; Montpellier in 1180 by students from Bologna; and Cambridge in 1223 by students from Oxford. Whilst philosophy, theology, law, science, mathematics and the arts were the subjects most often offered for study, Macdonald claims that at least ten universities set up before, or in, the twelfth and thirteenth centuries, included medicine in their offerings.[83]

University trained physicians were at the top of the medical hierarchy, and were the most expensive and least available health practitioners to the general population. These doctors were, in the main, educated to discourse learnedly to patients and their families, concentrating on dispensing advice, and appearing gentlemanly and discrete. They guarded their reputations by demonstrating that they knew universal truths, laws and purposes, such as medical mathematics, as well as the reason why disorders occurred. Such knowledge ensured that they were not mistaken for quacks or untrained healers. To be able to do this well they studied archaic and recent texts on the arts as well as medicine and, contrary to monastery-based physicians, adopted Aristotelian natural philosophy as the basis for that advice. However, they also had to know their "Galen". They felt the pulse, subjected urine to close scrutiny and considered the patient's history before estimating the number of critical days and giving a diagnosis of its probable consequences. It is unlikely that they learnt first hand about the structure and function of the human body, as dissections were not considered to be part of a medical curriculum. Indeed, it is claimed that it was at the University of Bologna, established in 1158, that public dissection was first done around 1300.[84'85] Scholastic medicine was not totally divorced from the church, ascribing to theories of body and soul, which provided some erroneous ideas about human anatomy.[86] People were placed within a scale between angels and "brutes", the latter not having souls so being available for "anatomies" at early Christian medical schools such as Salerno.

There are reported differences about how long it took to gain a medical qualification. Macdonald suggests that examinations to qualify students for medical practice were prepared for by 'eight year courses for physicians, and two year courses for surgeons'.[87] Others describe that the Bachelor of Medicine, which included Arts, took seven years to complete, and a medical doctorate about ten years. In Frederick II's 1231 regulations for Sicily it took five years including some surgery. The inclusion of surgery in Italian university medical training was not copied by northern European universities and in England surgery remained part of the guild system. Professional struggles for clients, territory, and superiority tended to grow as the number of healers increased with the rise in population and their 'dawning sense of civic status'.[88]

In most of the Italian Universities women were admitted as students and appointed as professors from at least the twelfth century. Indeed, the late Middle Ages were characterised by particular encouragement of women's education including admission to the study of medicine. Their academic role appears to have been little different from their male counterparts in that they taught medicine, wrote about it and consulted on medico-legal issues. There is a difference of opinion about how wide spread, or for how long, this relative freedom of access to medical careers existed. Some say that no century until the nineteenth was without women professors at Italian Universities. Others say that it was only until the thirteenth century, when medicine became almost exclusively a man's profession and women were, mostly, only able to practice as unlicensed healers.[89] In England they were known as "leech" or "medica", the latter being applied, for example, to a Sister Ann at St Leonard's Hospital, in York. However, in 1421 physicians petitioned English parliament to ban women practitioners, confining them to nursing, midwifery and home care.[90] Others argue that women continued to practice medicine for centuries, especially in Italy. In France, Nicaise in the introduction to his edition of Guy de Chauliac's, 1893, *Grande Chirurgie,* notes that it was in the sixteenth century that women doctors almost disappeared. He added as justification for this longer time span that whilst there was none who became distinguished, women 'could practise medicine in certain towns at least on condition of passing an examination before regularly appointed masters', and points to an 1311 edict of the corporation of Paris, and a similar one from King John in 1352, which recognised that right.[91]

Whilst it is heartening to know that earlier in history women were active in medical professions no record has been found that links them, particularly, with the application of occupation to health. This was even so in the Salernitan School of Women Physicians where the department of women's diseases was operated by them alone.[92] The best known of the university women physicians was Trotula (Dame Trott), from Salerno, who is attributed with a series of books on medical subjects,[93] but was, unlike Hildegard, her Monastic equivalent, essentially quiet on the matter of occupation. Trotula, some authorities believe, was possibly 'a male writing in drag'.[94]

Despite that disappointing fact, the medical school of Salerno deserves particular mention in this text, in part because it was the first medical faculty of the occidental world,[95] and also because it promulgated occupation as exercise as part of the *Regimen Sanitatis* which will be discussed in full, shortly. Packard described how 'on a hill just above the site of the present city of Salerno, 35 miles south-east of Naples, there was situated the ancient city of Salernum, which was first known as a Roman colony in 194 BC'. It became a health resort early in its history, because it stood on the route taken by crusaders to the Holy Land. Many stopped there, particularly on their way home, as it was not only renowned for the healing properties of the air and waters in which the returning crusaders bathed, but also miraculous cures associated with holy relics. Incidentally, the crusaders imported the wheelbarrow, which had been invented in China, as the earliest form of wheelchair used to transport people with physical disabilities.[96]

Recognising the significance of this health resort the monks of Monte Cassino extended their influence to Salerno some seventy miles away, establishing monastic settlements there and providing scholarly input to the medical school. The School, itself, is said to have been established by four scholars, a Jew, a Greek, a Latin, and a Saracen, in the 7th century.[97] Whatever the truth of that is, it was, of a certainty, a crossroads of many approaches, combining them and disseminating information from many corners of the Mediterranean world. One of the key players in that process was Alphanus, an 11th century Monte Cassino monk and Archbishop of Salerno. He became acquainted with Greek medical texts in Constantinople and introduced Galenian writings to Salerno, along with Byzantine medical interpretations of humoural physiology adapted to Christian belief systems.[98] Another monk of note was Constantinus Africanus who latinised Arabic translations of Galen, Hippocrates, and Johannitius' *Liber Isagogarum*, which broadened Galen's ideas of the six non-naturals and became a foundation text in Italian and French medical schools, setting the moulds for medieval therapeutics.[99] Such translations in combination resulted in the creation of the *Articella*, which Porter describes as "canonical" in 'the revival of medicine in Western Europe'. From that time, he says, 'medicine had a distinctly Galenic complexion'.[100]

The Regimen Sanitatis

A very important development during this period is the medico-literary phenomenon named the *Regimen Sanitatis* (rules of health), or *Tacuinum Sanitatis* (if in table form), which Porter describes as 'the first of the home health manuals'.[101] Along with other components that were described in the last chapter as "dietetics", the rules and tables directly related health to occupation as action, exercise or motion, and to rest, which is part of the occupation continuum. The Regimen and Tacuinum, which provided a way to understand health as a public and a private issue, addressed its preservation and the healing of the sick. Their content, which remained remarkably consistent for many centuries, developed from ideas held by Pythagorus, Hippocrates and others, augmented by later medical authorities such as Galen. Adopted within the Arabic medical tradition from the Greek, the ideas were reintroduced with classical medicine into Europe during the Middle Ages and continued well into the nineteenth century in Islamic, Jewish and Christian practices. The most famous was the verse *Regimen Sanitatis Salernitanum*, which came from the university medical school at Salerno about the end of the 11th century.

Regimens were based on the organisation of the medical knowledge of the time into three categories; the naturals, the contra-naturals, and the non-naturals as described in the last chapter on classical medicine. Reiterating, in brief: the naturals were factors of living beings such as the four humours; black bile, yellow bile, blood, and phlegm, and the four temperaments; the sanguine, the melancholy, the bilious, and the phlegmatic. The contra-naturals were factors harmful to life and health such as diseases and their causes and symptoms that were related to the humours and temperaments. The non-naturals were a group of factors regarded as necessary for life and health, and it is within these factors that occupation was recommended as action, exercise or motion, also, of course, according to the prevailing theory about how the humours acted on physiology.

In the writings of medieval medicine, and following the dictates of Galen, the doctrinal basis of the non-naturals was elaborated around the qualities of hot, cold, dry, and moist, and organised under the six headings of:

• Air and environment (and the climate)

- Motion (variously described as actions or exercise and including occupations) and rest
- Food and drink
- Sleep and waking (which occupational scientists would now include as an integral part of "doing and being")
- Evacuation and repletion (sexual release was regarded as necessary for humoural balance, and female orgasm for conception[102]), and
- Affections of the soul (psychological aspects which, in many ways, were also related to people's occupations).

These six non-natural factors were the activities of daily life characterised by a high degree of individual choice, which were deemed to determine health or disease according to their use or abuse and individual circumstance.

It was believed that illness occurred when the body's humoural or elemental balance was disturbed. If too hot and dry, fever was the result; if cold and damp, a "cold" could be foreseen; if the body lacked sufficient food then blood became thin and the person weak; if the person created an excess of blood by eating too much rich food it could be the cause of disorder such as a stroke. Whilst treatment consisted of altering or reversing the imbalance by, for example, the "cooling" use of cold baths, blood-lettings or herbal medicines, healthy lifestyle regimens could prevent illness and imbalance occurring in the first place. This view fitted well with an understanding of the "healing power of nature" (*medicatrix naturae*), and that many illnesses recovered following a natural course. The onus was on individuals to be sensible and avoid extremes, and on physicians to advise people appropriately about humoural balance.

Despite taking care, of course, some people did get sick and explanations for that followed the same argument. Illness may happen because of a person's particular constitution or temperament, which meant that he or she needed to take extra precautions with one or other of the humours. As well, it was common knowledge that illness quickly spread in over-crowded, airless environments, like poorer urban areas, and that sickness such as "ague", may be the result of "bad air" exhaled from marshy earth. Vigorous motion such as riding on horseback was one of the recommendations to dispel the effects of bad environments and accounts for some of its popularity amongst the occupation-based medical prescriptions of the time. It was also understood that people following particular forms of work occupations were more liable than others to particular diseases, such that many potters contracted lung disease and lead-workers experienced paralysis more commonly than others.[103]

The importance of the Regimen and Tacuinum Sanitatis' in the history of occupational regimes for health is twofold. First, it lies in the fact that the notion of occupation for health was encompassed as a preventive mechanism within the primary systems of monastic and secular medical care. The all embracing preventive doctrine, built on the six categories of the non-naturals, was very necessary as the limited medical knowledge at the time meant that even the most minor illnesses or disorders were potentially life threatening or could become ongoing impediments to normal living. So preventive medicine was paramount. Second, the inclusion of occupation as a curative agent was embedded in medical practice for centuries, for the six non-naturals not only provided the base for medieval preventive medicine, but also that of the pathology, diagnosis and therapeutics of medical services. The difference between what was pathologically unhealthy or healthy depended upon the correct quantity, quality and timing of the six non-natural activities. This required individuals to follow advice on regimen about the management of each.

The Regimen was manifest in, at least, three different forms. First, it was written as private and individualised prescriptions for the rich and well-to-do; second, as an essential component of medical texts; and third, as easy to learn verses capable of promulgating health information to a larger public. These different forms merit separate consideration.

Individualised regimens for health

Being able to order life in such a way that the health rules of the *Regimen Sanitatis* could be followed implies that this type of prescription could, in reality, only be directed to those people who had control over their lifestyles. In most cases this meant the rich of civil life, secular and ecclesiastical gentry and nobility, or royalty. Additionally, because of differences in cultural requirements, in socio-physical conditions, in lifestyles, and in the medieval views about the humours and temperaments of individuals there were perceived difficulties in the generic application of the rules.

Physicians, therefore, were commissioned to write individual regimens for their patrons based on all six non-naturals. As today, those tended to concentrate more on diet than the other rules. The regulation of occupations and lifestyles seems to have been as unpopular then as it is now, and as the intake of food to effect remediation was most similar to the taking of prescribed potions it seems to have been more acceptable. Physicians who could be seen to obtain rapid results through their diets, remedies and potions were most valued and therefore, also, the most materially advantaged. Despite that economic consideration, the creation of regimens flourished and a proliferation of texts emerged for particular individuals or groups living in special circumstances.

To stress just how influential the notion of *Regimen Sanitatis* was, a little time will be given to discussing the publication history of *Regimen Sanitatis Salernitanum* (also known as *Schola Salernitana*) which was written in verse and was, undoubtedly, the most popular and the most published version. Sinclair says in his 1806 account that:

> *Among the foreign books which have been printed on the subject of health, posterior to the destruction of Roman power and empire, a work in verse, written about the end of the eleventh century, for the use of Robert, duke of Normandy, or of his father, William the Conqueroe, deserves first to be mentioned …*
>
> *The work is supposed to have been drawn up about the year 1099, by Johannes de Mediolanus, or John of Milan, with the concurrence of the other physicians of Salerne, then reckoned the most celebrated school for medicine in Europe.*[104]

It was translated into various languages, including into English in manuscript form in 1530 and 1579. The latter, a translation by Paynell was also printed, in 1607. Only three of the nine English editions made before Ordronaux's in 1870 were different translations, which tells us that it was much copied. In Dr P. Holland's edition, a commentary and some additions by Arnold de Villanova were included.[105] Villanova was Montpelier's most distinguished professor and Walsh suggests that it was the next great medical school after Salerno. Like its predecessor, Montpelier was originally a health resort to which doctors were attracted because of the potential numbers of patients. Situated close to Marseilles, which had a strong Greek colony, that medical school, too, revisited the ideas of classical medicine, and attracted students from across the world.[106] Villanova, who was a medical translator and mathematician, as well as being physician to popes and the royalty of Aragon, is given the credit by some authorities for drawing together the work of several medical rhapsodists into the *Regimen Sanitatis Salernitanum.*[107,108]

Sir Alexander Croke (1758-1824), a distinguished English lawyer and scholar who provided another well respected edition published posthumously in 1830, notes that above one hundred and sixty editions of the *Schola Salernitana* are proof of its merit and popularity.[109,110] Ordronaux makes the tally 163,[111] and yet another interested scholar, 'Boudry de Balzac stated that to 1846, 240 editions of the poem were printed, and that there existed more than 100 manuscript copies in European libraries'.[112]

Although there is dispute about whether or not the Salerno Regimen was a general "medical rhapsody" of uncertain date or a "personal poem" of the late 11th century, the latter tells the most interesting story and has many authorities arguing for its authenticity. In that account the believed recipient of the *Regimen Sanitatis Salernitanum* was Robert, Duke of Normandy, older brother of William (Rufus) II, who was King of England between 1087 and 1100. Robert was injured in the Crusades and on his return journey to claim the throne upon his brother's death called at Salerno. He remained there for about a year, not only recovering his health but in dalliance with a lady whom he married. The romantic tale of the Duke's recovery has it that the fistulous wound in his right arm, which he had received when fighting in the Siege of Jerusalem, only recovered after his wife sucked the poison from it, against his wishes, when he was asleep. He was less fortunate in other matters. The English throne was taken by his younger brother Henry, whom he later fought. In the ongoing conflict between them, Robert was defeated and imprisoned for the last 28 years of his life.[113,114]

Despite his never, in fact, attaining the throne, Robert was referred to, at least on the Continent, as the King of England to whom the verses were addressed, and at the time of his long sojourn in Salerno could, with some justification, be so addressed. In his argument that the poem was addressed to Robert, Croke reveals that he was so called in many ancient writings, and quoted a passage from Peter Dianconus in which he refers to "Robertus Rex Anglicus". He also alludes to the version of the *Regimen* itself which he argues provides evidence that it was aimed at benefiting Robert's particular health concerns. The date of the poem's origin is also thought to support the claim.[115]

However apart from the romantic beginnings of this significant work, what is important is that *Regimen Sanitatis Salernitanum* was probably aimed at a particular person rather than being rules of health for a larger audience, although it has been used in that way for centuries. Despite that possible limitation, such was the poem's popularity that it was referred to over and over again as a useful source of rules for healthy living. It gave no recommendation for specific remedies, but contained other details such as the number of bones, veins, and teeth in the body, and descriptions of disorders such as the symptoms of excessive amounts of blood, bile, or phlegm that it was useful for people to know in order to maintain their own health. It was mainly composed of rules for the preservation of health through diet, and there is a disappointing sparsity of advice within it regarding "exercise" in general. However, as could be expected, fresh air, exercise, occupations, sleep and so on, were alluded to, very little of which advice has been entirely superseded in the intervening years.

Assuming that it was written for Robert, Duke of Normandy, the opening verse, after addressing him as England's King appears to prescribe his taking a relaxed attitude to his future occupation. I chose to use the word "prescribe" because it is made plain that what follows is a medical recommendation from the Salerne School, and hence a prescription for him to follow.

The Salerne Schoole doth by these lines impart
All health to England's King, and doth advise
From care his head to keepe, from wrath his harte.

The verse also suggests that although his position may result in him having the opportunity or need to eat and drink over much and for too long a period he should do so only in moderation of amount and time, whilst listening to his body's dictates:

Drinke not much wine, sup light and soon arise.
When meat is gone long sitting breedeth smart;
And after noone still waking keepe your eies,
When mou'd you find youre selfe to nature's need,
Forbeare them not, for that much danger breed.

Ordronaux, Professor of Medical Jurisprudence in the law school of Columbia College (now Columbia University, New York), who offered his own translation in 1870, cited these lines as additions provided by Arnold de Villanova.[116]

Use three physitians still - first Dr. Quiet,
Next Dr. Merryman, and Dr. Dyet[117]

For the Latin scholars amongst readers I provide the original:
Anglorum Regi scribit Scola tota Salerni.
Si vis incolumen, si vis te reddere sanum,
Curas tolle graves, irasci crede profanum.
Parce mero - coenato parum, non sit tibi vanum
Surgere post epulas; somne fuge merisianum;
Ne mictum retine, nec comprime fortitur anum;
Haec bene si serves, tu longo tenpore vives.
Si tibi deficiant medici, medici tibi fiant
Haec tria - mens laeta - requies - moderata diaeta[118]

One section discusses the four temperaments at length. These provide examples of "psychological types" in the way of early twentieth century psychologists. The descriptions presented also give an indication of the occupational natures as well as the kind of illnesses to which these types are prone. The version provided is from Paynell's 1607 English translation, and figure 1.4.5, which illustrates them, is from a 16th century German version:

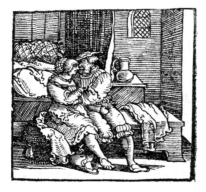

Figure 1.4.5: **The Sanguine Man, the Choleric Man, the Phlegmatic Man, and the Melancholy Man. Etchings from the old wooden cuts in the German edition of Curio, printed in 1559, 1568, and 1573**[119]

Complexions cannot vertue breed or vice,
Yet may they vnto both giue inclination,
The Sanguin gamesome is, and nothing nice,
Loues wine, and women, and all recreation.
Likes pleasant tales, and newes, plaies cards and dice,
Fit for all company, and euery fashion:
Though bold, not apt to take offence, nor irefull,
But bountifull and kind, and looking chearefull:
Inclining to be fat and prone to lafter,
Loues myrth, and musicke, cares not what comes after.

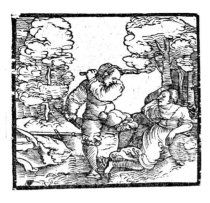

Sharpe Choller is an homour most pernitious,
All violent, and fierce, and full of fire,
Of quicke conceit, and therewithal ambitious,
Their thoughts to greater fortune still aspyre,
Proud, bountiful enough, yet oft malicious,
A right bold speaker, and as bold a lyer,
On little cause to anger great inclin'd,
Much eating still, yet euer looking pin'd,
In younger yeares they vse to grow apace,
In elder, hairy on their breast and face.

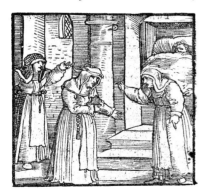

The Flegmatique are most of no great growth,
Inclining rather to be fat and square,
Giuen much unto their ease, to rest and sloth,
Content in knowledge to take little share,
To put themselues to any paine most loth,
So dead their spirits, so dull their sences are:
Still either sitting like to folke that dreame,
Or else still spitting, to avoid the flegme,
One quality doth yet these harms repayre,
That for the most part the Flegmatique are fair.

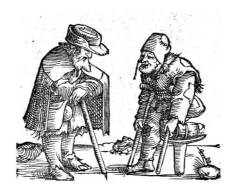

The Melancholy from the rest do vary,
Both sport, and ease, and company refusing,
Exceeding studious, euer solitary,
Inclining pensiue still to be and musing,
A secret hate to others apt to carry:
Most constant in his choice, tho long a choosing,
Extreme in loue sometime, yet seldome lustfull,
Suspitious in his nature, and mistrustfull.
A wary wit, a hand much giuen to sparing,
A heauy looke, a spirit little daring.[120]

The verses that follow those descriptions contain advice about the particular health difficulties the types might encounter, so that they can be avoided. If this poem was written for Robert, then the descriptions would be helpful in understanding his own temperament, inclinations and needs because:

Yet all men are of all participant,
But all haue not in quantity the same, …

The inclusion can also be seen as advice regarding the personality of his courtiers, advisers, and subjects in general, as it would be useful to understand the behaviour, the occupational drives, and the possible health consequences of such temperaments.

Ordronaux provided an appendix of all additions he thought 'foreign matter of questionable authenticity'. Of them the following appear relevant to this history. One on "Refreshment for the brain":

At early dawn, when first from bed you rise,
Wash, in cold water, both your hands and eyes.
With comb and brush then cleanse your teeth and hair,
And thus refreshed, your limbs outstretch with care.
Such things restore the weary, o'ertasked brain;
And to all parts ensure a wholesome gain.
Fresh from the bath, get warm. Rest after food,
Or walk, as seems most suited to your mood.

But in whate'er engaged, or sport, or feat,
Cool not too soon the body when in heat.[121]
And another about "Of Noontime Sleep"
Let noontide sleep be brief, or none at all;
Else stupor, headache, fever, rheums, will fall
On him who yields to noontide's drowsy call.[122]
And the last section of "Hygiene"
Food, labor, sleep, when moderate each day,
Do good - 'tis surfeits hurry on decay.
To rise betimes, at evening to walk late,
Keep man in health, contented and elate.

Two other examples of personal *Regimens* were those written in 1306-07 by Arnald of Villanova for King Jaume 11 of Aragon, and Maimonides' for al-Adil son of Saladin and Sultan of Egypt.

Medical texts

As medical schools became established, medieval physicians learnt that it was their primary task to interpret Galenism in order to regulate human life from their perspective. They learnt to call the management of the six non-naturals *regimen*. It is hardly surprising, therefore, that this provided the framework for medical texts concerned with health and its preservation along with the "natural principles" contained in books such as Avicenna's *Canon*.[123] Avicenna was a Persian physician of the 10th-11th century who is credited with Europe's re-adoption of much that classical medicine had to offer which had been forgotten in ensuing years. In order to link the art of medicine with the field of science and natural philosophy, the physician of the time had to unite his knowledge of the humoural qualities that defined the somatic constitution and temperament of individuals with that of the "climate"–their socio-physical environment, which was the first of the non-naturals. Avicenna's realm of practice was centred on how his patrons could live well and retain or regain health by giving advice on:

Medieval physiological ideas (which) not only provided a rational and ordered
account of the complexity of the human bodily function at any one moment but
also yielded a narrative of the progress of the human organism through time, from
conception and embryological development through various defined stages of life
to natural death.[124]

Despite considering that the *Regimen Sanitatis Salernitanum* was written in inferior Latin, it was, according to Ordronaux 'a Book of Proverbs among physicians'. Indeed, he said it was 'the medical Bible of all Western Europe', for ages holding 'undisputed sway over the teachings of the schools, next to the writings of Hippocrates and Galen'. He explained that in his view the Salerno regimen was a work of "transcendent merit" that took its place amongst the classics like Hippocrates' *Aphorisms* because no other secular work 'infused its canons so radically into the dogmas of any science'.[125] This was even though earlier versions of regimen had been promulgated. For example, Sir John Sinclair explained that 'two Jewish physicians had (previously) drawn up, at the desire of Charles the Great, a treatise called Tacuin, or Tables of Health, which is published under the name of *Elluchsem Elithimar*.[126]

> *The Tacuinum Sanitatis is about the six things that are necessary for every man in the daily preservation of his health, about their correct uses and their effects. The first is the treatment of air, which concerns the heart. The second is the right use of foods and drinks. The third is the correct use of movement and rest. The fourth is the problem of prohibition of the body from sleep or excessive wakefulness. The fifth is the correct use of elimination and retention of humors. The sixth is the regulating of the person by moderating joy, anger, fear, and distress. The secret of the preservation of health, in fact, will be in the proper balance of all these elements, since it is the disturbance of this balance that causes the illnesses which the glorious and exalted God permits. Listed under these six classifications are many useful varieties whose nature, God willing, we shall explain. We shall speak, further more, about the choices suitable to each person owing to his constitution and age, and shall include all these elements in the form of simple tables because the discussions of the sages and the discordances in many different books may bore the reader. Men, in fact, desire from science nothing else but the benefits, not the arguments but the definitions. Accordingly, our intention in this book is to shorten long-winded discourses and synthesise the various ideas. Our intention also, however, is not to neglect the advice of the ancients. (Rouen, f.1)[127]*

The popularity of the regimen points to the truth of Siraisi's suggestion that: 'From the early Middle Ages to the high Renaissance, medicinal recipes were the commonest form of medical writing'.[128]

One of the best known English physicians who used the Regimen was Somerset-born Roger Bacon (1214?-1294), a Franciscan monk, and a founder of English philosophy. He was educated in Paris where he studied with Albertus Magnus, an expert in experimental medicine, and in Oxford, where he is considered one of the University's most famous scholars. There, he lectured for many years, furthering his expertise in Arabian psychology and Aristotelian theories. Pictured in figure 1.4.6, Bacon was a man of great learning, who, despite his outlook being medieval and mystical, advocated, ahead of his time, for experience rather than authority being the basis of scholasticism and science. His tendency towards heretical propositions led to his being under suspicion, surveillance and confinement at various times during his life.[129]

Figure 1.4.6: Roger Bacon

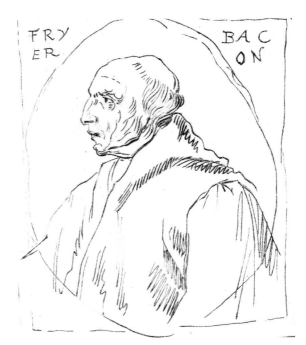

In his book *The Cure of Old Age and Preservation of Youth* he introduced the regimen listing the six causes 'prescribed by physicians and ancients as necessary to preserve and keep the body, and the true causes of health and strength'.[130] He recommended that 'the cheerful mind brings power, and vigour, makes a man rejoice, stirs up nature and helps her in her actions'[131] and in "occupation for health" terms encouraged people to engage in the many 'things that disperse and spread abroad the blood' such as:

> ... *if the soul be stirred by certain operations, actions and motions; of which sort are wrath, joy, mirth, anger, and whatever provokes laughter, as also instrumental musick, and songs, to converse with company which discourses facetiously, to look upon precious vessels, the heavens and stars, to be clothed with variety of garments, to be delighted with games, to obtain victory over ones enemies, to argue with ones most dear and beloved friends, as Aristotle saith in his epistle to Alexander.*[132]

With regard to the occupation of the elderly, Bacon referred to Aristotle's *Of the Secrets of Secrets*, which advised that they should reduce both physical and mental occupation to retain their strength, appearing to agree that:

> ... *they must abate of their labour and thoughtfulness, that the strength of their body may last a long time. And that they who are arrived at old age, avoid labour and thoughtfulness, and change, unless on great and urgent necessity.*[133]

However, somewhat later in his work, he suggested not cessation of "doing", but recommended 'they use moderate exercise, less there be any straitness or obstruction of the pores: let them avoid too violent labour and exercise'.[134]

In later centuries the trend amongst medical writers established during the Middle Ages continued, and it is obvious they based many of their arguments and recommendations on the Regimen.

Informative verses

As a strategy to disseminate information amongst a pre-literate population it was a custom in the Middle Ages to write in verse so that important messages were easier to promulgate, because people hearing them would remember them better, and so both use them and pass them on as common lore. Some writers have proposed that it was during the fourteenth century that the change occurred in consumers using the Regimen. What had been available for physicians and for the wealthy became the province of members of the urban bourgeoisie. These new consumers formed a relatively large market, and the importance of the Regimen began to grow. The Salerno Regimen was used in this way, and so too were other verses of the same ilk during the later part of the period. Particular attention was given to information on food and drink, which gained importance as a medical genre in their own right. Regimens were written for popular information in Latin verse with sub rhymes within as well as a rhyme at the end of each line, in a way similar to hymns. Perhaps faulty memories, in part, account for the many different versions of the Regimen in this form.

Sinclair, in his comments on the phenomena, suggests that its continuing popularity may have been because in the period immediately following the advent of the Regimen, very few literary works relating to health were produced. He points to Bacon as one exception, and to 15th century renaissance authors such as Antonius Gazius of Padua, and Marcilius Ficinus (1433-1499) who translated the works of Plato. The latter, who was born in Florence and worked under the patronage of the de Medici family, published a treatise on health and long life. In an interesting "dedication" he described Galen as the physician of the body and Plato the physician of the soul.[135]

In summary, Christian beliefs and monastic provision of services largely dominated health care during the medieval period. Searching for clues about the use of occupation as therapy depended on getting into the mindset of those days, which resulted in recognising two very different focuses.

The overwhelming direction for the use of occupations in health care was as a medium of spiritual well-being and recovery, not only via prayer, pilgrimages, and the like, but also by labour. As the spiritual base for medicine was the main stream approach at the time, occupation can be seen to have been central in medieval health care. In addition to the growth of secular medicine as universities were established and became involved in the promulgation of old and new medical knowledge, a preventive approach was accepted as underpinning all others. Within this, and the curative aspects of the same approach, whilst occupation did not play the most important role, which was given to "food," it was integral to more than one of the six rules of the regimen based on the humoural view of physiology. As this continued for several more centuries, different aspects of the preventive and curative use of occupation within the humoural view will be revisited in later chapters.

Despite acknowledging that the "air" in poor and crowded urban areas was unhealthy, the health sector was not powerful enough to effect major changes to those environments even if they had seen it as their role to do so. There is some evidence that they, or civic leaders, were beginning to think along those lines, when rising populations resulted in worsening sanitary conditions and contamination. In some places, for example, tanners were not allowed to wash their skins in public water sources, nor dyers their waste.[136] Additionally, and unfortunately, the preventive approach of the humoural system was not sufficiently advanced to appreciate that illness could be transmitted via other means than "air" and "human carriers". Indeed, the bubonic plague, Europe's most catastrophic epidemic, is believed to have been carried by rats through fleas to humans, and possibly by droplet infection.[137] 'At its peaks, (the plague) killed 10,000 people daily in Constantinople during the 6th and 7th century,[138] and in the 14th century, within only a few years, between a third and a half of the population in Europe and Britain.'[139][140] The latter epidemic, which was known as the "Black Death" was brought to Italy from the Near East in 1347, and then spread to the rest of Western Europe. It was to be instrumental in changes that occurred to Europe's social structure, and indirectly to its health care. This plus the spread of universities, contributed to a re-awakening in science known as the Renaissance which encompassed the study of medicine and its practice, as well as philosophy, the arts and culture.[141] The next chapter visits occupation for health regimes in the Renaissance.

[1]Walsh JJ. Medieval Medicine. London: A & C Black, Ltd., 1920. preface; vii. ('The Middle Ages are usually assumed to begin with the deposition of Romulus Augustulus, 476, and end with the fall of Constantinople, 1453.')
[2]Marti-Ibañez F, ed. Henry E. Sigerist on the History of Medicine. New York: MD Publications, Inc., 1960; 7.
[3]Marti-Ibañez. Henry E. Sigerist on the History of Medicine…; 27.
[4]Siraisi NG. Medieval and Early Renaissance Medicine: An Introduction to Knowledge and Practice. Chicago and London: University of Chicago Press, 1990; 7.
[5]O'Connor J. The Workhouses of Ireland: The Fate of Ireland's Poor. Dublin: Anvil Books, 1995.
[6]Macdonald EM. World-Wide Conquests of Disabilities: The History, Development and Present Functions of the Remedial Services. London: Bailliere Tindall, 1981.

[7]Macdonald. World-Wide Conquests of Disabilities…; 56.

[8]Macdonald. World-Wide Conquests of Disabilities…; 47-48.

[9]Girling DA, ed. New Age Encyclopedia. Sydney and London: Bay Books, 1983; vol 20: 242-243.

[10]Porter R. The Greatest Benefit to Mankind: A Medical History of Humanity from Antiquity to the Present. Harper Collins (first published 1997) paper back edition 1999; 108.

[11]Berger M. Hildegard of Bingen: On Natural Philosophy and Medicine: Selections from Cause and Cure. Cambridge: D.S. Brewer, 1999; 10-11.

[12]Macdonald. World-Wide Conquests of Disabilities…; 4 8-49.

[13]Macdonald. World-Wide Conquests of Disabilities…; 50.

[14]Macdonald. World-Wide Conquests of Disabilities…; 47.

[15]Walsh. Medieval Medicine…; 170.

[16]Macdonald. World-Wide Conquests of Disabilities…; 53.

[17]Marti-Ibañez. Henry E. Sigerist on the History of Medicine…; 12.

[18]Porter. The Greatest Benefit to Mankind…; 110.

[19]Marti-Ibañez. Henry E. Sigerist on the History of Medicine…; 8.

[20]Wright E, ed. History of the World: Prehistory to the Renaissance. Twickenham: Hamlyn Publishing Group, 1985; 325.

[21]Packard FR. (MD). History of the School of Salernum. In: The Schoole of Salernum: Regimen Sanitatis Salernitanum. (English version by Sir John Harrington). London: Humphrey Milford, 1922; 8.

[22]Berger. Hildegard of Bingen…; 9.

[23]Bettenson HS, ed. Documents of the Christian Church. New York: Springer, 1963.

[24]Bitel LM. Isle of the Saints: Monastic Settlement and Chritian Community in Early Ireland. Ithaca and London: Cornell University Press; 128-129.

[25]Bitel. Isle of the Saints…; 173.

[26]Fry T, ed and trans. The Rule of St Benedict. Collegeville, Minn: The Liturgical Press, 1981; 235.

[27]Packard. History of the School of Salernum…; 9.

[28]Macdonald. World-Wide Conquests of Disabilities.

[29]Bitel. Isle of the Saints…; 176, 182.

[30]Gasquet FA. Henry VIII and the English Monasteries. Volume II. 1888-9; 500.

[31]Price L. The Plan of St Gall in Brief. Based on the Work by Walter Born and Ernest Horn. Berkeley and Los Angeles: University of California Press, 1982.

[32]O'Connor. The Workhouses of Ireland…; 19.

[33]O'Connor. The Workhouses of Ireland…; 20.

[34]Macdonald. World-Wide Conquests of Disabilities.

[35]Porter. The Greatest Benefit to Mankind…; 110.

[36]Bitel. Isle of the Saints…; 175.

[37]Siraisi. Medieval and Early Renaissance Medicine…; 178.

[38]Porter. The Greatest Benefit to Mankind…; 110.

[39]Bitel. Isle of the Saints…; 176.

[40]Berger. Hildegard of Bingen.

[41]Macdonald. World-Wide Conquests of Disabilities…; 47-48.

[42]Bitel. Isle of the Saints…; 91, 176, 178.

[43]Bitel. Isle of the Saints…; 182.

[44]Wright. History of the World…; 327.

[45]Macdonald. World-Wide Conquests of Disabilities…; 56.

[46]Berger. Hildegard of Bingen…; 38.

[47]Berger. Hildegard of Bingen…; 38.

[48]Berger. Hildegard of Bingen…; 36.

[49]Berger. Hildegard of Bingen…; 37.

[50]Wilcock AA. An Occupational Perspective of Health. Thoroughfare, NJ: Slack Inc., 1998.

[51]Berger. Hildegard of Bingen…; 88.

[52]Porter. The Greatest Benefit to Mankind…; 112.

[53]Wright. History of the World…; 328.

[54]Porter. The Greatest Benefit to Mankind…; 127.

[55]Walsh. Medieval Medicine…; 199-200.

[56]Walsh. Medieval Medicine…; 203-204.

[57]Porter. The Greatest Benefit to Mankind…; 127.

[58]Porter. The Greatest Benefit to Mankind…; 113.

[59]Walsh. Medieval Medicine…; 171.

[60]Macdonald. World-Wide Conquests of Disabilities…; 55.

[61]Porter. The Greatest Benefit to Mankind…; 113.

[62]Walsh. Medieval Medicine…; 177-179.

[63]Packard. History of the School of Salernum…; 7.

[64]Porter. The Greatest Benefit to Mankind…; 113.

[65]Walsh. Medieval Medicine.

[66]Siraisi. Medieval and Early Renaissance Medicine…; 127.

[67]Bitel. Isle of the Saints…; 175.

[68]Berger. Hildegard of Bingen…; 10.

[69]Macdonald. World-Wide Conquests of Disabilities.

[70]Macdonald. World-Wide Conquests of Disabilities.

[71]Girling. New Age Encyclopedia…; 261.

[72]Girling. New Age Encyclopedia…; 181.

[73]Macdonald. World-Wide Conquests of Disabilities…; 48-49.

[74]Macdonald. World-Wide Conquests of Disabilities…; 58-59.

[75]Porter. The Greatest Benefit to Mankind…; 116.

[76]Macdonald. World-Wide Conquests of Disabilities.

[77]Paulus Aegineta. In: Walsh. Medieval Medicine…; 184.

[78]Walsh. Medieval Medicine…; 192-193.

[79]Walsh. Medieval Medicine…; 69.

[80]Macdonald. World-Wide Conquests of Disabilities…; 54.

[81]Porter R. Mind-Forg'd Manacles. London: The Athlone Press, 1987; 111.

[82]Porter. The Greatest Benefit to Mankind…; 113.

[83]Macdonald. World-Wide Conquests of Disabilities…; 52-53.

[84]Macdonald. World-Wide Conquests of Disabilities…; 56.

[85]Porter. The Greatest Benefit to Mankind…; 114.

[86]Porter. The Greatest Benefit to Mankind…; 132.

[87]Macdonald. World-Wide Conquests of Disabilities…; 56.

[88]Porter. The Greatest Benefit to Mankind…; 120.

[89]Berger. Hildegard of Bingen…; 11.

[90]Porter. The Greatest Benefit to Mankind…; 129-130.

[91]de Chauliac G. Grande Chirurgie. (Paris, 1893). In: Walsh. Medieval Medicine…; 166-167.

[92]Walsh. Medieval Medicine…; 158. (quote from Licence preamble. Archives of Naples).

[93]Walsh. Medieval Medicine…; 183-184.

[94]Porter. The Greatest Benefit to Mankind…; 129.

[95]Marti-Ibañez. Henry E. Sigerist on the History of Medicine…; 10.

[96]Covey HC. Social Perceptions of People with Disabilities in History. Springfield, Illinois: Charles C Thomas, 1998; 47.

[97]Packard. History of the School of Salernum...; 11,13.

[98]Porter. The Greatest Benefit to Mankind...; 107.

[99]Porter. The Greatest Benefit to Mankind...; 107.

[100]Porter. The Greatest Benefit to Mankind...; 108.

[101]Porter. The Greatest Benefit to Mankind...; 107.

[102]Porter. The Greatest Benefit to Mankind...; 129.

[103]Porter R. Disease, Medicine and Society in England 1550-1860. Basingstoke and London: MacMillan Education, 1987; 13-17.

[104]Sinclair J. The Code of Health and Longevity Volume III. Edinburgh: Printed for Arch. Constable and Co; London: T Cadell and W. Davies, and J. Murray, 1806; 3.

[105]Sinclair. The Code of Health and Longevity...; 4.

[106] Walsh. Medieval Medicine...; 61.

[107]Daremberg C. In: Ordronaux J. Regimen Sanitatis Salernitanum: Code of Health of the School of Salernum. J B Lippincott & Co., 1870; 32.

[108]Porter. The Greatest Benefit to Mankind...; 109.

[109]Croke Sir A. The Englishmans Doctor or, Schoole of Salerne, or, Physical Observations for the Perfect Preserving of the Body of Man in Continuall Health. London: Printed for John Helme, and John Busby Junior and are to be solde at the little shop, next to Cliffords Innegate, in Fleet-streete.

[110]Croke Sir A. Regimen Sanitatis Salernitanum: A Poem on the Preservation of Health in Rhyming Latin Verse Addressed by the School of Salerno to Robert of Normandy, Son of William the Conqueror, with an Ancient Translation: And an Introduction and Notes by Sir Alexandra Croke. Oxford: A.A. Talboys, 1830. Preface. (Printed editions detailed on pp. 67-94, and manuscript editions on pp. 95-99).

[111]Ordronaux J. Regimen Sanitatis Salernitanum: Code of Health of the School of Salernum. J B Lippincott & Co., 1870; 29.

[112]Packard. History of the School of Salernum...; 25.

[113]Packard. History of the School of Salernum...; 29.

[114]Ordronaux. Regimen Sanitatis Salernitanum...; 31-32.

[115]Packard. History of the School of Salernum...; 29.

[116]Ordronaux. Regimen Sanitatis Salernitanum...; 47.

[117]Paynell. Englishman's Doctor. London, 1607. In: Croke. Regimen Sanitatis Salernitanum.

[118]Ordronaux. Regimen Sanitatis Salernitanum...; 46.

[119]Conservadae bonae valetudinus praecepta integritati restituta et rhytmis Germanicus illustrata, cum Arnoldi, exegesi per J. Curionem. 1568. (Bibl. Bodl. and British museum) In: Croke. Regimen Sanitatis Salernitanum.

[120]Paynell. Englishman's Doctor...; 143-144.

[121]Ordronaux. Regimen Sanitatis Salernitanum...; 49.

[122]Ordronaux. Regimen Sanitatis Salernitanum...; 49.

[123]Gruner OC, Trans. A treatise on the Cannon of Medicine of Avicenna. London: Luzac & Co., 1930.

[124]Siraisi. Medieval and Early Renaissance Medicine...; 109.

[125]Ordronaux. Regimen Sanitatis Salernitanum...; 12.

[126]Sinclair. The Code of Health and Longevity...; 3.

[127]Sinclair. The Code of Health and Longevity ...; 3; Arano LC. The Medieval Health Handbook: Tacuinum Sanitatis. Barrie & Jenkins, Communica Europa.

[128]Siraisi. Medieval and Early Renaissance Medicine...; 141.

[129]Harvey P, ed. The Oxford Companion to English Literature. 4th ed. Oxford: Clarendon Press, 1967; 57.

[130]Bacon R. The Cure of Old Age and Preservation of Youth. Translated from latin by Richard Browne ML Coll. Med. lond. London: Printed for Thomas Flesher and Edward Evets, 1638; 20.

[131]Bacon. The Cure of Old Age...; 129.

[132]Bacon. The Cure of Old Age...; 128.

[133]Bacon. The Cure of Old Age...; 138.

[134]Bacon. The Cure of Old Age...; 142-142.

[135]Sinclair. The code of Health and Longevity...; 48.

[136]Porter. The Greatest Benefit to Mankind...; 120.

[137]Porter. The Greatest Benefit to Mankind...; 124.

[138]Procopius. Persian wars 23: 1. History of the Wars. 5 volumes. English translation by Dewing HB. Cambridge, Mass: Harvard University Press, 1914.

[139]Mumford L. The Condition of Man. London: Heinemann, 1944 and 1963.

[140]Wilcock. An Occupational Perspective of Health.

[141]Macdonald. World-Wide Conquests of Disabilities...; 57.

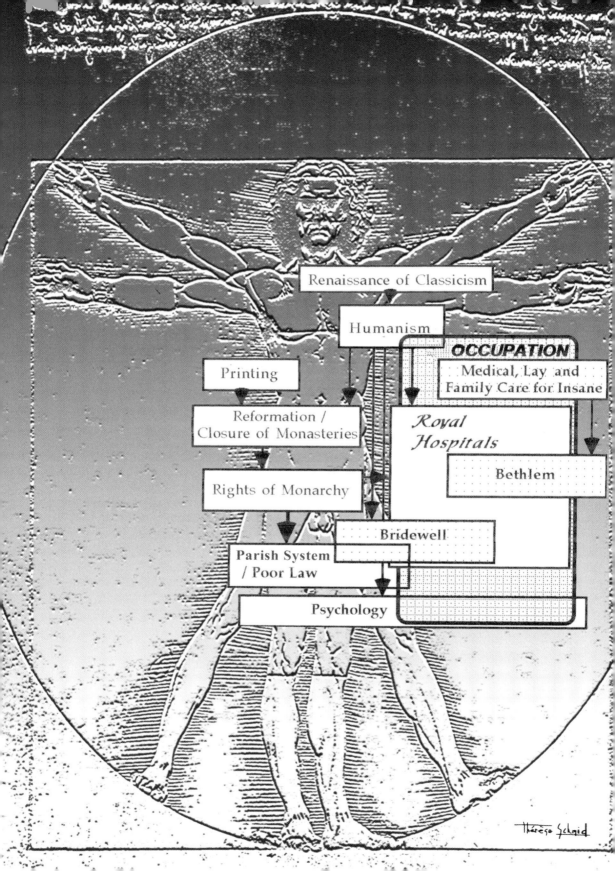

Renaissance of Classicism

Humanism

OCCUPATION

Medical, Lay and Family Care for Insane

Printing

Reformation / Closure of Monasteries

Royal Hospitals

Bethlem

Rights of Monarchy

Bridewell

Parish System / Poor Law

Psychology

Thérèse Schmid

Chapter 5

The Renaissance, Humanism and Beyond:
Occupational Regimes for Social and Mental Health

Contents

Humanism
Social context
Social health
    The Poor Law
    Bridewell Hospital
Mental health
    Bethlem Hospital
    Robert Burton: Occupation as a cause and cure for melancholy
    Parish and private care
Humanism and the advent of psychology

The story of the use of occupation for health told in chapters 5 and 6 is set in the era of the Renaissance which encompassed the 14th to 16th century, a period of great change and conflict across the western world. The impact of the Reformation, after centuries of monastic domination over the values and traditions of everyday life in many parts of Europe was overwhelming. Religious conflicts in Britain, for example, led to persecution, beheadings, public burnings, civil war, and emigration of members of recently established church sects to the New World. That, along with the humanist ideals of the Renaissance, which encouraged exploration and discovery, such as that of the Americas, impacted upon the way people went about their everyday lives. There was an earnestness apparent in the realisation that a new morality was emerging, which offered many who had not been eligible before to strive to better their own circumstances. Earnest endeavour and puritanical morals are reflected in the patterns of occupation for health that emerged during the Renaissance.

During the period humanism emerged as a dominant philosophy. As occupational therapy is often described as having a humanist orientation and approach, through a largely unwritten code aimed at human capabilities and dignity, it is important to appreciate the place of humanism in the scheme of history. It was a major conceptual change, which signalled a new secular order and a re-birth of opportunity for individual talent and interest. It could be expected that such a change would manifest in practical ways, in some spheres towards an understanding of the place of occupation in life and health. There are some indications in that direction but change was slow. Discussion will, therefore, range through the nature of the concept, as well as the shifts that occurred from an occupational therapy viewpoint, in social and mental health care in this chapter, and physical health care in the next.

Humanism

Humanism was the intellectual movement that provided the inspiration and the basis for the Renaissance or "revival of learning". It was a philosophical view and approach to life that centred on the importance of humans, stressing their dignity and potential. It was founded on the rediscovery of Classical Greek culture, the study of which was instigated in Italy by people such as Francesco Petrarch (1304-1374) who believed that it would restore virtue, culture, and order to disintegrating society.

Francesco Petrarca Petrarch was born at Arezzo but lived most of his early life in Provence where he enjoyed gardening for recreation. A poet, he is regarded as the father of Italian humanism and initiator of the revived study of Greek and Latin literature.[1] He had initially studied law and theology, which he abandoned for his new interest. In terms of health, his concern with humanism led to his denouncement of priests and unduly wealthy physicians, for spending more time on discussion and argument than on treatment. He was in favour of substituting exercises for other medical interventions.[2]

Although Petrarch was resolutely Christian, he and his scholarly colleague, Giovanni Boccaccio (1313-1375), turned from the theological explanations of the Middle Ages towards those provided by human achievement in the arts and sciences. They took a positive rather than negative view of people and regarded the world as for human use, rather than its renunciation. Literature, philosophy and history became known as "the humanities" and humanist ideas, according to many but not all historians, led the way forward to the scientific revolution, the Age of Reason and Enlightenment, and the great liberal tradition of modern Europe. For example, Michel de Montaigne's 16th century interest in self-knowledge, "the individual", and a fully humane and natural way of life is unthinkable without the Renaissance.[34] These ideas are also central to the conceptual stance of occupational therapy.

Montaigne (1533-1592), who was a magistrate in his early life and later became the mayor of Bordeaux, in his middle years travelled extensively and began writing "essais". When these were published they were found to express a mature humanist philosophy,[5] an insatiable intellectual curiosity, a kindly nature and a tolerant morality.[6] He linked his humanist views with occupation, recognising the value of engagement in a wide range, and 'described the social value of dancing, exercises, fencing, hunting, music, riding, wrestling, and other recreations'.[7]

The Renaissance, and humanism, impacted on other parts of Europe. Some English scholars, like priest John Colet (1467-1519), studied humanism in Italy. He, with others of like mind, including physician Thomas Linacre (c. 1460-1524) and statesman Sir Thomas More (1478-1535), became close friends with Desiderius Erasmus (1466-1536) of Rotterdam. Erasmus was the most noted humanist of northern Europe during the Renaissance and as an Augustinian monk combined Christianity and humanism, just as did the other three. He urged moderation but paved the way for the Reformation by his Greek version of the New Testament and comments on church abuses.[8] Macdonald claims that Erasmus held the view 'that household tasks were valuable as physical exercises'.[9]

Figure 1.5.1: **Sir Thomas More, after Hans Holbein, 1527**
(National Portrait gallery)

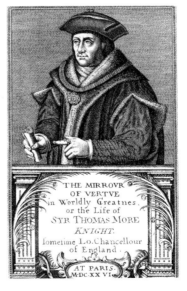

Sir Thomas More, pictured in figure 1.5.1, eventually became Lord Chancellor of England, and was the best known of the English humanists. He was born in Cheapside, gaining the first rudiments of education at the school said to be the best in the London, St Anthony's in Threadneedle Street. Following a few years in the household of the Archbishop of Canterbury, More studied at Oxford with Linacre, and there he acquired his interest in humanism. After studying law in London, he attracted the attention of the Royal House and became a Member of the Privy Council. More wrote his most famous work,

Utopia, in 1516. In this he tells the story of his vision of a people's commonwealth, in which humour and humanity abound. One section is called *Of Sciences, Crafts and Occupations* and from this it is possible to form some notion of More's humanist views on people's occupational nature and its impact on their well-being.

In Utopia, More explained, all people, regardless of sex or estate, were concerned in husbandry. Apart from this 'every one of them learneth one or other several and particular science as his own proper craft' which would usually be clothmaking, ironmongery or carpentry, with the division of crafts between male and female being with regard to strength. Whilst most commonly crafts were followed within families because of their natural bent or inclination, if this did not suit an individual's occupational interests and capacities, adopting into a family with another more suited craft followed.[10]

Recognising that people need to engage actively in occupation 'the chief and almost the only office of the Syphogrants is to see and take heed that no man sit idle, but that every one apply his own craft with earnest diligence'. One Syphogrant was chosen annually to represent thirty families, and those chosen 'who, though they be by the laws exempt and privileged from labour, yet they exempt not themselves, to the intent that they may rather by their example provoke others to work'. More also recognised, despite the customs of his times, the importance of each person enjoying a balance between obligatory and self-chosen occupations, and rest. He carefully divided the day up so that 'between the hours of work, sleep, and meat, that they be suffered to bestow, every man as he liketh best himself'.[11] In the same way he understood that community and individual well-being was a central issue of concern in social planning and custom.

> *Wherefore, seeing they be all exercised in profitable occupations, and that few artificers in the same crafts be sufficient, this is the cause that, plenty of all things being among them, they do sometimes bring forth an innumerable company of people to amend the high ways if any be broken. Many times also, when they have no such work to be occupied about, an open proclamation is made that they shall bestow fewer hours in work. For the magistrates do not exercise their citizens against their wills in unneedful labours. For why, in the institution of that weal-public this end is only and chiefly pretended and minded, that what time may possibly be spared from the necessary occupations and affairs of the commonwealth, all that the citizens should withdraw from the bodily service to the free liberty of the mind and garnishing of the same. For herein they suppose the felicity of this life to consist.*[12]

The factor which made time available for occupations of choice, More argued, resulted from there being few exemptions from this occupational regime, not by nature of gender, class, or other reason. He pointed to 'how great a part of the people in other countries liveth idle' and to the many clergy, rich men, 'which commonly be called gentlemen and noblemen', their servants, 'I mean all that flock of stout bragging rushbucklers', and 'sturdy and valiant beggars, cloaking their idle life under the colour of some disease or sickness'.[13] In Utopia only necessary work was obligatory, as More deemed that in a free and simple way of life filled with occupations which benefited both community and individuals, there was no place for the accumulation of wealth and its unnecessary trappings or the occupations they generated:

> *For where money beareth all the swing, there many vain and superfluous occupations must needs be used, to serve only for riotous superfluity and unhonest pleasure ... But if all these that be now busied about unprofitable occupations, with all the whole flock of them that live idly and slothfully, which consume and waste every one of them more of these things that come by other men's labour than two of the workmen themselves do, if all these (I say) were set to profitable occupations, you easily perceive how little time would be enough, yea, and too much, to store us with all things that may be requisite either for necessity or for commodity, yea, or for pleasure, so that the same pleasure be true and natural.*[14]

Some people were exempt from that regime, but very few:

> *... scarcely 500 persons of all the whole number of men and women that be neither too old nor too weak to work be licensed and discharged from labour. Among them be the Syphogrants ... The same vacation from labour do they also enjoy to whom the people, persuaded by the commendation of the priests and secret election of the Syphogrants, have given a perpetual licence from labour to learning*[15]

But learning was not the sole right of a separate class. More appreciated that any person may have the potential to scholarly and intellectual occupations:

> *... often it chanceth that a handicraftsman doth so earnestly bestow his vacant and spare hours in learning, and through diligence so profiteth therein, that he is taken from his handy occupation and promoted to the company of the learned. Out of this order of the learned be chosen ambassadors, priests, Tranibores, and finally the prince himself.*[16]

More's picture of Utopia illustrated the place of occupation in a healthy and just communal society. Some aspects of his picture clearly emanate from the social conditions of his time. Nonetheless, there are also pointers to the sorts of communities which the World Health Organisation of the present time recommends, if we are to achieve a healthy world and reduce unnecessary illness caused by the excesses of affluent societies on the one hand and deprived societies on the other. His picture also provides a view of how occupational therapy could be involved in political and social planning to maximise people's occupational health and well-being.

Other visionaries, later in the period covered by this chapter, had different Utopian ideas about improving societies. Peter Conelis-son, van Zurik-Zee proposed a Household-government or little Commonwealth in which husbandmen, handicraftsmen, mariners, masters of arts and sciences, and surgeons should live and work together.[17] Other idealist pamphleteers of the time, known as "Levellers" advocated changes to the state along communistic lines.

Social context

The re-awakening of thought about human value, as distinct from moral or religious values, led to a growing celebration of the abilities and talents of individuals. Traditional constraints no longer acted as fetters, so that people experimented, trod new paths, and found out about their capabilities through "doing". The Renaissance is typified by the genius of Leonardo da Vinci who appears to have gloried in, or been driven by, his occupational nature. Others, such as Giotto, Michelangelo, Botticelli and Titian, like da Vinci, brought "creativity" back into collective consciousness. It was a time when people, with newly found ideas, challenged the old order so that they might meet their needs in their own ways. It is not surprising, therefore, that medieval religious practices became a target for the great thinkers of the time.

The Renaissance was not essentially anti-Christian, and many of its principal followers were ardent churchmen. However, because humanists criticised the asceticism, dogmatism, and contemplative other-worldliness of religious and medieval scholarship, it became closely linked with religious reform. The Reformation of the 16th century, which led to the formation of Protestant religions and their separation from the Roman Catholic Church, with a concomitant rejection of the jurisdiction of the Pope, owed much to the Renaissance spirit. Another key factor was the dissemination of written argument assisted by the printing press, invented by Gutenberg in 1454.[18]

The Reformation impacted on the provision of health and welfare services in Northern Europe because before this, as seen in the previous chapter, many had been provided by religious institutions. The establishment of the Church of England, for example, resulted in the dissolution of monasteries that had over the centuries maintained medical scholarship and research. Their dissolution also resulted in the breakdown of long held traditions that supported the disadvantaged, aged, widowed, sick and poor. Whilst many monastic traditions have been criticised as adding to the state of poverty, it is irrefutable that they relieved much individual suffering and kept vagrancy and the numbers of wandering beggars in check.[19] For example the latter would probably have been the fate of the 34 sick and poor people resident in the monastic hospital at Bishopsgate at the time of its dissolution.[20] But, it was not only such poor unfortunates who swelled the ranks of the wanderers. It has been estimated that close to 10,000 clerics, and an even greater number of others who served in religious houses, also, in large part, became homeless and without resources. To give some credence to the latter point, in one nunnery, for example, where there were 16 of the order, there were 8 yeomen, 17 farm workers, and 9 women servants.[21] In London, few welfare establishments survived the Reformation however, in the case of almshouses, although there were not anywhere near enough, the early part of the 17th century was rich in new foundations.[22]

With the Renaissance of Greek ideals there was no revival of the Greek's love of hygiene because it tended to favour developing mental capacities rather than the Platonic notion of harmony and balance. So hygiene conditions remained appalling for centuries, along with morbidity and mortality due largely to devastating infectious diseases which reminded people of the plague.[23] Apart from the disappearance of religious traditions, the wide destruction of the Black Death had left an aftermath, particularly in rural areas, where landlords sought to re-establish the old order and labourers struggled for freedom from their traditional contracts. Neither was totally successful, but, in part, this lack of a common aim led to the emergence of 'a new antagonism between rich and poor'. It also contributed to the exodus of not a few rural labourers to towns to try their hand as artisans, the development of different methods of farming and husbandry, and the evolution of a "wool growing country" of yeoman farmers as enclosure changed the medieval system of the old open field. At the same time, even Protestants not in sympathy with monastic customs admitted that clerics had made better landlords than their successors, under whom 'the pore man that laboreth and toyleth upon it, and is hys slave, is not able to lyve'.[24] Dispossessed tenants, in large numbers, became weavers, fullers and dyers, and even farmers supplemented their labours and income with spinning and weaving.[25]

These secular changes also added to the alarming increase in the numbers of beggars and vagrants. The more enterprising and dishonest of those managed to survive by pilfering, threats, and other crimes, plus the occasional funeral "dole", but the numbers of these were but the tip of the iceberg in terms of the numbers affected by poverty.[26] Many of the honest poor became ill, physically or mentally as well as socially, and no provision was made for their relief as Robert Copland recounts:

I have sene at sondry hospytalles
That many have lyne dead without the walles,
And for lack of socour have died wretchedly,
Unto your foudacyon, I think, contrary,
Much people resort here, and have lodging,
But yet I marvel greatly of one thyng,
That in the night so many lodge without.[27]

Despite the advent of humanist philosophies governments of the day based their ideas on what they saw as good for the "state" rather than for individuals and, at that time, these did not necessarily coincide. The English Government took an active part in the regulation of trade according to the "Mercantile" system. All commercial questions were decided upon the lines of National power according to four major concerns: encouraging shipping so that the realm had many ships and sailors; protecting corn-growers so that the country was independent in terms of a basic supply of food; protecting and developing home industries to provide employment; and amassing and maintaining a large amount of money within the country. This protective, power driven system did not completely give way to free trade until the nineteenth century when Peel repealed the Corn-laws which were its last relics.[28]

Although, in this chapter, a division between social, mental and physical health is employed during the time of the Renaissance no clear-cut difference was made between them. People were much more holistic in their views enmeshing 'body and soul, flesh and spirit, mind and matter' and, indeed, as Porter maintains, bodily condition and the fluctuations between health and sickness interlocked with social ideas about identity, destiny, and moral and spiritual well-being.[29] This mix is reflected in the five Royal hospitals, which collectively provided for socially and occupationally disadvantaged children, adolescents and adults as well as for the poor suffering from physical or mental illness.

Social health

In other parts of Europe, help for the socially deprived was still largely the province of religious institutions. Vincent de Paul (c. 1580-1660) provides us with a model of the sorts of good works that could result from the older tradition coupled with a new humanistic view of mankind. A French priest, de Paul is most famous for his work amongst the poor and sick, which continues today in his name. In his time, little distinction was made between the deprived, whether it be caused by sickness or systems. He set up soup kitchens, homes for the aged, night shelters and workshops for the needy, as well as founding the Lazarists, a Congregation of Mission Priests and the Daughters of Charity, a nursing sisterhood.[30,31]

In England, with the closure of the monasteries, this ceased to be the case. This led to the necessity of establishing different social structures to meet the needs of those who had previously benefited from monastic and church assistance. In the main, such people had been of the poorer class, although the rich, too, could find sanctuary in monasteries when there was no obvious place for them in their world or, sometimes, when they experienced physical or mental illness. However, it was only gradually that the medieval systems of industry and charity were replaced with more humanistic ones. In Elizabethan times, the Statute of Apprentices helped to establish work opportunities and fair wages for labourers, and the Poor Law diminished the numbers of vagrants and provided State relief for the sick, disadvantaged and elderly poor through the Parish system.

It is within social health that most change of an occupational nature is found during this time, to the extent that Bridewell, a Royal Hospital, was established in London. Its purpose was to cater for those young people who were likely to experience occupational deprivation in the future, and to "rehabilitate" those whose occupations were considered sick, immoral or antisocial. The occupational nature of Bridewell is of great interest to this history. In many ways it links social and mental health problems, more that even at present, as well as providing an early example of occupational intervention for personal and community health prior to the establishment of the Poor Law. The stories of both the Poor Law and the history of Bridewell are particularly worthy of telling in the context of social health through occupation.

The Poor Law

In England, the change to a more humanistic view of mankind is evident in the legislation about "beggars". This group consisted of vagabonds and rogues, but also the poor, old, sick and disabled who had no one to look after their needs. During the period of Renaissance the earliest legislation in England concerning beggars occurred. An Act of 1349, during the reign of Edward III, forbad, under pain of imprisonment, the giving of alms to anyone who was able to work. That legislation provides some sort of context for the value given to occupation at that time. Over a period of approximately 150 years this view was extended to not only ensure that all who could work had the opportunity to do so, but also that those who were unable to work because of infirmity received succour in such a way that this also provided occupational opportunities for some people.

The first indication of this change occurred in 1388 when it was provided that beggars "impotent to serve" might be required "to draw them to the towns where they were born" so that, it can be surmised, they may conceivably be in a situation more conducive to help. It was not, however, until the Statute of 1531 that a distinction was clearly made 'between "aged, poor and impotent persons," who, under certain restrictions, are to be allowed to solicit alms, and those "whole and mighty in body and able to labour," who are to suffer punishment'. From that recognition that the State had some responsibility towards such unfortunates the whole system of poor relief was destined to grow.[32] However, the general result of the policy was, unfortunately, that 'the honest poor were punished and sometimes fed; the vagabond was fed and sometimes punished'.[33]

Five years later, the Act of 1536 applied a new principle - it made each parish legally responsible for the relief of its own poor. It required an authorised and systematic collection of voluntary alms, whereby:

> ... *the poor, impotent, lame, feeble, sick, and diseased people, being not able to work, may be provided, holpen, and relieved, so that in no wise they nor not of them be suffered to go openly in begging; And that such as be lusty or having their limbs strong enough to labour may be daily kept in continual labour, whereby every one of them may get their own substance and living with their own hands.*[34]

This was the first step towards the establishment of the Poor Law. Surprisingly, it was enacted before the Act of Dissolution of monasteries upon the Statute Book, although it was in the same year that dissolution of the smaller monasteries occurred. So whilst it can be suggested that the dissolution made a poor law more necessary, it was not a clear case of cause and effect.[35]

Some towns and cities such as Bristol, Exeter, Henley, Lyddington, Totnes, and York did attempt to set the poor to work,. At Thornabie, near York, with a gift of money provided for that purpose, wool, flax, and hemp was delivered for the poor of the parish to make into cloth at market rates.[36]

It was in the Act of 1563, during the reign of Elizabeth I, that the principle of compulsory collection of funds for poor relief was incorporated for the first time, and it was in 1601 that the Poor Law reached the final stage of its development. The Act was aimed at the suppression of begging, the setting to work of adults unable to support themselves and children whose parents were thought unable to maintain them, and at putting poor children into apprenticeships. It also included strategies to obtain, through parochial taxation, materials such as flax, hemp, wool, thread and iron for the provision of work, and money for the relief of the lame, impotent, old, blind and others unable to work.[37] The Poor Law also established parochial responsibility in that churchwardens or overseers were given the authority to decide what was "reasonable" in the way of relief, including the use of the House of Correction for 'those who refused or spoilt work or went abroad begging or lived idly'.[38] The Law recognised that in order to abolish the unhealthy personal and community results of social want, opportunities for occupation must be provided as well as sustenance for those unable to engage in self support and care. This Act was to determine the main features of National policy for the poor until the reforms of Poor Law Commission in 1834.[39] Aschrott summarised it:

> *Poor relief is recognised in principle as a public concern. It is to be administered by individual parishes through overseers, who are appointed and constantly controlled by the justices. The burden of relief is distributed by taxation. In the first instance, however, the nearest kin are made responsible for the maintenance of their relations; and in case a single parish is overburdened, the neighbouring parishes may be called upon to contribute proportionally. The persons to be relieved are divided into three classes: children, able-bodied, and*

infirm. The kind of assistance consists, in the case of children, in apprenticing them till their twenty-first or twenty-fourth year; in the case of the able-bodied, by setting them to work (which they must perform, under penalty for refusal); in the case of the infirm, in maintaining them, with power to place them in poor houses.[40]

This Act was supported by the *Statute of Charitable Uses*, passed around the same time, which had the intent of safeguarding charitable bequests for:

… relief of aged, impotent and poor people, some for maintenance of sick and maimed soldiers and mariners, schools of learning, free schools, and scholars of Universities, … some for education and preferment of orphans, some for or towards relief, stock or maintenance for houses of correction, some for marriages of poor maids, some for supportation, aid and help of young tradesmen, handicraftsmen, and persons decayed, and others for relief or redemption of prisoners or captives.[41]

Such legislation was deemed necessary as bequests did not always get used in the way originally intended, as John Stowe (1525?-1605), a contemporary chronicler, declared: 'the residue left in trust to their executors, I have known some of them hardly (or never) performed'.[42]

The matter of bequests for charitable purposes was not the only legislation to be adulterated by the greedy. Although a system of relief based on work appeared sensible to many of the wealthy farmers in the parishes and freeholders of the county, they petitioned James I, who became King in 1604, to keep down demands on parishes, and avoid some of the trouble of executing the Act of 1601. They proposed that 'if any person shall refuse to be so locked up and worked, he shall be entitled to no relief,' which, it was hoped, would 'prevent persons in distress from wanting relief and be the means of keeping down the poor rate'.[43'44]

In the 17th century, workhouses for the poor were established. An ordinance of 1647 divided the deprived from the depraved by requiring separate workhouses. After that time, this no longer occurred and both idle rogues and the honest, industrious poor were housed and engaged in work in the one place. Some people believe that this resulted in not achieving fully the purpose of either.[45] Certainly the distress caused by the thought of being committed to a workhouse appears to have been so overwhelming that strong feelings of antipathy have filtered down to the present day.

Any philanthropy was encouraged, as the parish system became quite costly for ratepayers. Food, medicine, and, in the last resort, funerals, were provided, as well as reimbursement of medical practitioner's fees. The recipients were commonly housed and cared for by other poor parishioners who were paid to nurse them.[46] An occupational policy was chosen in preference to a pecuniary policy. In terms of socially disadvantaged children and able-bodied adults the development of skills through apprenticeships, or the opportunity to regain self esteem through becoming self supporting must have appeared the obvious choice, instead of simply providing money which is the current, and probably less health giving, policy.

Bridewell Hospital

The modern use of the word "hospital" limits it to places where those with mental or physical sickness attend or stay when they require medical attention. Its earlier use was much broader as the word itself stems from the Latin noun *hospes*, meaning host or guest. In Renaissance times, before the compartmentalising of the sick according to medical interest, it was used for places were the unfortunate of all kinds might be housed and helped. So it was that the five Royal Hospitals of St Thomas, St Bartholomew, Bethlem, Christ's and Bridewell, which emerged during this period, addressed occupational and social needs as well as those of people with physical and mental illness.

Figure 1.5.2: **Bridewell Hospital in 1666, seen from the river. Wood engraving: probably the illustrated London news**
(The Wellcome Library)

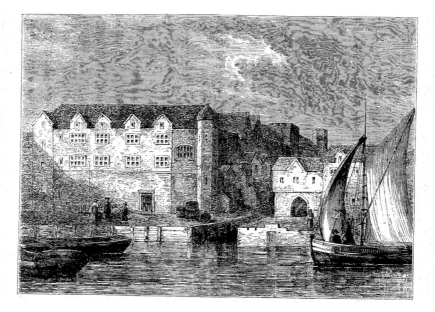

The original Bridewell was a hospital in Blackfriars, London, for the occupationally deprived or depraved. As other hospitals of a similar nature were established, they too became known as Bridewells, which name, in the longer term, became almost synonymous with "prison" or "gaol" because of the latter population. Before becoming a hospital, Bridewell had been a royal palace built close to a holy well once supposed to possess miraculous curative power. The well bore the saint's name, St Bride, as did the parish church, the only one in London dedicated to St Bridget, a Danish saint. Bridewell has 500 years of fascinating Royal history, such as, it was from there in 1528 that Henry VIII first disclosed his troubled conscience about his marriage with Catherine of Aragon. Incidentally, the third act of Shakespeare's *Henry VIII*, which addressed those issues, was correctly sited at Bridewell Palace.[47]

In 1551 Ridley, the Bishop of London, sent a petition to the boy King Edward VI, Henry's son, suggesting that 'a large, wide, empty house of the King's Majesty called Bridewell' might be put to better use. This was followed a year later by a supplication made in the name of the poor to the King to obtain the House of Bridewell. Part of that is quoted below:

> *For Jesu Christ's sake, right dear and most dread Sovereign Lord, we, the humble, miserable, sore, sick, and friendless people, beseech your gracious Majesty to cast upon us your eyes of mercy and compassion, who now, by the mighty operation of the Almighty God, the citizens of London have already so lovingly and tenderly looked upon, that they have not only provided help **for the maladies and diseases and the virtuous education and bringing up of our miserable and poor children, but also have in a readiness most profitable and wholesome occupations for the continuing of us and ours in godly exercises; by reason whereof we shall no more fall into that puddle of idleness which was the mother and leader of us into beggary, and all mischief, but from henceforth shall walk in that fresh field of exercise which is the guider and begetter of all wealth, virtue, and honesty.** But also, most gracious Lord, except we find favour in the eyes of your Majesty, all this their travail, and our hope of deliverence from that wretched and vile state, cannot be attained for lack of harbour and lodging, and therefore, most gracious Sovereign, hear us, speaking in Christ's name and for Christ's Sake, **have compassion on us, that we may lie no longer in the street for lack of harbour, and that our old sore of idleness may no longer vex us, nor grieve the commonweal.** Our suit, most dear Sovereign, is for one of your Grace's houses called Bridewell.*[48]

King Edward's schoolboy writings appear to point to his thinking about social failings in health terms and, as he was young, suggest that some of those ideas must have filtered through others such as his tutors and significant leaders who advised him. 'By the 1540s the many "faults" of the realm which needed to "be amended" could be translated … into "sores" that must "be cured".[49] All kinds of mischief, heresy and error were "pestilent", and the laws against them "medicines"'.[50] One of the most common of the ills to be identified during the period was idleness, and so the petition was granted, the gift being confirmed by charter only ten days before Edward's death.

It is evident from the charter that the citizens entered into a solemn and legal obligation to receive only two classes of inmates into the hospital: poor but virtuous youths to be taught some useful trade; and idle or disorderly vagabonds of any age for punishment and employment in what Edward termed 'the House of Occupations in Bridewell':

> *For as much as We mercifully considering the miserable Estate of the Poor, Fatherless, Lame, Aged, Sick, Sore, and Weak, inflicted with divers and sundry kinds of Diseases; and considering the honest and godly Endeavours of Our most humble and obedient Subjects, the Mayor and Commonality and Citizens of the City of London, who diligently, by all Manner of Means and Ways, study and travel for the good Provision of the aforesaid People, and for every Sort of them,* **... neither when they shall be of riper years shall they be destitute of honest Means and Occupations, wherein to exercise and occupy themselves, ... neither that the sick and diseased Persons, when they shall by their charitable Provisions and Means be recovered and restored unto health, shall then again as slothful and idle persons be permitted to beg and wander around as Vagabonds, to the displeasure of Almighty God and Grief of good People, but that they shall also be forced to practise and exercise themselves in honest and Profitable Sciences and Occupations.**[51]

Queen Mary I confirmed her brother's gift nearly two years later, but debated the issue of totally furnishing the means for housing and occupying its inmates which had been offered in the original charter:

> *Forasmuch as King Edward VI had given his house of Bridewell unto the city partly for the setting of idle and lewd people to work, and partly for the lodging and harbouring of the poor sick and weak and sore people of the city, and of poor wayfaring people repairing to the same; and had for this last purpose given the bedding and furniture of the Savoy to that purpose: therefore, in consideration that very great charges would be required to the fitting of the said house and the buying of tools and bedding, the money was ordered to be gotten up among the rich people of the Companies of London.*[52]

Two governors were appointed to oversee the occupations taught or carried out in Bridewell which included making gloves, coats, silk lace, yarn hose, candlewick, shoes, nails, knives, brushes, and tennis balls. Various methods were employed to inform the general population of Bridewell's existence, purpose and availability so that the relief of the "multitudes", who may, from time to time, be taken into the hospital could "so be preserved from perishing". Towards the end of the 16th century Bridewell employed men to teach trades whom were called Arts Masters, and also commenced a system of apprenticing.[53]

'Bridewell, "the house of labour and occupations" of 1552 where the poor were to be set to work in "sciences profitable to the common weal"' was, according to Paul Slack in the 1994-95 Ford Lectures, certainly unusual and perhaps unique. Its closest parallel was Trinity Hospital in Paris which was set up in 1545 by the French Parlement to provide "religious exercises, education, and work, chiefly for children". It was the Bridewell idea, however, which spawned offspring throughout Europe, and was adopted, in part, in other towns in the English provinces such as Ipswich and Coventry. In Oxford, the Earl of Huntingdon gifted the College of St Mary for multiple purposes: a hospital for the sick poor, for the education of ten poor children, and for setting to work of ten poor adults. Unfortunately, Bridewell was torn between its two functions, and its provincial copies increasingly became houses of correction, physically separated from workhouses by only a dividing wall.[54]

The establishment of other poorhouses somewhat later appears to have affected the numbers in the original Bridewell Hospital. In *A True Report of the Great Costs and Charges of the foure Hospitals in the City of London* the figures for the numbers maintained there in the decade between 1644-1655 are given. See table 1.5.1.

Year	1644	1645	1647	1648	1649	1650	1655
Bridewell	1128	793	575	545	521	725	668

Table 1.5.1: Number of inmates in Bridewell 1644-1655[55]

Bridewell was closely linked to Bethlem Hospital for the mentally ill. Indeed, in 1557 both were placed under the same governorship. As the administrative headquarters, including the Governor's meeting place, were at Bridewell, it is perhaps not surprising that that hospital received the greater share of attention during the early days. An additional element that may have led to that unequal state of affairs was the Lay Governor's comfort with matters occupational and discomfort with matters of the mind and insanity. It is therefore appropriate that this history now proceeds to a discussion of mental health during the period, starting with the story of the establishment of Bethlem.

Mental health

Bethlem Hospital

It was during the early years of the Renaissance that Bethlem Hospital for the insane was established. The Priory of St Mary of Bethlehem, in which it was housed, was founded in Bishopsgate in 1247 by Simon Fitzmary. It is thought to bear that name, perhaps, to celebrate Fitzmary's devotion to Mary the mother of Jesus, whose name he bore, or as the result of a visit during that year by the Bishop of Bethlehem who was on a fund raising tour for his Order.[56]

The Priory was built on the site now occupied by Liverpool Street Station in London, and there, as well as at other later sites, the Asylum was known by the names Bethlem, or Bedlam, both of which were medieval variations of Bethlehem. The earliest surviving reference to it as a hospital was in 1330, which gives Bethlem the distinction of being, probably, the oldest surviving institution of its type. The reference was in a letter from the Archbishop of Canterbury to the clergy, which mentioned the "poor infirm dwelling in the said hospital of Bethlem".[57] Additionally, records of the same year report that the King did not like 'such kind of people to remaine so near his palace' so gave orders for the removal of 'certain lunatics from Charing Cross (London's original lunatic house) to Bethlehem in the Bishopsgate'.[58] In 1403 an inquisition precipitated by misconduct of Peter, the porter at the Priory, further identified its use as a hospital for the insane when it was noted that, resident at that time, there were *"sex viri menti capti"*, that is, six men whose "minds had been seized".[59]

Figure 1.5.3   Bethlem Hospital location in Bishopsgate
(The Bethlem and Maudesley NHS Trust)

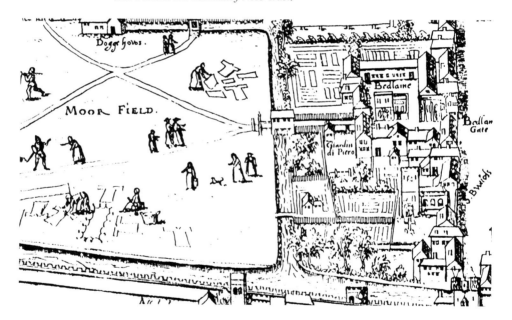

Before this, in 1346, some financial support and governance was supplied by the City of London to what was described as a "miserably poor" establishment, which was the start of a close and ongoing association between City and hospital. However, during the reign of Edward III, in 1375, the hospital was seized by the Crown and the religious order of St Mary of Bethlehem ceased to be involved. However, it was not until the suppression of the Monasteries in 1539 that it came to be known only as Bethlem Hospital and not as a priory.[60,61]

From the late 14th century therefore the City as well as the Crown had an interest in the management of the Hospital's affairs. This entailed some ongoing dispute about which of them had the right to appoint the "Keeper". That was resolved in 1547 when Henry VIII appointed the Mayor and the citizens of London appointed 'masters, keepers and governors' granting them the 'custody order and government of our house and hospital called Bethlem'.[62] This remained the case until 1948 when the National Health Service took over the management.[63]

No mention has been found of the inmates being engaged in occupation. Indeed they were called "prisoners", and their accommodation was sparse and hardly conducive to productive activity. It contained 'below stairs a parlor, a kitchen, two larders, a long entry throughout the house, and twenty-one rooms wherein the poor distracted people lie, and a long anteroom now being contrived to make eight rooms more for poor people to lodge'.[64] Confinement and, probably, brutality were used, particularly after unruly behaviour, which the keepers quelled with the assistance of local shopkeepers. An early inventory records 'six chains of iron with six locks, four pairs of manacles of iron, and two pairs of stocks'.[65]

In 1676 a new baroque Bethlem was built at Moorfield on the site of the ditch outside London's Northern City wall. The first custom-built hospital for the insane in the Country, it was an impressive building, between 550-600 feet long, and somewhat reminiscent of Versailles. The hospital was planned for about 120 patients.[66] It was, however, an unsuitable "dreary" place. Each patient had a bed and clean straw in their individual cells, which were about 8 by 12 feet, with little windows set into the doors which opened onto a long gallery. Those patients not considered dangerous could use the gallery as a day room. Iron grilles in the central area separated the men from the women.[67]

Figure 1.5.4:   Bethlem Hospital at Moorgate
(Bethlem Royal Hospital Archives and Museum)

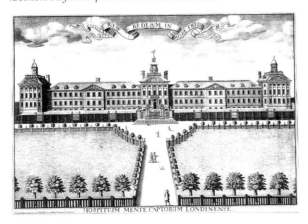

Bethlem, as the only public hospital for the insane, was open to applicants from the whole country and they were examined by a court of governors to ensure their curability. Those considered to be incurable were not admitted. Although in later times a patient was standardly admitted for a year, in Bethlem's early period those who proved difficult to cure sometimes stayed for many years. In 1558, for example, when the earliest known full list of patients was compiled, one of the twenty one patients had been there for 25 years, in contrast to ten others who had been there for less than 10.[68] It was claimed 'that from the Year 1648 to 1703 … there had been in this Hospital 1294 Patients; of which Number had been cured and discharged 890, which is above two Patients in three'.[69]

It is possible that early patients were cared for by a secular brotherhood following the disbanding of the Order of St Mary of Bethlehem. Officially, a physician was appointed from 1634. Attendants, known until the 19th century as "Basketmen", were employed from the 17th century. By that time there was also a matron who was in charge of the female patients and servants. The role was undertaken by the Porter's wife for no additional remuneration. Later the post became one of extreme responsibility, and of interest to this history as the occupations of female patients were listed as one of the matron's duties. This responsibility may well have been instituted some time earlier, as it was held to be important in the general population and was the central mission of Bridewell Hospital with which it was closely associated.

There appears to be a good deal of debate in the literature about whether or not other hospitals existed which cared for the insane. Walsh believes there were and reports that a chaplain, Robert Denton, paid King Edward III forty shillings for a licence to establish a hospital in the parish of Berking Church, London. Berking Church Hospital was for 'poor priests, and for men and women in the said city who suddenly fall into a frenzy and lose their memory, who were to reside there till cured'.[70] He also asserts that at the close of the fourteenth century "mad" people (furiosi custodiantur donec sensum adipiscantur) were admitted to general infirmaries such as the Holy Trinity at Salisbury. In a 1414 petition for the Reformation of hospitals, one reason given was 'to maintain those who had lost their wits and memory (hors de leur sennes et memoire)'.[71] Certainly in other parts of Europe there were asylums, such as at Metz (1100) Elbing, near Danzig (1320) and Valencia (1409).[72]

> *By the fourteenth century non-military brotherhoods, such as the order of the Holy Spirit, were also running infirmaries from Alsace to Poland, while the Order of St John of God appeared in Spain in the sixteenth century, building insane asylums and putting up about 200 hospitals in the New World.*[73]

Apart from the issue of the establishment of hospitals for the insane, there was, at the time, recognition of mental ill health as a medical problem. Many medical authorities believed it was closely associated with the humoural system of physiology. Paracelsus, or Theophratus Bombastus von Hohenheim, (1493-1541) who was born in Salzburg, was not one of those. He chose instead to analyse possible types of psychiatric illnesses in terms of mania, melancholia, mental defectiveness, and changes of character and personality. He advised treatment, which included suggestion and analysis. Another was Thomas Sydenham (1624-1689) who gave accounts of neurological and mental disorders, such as chorea, St Vitus' dance, hysteria, and hypochondria. For those conditions he recommended thoughtful and kindly treatment, whilst prescribing horse riding particularly for depression. Andrew Boarde, a Winchester doctor, also pleaded for the proper care of the mentally ill, whilst quite sensibly advising that acute cases should be prevented from having sharp edged objects.[74]

Sanctorius Sanctorius (1561-1636), a well-known Italian physician who studied at Padua also recommended occupation for mental disorders. In his rules for health, as they are concerned with the affections of the mind, a link with perspiration is made in the tradition of humoural physiology:

Of the Affections of the Mind: Section VII

II. In grief and fear that which is lighter perspires, but what is more ponderous is left behind; in gladness and anger there is a perspiration of both.

IIV. Such as are angry or joyful feel no weariness in travelling, for their bodies easily perspire the gross matter; which happens not when they are troubled with grief or fear.

V. The ponderous part of perspirable matter being more than usually retained in the body, disposes a man to sadness and fear, but the light part disposes him to gladness and anger.

XLVII. They who are sometimes merry, sometimes sad, sometimes angry, sometimes timorous, have a more healthful perspiration than they who continue in one and the same, though that a constantly-good affection.

Perspiration and feelings are linked with occupational nuances, such as in:

VI. Nothing contributes more to freedom of perspiration than satisfaction and consolation of mind.

This brings to mind the likelihood that satisfaction and consolation often result from engagement in meaningful occupation. Other examples of similar links include:

XVII. Melancholy is two ways overcome, either by a free perspiration, or some continual satisfaction of the mind.

XIX. The consolation of the mind, from whatsoever cause it proceeds, opens the passages, and very much promotes perspiration.

XLII. Let those forbear gaming whose thoughts are altogether upon winning; because if they always have good fortune, out of excessive joy, they will hardly sleep in the night, and, in time, will find the want of the exhalation of the concocted perspirable matter.[75]

In this last citation, Sanctorius recognised that feelings could affect health status in a way not possible through medicine, just as feelings engendered by occupations could have far reaching health effects apart from medicine:

> *XII. Anger and hope take away fear, and joy taketh away sadness: for a passion of the mind is overcome, not by medicines, but by some contrary passion; for contraries are under the same genus.*[76]

The first major English tract on depression was Timothy Bright's *A Treatise on Melancholy* (1586).[77] Written by a sufferer, addressed to a sufferer, and urging sympathy and gentleness, the writing of it was surely a form of self-prescribed occupational therapy. Another text, by Timothy Rogers in 1691, *A Disease Concerning Trouble of Mind and the Disease of Melancholy,*[78] similarly, urged kindness rather than severity, and condemned as counter therapeutic the notion that melancholy should be regarded as different from regular somatic disease.[79]

Robert Burton: Occupation as a cause and cure for melancholy

One very famous work of the same genre that requires close attention is that by Robert Burton (1577-1640) on *The Anatomy of Melancholy*. Burton was a clergyman, educated at Christ Church, Oxford. Although not a physician, Burton's work is scholarly, of immense proportions and particularly interesting to this history in that it discusses occupation as both a cause of and a cure for what would now be termed depression. The substantial extracts provided below reflect his thinking on both issues, and must be one of the clearest and most lengthy documents of the Renaissance, and, indeed, of any time prior to the genesis of the profession itself, about using occupation in the treatment of a particular illness. In some ways, many of his ideas about remediation are not dissimilar to those held early in occupational therapy's twentieth century history. His views on occupational causes of melancholy are also included at length. As modern medicine tends to take more seriously those health professions that are clearly shown to have an integral role in illness or death, rather than enabling health and well-being, it can be suggested that failure to consider the relationship between occupation and health from a negative as well as positive perspective could have been a major deterrent to a more central role for the profession in modern medicine. The frontispiece of the text is shown as figure 1.5.5.

Figure 1.5.5 **Frontispiece of**
The Anatomy
of Melancholy
(British Library)

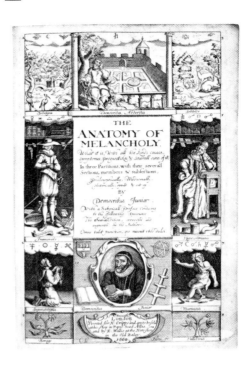

In his discussion about the causes of melancholy Burton included a strong view about what he terms "immoderate exercise":

Nothing so good, but that it may be abused: Nothing better then Exercise (if opportunely used) for the preservation of the Body: Nothing so bad, if it be unseasonable, violent, or overmuch. Fernelius out of Galen, Path. lib. 1. c. 16. saith, "That much exercise and weariness consumes the spirits and substance, refrigerates the body; and such humors which Nature would have otherwise concocted and expelled, it stirs up, and makes them rage: which being so inraged, diversly affect, and trouble the body and minde"… Not without good reason then, doth Salust Salvianus, l. 2. c. 1. and Leonartus Facchinus in 9 Rhasis. Mercurialis, Arculanus, and many others, set down immoderate exercise, as a most forcible cause of melancholy.[80]

Then, at much greater length, he put his case about, "idleness" and lack of occupation being a major cause:

Opposite to Exercise, is Idleness (the badg of gentry) or want of Exercise, the bane of body and minde, the nurse of naughtiness, stepmother of discipline, the chief author of all mischief, one of the seven deadly sins, and a sole cause of this and many other maladies, the devils cushion, as Gaulter calls it, his pillow and chief reposal. For the minde can never rest, but still meditates on one thing or other, except it be occupied about some honest business, of his own accord it rusheth into melancholy. As too much and violent exercise offends on the one side, so doth an idle life on the other, (saith Crato) it fills the body full of flegm, gross humors, and all maner of obstructions, rheumes, catars, etc. Rhasis, cont. li. 1. tract. 9. accounts of it as the greatest cause of melancholy. I have often seen (saith he) that idleness begets this humor more than anything else. Montaltus, c. 1. seconds him out of his experience. They that are idle are far more subject to melancholy, then such as are conversant or imployed about any office or business. Plutarch reckons up idleness for a sole cause of a sickness of the soul: There are they (saith he) troubled in minde, that have no other cause but this. Homer, Iliad. 1. brings in Achilles eating of his own heart in his Idleness, because he might not fight. Mercurialis, consil. 86. for a melancholy young man urgeth it is a chief cause; why was he melancholy - because he was idle. Nothing begets it sooner, encreaseth and continueth it oftner then idleness. A disease familiar to all idle persons, an inseparable companion to such as live at ease. Pingui otio defidios agentes, a life out of action, and have no calling or ordinary imployment to busie themselves about, that have small occasions; and though they have, such is their laziness, dullness; that they will not compose themselves to do ought, they cannot abide work, though it be necessary, easie, as to dress themselves, write a Letter, or the like; yet as he that is benummed with cold, sits still shaking, that might relieve himself with a little exercise or stirring, do they complain, but will not use the facile and ready means to do themselves good; and so are still tormented with melancholy. Especially if they have been formerly brought up to business, or to keep much company, and upon a sudden comes to lead a sendentary life, it crucifies their souls, and seazeth on them in an instance; for whilst they are any ways imployed, in action discourse, about any business, sport or recreation, or in company to their liking, they are very well; but if alone or idle, tormented instantly again; one days solitariness, one hours sometimes, doth them more harm, then a weeks physick, labor and company do good. Melancholy seazeth on them forthwith being alone, and is such a torture, that as wise Seneca well saith, malo mihi male quam molliter esse, I had rather be sick than idle. This idleness is either of body or minde. That of body is nothing but a kinde of benumming laziness, intermitting exercise, which if we may believe Fernelius, causeth crudities, obstructions, excremental humors, quencheth the natural heat, dulls the spirits, and makes them unapt to do anything whatsoever.[81]

The number of references which Burton draws upon leads the reader to understand that he was not alone in his view that lack of worthwhile occupation was a major cause of depressive illness, even if it was a self chosen lack as in the case of the "idle rich". He continued with more argument of a similar nature, which is included here so that the reader becomes aware, to some extent, of the depth of his conviction. In this next extract Burton clearly differentiates against recreational occupations without purpose, in favour of vocational occupations, linking the former with idleness and resultant depression. Whilst expressing his ideas in a different way to present day occupational therapists he obviously believed, as they do, that meaning and purpose are necessary for both mental and physical health. But in his opinion, lack of occupation that results from "idleness of the mind" results in a much worse type of disorder than melancholy from physical deprivation which can also result from idleness:

Idleness of the minde, is much worse then this of the body; wit without employment, is a disease, Aerugo animi, rubigo ingenii: the rust of the soul, a plague, a hell it self, Maximum animi nocumentum, Galen calls it. As in a standing pool, worms and filthy creepers increase, (vitium cappiunt ni moveantur aquae, the water it self putrifies, and air likewise, if it be not continually stirred by the wind) so do evil and corrupt thought in an idle person, the soul is contaminated. In a common-wealth, where is no publike enemy, there is likely civil wars, and they rage upon themselves: this body of ours, when it is idle, and knows not how to bestowe itself, macerates and vexeth it self with cares, griefs, false-fears, discontents, and suspicions; it tortures and preys upon its own bowels, and is never at rest. Thus much I dare boldly say, He or she that is idle, be they of what condition they will, never so rich, so well allied, fortunate, happy, let them have all things in abundance, and felicity, that heart can wish and desire, all contentment, so long as he or she, or they are idle, they shall never be pleased, never well in body and minde, but weary still, sickly still, vexed still, loathing still, weeping, sighing, grieving, suspecting, offended with the world, with every object, wishing theselves gone or dead, or else carried away with some foolish phantasie or other. And this is the true cause that so many great men, Ladies and Gentlewomen, labor of this disease in Countrey and City; for idleness is an appendix to nobility, they count it a disgrace to work, and spend all their days in sports, recreations and pastimes, and will therefore take no pains; be of no vocation; They feed liberally, fare well, want exercise, action, employment, (for to work, I say, they may not abide) and company to their desires, and thence their bodies become full of gross humors, wind, crudities, their mindes disquieted, dull, heavy, etc. care, jealousie, fear of some diseases, sullen fits, weeping fits seize too familiarly on them.[82]

When you shall hear and see many discontented persons, in all places where you come, so many several grievances, unnecessary complaints, fear, suspitions, the best means to redress it, is to set them to work, so to busie their mindes; for the truth is, they are idle. Well may they build up castles in the air for a time, and sooth up themselves with phantastical and pleasant humors, but in the end they will prove as bitter as gall, they shall be still I say discontent, suspicious, fearful, jealous, sad, fretting and vexing of themselves; so long as they be idle, it is impossible to please them. Otio qui nescit uti, plus habet negotii quam qui negotium in negotio, as that Agellius could observe: he that knows not how to spend his time, hath more business, care, grief, anguish of minde, then he that is most busie in the midst of his business. Otiosus animus nescit quid volet: An idle person (as he follows it) knows not when he is well, what he would have, or whither he would go, Quum illuc ventum est, illinc lubet, he is tired out with everything, displeased with all, weary of his life.[83]

Burton added solitariness, which he saw as one of the probable consequences of idleness to his list of causes of depression 'cozen german to Idleness, and a concomitant cause, which goes hand in hand with it, is nimia solitudo, too much solitariness, by the testimony of all Physicians, Cause and Symptom both'.[84] In his discussion of that, he provides an example of how Mercurialis remonstrated with his patients, presumably to increase their awareness of the cause and potential remedy of their disorder. The remonstration illustrates a "victim blaming" technique:

> *So that which Mercurialis consil. 11. sometimes expostulated with his melancholy patient, may be justly applyed to every solitary and idle person in particular. Natura de te videtur conqueri posse. etc. Nature may justly complain of thee, that whereas she gave thee a good wholesome temperature, a sound body, and God hath given thee so divine and excellent a Soul, so many good parts, and profitable gifts, thou hast not only contemned and rejected, but hath corrupted them, polluted them, overthrown their temperature, and perverted those gifts with riot, idleness, solitariness, and many other wayes, thou arte a traitour to God and Nature, an enemy to thyself and to the world. Perditio tua ex te; thou hast lost thyself wilfully, cast away thy self, thou thy self art the efficient cause of thine own misery, by not resisting such vaine cogitations, but giving way unto them.*[85]

Yet another of the multiple possible causes of melancholy which Burton elaborates upon is sleep. As sleep is part of the activity / rest cycle of a present day occupational perspective of health it is useful to appreciate that it was also considered some 500 years ago. It was, of course, one of the six non-naturals upon which the humoural system of health was based:

> *What I have formerly said of exercise, I may now repeat of Sleep. Nothing better than moderate sleep, nothing worse than it, if it be in extremes, or unseasonably use. It is a received opinion, that a melancholy man cannot sleep overmuch: ... yet in some cases sleep may do more harm then good in that flegmatick, swinish, cold and sluggish melancholy, ... It duls the Spirits, if overmuch, and senses, fils the head ful of gross humors, causeth distillations, rheumes, great store of excrements in the brain, and all other parts.*[86]

Taking a more social view of the possible causes of melancholy, Burton enlarged upon some people's engagement in particular types of occupation, which he claimed were at fault.

> *It is a wonder to see, how many poor, distressed, miserable wretches, one shall meet almost in every path and street, begging for an almes, that have been well descended, and sometimes in flourishing estate, now ragged, tattered, and ready to be starved, lingring out a painful life, in discontent and grief of body and minde, and all through immoderate lust, gaming, pleasure and riot. Tis the common end of all sensual Epicures and brutish prodigals, that they are stupified and carried away headlong with their several pleasures and lusts. Cebes in his table, S. Ambrose in his second book of Abel and Cain, and amongst the rest Lucian in his tract de Mercede conductis, hath excellent well deciphered such mens proceedings in his picture of Opulentia ...*[87]

> *The ordinary rocks upon which such men do impinge and precipitate themselves, are Cardes, Dice, Hawkes, and Hounds, ...*

Some men are consumed by mad, phantastical buildings, by making Galleries, Cloisters, Tarraces, Walkes, Orchards, Gardens, Pooles, Rillets, Bowers, and such like places of pleasure …

Others, I say, are overthrown by those mad sports of Hawking and hunting; honest recreations, and fit for some great men, but not for every base inferior person … They persecute beasts so long, till in the end they themselves degenerate into beast …. so do they devour themselves and their patrimonies, in such idle and unnecessary disports, neglecting in the mean time their more necessary business, and to follow their vocations. Over-mad too sometimes are our great men in delighting and doting too much on it. When they drive poor husbandmen from their village, as Sarisburiensis objects, polycrat. l. 1. c. 4. fling down countrey Farmes, and whole Townes, to make Parkes, and Forests, starving men to feed beasts, and punishing in the mean time such a man that shall molest their game, more severely then him what is otherwise a common hacker, or a notorious thief. But great men are some wayes to be excused, the meaner sort have no evasion why they should not be counted mad.[88]

Apart from "Wine and Women", other potential causes which Burton identified were those frequently associated with the pursuit of occupations for perceived egotistical rewards such as "self-love", "vain glory", and "pride". Taking a different tack, he then went on to consider melancholy resulting from scholarly occupations, such as the love of learning or overmuch study:

Fernelius lib. 1. cap. 18. puts Study, contemplation, and continual meditation, as an especial cause of madness: … Marcilius Ficinus de sanit. tuenda. lib. 1. cap. 7. puts Melancholy amongst one of those five principle plagues of students, 'tis a common Maul unto them all, and almost in some measure an inseparable companion. … For (as Machiavel holds) Study weakens their bodies, dulls the spirits, abates their strength and courage; … The Turks abdicated Cornutus the next heir, from the Empire, because he was so much given to his book: and 'tis the common Tenent of the world, that Learning duls and diminisheth the spirits, and so per consequens produceth melancholy.

Two main reasons may be given of it, why Students should be more subject to this malady than others.

• The one is, they live a sedentary solitary life, fibi and musis, free from bodily exercise, and those ordinary disports which other men use …

• but the common cause is overmuch study; too much learning (as Feltus told Paul) hath made thee mad.[89]

Burton points to several aspects of "overmuch study", such as the effects of contemplation, and a scholar's failure to care for the tools of his occupation: that is his intellectual capacities. Of that he wrote:

… other men look to their Tools, a Painter will wash his Pencils, a Smith will look to his Hammer, Anvil, Forge: an Husbandman will mend his Plough-Irons, and grinde his Hatchett if it be dull; a Faulkner or Huntsman will have an especial care of his Hawks, Hounds, Horses, Dogs &c. A Musician will string

and unstring his Lute, &c. onely Scholars neglect that instrument, their brain and spirits (I mean) which they daily use, and by which they range over all the world.[90]

Of the dangers of excessive contemplation, Burton recorded that it:

… dries the brain and extinguisheth natural heat; for whilst the spirits are intent to meditation above in the head, the stomack and liver are left destitute, and thence come black blood and crudities by defect of concoction, and for want of exercise, the superfluous vapours cannot exhale, … Students are commonly troubled with Gouts, Cattarrhes, Rhumes, Cacexia, Bradiopepsia, bad Eyes, Stone and Collick, Crudities, Oppilations, Vertigo, Windes, Consumptions, and all such diseases as come by overmuch sitting; they are most part lean, dry, ill coloured, spend their fortunes, lose their wits, and many times their lives, and all through immoderate pains and extraordinary studies,' and all 'to gain knowledge for which, after all their pains in their worlds esteem they are accounted ridiculous and silly Fools, Idiots, Asses, and (as oft they are) rejected, contemned, derided, doting and mad. [91]

Now because they are commonly subject to such hazards, and inconveniences, as dotage, madness, simplicity, &c. 10. Voschius would have good Scholars to be highly rewarded, and had in some extraordinary respect above other men, to have greater priviledges than the rest, that adventure themselves and abbreviate their lives for the publike good. But our Patrons of Learning are so far now adays, from respecting the Muses, and giving that honor to scholars, or reward which they deserve … that their familiar attendants are

"Grief, labor, care, pale sickness, miseries,

Fear filthy-poverty, hunger that cries,

Terrible monsters to be seen with eyes" (Virg. 6 Aen.)

If there were nothing else to trouble them, the conceit of this alone were enough to make them all melancholy.[92]

In arguing that because all who try to do studious work are not necessarily wise or competent scholars despite training, and indeed, 'it is not so easily performed to finde out a learned man', Burton demonstrated his appreciation that individuals need to find meaning in their occupation. He implied that individuals might not be fitted for the tasks associated with scholarship because of lack of innate capacity. It may be a reason for some of this group's proneness to sickness and melancholy. On the other hand, he still questioned why, even if people were 'studious, industrious, of ripe wits, and perhaps good capacities, then how many diseases of body and minde must they encounter?' This led to his conclusion that there was 'no labor in the world like unto study' for its potential detriment to health.[93]

Burton also considered aspects of loss of liberty and subsequent types of deprivation as a cause of depression. Interestingly he refers to Robert, Duke of Normandy, mentioned in the previous chapter, as a case in point. Following Robert's imprisonment by his younger brother Henry I of England, 'saith

Matthew Paris (13th century chronicler to the monastery of St Albans): from that day forward (he) pined away with grief.' Burton wrote:

> To this Catalogue of causes, I may well annex loss of liberty, servitude, or imprisonment, which to some persons is as great a torture as any of the rest. Though they have all things convenient, sumptuous houses to their use, fair walkes and gardens, delicious bowers, galleries, good fear and diet, & all things correspondent: yet they are not content, because they are confined may not come and go at their pleasure … As it is in meates so it is in all other things, places, societies, sports; let them be never so pleasant, commodius, wholesome, so good; yet omnium reru est satietas, there is a loathing satiety of all things.

Basically, Burton's argument was that however good a situation may seem from the outside, people are never content with their lot if they do not have choice, change, and new challenges. He reflected on this not only with regard to noble or political prisoners, to which the paragraph above alludes, but also to men working in mines or condemned to the "gallies", and women in harems, or subject to the jealous needs of their husbands. 'Now it be death it self, another Hell, to be glutted with one kind of sport, dieted with one dish, tied to one place … worse than death is bondage.'[94]

Turning from cause to cure, Burton considered "occupational" remedies or "therapy" for melancholy, and wrote extensively about it. For example in a section titled *Exercise rectified of Body and minde* he began by stating:

> To that great inconvenience, which comes on the one side by immoderate and unseasonable exercise, too much solitariness and idleness on the other, must be opposed as an antidote, a moderate and reasonable use of it, and that both of body and minde, as a moste material circumstance, much conducing to this cure, and to the general preservation of our health.[95]

That statement points to the central tenet of Burton's whole epistle about depression, that moderation is primarily important and that a balanced mix in all areas of endeavour is essential to health and the prevention of illness, and now it seems it was his view, that remained the case with regard to cure.

Apart from that foresight, Burton obviously saw occupation and activity as a general rule of the natural world as he observed that:

> The heavens themselves run continually around, the Sun riseth and sets, the Moon increaseth and decreaseth, Stars and Planets keep their constant motions, the aire is still tossed with the winds, the waters eb and flow to their conservation no doubt, to teach us that we should ever be in action.[96]

He reinforced his argument with reference to many authorities who had similar points of view, and to flourishing Nations, which developed policy along these lines. Of interest in itself is the number of references, which point to a very widely held understanding, at that time and earlier, of the need for occupation as part on ongoing mental, physical, spiritual and social health. While this is not immediately apparent in most medical texts, it does equate well with the spiritual regimes discussed in the last chapter and with the era of Renaissance and the growth of humanistic beliefs. Some of those he mentioned, like Seneca or Xenophon, expressed the notion that any activity was better than none at all, whether or not it had purpose, although, of course, that was of most benefit. Additionally, an implication was made that 'our (English) Divines, Physicians, and Politians' exhorted those who foreswore occupation as beneath them to mend their ways by 'so much (serious) labour'.[97]

For depression particularly he prescribed:

> ... there can be no better cure then continuali business, as Rhasis holds, to have some employment or other, which may set their minde at work, and distract their cogitations. Riches may not easily be had without labour and industry, nor learning without study, neither can health be preserved without bodily exercise ...[98]

although, like most other authorites he argued that the activity should be moderate. The reason for such confidence in the effectiveness of occupations was, in accordance with humoural theory, that they added 'strength to the whole body', and that by:

> ... increasing naturall heat, by means of which, the nutriment is well concocted in the stomacke, liver and veines, few or no crudities left, is happily distributed over all the body. Besides it expells excrements by sweat, and other insensiblle vapours; in so much, that Galen prefers Exercise before all Physicke, Rectification of diet, or any regiment in what kinde soever; 'tis Natures Physician.[99]

The actual occupations which Burton and his authorities recommended, often to the level of 'a beginning sweat', were extensive and inclusive of many of those seen as responsible for the melancholy state, presumably, of others. The key to the choice of therapeutic occupations was that they were antidotal, moderate, and balanced, as well as having interest, choice, change, and purpose.

> This which I aim at, is for such as are fracti animis, troubled in mind, to ease them, over toiled on the one part, to refresh, over idle on the other, to keep themselves busied. And to this purpose, as any labour or imployment will serve to the one, any honest recreation will conduce to the other, so that it be moderate and sparing, as the use of meat and drink, not to spend all their life in gaming, playing and pastimes, as too many gentlemen do; but to revive our bodies and recreate our souls with honest sports: of which there be divers sorts, and peculiar to several callings, ages, sexes, conditions, ... (seasons,) ... some gentle, some more violent, some for the mind alone, some for the body and mind.[100]

Of Burton's suggestions for therapeutic 'labours, exercises and recreations', 'some properly belong to the body, some to the mind, some (are) more easy, some hard, some with delight, some without, some within doors, some naturall, some artificiall'.[101] The following list includes many but not all of those identified by Burton, and certainly is not inclusive of the detail:

1. Wholesome business, as to dig long in his garden, to hold the plough and the like
2. Frequent and violent labour and exercises, as sawing every day
3. To play at ball, be it with hand or racket, in Tennis courts or otherwise

4. 'The ordinary sports which are used abroad, (such as) Hawking, Hunting, ... because they recreate body and minde'. Some call them 'the best exercise that is, by which alone many have been freed from all ferall diseases'.

5. Fowling, and fishing, and *'many other sports and recreation ... much in use, as Ringing, bowling, shooting ... Keel-pings, tronks, coits, pitching bars, hurling, wrestling, leaping, running, fencing, mustring, swimming, wasters, foiles, football, baloon, quintan &c. and many such ... common recreations of the country folks. Riding of great horses, running at rings, tilts and turnaments, horseraces, wilde-goose chases ... '*

6. Visits and holidays such as *'a merry journey now and then with some good companions, to visit friends, see Cities, Castles, Towns ... To walk among Orchards, Gardens, Bowers, Mounts and Arbours, artificiall wildernesses, green thickets, Arches, Groves, Lawns, Rivulets, Fountains and such like pleasant places.'* 'To take a boat in a pleasant evening, and with musick to row upon the waters.' To watch combats or to read about them or about 'feasts, triumphs, interviews, nuptials, tilts, turnaments, combats and monochamies.'

7. Playing with domestic animals. Ordinary recreations of winter such as 'Cardes, Tables and Dice, Shovelboard, Chess play, the Philosophers game, small trunks, shuttle-cock, balliards, musick, masks, singing, dancing,' etc.

8. Study. *'Among those exercises, or recreations of the minde within doors, there is none so general, so aptly to be applyed to all sorts of men, so fit and proper to expell idleness and melancholy ... provided always that his malady proceed not from overmuch study.'*

9. *For women, instead of laborious studies they have curious needleworks, Cut-works, spinning, bone-lace, and many pretty devices of their own making, to adorn their houses, Cushions, Carpets, Chairs, Stools, confections, conserves, distillations, ... houshould offices, &c. neat gardens, full of exotick, versicolour, diversly varied, sweet-smelling flowers and plants ... curious to preserve and keep, proud to possess.*

10. 'Strong drink, mirth, musick, and merry company.'[102]

Burton explained the choice of occupation in more detail. For example, included here are the circumstances in which chess was useful as a cure for melancholy, and when it was not:

> *Chess-play, is a good and witty exercise of the minde, for some kinde of men, and fit for such melancholy, Rhasis holds, as are idle, and have extravagant impertinent thoughts, or troubled with cares; nothing better to distract their mind, and alter their meditations. ... but if it proceed from over much study, in such a case it may do more harm then good; it is a game too troublesome for some mens braines, too full of anxiety, all out as bad as study; besides it is a testy cholerick game, and very offensive to him who looseth the Mate.*[103]

Burton even advocates occupation as a cure for love-melancholy, citing Avicenna, Savanarola, Iason Pratensis, Laurentius, Arnoldus, Valleriola, Montaltus, Hildesheim, and Langius in this regard. The first rule to be observed 'in this stubborn and unbridled passion', he said, was exercise and diet, prescribing 'labour, slender and sparing diet, with continual business,' as 'the best and most ordinary means to prevent it':

For if thou do'st not ply thy book,
By candle-light to study bent.
Imploy'd about some honest thing,
Envy or Love shall thee torment.
No better physick then to be alwaies occupied, seriosly intent.[104]

Parish and private care

In Europe, Michel Foucault contends, mass confinement of the mentally ill occurred.[105] Confinement was often in religious institutions. Tsarist policy, in Russia, provides a case in point, as those of the nobility considered to be mentally incapacitated in any way were entered into monastic life in order to avert potential threats to the crown and government.[106] In Britain, the situation was different, and although a small number were locked up, as in earlier times it was not general policy to routinely constrain the mentally disturbed within institutions and no state asylums were built apart from Bethlem. Many were incarcerated with other disadvantaged people in gaols or almshouses, and one can imagine that many were expected, or perhaps forced, to engage in some forms of occupations appropriate to the district, family or social situation. Some almshouses forbad the admission of the insane. Clay, for example, reports:

> *A regulation concerning an endowed bed in St John's, Coventry (1444)*
> *declared that a candidate must be "not mad, quarrelsome, leprous, infected." At*
> *Ewelme "no wood man" (crazy person) must be received; and an inmate*
> *becoming "madd, or woode," was to be removed from the Croydon almshouse.*[107]

The period, though, can be said to be characterised by diverse *ad hoc,* local arrangements. Social regulation and welfare initiatives were devolved to shires and parishes, with management, in the main, remaining under the watchful eyes of family, community or appointed guardians, like clergy or doctors. Most people with mental disorder, therefore, were maintained in their own locality with people whom they knew.[108]

In Scotland, similar rules applied. In a fourteenth century statute, Robert I, put people with mental disorder in the charge of the nearest male relatives on the father's side of the family. He made differentiation between those, who he described as "fatuous", and the "furious" (the manic) who could be fettered but only according to the direct authority of the crown. In the 17th century "the better sort of mad people" were committed to the care and training of "chirurgeons", and others, less fortunate to the "scourge" or lash.[109]

There was minimal government legislation regarding the management of insanity. What legislation there was had a long history such as trusteeships established in the Middle Ages for idiots or lunatics of all classes with regard to legal matters. The Court of Wards, and later the Chancellory, handling these tended to appoint responsible and respected people as trustees. They also devised practical, rather than medical tests, to assess competence and mental capacity to manage what today we would describe as activities of daily living. In some ways the tests were not dissimilar to those used by occupational therapists and others in present times to quickly evaluate orientation, such as asking the subject to give his or her name, to recognise familiar people, to count out loud or to add up a sum of money.[110] It was on the basis of such evaluations that future plans were based.

The practice of using private houses as places to board and care for lunatics was well established during this period although it developed into a substantial trade in the eighteenth century, and will be discussed in more detail in a later chapter. In the same way that most other private, profit making institutions with social benefits, such as schools, were small and informal family businesses, so too were private asylums. Knowledge of their fairly wide spread use comes from glimpses in the literature. Porter, in *Mind-Forg'd Manacles*, provides a number of examples:

"When George Trosse went out of his mind in mid-century, he was boarded in Glastonbury with a family experienced in handling the mad." At about the same time the Revd John Ashbourne, a high Anglican, was keeping lunatics in Suffolk; in 1661 he was slain by one of his charges, thus becoming an early psychiatric martyr. Contemporaneously, Thomas Willis was casually referring to a lunatic being placed "in a house convenient for the business", presumably a reference to a private madhouse. About then, John Newton of Clerkenwell Green was keeping a house for lunatics "in an excellent air, nere the City", so surviving advertisements assure us.[111]

Owners or keepers seldom kept written records. Sometimes short-lived, other family "madhouses" passed from generation to generation. A few were maintained by physicians, two of which were associated with Bethlem Hospital, such as Dr Allen, who owned a private asylum at Finsbury and Dr Helkiah Crooke, of somewhat doubtful reputation, who used his home for private patients.[112]

Humanism and the advent of psychology

It appears appropriate, under the major heading of mental health, that the early beginnings of psychology are recognised. People at this time did not describe themselves as psychologists but rather as philosophers, influenced, no doubt, by the humanist ideas that flourished. Ludovicus Vives (1492-1540), a contemporary of Erasmus, was one such. A Spanish humanist, who taught at Louvain and Oxford, Vives was concerned for people with social and medical problems and, with what would now be called a psychological approach, recommended benign treatment for the mentally ill. He advocated problem-solving schemes to prevent difficulties, and rehabilitation to follow any that ensued. Vives was particularly interested in child psychology, advising that education and future vocations should be according to the child's interests and attitudes.[113]

One of the most respected and influential of the new age philosopher-psychologists was John Locke(Figure 1.5.6). Locke (1632-1704) was an English philosopher educated at Westminster and Oxford, where he later held various academic posts. He was also a physician (untrained) and in that capacity, and as secretary, he took up residence with the first Earl of Shaftsbury. Following suspected complicity in Shaftesbury's plots, he went to live in Holland, but returned to take up posts as Commissioner of Appeals and member of the Council of Trade during William III's reign. He greatly influenced modern concepts of liberal democracy in his works, such as *Of Government* (1690). In this he proposed that it was the function of those in power to preside over the exchange of "natural" for "civil" rights.[114] Locke also wrote *On Education, Religious Liberty and Tolerance* in which, Macdonald reports, he considered that children should acquire more than knowledge during their education. He advised a broad curriculum which demonstrated an understanding of the breadth of human occupational capacities, and the need to enable children to learn to balance their own particular talents. Indeed, well ahead of his time, he recommended the inclusion of artistic, cultural, domestic and handiwork subjects, and physical exercise, whilst children were assisted to develop 'satisfactory characters, and good judgments, habits and manners'.[115]

Figure 1.5.6: **John Locke by Lecoeur, 1800, after J.M.Rysbrack(?)**
(The Wellcome Library)

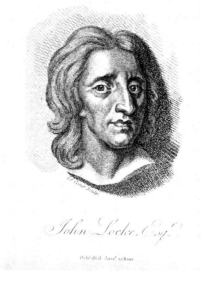

In his greatest work, *An Essay Concerning Humane Understanding* (1690), which reveals him as a pioneer empiricist,[116] he makes statements such as 'Experience must teach me what Reason cannot'.[117] That led John Stuart Mill to describe him as the 'unquestioned founder of the analytical philosophy of mind'.[118] Some idea of the breadth of Locke's subject matter is apparent in the first page of the book's contents, shown in figure 1.5.7.

Figure 1.5.7:
Contents page of
Locke's *An Essay*
concerning
Humaneeeee
Understanding.

(British Library)

THE
CONTENTS.

BOOK I.

Of Innate Notions.

CHAP.
1. Introduction.
2. No innate speculative Principles.
3. No innate practical Principles.
4. Other Proofs against innate Principles.

BOOK II.

Of Ideas.

CHAP.
1. Of Ideas in general.
2. Of simple Ideas.
3. Of Ideas of one Sense.
4. Of Solidity.
5. Of simple Ideas of more than one Sense.
6. Of simple Ideas of Reflexion.
7. Of simple Ideas both of Sensation and Reflexion.
8. Other Considerations concerning simple Ideas.
9. Of Perception.
10. Of Retention.
11. Of Discerning.
12. Of complex Ideas.
13. Of Space, and its simple Modes.
14. Of Duration.
15. Of Extension and Duration considered together.
16. Of Number.

17. Of Infinity.
18. Of other simple Modes.
19. Of the Modes of Thinking.
20. Of the Modes of Pleasure and Pain.
21. Of Power.
22. Of mixed Modes.
23. Of the complex Ideas of Substances.
24. Of the collective Ideas of Substances.
25. Of Relation.
26. Of Cause and Effect, and other Relations.
27. Of other Relations.
28. Of clear and distinct, obscure and confused Ideas.
29. Of real and phantastical Ideas.
30. Of adequate and inadequate Ideas.
31. Of true and false Ideas.

BOOK III.

Of Words.

CHAP.
1. Of Words and Language in general.
2. Of the Signification of Words.
3. Of general Terms.
4. Of the Names of simple Ideas.
5. Of the Names of mixed Modes and Relations.
6. Of the Names of Substances:
7. Of abstract and concrete Terms.
8. Of the Imperfection of Words.
9. Of the Abuse of Words.
10. Of the Remedies of the foregoing Imperfections and Abuses.

Aaa 2   BOOK

Locke obviously studied his subject in terms of day to day life, making rare but commonsense recommendations to do with people accepting themselves as they are, making the most of their talents and skills, and not hankering after what is out of reach and impossible to attain. He advised:

… it will become us, as rational Creatures, to employ our Faculties about what they are most adapted to, and follow the direction of Nature, where it seems to point us out the way. For 'tis rational to conclude, that our proper Imployment lies in those Enquiries, and in that sort of Knowledge, which is most suited to our natural Capacities, and carries in it our greatest interest.[119]

Men have Reason to be well satisfied with what God hath thought fit for them since he has given them ... whatsoever is necessary for the Conveniences of Life, and Information of Vertue; and has put within the reach of their Discovery the Provisions, that may support, or sweeten, this Life, and the Way that leads to a better ...

Men may find Matter sufficient to Busie their Heads, and employ their Hands with variety, Delight, and Satisfaction; if they will not boldly quarrel with their own Constitution, and throw away the Blessings their Hands are fill'd with, because they are not big enough to grasp every thing. We shall not have much Reason to complain of the narrowness of our Minds, if we will but employ them about what may be of use to us; for of that they are very capable: And it will be unpardonable, as well as Childish peevishness, if we undervalue the Advantages of our Knowledge, and neglect to improve it to the ends for which it was given us, because there are some Things that are set out of the reach of it ...

If we will disbelieve everything, because we cannot certainly know all things; we shall do much-what as wisely as he, who would not use his Legs, but sit still and perish, because he had no Wings to fly.[120]

In trying to tease out the issues of human understanding, Locke links thought and action in some ways similar to late 19th, early 20th century pragmatists such as William James, who was influential in the ideas of the modern occupational therapy profession at the time of its development in the United States of America. Additionally, a recurring theme throughout the text is the way he drew people back to the practical and the possible:

Our Business here is not to know all things, but those which concern our Conduct. If we can find out those Measures, whereby a rational Creature put in that State, which Man is in, in this World, may, and ought to govern his Opinions and Actions depending thereon, we need not be troubled, that some things scape our Knowledge.[121]

Locke, made a plea for what he considered to be the right approach for the acquisition of knowledge and "scientific" understanding which would eventually benefit humankind. He argued:

We are able, I imagine, to reach very little general Knowledge concerning the Species of Bodies, (not, human bodies, but what would later be termed "matter") and their several Properties, Experiments and Historical Observations, we may have, from which we may draw Advantages of Ease and Health, and thereby increase our stock of Conveniences for this Life; but beyond this our Talents reach not, our Faculties cannot attain.[122]

He goes on to say:

I would not therefore be thought to dis-esteem, or dissuade the Study of Nature. I readily agree the Contemplation of his Works gives us occasion to admire, revere, and glorifie their Author: and if rightly directed, may be of greater benefit to Mankind, than the Monuments of exemplary Charity, that have at so great Charge been raised, by the Founders of Hospitals and Alms-houses. He that first invented Printing; discovered the Use of the Compass; or made publick the Virtue and right Use of Kin Kina; did more for the propagation of Knowledge, for the acquisition of Conveniences of Life; and saved more from the Grave, than those who built Colleges, Work-houses, and Hospitals.[123]

In the last chapter of the four volumes, Locke discussed his view "of the Division of the Sciences". He argued that science, which he recognised as the means to explore, discover and understand the whys and wherefores of the world as far as it was possible, could be divided into three distinct fields. His ideas differed somewhat from what would be considered mainstream science in the present day, but points to his awareness of the interaction between doing and being, the importance of human occupation, and the need to understand that as a foundation science. His choice also underlines his basic rationale, which was that science should add to knowledge in a way which betters the human experience: a view not surprising at a time when humanist values held sway. The three sciences he recommended included, in closest to modern day terms, biological science, communication science, and occupational science. As the latter is of particular interest to this history, Locke's words alluding to it are bold in the following extracts.

*All things that can fall within the compass of humane Understanding, being either, First, The Nature of Things, as they are in themselves, their Relations, and their manner of Operation: Or, **Secondly, that which Man himself ought to do, as a rational and voluntary Agent, for the Attainment of any Ends, especially Happiness**: Or, Thirdly, The ways and means, whereby the Knowledge of both the one and the other of these, are attained and communicated; I think, Science may be divided properly into these Three sorts.*[124]

It is the second of the three that resembles the newly emerging occupational science, but which Locke called ethics. Ethics are defined in current times in the *Hutchinson Dictionary of Ideas* as a 'branch of philosophy concerned with the systematic study of human values. It involves the study of theories of conduct and goodness, and of the meanings of moral terms.'[125] Locke described it this way:

The skill of Right applying our own Powers and Actions, for the Attainment of Things good and useful. The most considerable under this Head, is Ethicks, which is the seeking out those Rules, and Measures of humane Actions, which lead to Happiness, and the Means to practice them. The end of this is not bare Speculation, and the Knowledge of Truth; but Right, and a Conduct suitable to it.[126]

He concluded (points are bolded which relate to his "occupational science"):

*This seems to me the first and most general, as well as natural division of the Objects of our Understanding. For since a Man can employ his Thoughts about nothing, but either the Contemplation of Things themselves for the discovery of Truth; **Or about the Things in his own Power, which are his own Actions, for the Attainment of his own Ends**; Or the Signs the Mind makes use of, both in the one and the other, and the right ordering of them for its cleare Information. All which three, viz. Things as they are in themselves knowable; **Actions as they depend on*** *us, in order to Happiness;* and the right use of Signs in order to Knowledge, being tota caelo different, they seemed to me to be the three great Provinces of the intellectual World, wholly separate and distinct one from another.[127]

In summary, the Renaissance embraced humanism as a dominant philosophy that presaged a new secular order and a re-birth of opportunity for individual talent and interest. As such it provided a conceptual base for thinking about the place of occupation in life and health. That led, centuries later, to the development of the profession of occupational therapy, which is often described as having a humanist approach to restoring human capabilities and dignity following disorder or disability.

Although, during the 14th to 17th centuries, practical manifestations of change were slower to develop than the ideas, some exciting shifts did occur from an occupation for health viewpoint, in terms of social and mental health. The slowness was, in part, due to the monumental change of service deliverers, from monasteries and monks to secular authorities and private entrepreneurs. The exciting shifts included the development of ideas about the centrality of occupation within social health, and the beginning of communally based institutions to rectify problems and provide remedial services for the occupationally derived and depraved. Even though those services did not survive over the centuries, a precedent was set which could be revisited and updated according to modern thought.

In mental health, although the state did not provide leadership in the provision of treatment using occupation, it was apparently, part of common understanding of, at least, some members of the intelligentsia. That is clear from the work of Burton, and the thrust of some of Locke's philosophies, and the numerous references they called upon to support their arguments. Because of the trends just alluded to, it may be possible to find similar ones with regard to the provision of physical health during the Renaissance, which will be addressed in the next chapter.

---

[1] Harvey P, ed. The Oxford Companion to English Literature. 4th edition. Oxford: Clarendon Press, 1967; 637.
[2] Macdonald EM. World-Wide Conquests of Disabilities: The History, Development and Present Functions of the Remedial Services. London: Bailliere Tindall, 1981; 58.
[3] Montaigne ME de. Les Essais. Paris: A L'Angelier, 1580-1588. (first translated into English by John Florio in 1603).
[4] Girling DA, ed. New Age Encyclopaedia. 7th edition. Sydney & London: Bay Books, 1983.
[5] Isaacs A, ed. Macmillan Encyclopedia. London: Macmillan, 1990; 829.
[6] Harvey. The Oxford Companion to English Literature…; 554.
[7] Macdonald. World-Wide Conquests of Disabilities…; 67.
[8] Isaacs. Macmillan Encyclopedia…; 594-595.

[9]Macdonald. World-Wide Conquests of Disabilities…; 60.

[10]More T. Utopia. (first published 1516). Abridged edition. London: Phoenix, 1996; 12-13.

[11]More. Utopia…; 14, 17.

[12]More. Utopia…; 20.

[13]More. Utopia…; 16.

[14]More. Utopia…; 16-17.

[15]More. Utopia…; 17.

[16]More. Utopia…; 18.

[17]Conelis-son, van Zurik-Zee P. A Way Propounded to make the Poor… Happy. 1659.

[18]Girling. New Age Encyclopaedia…; vol 24: 153.

[19]Kirkman Grey B. A History of English Philanthropy. London: P. S. King and Son. 1905.

[20]Gasquet FA. Henry VIII and the English Monasteries. Volume II. (originally 1888-9). London: George Bell, 1920.

[21]Gasquet. Henry VIII and the English Monasteries. Volume II.

[22]Kirkman Grey. A History of English Philanthropy…; 15.

[23]Marti-Ibañez F, ed. Henry E. Sigerist on the History of Medicine. New York: MD Publications, Inc., 1960; 21.

[24]Kirkman Grey. A History of English Philanthropy…; 7.

[25]Warner GT. Landmarks in English Industrial History. 1899. Revised and extended by Marshall TH. London and Glasgow: Blackie & Son Ltd., 1924.

[26]Kirkman Grey. A History of English Philanthropy.

[27]Copland R. Quoted by Furnival in: Notes to Stubbes P. Anatomie of Abuses: Containing, A Discoverie or Brief Summarie of such Notable Vices and Imperfections as now Raigne in many… Countreyes of the Worlde: but (especially) Ailgna (Anglia). Together with most Fearful Examples of Gods Judgements. London: J. R. Jones, 1583.

[28]Warner. Landmarks in English Industrial History…; 143.

[29]Porter R. Disease, Medicine and Society in England 1550-1860. Basingstoke and London: Macmillan Education, 1987; 13-17.

[30]Isaacs. Macmillan Encyclopedia…; 1269.

[31]Macdonald. World-Wide Conquests of Disabilities…; 67.

[32]Tanner JR. Tudor Constitutional Documents AD 1485-1603, With a Historical Commentary. Cambridge: Cambridge University Press, 1951; 469-470.

[33]Kirkman Grey. A History of English Philanthropy…; 25.

[34]Beggars Act of 1536: An Act for the punishment of sturdy vagabonds and beggars. In: Tanner JR. Tudor Constitutional Document…; 480.

[35]Beggars Act of 1536. In: Tanner. Tudor Constitutional Documents…; 480.

[36]Kirkman Grey. A History of English Philanthropy.

[37]Kirkman Grey. A History of English Philanthropy.

[38]O'Connor J. The Workhouses of Ireland: The Fate of Ireland's Poor. Dublin: Anvil Books, 1995; 28.

[39]Tanner. Tudor Constitutional Document…; 469-470.

[40]Aschrott PF. The English Poor Law System. Translated Preston-Thomas H, 1st edition 1888; 7.

[41]Statute of Charitable Uses. In: Kirkman Grey. A History of English Philanthropy…; 37.

[42]Stowe J. A Survey of London. Contayning the Originall. Increased. Moderne Estate, and Government of that City. Methodically Set Down. London: Thoms, 1842; 44. (Originally printed by Elizabeth Purslow, sold by Nicholas Bourne, 1598 and 1603).

[43]Blakey R. The History of Political Literature. London: 1858; vol II; 84-85.

[44]O'Connor. The Workhouses of Ireland…; 28.

[45]Kirkman Grey. A History of English Philanthropy.

[46]Porter. Disease, Medicine and Society in England 1550-1860.

[47]A Short History of Bridewell and Bethlem Royal Hospitals. The Bethlem Art and History Collections Trust 1899; 2.

[48]A Short History of Bridewell and Bethlem Royal Hospitals…; 3-4.

[49]Jordan WK, ed. The Chronicle and Political Papers of King Edward VI. Ithaca, New York: Cornell University Press for Folger Shakespeare Library, 1966; 165.

[50]Slack P. From Reformation to Improvement: Public Welfare in Early Modern England. The Ford Lectures Delivered in the University of Oxford 1994-1995. Oxford: Clarenden Press, 1999; 9.

[51]The Charters of the Royal Hospitals of Bridewell and Bethlem. London: Printed by H. Bryer, Bridewell Hospital, 1807; 5.

[52]Abstract: Act of Common Council in the second and third year of Philip and Mary. In: A Short History of Bridewell and Bethlem Royal Hospital…; 5.

[53]A Short History of Bridewell and Bethlem Royal Hospitals…; 5, 7.

[54]Slack. From Reformation to Improvement…; 20-25.

[55]A True Report of the Great Costs and Charges of the Foure Hospitals in the City of London 1644. Cited in: Kirkman Grey. A History of English Philanthropy…; 67.

[56]Alldridge P. The Bethlem Royal Hospital: An Illustrated History. London: The Bethlem and Maudesley NHS Trust, 1995.

[57]Archbishop of Canterbury. Copy of letter. British Museum Harleian Manuscripts. 1330. Cited in: A Short History of Bridewell and Bethlem Royal Hospitals…; 3.

[58]Stowe. Records. 1330. Cited in: A Short History of Bridewell and Bethlem Royal Hospitals…; 2-3.

[59]Alldridge. The Bethlem Royal Hospital: An Illustrated History.

[60]A Short History of Bridewell and Bethlem Royal Hospitals.

[61]Alldridge. The Bethlem Royal Hospital: An Illustrated History.

[62]The Charters of the Royal Hospitals of Bridewell and Bethlem…; 37.

[63]Alldridge. The Bethlem Royal Hospital: An Illustrated History…; 5.

[64]Muniment book of 1644. Cited in: A Short History of Bridewell and Bethlem Royal Hospitals…; 6.

[65]Inventory. Cited in: A Short History of Bridewell and Bethlem Royal Hospitals…; 5.

[66]Alldridge. The Bethlem Royal Hospital: An Illustrated History…; 6-7.

[67]Alldridge. The Bethlem Royal Hospital: An Illustrated History…; 9.

[68]Alldridge. The Bethlem Royal Hospital: An Illustrated History…; 22.

[69]Porter R. Mind-Forg'd Manacles. London: The Athlone Press, 1987; 127.

[70]Dugdale. In: Walsh JJ. Medieval Medicine. London: A & C Black, Ltd., 1920; 191.

[71]Walsh. Medieval Medicine…; 190.

[72]Burdett HC. History of Hospitals. Vol. 1. London: J & A Churchill, 1891-93; 42.

[73]Porter R. The Greatest Benefit to Mankind: A Medical History of Humanity from Antiquity to the Present. Harper Collins (first published 1997) Paper back edition 1999; 113.

[74]Macdonald. World-Wide Conquests of Disabilities…; 60.

[75]Sanctorius Sanctorius. Medicina Statica. In: Sinclair, Sir J. Code of Health and Longevity. Edinburgh: Arch Constable & Co, 1806; 184-189.

[76]Sinclair. Code of Health and Longevity…; 185.

[77]Bright T. A Treatise on Melancholy. 1586.

[78]Rogers T. A Disease Concerning Trouble of Mind and the Disease of Melancholy. 1691.

[79]Porter. Mind-Forg'd Manacles…; 171.

[80]Burton R. The Anatomy of Melancholy. Oxford: Printed for Henry Cripps, 1651; 84-85.

[81]Burton. The Anatomy of Melancholy…; 85-86.

[82]Burton. The Anatomy of Melancholy…; 86.

[83]Burton. The Anatomy of Melancholy…; 87.

[84]Burton. The Anatomy of Melancholy…; 88.

[85]Burton. The Anatomy of Melancholy…; 90.

[86]Burton. The Anatomy of Melancholy…; 90.

[87]Burton. The Anatomy of Melancholy…; 117.

[88]Burton. The Anatomy of Melancholy…; 118.

[89]Burton. The Anatomy of Melancholy…; 127.

[90]Burton. The Anatomy of Melancholy…; 128.

[91]Burton. The Anatomy of Melancholy…; 128-129.

[92]Burton. The Anatomy of Melancholy…; 130.

[93]Burton. The Anatomy of Melancholy…; 131.

[94]Burton. The Anatomy of Melancholy…; 152.

[95]Burton. The Anatomy of Melancholy…; 265.

[96]Burton. The Anatomy of Melancholy…; 265.

[97]Burton. The Anatomy of Melancholy…; 265.

[98]Burton. The Anatomy of Melancholy…; 266.

[99]Burton. The Anatomy of Melancholy…; 266-267.

[100]Burton. The Anatomy of Melancholy…; 277.

[101]Burton. The Anatomy of Melancholy…; 267.

[102]Burton. The Anatomy of Melancholy…; 267-298.

[103]Burton. The Anatomy of Melancholy…; 275.

[104]Burton. The Anatomy of Melancholy…; 545.

[105]Foucault M. Folie et Deraison a la Renaissance. Bruxelles: Editions de l'Universtite de Bruxelles, 1976.

[106]Porter. Mind-Forg'd Manacles…; 113.

[107]Clay. Medieval Hospitals. In: Walsh. Medieval Medicine…; 190.

[108]Porter. Mind-Forg'd Manacles…; 111, 120-21.

[109]Henderson DK. The Evolution of Psychiatry in Scotland. Edinburgh and London: E & S Livingstone Ltd, 1964; 41, 42.

[110]Porter. Mind-Forg'd Manacles…; 112.

[111]Porter. Mind-Forg'd Manacles…; 137.

[112]Porter. Mind-Forg'd Manacles…; 137.

[113]Macdonald. World-Wide Conquests of Disabilities…; 60.

[114]Isaacs. Macmillan Encyclopedia…; 734.

[115]Macdonald. World-Wide Conquests of Disabilities…; 73.

[116]Isaacs. Macmillan Encyclopedia…; 734.

[117]Locke J. An Essay Concerning Humane Understanding. London: Printed for Tho, Basset, and sold by Edw. Mory at the sign of the Three Bibles in St Paul's Church-Yard. MDCXC (book IV); 326.

[118]Harvey. The Oxford Companion to English Literature…; 484.

[119]Locke. An Essay Concerning Humane Understanding…; 327.

[120]Locke. An Essay Concerning Humane Understanding…; 2-3.

[121]Locke. An Essay Concerning Humane Understanding…; 3.

[122]Locke. An Essay Concerning Humane Understanding…; 326-327.

[123]Locke. An Essay Concerning Humane Understanding…; 327.

[124]Locke. An Essay Concerning Humane Understanding…; 361.

[125]Norton AL, ed. Hutchinson Dictionary of Ideas. Oxford: Helicon, 1994; 178.

[126]Locke. An Essay Concerning Humane Understanding…; 361.

[127]Locke. An Essay Concerning Humane Understanding…; 362.

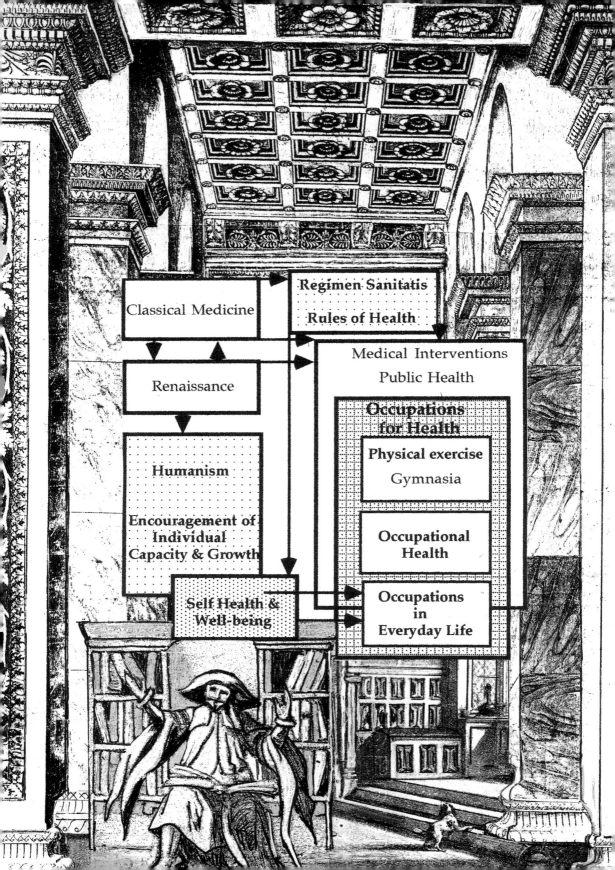

Classical Medicine

Regimen Sanitatis
Rules of Health

Renaissance

Medical Interventions
Public Health

Humanism

Encouragement of
Individual
Capacity & Growth

Occupations
for Health

Physical exercise
Gymnasia

Occupational
Health

Self Health &
Well-being

Occupations
in
Everyday Life

Chapter 6

The Renaissance, Occupational Regimes and Physical Health

Contents

Medical intervention
Public health and health promotion
Occupation for health
Anatomy and physiology, iatro-mechanical doctrines, gymnastics and spas
Occupational health
Occupations in every day life: Preventive and remedial care
Mobility

The story of the use of occupation for the maintenance and restoration of health during the Renaissance is continued in this chapter, which concentrates on aspects of physical health. It does so by, first of all, outlining the provision of medical services during that time. These services provide some indication of the beginnings of the development of interest in public health, as well as the ongoing prescription of occupation as "exercise," largely with a health promotion and illness prevention focus but sometimes for remediation. Such prescriptions continued the tradition of the rules for health, which were first articulated in classical times and reinvented during the Middle Ages. Interest in the physical health giving effects of occupation once more began to focus on the use of gymnastics and spas. While several physicians developed a fascination about occupational diseases, lay experts continued the self health tradition by articulating an appreciation of occupations for health in everyday life. This was a time of encouragement of individual capacities and growth. The work of Paré and Ramazzini is featured in particular, not only because of their importance in general terms, but because they had something of value to say about the place of occupation within their specialties. The chapter will close with a brief section on mobility aids to daily living that were used during the period.

Medical intervention

In London, few medical institutions of any note survived the Reformation. St Bartholomew's, St Thomas's, and Bethlem Hospital were the exception. Having grown from monastic beginnings, these were three of the five Royal Hospitals established, and were for those with physical or mental illness. In the matter of creating more hospitals for the sick, no immediate State provision was made to replace what was lost with the demise of monasteries around the country. Although there were 'hospitals, spittles, lazar houses, and almshouses in some cities, towns and other places' there were not anywhere near enough.[1] Such lack of that type of facility would make one suspect that people, when sick, relied on private care. Although nowadays people call upon doctors in their premises or are visited by a doctor in their home, whilst possible, then, for some people, it was not the reality for most.

During the Renaissance and subsequent years the three principal types of specialist in health care remained physicians, surgeons, and apothecaries. Despite limited success, the most elite and expensive were the university-educated physicians who, with gentlemanly bearing, attended, diagnosed, advised and prescribed. However they had a reputation of being monopolistic and self-serving and were, on the whole, out of the reach of everyday folk. As well, what they could offer was restricted by the knowledge of the times. The limit of their expertise is, perhaps, demonstrated by the fact that doctors were rarely present at either birth or death, these being the province of either midwives or clergy. Many physicians practised in London, some were scattered in major towns and cities, but only a few were to be found in the country, which was less lucrative. Linacre, a humanist, was the physician who, concerned about the indiscriminate practice of medicine, founded the Royal College of Physicians in 1518, to act as both a licensing agency and to develop a system of examination.[2,3]

Surgeons, in contrast to physicians, served indentured apprenticeships of some seven years. They became essentially, craftsmen, or occasionally craftswomen, who set bones; performed operations; treated wounds, injuries, boils, and so forth. Part of the guild-system, the Barber Surgeons Company of London dated from 1540. Apothecaries also served an apprenticeship and made up the "remedies" that the physicians prescribed. They were legally subject to supervision from the College of Physicians from the time of their foundation, although many apothecaries prescribed on their own authority. In the country, the forerunner of the general practitioner was often a "surgeon-apothecary" whether trained in both or not.[4]

If those were largely out of the reach of the masses, what other options were available? There were other types of licensed medical practitioners such as midwives and at least some of the "quacks". Midwives were female, and despite the popular image of them as gin drinking, unhygienic, uneducated women, many were from respectable families and literate. To practise they had to obtain a licence from the local bishop, obviously to ensure that midwifery was carried out by those of good character. Quacks, too, could get a license to patent and vend their proprietary "cures" by purchasing a "royal privilege"–a money making scheme of the monarchs. Apart from those, unlicensed, itinerant quacks and pedlars went from place to place selling their nostrums. Grocers, too, sold drugs, and blacksmiths or farriers acted as dentists and orthopaedic surgeons for people as well as animals. Additionally, in most places, there were women "nurses" and "wise-women" skilled with herbs and secret remedies from earlier days.[5]

With those facts in mind it is possible to surmise that "proto-occupational therapy" could have been carried out by a range of people with different types of expertise, as many people, apart from those already named, practised "physic" activated by neighbourliness, paternalism, religious charity, or to demonstrate good housekeeping. The wives of the affluent class, for example, often played "lady physician" to the sick, taking as great a pride in their homemade medicines as in other forms of housewifery skills. Neither was it unknown for their men folk to "doctor" members of their households or their tenants, in the same way that members of the clergy, as part of their pastoral care, often assumed a doctoring role with parishioners. Such lay practitioners were necessary because of scarcity of trained people and their cost, so that it was only occasionally that regular doctors denounced "lay" medicine, especially as the profession as a whole had very limited corporate power.[6]

This "live and let live" approach was partly due to a common belief at the time that doctors did not have the monopoly on medical reasoning, so they were not routinely sent for when people were sick. Most people diagnosed themselves before deciding whether or not to seek help, and frequently they would treat themselves with kitchen-physic, the making of which could be regarded as a form of occupational therapy. This is not surprising, for doctors, quite possibly, had no remedies that worked any better, especially as all drugs, even such as opium, could be bought over the counter. If people sought help it was not necessarily from professionals. Furthermore, if the well-to-do called a doctor, the physician was often expected to agree with the patient's own diagnosis and suggested treatments. His advice was often disregarded, or second and third opinions called for, and sufferers mixed and matched his remedies with their own and those of quacks or others.[7]

This approach was also due to the beliefs held about the causes of sickness. Unlike the modern day, when illness is largely understood as the result of physiological processes that can be cured by medical intervention, then it was still widely held that disease might be the result of evil spirits, satanic possession, punishment for original sin, natural justice, or the finger of Providence. It was supposed that God may use illness to deliver moral or spiritual messages, and to remind people of the torments of Hell should they sin. In more modern vein, yet not totally inconsistent with those other beliefs, health was understood by physicians and many others as the product of a properly functioning body, so common sense held that illness resulted from its malfunctioning.[8]

The latter belief resulted in notice being taken of the ongoing message of the *Regimen Sanitatis*, which was reiterated in many medical texts of the day. Indeed, learned medicine still leant heavily on the Classical School of Galen by basing its prescriptions on those earlier ideas about the constituents of a healthy life–diet, exercise and moderation in all things, which are little different from today. What did differ was ongoing adherence to the humoural theory of medicine, which resulted in an emphasis on purging, sweating, blood-letting, vomiting, and the prescription of a host of medicaments to expel toxic substances from the body and to restore its "balance". Those views were so widely held that it was commonly understood that evacuations, the right environment, adequate sleep, and temperance as well as proper diet and exercise were important to maintain an ideal balance between the "humours," which were central to the experience of health and to prevent sickness from occurring. Whilst this placed the responsibility with individuals rather than medical practitioners, doctors were still in demand when they could be afforded, and commanded respect. Their public health initiatives, particularly those aimed at socio-environmental improvement, as well as advice to prevent illness were probably, at that time, their most useful measures against disease, and it was here that occupational regimes were also advised.

Public health and health promotion

An increasing interest in public health, the prevention of disease and promotion of health during the Renaissance is easy to understand. Many people lived and worked in environments or at types of employment that were conducive to disease. For example, potters frequently succumbed to lung diseases, and leadworkers to paralysis. It had long been understood, and part of the humoural doctrine that environments were the cause of much ill health. Marshy areas were blamed for "ague" or malarial fever and shivering, and overcrowded, airless, urban developments were regarded as the seat of epidemic diseases. Miasmas, poisonous gases that were exhaled from the earth, were blamed and so, it follows that vigorous activity, free currents of air and fast flowing water were regarded as antidotes.[9]

Public health boards were established in various places around Europe, mainly to stop the spread of disease by imposing compulsory isolation or quarantine on people arriving from plague or similar epidemic infested areas. In

Milan, as elsewhere in Italy, for example, a permanent body of magistrates was established about 1410 "for the preservation of health". Within forty years it had a staff of a physician, surgeon, notary and barber, two horsemen, three footmen, and two grave diggers. Northern European towns did not establish similar authorities for at least another century. As health workers began to acquire roles within the public sphere, midwives, too, became involved. In order to acquire a bishop's licence, which permitted them to engage in their work, they were required to swear an oath that they would report illegitimate births and extract paternal names. They were also called upon to ascertain sterility or virginity, and to certify infant deaths.[10]

Occupation for health

Anatomy and physiology, iatro-mechanical doctrines, gymnastics and spas

The lightening of religious taboos at the same time as renewed interest in the classical world and the physical body, led to a break through in terms of dissection, to understand anatomy and physiology for medical purposes. Leonardo da Vinci, (1452-1519) who, to many, typifies the Renaissance man took advantage of an easing of legislation regarding human dissection in order to understand the form and function of the human body which he drew, painted and sculptured. His anatomical drawings, which he kept in his famous notebooks, were enhanced by his experiences with dissection and instruction in experimental physiology, both of which he undertook with a medical lecturer from Padua. The famous Italian was not only a Renaissance man but also a prime example of the occupational nature of humans. He had numerous occupational interests and great capacity for most of them. As well as being an artist he was a physicist, philosopher, geographer, astronomer, engineer, writer, and mechanic interested in music, medicine, and anatomy.[11]

Marcantonio della Torre (1475-1506), a lesser known figure of the period, was also interested in anatomy. He was an expert draughtsman and illustrated the textbook on anatomy and physiology that he produced with details of the muscular system along with descriptions of movement, leverage and gravity. He investigated and illustrated the anatomy and physiology of speech organs, and taking the pursuit of anatomy and physiology a step further, like industrial engineers and occupational therapists centuries later, he analysed the rhythm of various trade activities. Like da Vinci he had multiple skills and interests in devising industrial machinery, flying machines, and glasses for detecting and drawing very small items.[12]

Interest in anatomy began to be more acceptable in scientific medical circles. Flemish born Andreas Vesalius (1514-64) was the best known medical expert in anatomy of the early part of the 16th century. He originally attended Louvain University, moved to Paris where he continued his studies with Jacobus Sylvius (1478-1555), and later went to Venice where he graduated as a physician. He was appointed professor of surgery and anatomy at Padua. His major work, *De Humani Corporis Fabrica* (Seven Books of the Human Body), published in 1543, included accurate descriptions of the form and action of the human body. They were illustrated by Jan Calcar, an expert artist, and based on human and animal dissection and vivisection, and on careful observation of movement. At first he followed the works of Galen which prevailed at the time. Later, he made observations that challenged Galen's theories and thereafter confined his lectures at Padua to his own findings. Considered the founder of modern theories of anatomy and physiology, his replacing of traditional views about anatomy with observation and experiment paved the way for experimental medicine like that of Harvey (1578-1657), and opened up "a new era of scientific investigation".[13][14][15]

The re-emergence of interest in the physical body led to a resurgence of the doctrine and practice of physical exercise and occupations in gymnasia. Not surprisingly, as the Renaissance was a rebirth of classical culture, the use of physical activity in gymnasia again gained popularity. Paulus Vergerius (1348-1419) was one of the first of that period to demonstrate interest in physical activity. He proposed that, for adolescents, intellectual studies should alternate with exercises and recreation, which he suggested should include enjoyable occupations such as board and ball games, walks, music, singing and dancing. A little later, Vittorino da Feltre (1378-1446), a humanist-physician with an interest in education operated a school where, in addition to the usual intellectual pursuits, the students were provided with physical exercises and games in the fresh air, "happy occupations" and mountain climbing.

As the interest in physical exercise increased, studies became more sophisticated, with Maffeus Vegius (c. 14-15th) propounding a distinction between light exercise for intellectuals, and strong exercise for physical improvement; Giovanni Savaronala (1452-1498), a surgeon of Padua and Ferrara, included his ideas about movement, rest and hydrotherapy spas in his treatise on hygiene; and Laurent Joubert (1529-1583) introduced gymnastics to the medical school at Montpellier, arguing that they should be prescribed as medical treatment. Nicholas Andre, mentioned earlier for his prescription of occupations, authored the first work on orthopaedics, which included an analysis of exercises. He recommended exercises to improve children's posture, and as treatment for fractures, paralyses and similar disorders, and provided careful instructions for massage.

Another leading figure at that time was Hieronymus Mercurialis (1530-1606), a professor of medicine at Bologna and Pisa with expertise in paediatrics. He is pictured in figure 1.6.1. Mercurialis also addressed the value of occupation and gymnastics as exercise to be used as medical treatments. He advanced his views in *De Arte Gymnastica,* a treatise in six books in which he analysed the action of muscles during movement and divided exercises into three types: military, preventive, and therapeutic. For the latter he stressed the need for exact diagnosis, for consideration of each patient and their particular disability, and the need to obtain the patients' cooperation. His interest was wide ranging; from speech problems such as stammering to respiration problems and eye diseases; from paralysis to mental illness; and for each he recommended exercise through engagement in particular occupations.

Figure 1.6.1: **Hieronymus Mercurialis: Engraving attributed to A. Bosio, 1666**
(The Wellcome Library)

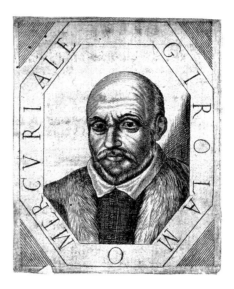

Mercurialis believed in graded activity so, for example, recommended walking according to three grades: the first was walking to and fro; the second, walking further and for longer periods; and the third, mountain climbing, running and jumping. When he recommended playing games with balls, such as football or punch ball, he graded the work by varying the weight of the ball by filling them with feathers or sand. For arthritic patients he prescribed a wide range of occupations from passive exercise in vehicles or hammocks, exercises accompanied by music, climbing ropes, wrestling, throwing and riding. For preventive, health-giving occupations Mercurialis advised hunting, rowing, swimming, and boxing.[16]

From Blundell's 19th century translation of Mercurialis's work we learn:
… that there are 2 parts to the maintenance and restoration of health, namely "prophylactics or matters of Hygiene, and the other as therapeutics or the application of remedies to cure disease". Whilst the curative takes properly the highest place in medicine, the conservative, as an adjunct to it, is no less necessary to the perfection of the science that disposes of our lives and our persons …

... Conservative medicine or Hygiene may be said to possess three special qualities, namely the phophylactic, which comprises any means made use of to prevent disease; the preservative, if it may be so called, which maintains present health; and the analeptic, that recruits or recovers strength lost by sickness. To secure these advantages there appears to have been in ancient times an almost incredible number of appliances, which were deemed guardians of health, ...

... public writers [of Rome] then, one and all, bear witness to the value of the art of exercise in averting future diseases, preserving present health, and reinvigorating convalesents![17] See figure 1.6.2.

Figure 1.6.2: **Flow chart of occupation as exercise for health according to Mercurialis**

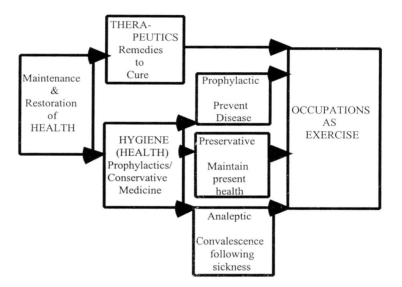

Towards the end of the sixteenth century the interest in physical occupation and gymnastics led to the notion of an *"iatro-mechanic"* doctrine which was introduced by several experts in physical treatments and was adopted by some eminent physicians and physiologists.[18] It attempted to explain medicine and the phenomena of life from a mechanical point of view. Sigerist went so far as to describe the seventeenth as the century of the iatromechanists. He described, how in attempting to explain the functions of the human body mechanically, they liked to compare the organs to tools and therefore were interested in tools and machines,[19] in a way similar to the present day when explanations are often couched in computer terms. That interest triggered attention into issues of occupational health. Iatro-mechanics were probably the forerunner of the speciality of physical medicine with which occupational therapists have been closely associated.

Gymnasia and baths were linked in the classical period, so resurgence in the use of public baths in spa towns was to be expected. Hydrotherapy certainly came back into vogue, which led to considerable competition between the various spas, with many of them publicising the treatment they offered as well as the recreations, and entertainments that were provided for visitors. Some waters were considered to be holy, while others were favoured for having mineral and therapeutic properties. Health authorities, like Robert Pierce (1622-1710) and Sir John Floyer (1649-1734), varied in their prescriptions, the former recommending all forms of bathing as therapeutic, and the latter only cold baths.[20]

In Bath, the most famous of the spa towns, the hospital of St John, having fallen into decay, was rebuilt. It was established around the Roman baths, and the poor were assisted to utilise the health giving nature of the waters by being allowed to beg in Bath. Any diseased or impotent person journeying to Bath, or to Buxton where there was a more recent spa, for treatment must obtain a permit from two justices which allowed them to beg on journeys to and from the towns, as well as during their watery cure.[21] The permits that entitled them to 'travell to Bathe or Buxstone for remedie of their griefe' were supported by a 1597 Act of Parliament. This encouraged others who were not entitled to beg to do so under pretence and resulted in a licensing requirement.[22]

Elizabeth I, who herself went to Bath for treatment of rheumatism and toothache, authorised local authorities to help finance the visits of poorer subjects to spas for treatment of cramp, gout, rheumatism, sciatica, paralyses, lung troubles, jaundice, apoplexy, epilepsy, oedema, lethargy, deafness, forgetfulness, and shivering and shaking.[23] So, it was not unknown for a parish to pay for a sick person to visit a spa or alternatively to visit London for treatment. It was always possible that such outlays would prove less expensive than permanent parish relief.[24] Not only the poor visited spas such as at Bath and Buxton, but also those able to afford it of their own accord, and spa towns became increasingly fashionable places to visit for the well to do.

Occupational health

With its emphasis on the spiritual, the Middle Ages had scarcely made any contribution to the subject of occupational health. It should not be surprising, however, that during the time of Renaissance, when human capacities began again to be recognised and celebrated, and the ideas of classical medicine studied with greater intent, that occupational health re-emerged as a concern within medicine. There was a difference to that earlier time. Instead of "workers" being regarded as lesser human beings, or expendable, as had sometimes been the case, they began to be of interest, at least in research terms. The noxious elements experienced, and the skills required by men and women as they engaged in their various trades and crafts became the subject of analysis by some physicians. A few even recognised the economic needs of poorer people, the unpleasantness of some jobs which were essential to societal health, and understood that workers could not be arbitrarily grouped according to their occupation, as they were each different.

Towards the end of the fifteenth century medical literature devoted to occupational diseases began to surface. One reason for that was that medicine was once more in the hands of the progressives rather than the charitable, and physicians were keen to describe new diseases. However, it was not only physicians who were interested in the topic. Italian, Marcilio Ficino (1433-1499), was a case in point, although rather than describe disease he offered his advice on preventing occupational disease. A philosopher and writer, who lived quietly under the patronage of the Medici, he wrote *On Caring for the Health of Learned People,* to which he referred in *On a Long Life,* one of a trilogy. He recommended effort as a requisite for a long life, and argued that with adequate care and attention to health regimes it was possible for the "weak" to live lengthy lives.[25]

For those whose occupation was of a studious nature he recommended that the day's work should start at or before sunrise. However before rising 'first massage all of your body for a while pleasantly with your palms, then massage your head with your nails, but a little more lightly'. On rising 'give over at least half an hour for expurgation; right after this, prepare yourself carefully for meditation' which would last for about an hour. That was followed by a period of relaxation when the head was combed, with an ivory comb, from forehead to neck about forty times, then the neck was rubbed with a rough cloth before returning to meditation and study for one to two hours. The maximum period he thought permissible to continue work, including regular relaxation breaks, was until two hours after noon. Reading 'the work of other scholars' could be pursued at later times, rather than using that 'for thinking new thoughts of one's own'. His advice was–'we ought always to remember, however, that in any hour, once at least, the mind's intentness should be relaxed for a little while'.[26]

The interest in occupational health can be said to have coincided with economic changes. As rural workers in many countries lost their traditional livelihoods with enclosures and evictions, many moved to urban areas to sell their labour. As well, iron, copper, and lead were needed for firearms, which were being used with ever increasing frequency. However as shallow deposits became exhausted it was necessary to mine deeper, which obviously created different, and usually increased, hazards. Additionally, a demand for gold and silver as a medium of exchange resulted from an increase of trade, which, in turn, led not only to voyages of discovery, but increased mining activity in search of precious metals.[27]

The occupational diseases of metal workers were the first to be set down by medical writers. Ulrich Ellenbog, a German physician, wrote a seven-page pamphlet, in 1473, *On the Poisonous Wicked Fumes and Smokes.* Augsburg, where he lived, was famous for its goldsmiths, and Ellenbog's contribution was prompted by the diseases he noted amongst his patients who were goldsmiths, and was circulated amongst their workshops. Believing some symptoms were due to their working conditions he described the dangers of coal, nitric acid, lead, and mercury fumes among others, and advised the goldsmiths to work, as much as possible, in the open air covering their mouths when there were fumes. He also recommended the inhalation of various nostrums.[28]

A well-known physician with an interest in occupational health was Paracelsus. Theophratus Bombastus von Hohenheim (1493-1541), known as Paracelsus, was born in Salzburg, the son of a doctor of medicine.[29] He trained at Basle and travelled within Italy and Germany before being appointed Professor of Medicine at Basle University where his radical ideas became very influential within medicine. As an alchemist he is also attributed with being the founder of medical chemistry. He, somewhat arrogantly, challenged classical theories including the humoural, publicly burning the works of Avicenna and Galen. He insisted that medicine, as a science, should be based on the study of nature, and that practising physicians should depend on their own experience and judgement rather than the views of others.[30]

He expressed his own views about occupational health issues strongly, arguing that medicine was an art concerned with all the various aspects of life, and that particular occupations, such as mining, caused particular diseases. He had spent some time in the Tyrol studying the mechanics of mining, mineralogy, and the diseases of miners in which he was greatly interested because of his involvement in chemistry. He visited many mines, particularly those of Villach in Karnten where his father had settled. He wrote the first text devoted to occupational diseases, based on first hand experience as he had lived and worked with the miners, seen the appalling conditions under which they laboured, and the hazards to which they were exposed. Since Paracelsus' work, every writer on mining touched on the diseases peculiar to the industry.[31]

Despite his obvious talents Paracelsus aggravated many of his contemporaries and was driven from Basle in 1529 after only three years. He became a travelling physician, visiting various treatment spas, like Baden-Baden, Lorenz, and Heister, and recommending this form of therapy as he journeyed.[32,33]

Georgius Agricola (1494-1555) became another eminent authority on mining diseases. A German physician and mineralogist, he worked as a doctor in several mining towns and described the observable physical properties of minerals, in a systematic study which discounted their "long held" magical properties. His subsequent publication *De Re Metallica,* published in 1556 became the standard text for two centuries.[34] In book VI of the text he wrote:

It remains for me to speak of the ailments and accidents of miners, and of the methods by which they can guard against these, for we should always devote more care to maintaining our health, that we may freely perform our bodily functions, than to making profits. Of the illnesses, some affect the joints, some the eyes, and finally some are fatal to men.

He described the various hazards such as:

- Water which often collected in shafts making miners cold,
- Dust with corrosive qualities which ate away the lungs, and implanted consumption,
- Stagnant air which caused difficulty in breathing,
- Poisonous air which caused swellings and paralysis,
- Frequent accidents such as workers breaking their arms, legs, or necks after slipping from ladders in the shafts, or being drowned from falling into sumps,
- Mountain slides,
- Venomous ants which were found in several mines, and
- Demons of ferocious aspect which were pernicious pests in a few mines, and which were "expelled and put to flight by prayer and fasting".

Agicola recommended ventilating machines to overcome some of the hazards.[35]

He illustrated some of his findings with stories. Apparently in the mines situated in the Carpathian Mountains some women were known to have been married seven times because consumption caused their husband's premature death. Another told of how, in Rammelsberg, mountain slides occurred. In one day four hundred women lost their husbands.[36]

Without doubt, mining was the most dangerous of all jobs at that time, and so received primary attention. Indeed, several monographs were written on the diseases of miners by other German physicians, such as *Consilium Peripneumoniacum* by Martin Pansa in 1614, *De Morbis Metallariorum* by Leonardus Ursinus in 1652, *De Lythargyrii Fumo Noxio Morbico* by Samuel Stockhausen in 1656, and *De Paralysi Metallariorum,* by Suchlandius in 1693.[37] In the next century the interest continued and broadened to include other trades and diseases, with many scattered observations in the medical literature on soldiers and sailors and, perhaps surprisingly, on scholars, men of letters, and courtiers.[38] The best known of such physicians was undoubtably Bernadino Ramazzini (1633-1714), who is pictured in figure 1.6.3.

Ramazzini was born at Carpi, a small town near Modena, in Italy. Despite being a sickly youth, he achieved acclaimed success throughout his education, which continued until his nineteenth year. This included classical studies at the College of Jesuits, and three years of philosophy followed by a further three years of medicine at the University of Parma. After his graduation with a Diploma of Master of Arts and Doctor of Medicine, and convinced that "theory without practice could never constitute a genuine physician" he went to Rome

Figure 1.6.3: **Bernadino Ramazzini (1633-1714)**

(The Wellcome Library)

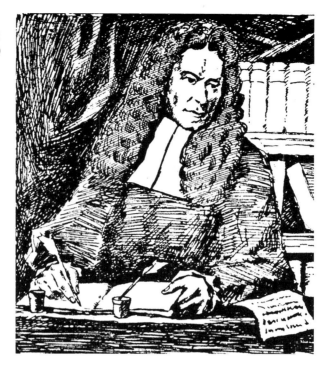

to study the practice of medicine. However, his health remained poor, and he determined that it would be best to return to his native clime. Back in Carpi he gradually recovered and married a woman of "considerable note".[39]

Ramazzini was appointed to the Chair of Practical Medicine at Padua, and in 1700 published his great work *De Morbis Artificum Diatriba*. (An English translation appeared in 1705 under the title: *A Treatise of the Diseases of Tradesmen, Shewing the Various Influence of Particular Trades upon the State of Health; with the Best Methods to Avoid or Correct It, and Useful Hints Proper to Be Minded in Regulating the Cure of all Diseases Incident to Tradesmen.*) This is considered by many to be the earliest substantial work on matters of occupational health, about which he lectured at the University. From Ramazzini's mention of his colleagues working in the field, whose material he was able to draw on in his text, the interest in occupational health was obviously part of the practice for many physicians at that time. Sigerist described it as 'a fine book, a real medical classic. It is to the history of occupational diseases what Vesalius' book is to anatomy, Harvey's to physiology, Morgagni's to pathology'.[40]

Because of occupational therapists' interest in occupational health and safety, and the importance of Ramazzini's treatise, numerous extracts are provided below to illustrate how he analysed a large variety of trades, industries and occupations, and the diseases and disabilities which commonly occurred in those engaged in them. In common with modern day occupational therapists working in occupational health, he considered it important for physicians to observe workers in their employment environments, as well as investigating the patterns of movements and postures maintained in particular occupations, along with the materials used. Ramazzini identified three major causes of occupational disease. The first was from emission of harmful substances such as noxious vapours or fine particles and the second was from demands imposed on the body's structure, such as unaccustomed or violent movement, static or unnatural postures and lack of exercise. The third was from social factors, such as of a pecuniary nature that might lead people to living a life of boredom and self-indulgence on the one hand, and continuance in a deadly trade on the other. He followed those findings with detailed analysis and a range of recommendations for prevention or cure.

Ramazzini attributed occupational diseases to two major causes; dangerous or toxic materials, and the postural or movement requirements of the occupation.

> *The various and numerous Train of Diseases that accrues to the Artificers from the Exercise of their respective Trades, is in my Opinion owing chiefly to two Causes: namely, first the noxious Quality of the Matter that goes thro' their hands, which by breathing out nocive Steams and thin Particles offensive to human Nature, gives rise to and particular Diseases; and in the next place certain violent and disorderly Motions, and improper Postures of the Body, by which the natural structure of the vital Machine is so undermin'd as gradually to make way for grievous Distempers.*[41]

For at least a century, he recorded, it had been recognised that there were 'workers who habitually incur serious maladies from the deadly fumes of metals', and that this was a cause for grave concern and specific action on the part of the medical profession:[42]

> *To shorten the treatment for workers who must use metals and other minerals, we must as I have said employ first of all remedies derived from the mineral world, next emollients from the vegetable class, also the common antidotes such as theriac and Mithridate and those that are supposed to blunt the malignant onslaughts of poisons by their specific force. We must use purgatives and emetics and prescribe them in liberal doses, in fact twice as large as usual. I say this on account of the stubborn and unyielding nature of metallic substances.*[43]

Ramazzini's notes of the diseases of potters provide an example from the many trades of this nature that he discussed. He provided detailed understanding of the processes he has observed as part of the occupation:

> *Now, the Potters muake use of burnt roasted or calcin'd Lead for glazing their Ware; and for that end grind their Lead in Marble Vessels, by turning about a long Piece of Wood hung from the Roof, with a square Stone fastenede to it at the other end. While they do this, as well as when with a pair of Tongs they daub their Vessels over with melted Lead before they put 'em into the Furnace; they receive by the*

mouth and Nostrils, and all the Pores of the Body all the virulent Parts of the Lead thus melted in Water and dissolv'd, and thereupon are seiz'd with heavy Disorders. For first of all their Hands begin to shake and tremble, soon after they become Paralytick, Lethargick, Splenetick, Cachetick, and Toothless...[44]

In his practice he sometimes found mercurial purgatives to be beneficial, as well as rubbing the patients hands and feet with petroleum[45]. He suggested that:

> *As for the Cure of such Workmen as fall under the above-mention'd Disorders, 'tis a hard matter to light upon such Remedies as will restore them to perfect Health. For they seldom have recourse to the Physicians, 'til the use of their Limbs is taken from 'em, and their Viscera grown hard. ... In the meantime we must take Notice, that there are several different Sorts of Workmen in a Potter's Workhouse; some of whom are imployed in Working of Chalk with their Hands and Feet; and others in forming the Vessels by Sitting and Turning a Wheel. So that all who go by the Name of a Potter are not subject to the Disease before mention'd, and therefore care must be taken that when ever the Name of a Potter is heard, we do not presently administer the remedies calculated to correct the injuries of the Mineral Matter. However, this may be said of 'em all in General, that as they all spend their Lives in moist Places, and are still imploy'd in Handling moist Earth, so they are for the most part wan Complexion'd and Cachectick, and a'most always complaining of some illness or other. Those who sit at the Wheel and form the Vessels by turning it with their Feet, are apt to have swimming in the Head, if their Eyes are otherwise weak; and often-times the over tyring of their Feet makes 'em subject to the Sciatica; and therefore we ought to assist 'em with the Remedies prescrib'd by Practitioners in such Cases; which if they do not extirpate, will at least soften and mitigate the Disease.*[46]

He noted, as part of his treatment plans the social situation and economic position of his patients 'they are commonly pinch'd with another Evil, viz.. Extream Poverty. So we are forc'd the flye to the 'Medicina Pauperum', and prescribe such things as at least will mitigate the Illness...advising 'em withal to give over Working at their Trade...,'[47] and, because of this recommended that speedy intervention and solutions are necessary:

> *For upon these occassions the chief Bussiness of a Physician is to restore the Patients to Health with all possible Expedition with proper and generous remedies; Oftentimes you'll hear the miserable Wretches begging thc Physician either to kill 'em or cure 'em out of hand. This then is the chief Caution to be observed in the Cure of such Workmen, that it must be short and expeditious, otherwise the tedious Weight of the disease joyn'd to the Grief of their Mind, pointed to the necessitous Circumstances of their Families, will throw 'em into mortal Consumptions.*[48]

Recognition of the economic constraints and the consequences of these on the health of the poor, led Ramazzini to be critical of the practices of some of his colleagues who failed to take this into account, or who were motivated by greed rather than professional ethics. Despite the fact that some colleagues chose a slow method of treatment, for their own benefit Ramazzini had frequently observed that :

> *if Tradesmen do not recover speedily, they will return to their Shops with the Sickness upon 'em, and oftentimes elude the prolix ('roundabout' in later translation) Cures of Physicians. Tho' these prolix Methods will not do with Handicrafts-men, yet they'll suit a Rich man well enough; for they have a great deal of time on their Hands to be sick in, and sometimes the Ostentation of Riches moves 'em to counterfeit a Fit of Sickness,..*[49]

He continued that moral tone by also recognising the duty of physicians to help people despite their role or status. He argued particularly for the rights of people who undertake unpleasant occupations which benefit large numbers of others. For example, in the case of laundresses because "these women keep us clean, so we must see what benefit the medical profession can provide that may protect them "from lung disorders and brain contamination caused by inhalation of harmful vapours, and from inflammation of the hands:

> *I usually advise 'em, as soon as their Work is over, to throw off their wet things and put on dry Cloathes; in which point they are generally very careless: I advise them likewise to use Frictions (rub themselves); to turn away their Faces as much as they can from the Smoak of the hot Lye, to annoint their hands with Oyntment of Roses or butter, and to observe a regular Diet*[50]

In some ways similar to modern practice, Ramazzini advocated protective or adaptive measures to prevent illness occurring, for example, for the sewer workers:

> *I have advised them to put transparent Bladders over thcir Face, as those do who polish Red Lead, or to spend less time at once at in cleaning the Jakes; or if their Eyes are weak, to leave off that Business and apply themselves to some other Trade, for fear of being oblig'd, for the sake of sordid Lucre to lose their Eyes and so beg for their Bread.*[51]

He argued that it was right and proper that medicine should provide protection for workers whose labour was essential in every city. Indeed, he may have felt a special interest in that group of workers himself as, it was they who first roused his interest in occupational health and safety issues. Ramazzini described how, in the large city in which he lived, dense, high rise housing was the norm, in which it was the custom to have the 'Houses of Offices' (the depository of human waste within buildings) cleaned every third year. He observed one man engaged in the task at his own home, and asked him why he appeared to be rushing and, potentially, straining himself at the work. The man told him that those who took longer than four hours at the task became blind. Subsequent to the work his eyes were found to be 'red and dimmed' when he had finished. The only remedy, he said, was to lie in a darkened room for a day and wash the eyes with warm water. Ramazzini subsequently noted the number of blind beggars who had previously been sewage workers, and became intrigued why it was the eyes rather than other parts of the body, like the lungs, that were affected.

When considering the second major cause of occupational diseases which, it will be recalled, he considered due to 'certain violent and disorderly Motions, and improper Postures of the Body' he observed that some people 'stand all Day, some sit, some have their Faces bended to the Ground, some sit double with their Backs bended, some are oblig'd to run, others to ride, and others again to various sorts of Exercises'[52]. Ramazzini analysed and discussed body physiology as a cause of particular problems. Of the physiological effects on those who work standing he wrote:

> 'Tis worth the while to enquire how it comes to pass, that standing for a little while tires us more than either walking and running for a longer space of time. The common Opinion is that 'tis owing to the tonic Motion of all the antagonist Muscles, whether extended or bended. But this opinion is reputed by the Learned Borelli, who demonstrates, that the Arm is stretched out without the Action of the Flexors or bending Muscles, only by the Active Force of the Extenders; and that the Case is the same in the erected Posture of the Body where all the Benders lie by, and only the Extenders are call'd to act. This Ingenious Author imputes the cause of our being so soon tir'd with standing to the continual and uninterrupted Action of the same muscles; for, he says, Nature delights in alternate and interpolated Actions; and for that reason walking do's not tire us so much; and those who stand alternately on one Foot at a time, are less tir'd than if they stood upon both at once.... This alternate Succession of Action is Agreeable to Nature not only in the Motions of the body, but in most all the natural Functions. For if we look steadily upon one Object, if we listen with our Ears to one Sound, if the same Meat be often serv'd up at Table , if our Nostrils be often expos'd to the same Smells, we are uneasy; so much do' Nature delight in Vicissitude and Change.[53]

Although Ramazzini bemoaned the 'disuse' of running generally when compared to earlier times, he recognised that:

> Those who run are oftentimes liable to acute and grievous Disease of the Breast (Lungs) such as Pleurises and Peripneumonia's.
>
> Motion and Running strengthen the Joynts, as idleness infeebles 'em: But 'tis not so with the lungs, which are heated by the violent Motion, and lose their natural Spring. [54]

For those who did sedentary work:

> Since to do their work they are forced to stoop, the outermost vertebral ligaments are kept pulled apart and contract a callosity, so that it becomes impossible for them to return to the natural position. Wedel noted these simian round shoulders in the case of an aged cobbler, and says it was incurable because the trouble was neglected in his youth. Tailors are often subject to numbness of the legs, lameness, and sciatica, because while they are sewing garments they are almost of necessity obliged to keep one of the legs back against the thigh ... It is a laughable sight to see those guilds of cobblers and tailors on their own special feast-days when they march in procession two by two through the city or escort to the tomb some member of their guild who has died; yes, it makes one laugh to see that troop of stooping, round-shouldered, limping men swaying from side to side; they look as though they had all been carefully selected for an exhibition of these infirmities.[55]

He named the illnesses acquired by workers who stand as ulcerated legs, weakened joints, kidney trouble, bloody urine, and weakness of stomach, and, found them to be:

...subject chiefly to Varices or swellings in the veins; for the tonick motion of the Muscles retards the course of the Blood, upon which it stagnates in the Veins and Valves of the Legs, and makes those Swellings which we call Varices. How much the Distention of the Muscles contributes to retard the Natural Motion of the Blood is apparent to any one that does but feel his own Pulse when his arm is stretch'd out;for then he'll find it very low and small. In the Case now before us, the muscular Fibres of the Legs and the Loyns being stretch'd out, the Arteries that run downwards are therby press'd and straitn'd; so that their Cavity being narrower they don't push forward against the Blood with that Force that takes place in walking, where the alternate Motion of the Muscles conspires to assist 'em: Hence the blood that returns from the Arteries into the Veins do's not receive the necessary Force from the Impulse of the Arteries to make it rise in a perpendicular Line; so that for want of the due Impulse to back it, it stops and makes Varices in the Legs.[56]

Upon the whole, such Tradesmen who are oblig'd to stand when they are at Work, ought to shift their standing Posture as often as they can, either by sitting now and then, or walking or moving the Body any other way.[57]

Ramazzini also discussed the problems that sedentary workers were subject to as a result of lack of exercise:

The Tradesmen that lead a sedentary life, such as Shoemakers and Taylors, are likewise disposed to peculiar Diseases. Both these and other Artifisers, whether Men or Women, who work in a sitting Posture, are, by the sendentary and bending Posture of their body, so form'd, as to have their Backs bended or bow'd, with wry Necks, or their heads hanging down as if they were looking for somewhat on the ground... The Sedentary Trades People use likewise to be Scabby and ill Complexion'd, especially Taylors and Needle-women that work at Home Night and Day; for if the body is not mov'd the Blood grows foul, its Ecrements stick in the Skin, and the whole Habit of the Body is defiled. They are likewise more soluble in the Body than those who follow Exercise. For as Hippocrates informs us, the excrements of the latter are scanty, yellow, and hard...[58]

In time, their sedentary Life exposes 'em to an ill Habit of Body, and manifold Redunancy of vicious Humours. But all sitting Tradesmen are not equally expos'd; for your Potters, Weavers and others who exercise their Hands and Feet and the whole Body, are of a healthier Constitution; the Impurities of their Blood being more easily discuss'd by Vertue of the Motion. The Weavers indeed are wont to complain of a Pain in the Loyns, which proceeds from the violent Motion and Great Force that they are obliged to use in weaving Coarser Cloathe, and that which is made of Hemp:[59]

A separate group of workers with similar problems to those of sedentary or standing workers were those Ramazzini described as "learned men" and about whom he wrote a separate dissertation.

> For your learned men, to use Ficinus's Words, are as as Slothful and Idle in their Body, as they are Active and Busie in their Mind and Brain, and so almost all of 'em, excepting the Practioners of Physick, undergo the Inconveniencies of a sedentary Life inactive in proportion to the activity of their minds and brains," 'Tis a known Saying That a Man grows Wise by sitting; and accordingly they sit Night and Day among the Trophies Inconveniences accruing to their Bodies, till the hidden Causes of Diseases have gradually crept in upon 'em and confined them to their Beds. I have already shewn the Inconveniencess of a sedentary life, and therfore shall not insist upon 'em now.

> The Professors of Learning are likewise not unfrequently subject to the Inconveniences of a standing Life; for to avoid the Injury of a sedentary life, that's so much cry'd down, many of 'em run to the contrary Extream, and stand turning over their books for several Hours and even whole Days, which is not less, nay perhaps more hurtful than constant sitting.

> All the men of learning use to complain of a weakness in the Stomach...
> They likewise contract a Weakness of the Eye-sight by Degrees...[60]

> The Professors of Learning ought therefore to pursue the Study of Wisdom with moderation and Conduct, and not to be so eager upon the Improvement of their Mind, as to neglect the Body: they ought to keep an even balance, so that the Soul and the Body may like Landlord and Guest observe the the dure Measures of Hospitality, and do mutual Offices, and not trample one another under Foot.[61]

Ramazzini advised sedentary workers to exercise and be more balanced in the use of the muscles as a means of maintaining health:

> I can't see what preservatory Cautions can be given to these Tradesmen, as long as the occasional Cause is in Force, and Necessity obliges them to work at their Trade... They must be sure to exercise their Body on Holy Days, and repair the Dammage of many Days sitting by the exercise of some.[62]

and

> In order to avoid the risks or a life of sitting or standing they ought to take moderate exercise every day, but only if the air is bright and calm and there is no wind; gentle rubbing to maintain and to stimulate transpiration should be applied rather often; also bathing in fresh water would be very beneficial, especially in summer, when scholars are particularly liable to become atrabilious; for baths modify thc acrimony of the humors and soften dry, hard viscera; thc best time for the bath will be in the evening, then take food and go to bed. This was the custom and order followed by the ancients; Homer says: "When he had bathed and taken food, he relaxed his limbs in sleep.[63]

and "advice that will help to preserve the health" despite the suggestion that:

> ... they never ask for Advice till they are actually laid upon a sick Bed, or brought under by some of the above-mention'd Disorders; in the Cure of which 'twill still be necessary to have a regard to the occasional Cause. [64]

For those who did fine work, Ramazzini advised them to take regular breaks, similar to advice now given to people who work constantly with visual display units :

> *So injurious is the effect of their occupation on men who do fine work and make the ornate and elaborate objects so much in vogue, timepieces above all, and they incur such grave defects of vision that before they are old they become practically blind. ...*
>
> *... it would help such workers very much if besides wearing spectacles they would give up that habit of keeping the head constantly bent and the eyes fixed on what they are making; if they would now and again drop their work and turn their eyes elsewhere or snatch a respite of several hours from their task and rest their eyes by looking at a number of different things. You would hardly believe how much it helps to preserve the mobility of the membranes of the eye and the natural fluidity of its humors if you gaze at a great variety of objects, some near, some distant, looking now straight ahead, now sideways, in short in every direction. By this method the eye retains the habits that nature gave it, so that the pupil is now contracted, now dilated; and the crystalline humor can when necessary move nearer to the pupil and again recede according as required by the ordinary need to see clearly things distant or close. Otherwise the eye will suffer the same fate as other parts of the body which if kept too long in the same position become stiff.*[65]

Ramazzini gives warning, though, that when providing advise about occupational health it is necessary to consider all people and patients as unique individuals, saying that "we must allow for each man's habits".

His treatise was very wide-ranging and thorough, covering many trades, and applying his discoveries to other types of prescription. In some cases those reflect the prescription of specific occupations for particular purpose or disorder which has formed part of the practice of occupational therapy during much of the twentieth century. For example he recommended that bellringing would assist nuns to keep in health, and that the movements involved in weaving were valuable for treatment of women's menstruation. Indeed, he added that when 'Women complain to me of irregular or inordinate Discharge of their Menses, I generally advise them to consult with working Women or those employ'd in Weaving, rather than with Physicians'.[66] It is doubtful that modern occupational therapists would prescribe the same activities.

In the year 1710, Ramazzini published another book entitled *De Principum Valetudine Tuenda Commentatio* solely for the use of Raynald, Duke of Modena, apparently believing that the health of a good prince was the greatest blessing imaginable to the public. However, with true medical caution, he advised the Duke that if he had regard for his health he should permit his physician to remind him about:

- Changing his clothes, palace, furniture, and method of living according to the seasons,
- Moving into a healthier environment at the start of any epidemical distemper,
- Partaking only a moderate quantity of the delicacies which cover the tables

of the rich, and to resist the temptation to inbibe anything other than that known by experience to agree with their constitution,

• Not engaging in business soon after dinner, nor at all after supper,[67]
• Not being a drunkard,
• Engaging in manly exercises and occupations, appropriate to rank and custom, and especially riding on horse back,
• Indulging in other innocent and genteel recreations, and never failing to admit young people to partake of their diversions,
• Regulating diet, exercise, and evacuations according to the understanding of his physician who knew his constitution through careful study, and
• Avoiding violent passions, since anger, fear, grief, and even excessive joy, have been the causes of death to many.[68]

Figure 1.6.4: Ramazzini's occupational health approach

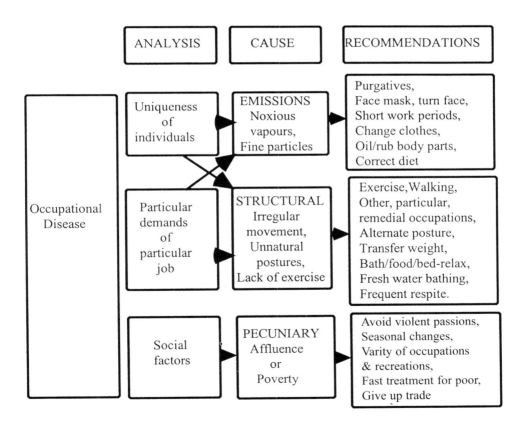

Occupations in every day life: Preventive and remedial care

The third type of intervention of an occupational nature was concerned with everyday living, which drew heavily upon the classical rules for health as set down by Galen and re-articulated by medieval university physicians. Thomas Paynell's original English version of the *Regimen Sanitatis Salerni* of 1528 set the tone for health interventions that made use of the occupations of everyday life. The introduction is reproduced below:

TO THE RYGHT EXCELLENT AND HONORABLE LORDE JOHU ERLE OF OXFORDE, AND HYGH CHAMBERLAYNE OF ENGLANDE THOMAS PAYNELL GREETYNGE.

Redynge of olde authors and stories my most honorable lorde, I fynde, that men in tyme past were of longer lyfe, and of more prosperous helthe, than they are nowe adayes. Whiche thynge as hit greued me, so in maner hit enforced me, to leke the cause of this sodeyne and strage alteracion. For why, it is written, y Adam Iyued. 930. yere. The Sibyls of Cumane liued. iii C. Wynters: Neltor. iii. C. Wynters: Arganton, kynge of Tartesses. iii. C. yeres: and Galen that famous doctor. C. and xl. yeres: but nowe adays (alas) if a man may aproche to. xl. or. lx yeres, men repute hym happy and fortunate. But yet howe many come therto: To serche (gpue) very true reason hereof passeth my small capacite: without I may say hit be, bicause we fulfyll nat the commandementes of almyghty god: whiche to well wyllyng psones are very lyght, and of no burden. For our lorde sayth: My yocke is lwete, and my byrden lyght to be borne.

(Mat. pla. 127) Sayth not the prophet David: that who feareth god, and walketh in his wayes and precept is, shall so his childers children: And Salomon sayth: O my childre, forget nat my preceptes or lawes: for they shall kepe you ploye your days and yeres.

(Prouer. 3) And I will saith our lorde god by David lengthen his dayes. Than may nat this be a reasonable cause of this our so shorte and wretched lyfe: Trewely I suppose hit be by our myslyuynge and fylthy synne: whiche beynge so abominable and so horrible is at som tyme the very cause of corporall infirmite, and of short lyfe. Sayd nat our lorde, the physician of all physicians, to the sicke man: Nowe I have heled thee, depart thou from hens: and loke though syn no more, lest a worse harme happe upo the. Or ther shall I say, y hit chanceth by our mys diete: and to moche surfettynge: Truely the prouerbe sayth, that there dye many mo by surfet, than by the sworde. Accordyng whereto which wyse man sayth: Surfet sleeth many a one: and temperance prolongeth the life. Surfet and diuersites of meates and drynkes, lettyng and corruptyng the digestion febleth man, and very oft causeth this shortnes of lyfe. What other thyng but mys diete caused Ptolomeus Philadelphus to be so miserably and peynefully vexed with the goute: and so (as hit is written) that nothyng could releffe his peyne, sauying dethe. What caused Antipater, and that noble man Mecenas, to be contynually vexed with the feuer, but yll diete. What other thynge infected Aristarcus with the

dropsy, but yll diete. Yll diete (as me thynketh) is chief cause of all dangerous and intollerable diseases: and of the shortenes of mans life. Than hit must nedes folowe, that a teperate and a moderate diete prolongeth mans lyfe: and saueth hym from all suche peynfull diseases. And therefore Alclepiades that noble physician professed. There are 4 necessarie thynges to conserue and prolonge mans prosperite and helthe: that is abstinence from meate, abstinence from wyne, rubbyng of the body, exercise and digestion. O howe holsome is hit than to use good diete, to lyue temperatly, to eschewe excesse of meatis and drinkes. Yea howe greatly are we English men bounde to the maisters of the universite of Salerne (Salerne is in the realme of Naples) which vouchesafed in our behalfe to compile thus necessari, and thus holsome a boke. But what auayleth hit, to haue golde or abundance of riches, if one can nat use hit. What helpeth costely medicines, if one receyue them nat. So what profiteth us a boke, be hit neuer so expedient and frutefull, if we understande hit nat. Wherefore I consydryng the frute which myght come of this boke if hit were translated in to the englishe tongue (for why euery man understandeth nat the latine). I thought hit very expedient at some tymes, for the welthe of unlerned psones to busy my selfe there in: For lerned psones, and such as hauue great experience, nede no instructions to diete them selfe nor to conserue theyr helthe. Yet if suche other wyse and discrete parsons, as if your lordshippe by chance rede this boke: they may pauenture fynde that shall please them: and that besides theyr owne diete and custome of lyuynge, shall be for theyr corporall welfare and good helthe.[69]

Although Paynell's introduction centred mainly on the health consequence of diet, he did mention "exercise" as another necessity, and it was spelt out somewhat further in the work itself as discussed in the last chapter. In its entirety, the work provided the starting point for interest in the occupations of everyday life, particularly as exercise. How they were thought to be related to health was evident in the work of self health adherents, lay and medical practitioners. Amongst the latter, there are some examples of noted practitioner's use of occupation within preventive and remedial care. Because they were leaders in the field, it can be suggested that they are representative of other, less well-known medical men, and that occupation had its place in Renaissance medicine. It can be noted from their recommendations that they recognised a difference between available choices for affluent or poor people and prescribed accordingly. Because of the interest in exercise, the occupations were usually of a gross motor nature and included recognition of work as therapy.

A brief but interesting occupational view was provided by Girolamo Fracastoro of Verona (1478?-1553), a physician, poet, mathematician, astronomer, and geologist of the Italian Renaissance. He is best known for the poem *Syphilis, sive Morbus Gallicus* published in 1530, and which gave the name "syphilis" to a disease which was new, malignant, and of epidemic proportions in his day.[70] He prescribed hard physical exercise, muse and dance for its cure:

Especially guard yourself against laziness and nonchalance. Go, go drive in their dens the bear and the boar; hunt the deer from the crests of the mountains to the foot of the valleys and into the depths of the woods. As a fact, I have often seen the disease clear up by the sweating and cure after long runs in the forests. This is not all. Without false shame, take in hand the plough and turn its share in the bosom of the earth; armed with a hoe tear up the underbrush, strike with an axe the towering oak, uproot the sycamore.

Drive away far from you the anxieties, preoccupations, and regrets; far from you the trouble of passions and the assiduity of serious study! What suits your state is the mild business of the muses, it is joyous complete and frolicsome dances.[71]

Girolamo Cardano (1501-76) of Pavia, a famous Italian mathematician, philosopher, physicist, writer on medical and occult sciences, and physician recommended cold sea baths for skin diseases. Such was his fame, he travelled from Italy to Edinburgh to treat the asthmatic Archbishop of St Andrews, John Hamilton. Cardano recommended to him exercises, sleep, a special diet, and the removal of feathers from his bed. In another sphere he became involved in how to teach people who were blind to read and write, and how to enable people who were deaf-mute to understand a sign language.[72]

Thomas Sydenham, one of the most eminent British physicians of the 17th century, was another who prescribed some occupations for the treatment of physical disorders. Having studied medicine at both Oxford and Cambridge he later practised in London where he became known as the local "Hippocrates", although, apparently in spite of his reputation and skill some colleagues considered him dogmatic and difficult.

In modern times Sydenham is still held in respect, being considered a founder of clinical medicine. He argued for variation in treatment according to disease symptoms, differences in patients' ages and personalities. He was much influenced, in the latter, by the work of John Locke. Sydenham is particularly well known for his work on London epidemics, fevers, dropsy and gout, and had several publications the best known of which is *Observationes Medicae.*[73] He instigated the use of some treatment regimes still in use today, like quinine for malaria, iron for anaemia, and the medical use of opium. For treatment he also followed the rules of the *Regimen Sanitatis*, recommending exercise as well as moderate diet and hydrotherapy. He prescribed carriage riding for the weak, aged and gouty, and horse-riding for phthisis, colic, diarrhoea, constipation, gout and rheumatism, lending his own horses to those without.[74]

Andrew Boarde was another well-known English physician. He worked in Winchester, after graduating from Montpellier, and having studied the medicine of antiquity there, recommended occupations as exercise such as walking, tennis, bowling, or employment. As well as providing exercise, he argued that the chosen occupations should hold interest, probably because it was also his belief that the heart and mind should be happy. In the tradition of the *Regimen*, he warned against incorrect diets, but also over exposure to the sun, and extravagance. Nicholas Andre (1658-1742), Professor of Medicine at the Royal College, Paris, also prescribed occupations for his patients. He favoured riding and hunting for children of upper strata, and rural occupations, such as ploughing, digging, and carrying loads, for their poorer counterparts.[75]

More precise recommendations for various occupations as exercise are provided by Ambroise Paré (1510-90), a well-known French military surgeon regarded by the French as a father of modern surgery,[76] who treated wounds with cleansing, ointments, and surgery to tie major arteries. He trained under a barber-surgeon and before his military career, was a Master Surgeon practising at the "Hotel Dieu", a Paris Hospital. He stressed the need for medical experts to have a sound knowledge of anatomy, but also considered that nature contributed to healing and recovery.[77] He is pictured in figure 1.6.5.

Figure 1.6.5: **Ambroise Paré: Pencil drawing after J. Le Royer, 1561**

(The Wellcome Library)

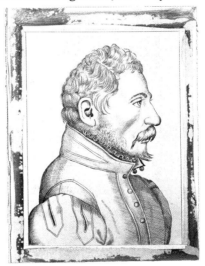

Paré dedicated his *Workes* to King Henry III of France and in the dedication he demonstrated, in a few words, his understanding of the occupational nature of people as individuals and as important contributors to community health:

Even as (most christian King) we see the members of mans body by a friendly consent are always busied, and stand ready to perform those functions for which they are appointed by nature, for the preservation of the whole, of which they are parts; so it is convenient that we, which are, as it were, Citizens of this earthly Common-weale should be diligent in the following of that calling which (by Gods appointment) we have once taken upon us.[78]

In the tradition of the *Regimen Sanitatis*, Paré discussed occupations as exercise under the "non-naturals" of motion and rest. He described the physiological benefits as improved digestion, nourishment, "expulsion" of wastes, internal cleansing, strengthening of respiration and body-limb function and increased tolerance. Even though that explanation no longer fits with current physiological understanding, much of his advice remains relevant and, in many cases, is still valid.

Of motion and rest.

> *Here physicians admonish us, that by the name of motion, we must understand all sorts of exercises, as walking, leaping, running, riding, playing at tennis, carrying a burden, and the like …*

> *The benefit of exercise is great, for it increases naturall heate, whereby better digestion followes, and by that meanes nourishment, and the expulsion of the excrements, and lastly, a quicker motion of the spirits, to performe their offices in the bodie, all the wayes and passages being cleansed. Besides, it strengthens the respiration, and the other actions of the body, confirmes the habite, and all the limbes of the body, by the mutual attrition of the one with the other; whereby it comes to passe they are not so quickly wearied with labour. Hence we see that country people are not to be tired with labour.[79]*

Paré also identified the undesirable consequences of lack of exercise:

> *But, as many and great commodities arise from exercise conveniently begunne and performed, so great harme proceeds of idleness; for grosse and viscious juyces heaped up in the body commonly produce crudities, obstructions, stones both in the reines and bladder, the goute, apoplexie, and a thousand other diseases.[80]*

He goes on to discuss moderation and timing of exercise in terms of bodily benefit or misuse:

> *If any will reape these benefits by exercise, it is necessary that he take opportunity to beginne his exercise, and that he seasonably desist from it, not exercising himself violently and without discretion; but at certain times according to reason.*

> *Wherefore the best time for exercise will be before meate (that the appetite may be encreased by augmenting the natural heate) all the excrements being evacuated, lest nature being hungry and empty, doe draw and infuse the ill humors contained in the guts, and other parts of the body, into the whole habits, the liver, and other noble parts. Neither is it fit presently, after meate, to runne into exercise, lest the crude humors and meats not well concocted be carried into the veines. The measure and bounds of exercise must be, when the body appeares more full, the face lookes red, sweat beginnes to break forth, we breathe more strongly and quicke, and begin to grow weary; if any continue exercise longer, stiffness, and weariness assayles his joints, and the body flowing with sweate suffers a losse of the spirituous and humid substance which is not easily repaired; by which it becomes more cold, and leane even to deformitie.*

> *The qualitie of exercise which we require, is in the midst of exercise, so that the exercise must be neither too slow and idle, neither too strong, nor too weake,*

neither too hasty, nor remisse, but which may move all the members alike. Such
exercise is very fit for sound bodies.[81]

Paré went on to discuss exercise in terms of remediating illness. This is, of
course, described according to the prevailing view of how the humours are
activated by the occupation:

But if they be distempered, that sort of exercise is to be made choice of, which
by the qualitie of its excesse, may correct the distemper of the body, and reduce it
to a certaine mediocritie. Wherefore such men as are stuffed with cold, grosse, and
viscious humors, shall hold that kinde of exercise most fit for them, which is more
laborious, vehement, strong and longer continued. Yet so, that they doe not enter
into it before the first and second concoction, which they may know by the
yellownesse of their urine. But let such as abound with thinne and cholericke
humors chuse gentle exercises, and such as are free from contention, not
expecting the finishing of the second concoction, for the more acride heate of the
solid parts delights in such halfe concocted juices, which otherwise it would so
burne up, all the glutinous sustance there of being wasted, that they could not be
adjoyned, or fastened to the parts. For the repeating, or renewing of exercise, the
body should bee so often exercised, as there is a desire to eate. For exercise stirres
up and revives the heat which lies buried and hid in the body: For digestion
cannot be well performed by a sluggish heate; neither have we any benefit by the
meate we eate, unlesse wee use exercise before.[82]

As in the present day, Paré understood that "cooling down" was an essential
part of exercise regimes:

The last part of exercise begun and performed according to reason, is named
"the ordering of the body", which is performed by an indifferent rubbing, and
drying of the members; that so the sweat breaking forth, the filth of the body, and
such excrements lying under the skinne, may be allured and drawne out; and also
that the members may be freed from stiffness and wearinesse. At this time it is
commonly used by such as play tennis.[83]

He also understood that occupation and rest are parts of a continuum that
cannot be thought about with any thoroughness unless both are taken into
consideration. Sleep and rest are central to the notion of occupational balance,
which in turn is essential to health. Paré said:

Sleepe is nothing else than the rest of the whole body, and the cessation of the
animall facultie from sense and motion. Sleepe is caused, when the substance of
the braine is possessed, and after some sort overcome and dulled by a certaine
vaporous, sweet and delightsome humidity; or when the spirits almost exhaust by
performance of some labour, cannot any longer sustain the weight of the body, but
cause rest by a necessary consequence, by which meanes nature may produce
other from the meate by concoction turned into bloud …

The night is a fit time to sleepe and to take our rest in, as inviting sleepe by
its moisture, silence and darkness.[84]

Figure 1.6.6: **Paré's indications, type, and prescription details of occupations for health**

OCCUPATIONS AS EXERCISE	RESULTS OF IDLENESS	OCCUPATIONS	PRESCRIPTION
* Improved digestion, * Nourishment, * Expulsion of wastes, * Internal cleansing, * Strengthened respiration, * Strengthened body/limb function, * Increased tolerance.	* Crudities, * Obstructions, * Renal stones, * Bladder stones, * Gout * Apoplexy	* Walking, * Leaping, * Running, * Riding, * Playing tennis, * Carrying a burden, *Etc	* Before food, * Involve all body parts, * Moderate, * Cooling down exercises, * Nightime rest, *Cease when red, perspiring, weary, breathing heavily.

Paré prescribed occupation as exercise, especially after fractures, and for leg deformities.[85] He used splints, prostheses, and other orthopaedic aids to assist with problems he was not able or willing to tackle surgically, providing his patients with advice and instructions on their use. The design of some of these is remarkably similar to those of today, despite a difference in materials used. Based on a real case in which the median nerve was severed, Paré described how such an injury could be sustained, the occupational consequences on physical and psychological functioning, and of the need for, and design of a thumb (or finger) stall shown in figure 1.6.7:

> When a synew or tendon is cut cleane asunder, the action of that part, whereof it was the author, is altogether abolished, so that the member cannot bend or stretch out it selfe, unlesse it bee holpen by art: Which thing I performed in a certain French horseman, who in the battle of Dreux received so great a wound with a back sword, upon the outside of the wrest of the right hand, that the tendons that did erect or draw up the thumb were cut cleane insunder, & also when the wound was throughly whole and consolidated, the thumb was bowed inwards, and felle into the palme of the hand, so that he could not extend or lift it up, unlesse it wer by the helpe of the other hand, and then it would presently fall downe againe; by reason wherof he could hold neither sword, speare or javeline in his hand, so that he was altogether unprofitable for war, without which he

supposed there was no life. Therefore he consulted me about the cutting away of his thumbe, which did hinder his griping, which I refused to doe, and told him that I conceived a meanes how it might bee remedied without cutting away. Therfore I caused a case to bee made for it of latine, whereinto I put the thumb: this case was so artificially fastened by two strings that were put into two rings, made in it above the joint of the hand, that the tumbe stood upright, and straight out, by reason whereof he was able afterwards to handle any kinde of weapon.[86]

Figure 1.6.7: **Paré - 'The forme of a thumbe or finger-stall of iron or latine, to lift up or erect the thumb, or any other finger that cannot be erected of itselfe'**[87]
(British Library)

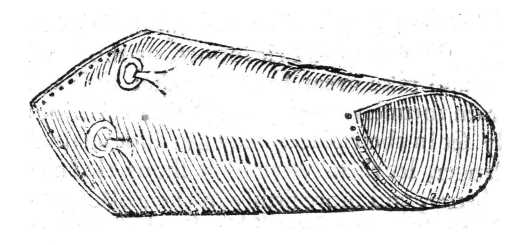

He also described the manufacture of what would now be known as a radial nerve, or "wrist cock up" splint shown in figure 1.6.8:

If that in any man the sinews or tendons which hold the hand upright, be cut asunder with a wound, so that he is not able to lift up his hand, it may easily bee erected or lifted up with this instrument that followeth, being made of an equall, streight, thin, but yet strong plate of latine, lined on the inner side with silke, or any such like soft thing, and so plac't in the wrest of the hand, that it may come unto the palme, or the first joints of the fingers, and it must bee tyed above with convenient stayes, and so the discommodity of the depression, or hanging of the hand, may bee avoyded; therefore this instrument may be called the erector of the hand'.[88]

Figure 1.6.8: **Paré - "The erector of the hand"**[89]
(British Library)

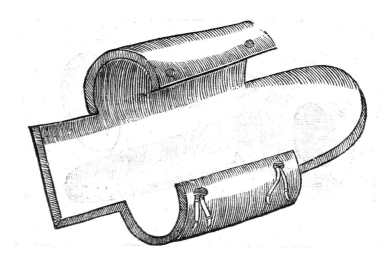

Whilst prevention of disease was becoming part of the public domain, the promotion of health, in general, appears to have continued to be a subject which many educated people chose to consider as important, and some to write about. Sir John Sinclair republished a number of such writings in *Code of Health & Longevity*. Included in the collection was the work of Lewis Cornaro, a noble Venetian, who wrote four parts of the lengthy *A Treatise on a Sober Life* from 1558 onwards.

Cornaro had suffered illness as a result of his 'intemperance until he was about 40 years old', when he became 'a man of sound understanding, determined courage and resolution'. Realising the consequences of 'his passion and inordinate appetites' he recovered his health and vigour by sobriety and a healthy dietary regime. Living to extreme old age he wrote the first of his treatises at the age of eighty-three, and the second, at eighty-six, in which he discussed the means of mending a bad constitution. 'He says that he came into the world with a choleric disposition, but that his temperate way of life had enabled him to subdue it.' His third and fourth treatises he wrote at ninety-one and ninety-five, the latter containing a lively description of the health, vigour, and perfect use of all his faculties which he enjoyed in his advanced years.[90]

He was certainly not occupationally deprived, mentioning many occupations in which he engaged as part of his healthy "sober" life. These included horse riding, walking and hill-climbing, discourse with men of letters, reading, writing comedy, travelling, hunting, gardening, playing with his grandchildren, and singing:

I will therefore give an account of my recreations, and the relish which I find at this stage of life, in order to convince the public (which may likewise be done by all those who know me) that the state I have now attained to is by no means death, but real life; such a life as by many is deemed happy, since it abounds with all the felicity that can be enjoyed in this world.

And this testimony they will give, in the first place, because they see, and not without the greatest amazement, the good state of health and spirits I enjoy; how I mount my horse without any assistance, or advantage of situation and how I not only ascend a single flight of stairs, but climb up a hill from bottom to top, afoot, and with the greatest ease and unconcern; then how gay, pleasant, and good-humoured, I am; how free from every perturbation of mind, and every disagreeable thought; in lieu of which, joy and peace have so firmly fixed their residence in my bosom as never to be part from it. Moreover, they know in what manner I pass my time, so as not to find life a burden; seeing I can contrive to spend every hour of it with the greatest delight and pleasure, having frequent opportunities of conversation with many honourable gentlemen, men valuable for their good sense and manners, their acquaintance with letters, and every other good quality. Then, when I cannot enjoy their conversation, I betake myself to the reading of some good book. When I have read as much as I like, I write; endeavouring in this, as in every thing else, to be of service to others, to the utmost of my power. And all these things I do with the greatest ease to myself, at their proper seasons, and in my own house.[91]

Cornaro enjoyed sufficient affluence to indulge his interests:

Besides this house, I have my several gardens supplied with running waters, and in which I always find something to do that amuses me. I have another way of diverting myself, which is, going every April and May, and likewise every September and October, for some days, to enjoy an eminence belonging to me in the Euganean mountains, and in the most beautiful part of them, adorned with fountains and gardens; and, above all, a convenient and handsome lodge, in which place I likewise now and then make one in some hunting party suitable to my taste and age … I see the palaces, gardens, antiquities; and with these the squares and other public places, the churches, the fortifications, leaving nothing unobserved, from whence I may reap either entertainment or instruction[92]

He described indulging in occupations that he associated with children or youth:

I will further venture to say, that such are the effects of this sober life, that, at my present age of eighty-three, I have been able to write a very entertaining comedy, abounding with innocent mirth and pleasant jests. This species of composition is generally the child and offspring of youth, as tragedy is that of old age; the former being, by its facetious and sprightly turn, suited to the bloom of life, and the latter, by its gravity, adapted to riper years.[93]

As part of his health giving occupations of older age Cornaro explained his enjoyment of his grandchildren with whom he played:

I find there, before me, not one or two, but eleven, grandchildren, the oldest of them eighteen, and the youngest two; all the offspring of one father and one mother; all blessed with the best health; and, by what as yet appears, fond of learning, and of good parts and morals. Some of the youngest I always play with, and, indeed, children from three to five are only fit for play. Those above that age I make companions of; and, as nature has bestowed very fine voices upon them, I amuse myself, besides, with seeing and hearing them sing, and play on various instruments. Nay, I sing myself, as I have a better voice now, and a clearer and louder pipe, than at any other period of life. Such are the recreations of my old age.[94]

He boasted that 'indeed, if I may be allowed to be an impartial judge in my own cause, I cannot help thinking that I am now of sounder memory and understanding, and heartier, than (Sophocles) was when ten years younger'.[95] Cornaro was over 100 when he died 'without pain or agony, and like one who falls asleep'.[96]

Sinclair also republished the work of Guilielmus Gratarolu, a Piedmontese whose book *De Literatorum, et Eorum qui Magistratum Gerunt, Conservanda Valetudine* was published in 1555. Gratarolu urged moderation in five activities; namely, eating, drinking, labour, sleep, and concubinage affirming that those great fathers of physic, Hippocrates and Galen recommended the same moderation as the principal means to secure health.[97] In contrast, Hieronimus Cardan who was born in Pavia in 1550 wrote about his many contrary views. For example, he criticised Hippocrates and Galen for their prescriptions of exercise as health giving:

He exclaims … against using any exercise that can fatigue a man in the smallest degree, or throw him into the most gentle sweat, or in the least accelerate his respiration; and gravely observes, that trees live longer than animals, because they never stir from their places.[98]

Another in Sinclair's collection was work by Sanctorius Sanctorius, an Italian physician mentioned in the last chapter. Sanctorius spent a few years as physician to the King of Poland, practised physic at Venice where he was held in high esteem, and was a celebrated professor at Padua. The founder of the physiology of metabolism, he is regarded as an originator of quantitative medical research because of his introduction of exact methods of measurement such as pulse taking, weight taking, and determining temperature using a thermometer.[99] He establishing several laws which were useful to physicians and for the preservation of health generally. Some excerpts from Sanctorius' major work, *Medicina Statica* (Rules of Health), are provided below.[100] The first sections quoted from the chapter on exercise and rest provide an indication of the health giving function of perspiration as a means of eliminating excessive humours, which was deemed essential by the humoural physiologists. They suggest a different role for occupation in the promotion and restoration of health to that suggested by modern therapists:

IV. The body perspires much more lying quietly in bed than turning from one side to another by frequent agitation.

V. Cheerful and angry persons are less wearied by long travelling than the fearful and pensive: for the former perspire more healthfully, but the other less.

VI. Those bodies which are admitted to refection, (defined as refreshment with food and drink or a light meal) *after immoderate exercise, receive much prejudice; because, as they are wearied and burthened with meat, they perspire less.*

VII. Exercise from the seventh hour to the twelfth after refection, does insensibly dissolve more in the space of one hour than it does in three hours at any other time.

XV. An excessive rest of the mind does more obstruct perspiration than that of the body.

XXI. By exercise the body perspires less, by sleep, more, and the belly is more loosened.

XXIV. Swimming immediately after violent exercise, is hurtful; for it very much obstructs perspiration.

XXXII. The exercise of the top, consisting of moderate and violent motion, to-wit, walking and the agitation of the arms, promotes perspiration.

XXXIII. Moderate dancing, without any capering or jumping, comes near the commendation of moderate walking; for it moderately expels the concocted perspirable matter.[101]

Sanctorius offered other rules concerned with types of exercise or occupations and the timing of them:

XIII. If a person who has kept his bed long be troubled with pain in the feet, the remedy is walking; if one that is upon a journey be so troubled, the remedy is rest.

XIV. There are two kinds of exercises, one of the body, the other of the mind: that of the body evacuates the sensible excrements: that of the mind the insensible rather, and especially those of the heart and brain, where the mind is seated.

XVI. The exercises of the mind which most conduce to the cheering up of the spirits, are anger, sudden joy, fear, and sorrow.

XVII. Men's bodies resting in bed, and agitated with a vehement motion of the mind, for the most part become more faint, and less ponderous, than if there be a tranquility of mind, with a violent motion of the body, as it happens at tennis, or any game at ball.

XIX. Violent exercise of mind and body renders bodies of lighter, hastens old age, and threatens untimely death: for, according to the philosopher, those persons that are exercised die sooner than such as are not.

XXV. Violent exercise in a place where the wind blows is hurtful.

XXVI. From the wind proceeds a difficulty of respiration, from the motion, acrimony.

XXVII. Riding relates more the perspirable matter of the parts of the body from the waist upwards, than downwards, but in riding, the amble is the most wholesome, the trot the most unwholesome, pace.[102]

He gave particular attention to "study", perhaps because he, himself, must have experienced many hours of "exercising his mind" engaged in what is most usually a fairly static occupation. Other health practitioners who subscribed to the theories of the *Regimen Sanitatis* were also fascinated by the health outcomes that resulted from studious occupations, often recommending, for example, that "princes" avoid study at particular times of day. Sanctorius proclaimed that:

> *XLV. Study, without any affection, hardly endures an hour; with any one affection, hardly four hours; with vicissitude of affections, as at dice, at which kind of gaming men feel, one while the joy for winning, another, sadness for losing, it may continue night and day.*
>
> *XLVI. In all study continual sadness disturbs the good constitution of the heart, and excess of gladness hinders sleep; for every excess is destructive to nature* [103]

Surprising to many modern practitioners, Sanctorius also linked study and emotions with perspiration.

Maybe, one could expect that in Italy there would be continued observation, application and up dating of the rules generated in the *Regimen Sanitatis*. In Scotland too, however, it was used during the Renaissance. A Gaelic manuscript, containing 62 vellum folios making up the early 16th century version, was owned by John Macbeath whose family were 'hereditary physicians to the Lords of the Isles and to the Kings of Scotland for several centuries'. [104] Figure 1.6.9 is a copy of the hand written first page of the Regimen.

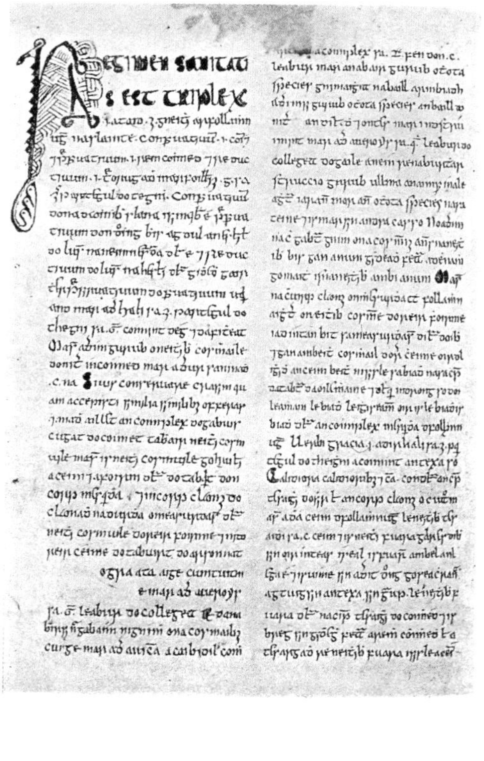

Figure 1.6.9:   **Regimen Sanitatis est triplex: Early 16th century Gaelic manuscript** [105]

In English, the start of the chapter begins with clarifying notions about the prevention of illness, and the maintenance and restoration of health, using three divisions of health care similar to Mercurialis illustrated in figure 1.6.2:

> *Regimen Sanitatis est triplex, that is, there are three aspects of the Regulation of the health. Conseruatiuum, that is, guarding, (or maintaining the healthy state); and Preseruattiuum, that is, fore-seeing; and Reductiuum, that is guiding backwards (restoration) as Galen shows in the third Particle of his Tegni. Conseruatiuum to the healthy men, it is right. Preseruattiuum to those who are going into unhealth and to those of debility, it is a duty. And Reductiuum to such as are in illness, it is necessary.*[106]

Whilst this version, like those discussed in the last chapter, has much about nutrition, it too links nutrition with occupation, as for example in the seventh chapter on age and temperament:

> *And those given to study should be nourished like old people, for the studying dries them; so let them eat tender things according to their sufferance (as they can bear them) so that their blood is replenished quickly and well. Those who labour, however, let them eat roasted fat things for these are the things that resist (the waste) of labour.*[107]

> *… Galen said Commedo ut uiuam non uiua commedam, that is, it is said to be in life that I eat and not for eating that I am in life.*[108]

> *… And those of black humours bear it (hunger) better than those of red humours for the heat is less which they set free within them, and they spend more upon the thing (or work) upon which they employ themselves.*[109]

> *… do not think it foolish to have a walk after the meal, and avoid the sleep of the middle-day.*[110]

Mobility

'Before the advent of adaptive devices to help with mobility, many people with severe disability had to crawl about', if they survived. Such crawling or creeping resulted in them being known as "creepples"–cripples. Covey suggests that 'societies generally looked upon crawling as a means of human mobility with disfavour' because historically it is associated with animals. It was also a much less functional method of mobility for humans, whose arms and legs differ in length, and who need hands free to engage in the other everyday occupations of life. Perhaps for that reason, other means of mobilising with an upright stance have been sought.

Although relatively rare, particularly in early examples, in both art and literature the most frequently depicted or mentioned aid for people with disability was a staff, cane or crutch. A few Renaissance painters included such aids in their works, such as Hieronymus Bosch (1450-1516), Pieter Bruegel the Elder (1525-1569), and the Flemish artist Hieronymus Cock (1520-1570). In Cock's engraving of 31 disabled "Beggars" many devices are illustrated which were used to assist mobility. Additionally some of the subjects clearly demonstrate that begging was carried out as, perhaps, the major occupations open to people with physical disability. At least a couple are dressed in fools costumes, a few carried lutes and one a harp, as well as begging bowls in the way of present day buskers who are socially disadvantaged.[111]

Figure 1.6.10: **Detail from 'A Variety of Crippled Beggers' Wood engraving by A Rivaud, 1892, after a tapestry in Reims.**

(The Wellcome Library)

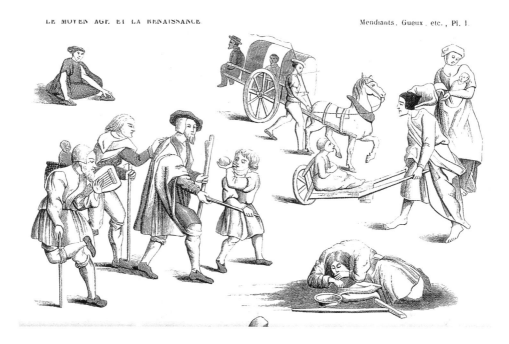

Paré described and illustrated a crutch to assist with 'amending or helping lamenesse or halting' which he described as 'not onely a great deformity, but also very troublesome and grievous'. He attributed the design of the crutch to Nicholas Picard, chirurgian to the Duke of Loraine. The crutch, featured as figure 1.6.11, is ingenious, in assisting a user with one leg shorter than the other to stand and walk upright 'more easily and with little labour or no pain at all'.

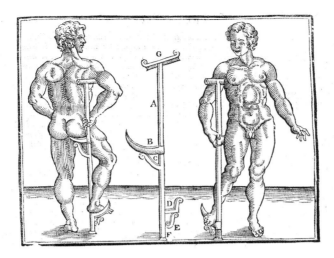

Figure 1.6.11: **Paré's crutch, attributed to Nicholas Picard, to amend "halting"**[112]
(British Library)

Adaptive wheeled devices were also used during the period. The painting by Lucas Cranach the Elder (1472-1553) of the *Fountain of Youth* depicts a wheelbarrow, a litter, and a cart transporting people for rejuvenation and, perhaps, miracle cures, along with fertility and fecundity. Furniture makers, too occassionally modified furniture to assist mobility, by adding wheels or rollers to chairs. Some even had cogwheels included in their design to allow people to propel themselves.

Figure 1.6.12: **A crippled dwarf being helped to a wheelchair by a monk. Pen and ink drawing after a design attributed to P.L.Ghezzi.**
(The Wellcome Library)

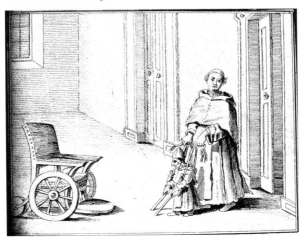

Perhaps an example of the ultimate of sophistication of the day is "the flying chair" invented by Jean Jacques de Renouard which lifted people from one level to another.[113]

In summary, the Renaissance was a time of change from charitable services for the physically sick being provided by the church and considered as a secondary consideration to the soul, to them being more and more the province of medical experts and of importance in their own right. It was a period of earnest endeavour and exploration. The humanist ideas, which encouraged individuals to recognise and develop their capacities and potential, assisted medically trained personnel and others to follow an interest in matters relating to health. That facilitated a growth of basic scientific exploration, some resulting in specialties that provide foundation knowledge in the education of occupational therapists.

More than that, the period was one in which occupation was used as therapy by leading medical authorities and self health practitioners as exercise within daily life for both the affluent and, although one suspects only occasionally, for the poor. Gross motor occupations appear to have been most often prescribed, but following an analysis of both scientific and popular current literature, the same would be found to be the case nowadays. However, there is some evidence that during the Renaissance how and when the occupations should be used was carefully prescribed, within the context of other daily events.

It was also the historical period when illness-causing occupations were recognised and their study developed as a speciality. Although some occupational therapists work in the sphere of occupational health and safety, it is the ergonomic aspects that have claimed most of their attention rather than the negative effects of some occupations on health. It could be argued that for occupational therapists to be regarded as experts in occupation for health they need to be as knowledgeable about the negative as well as the positive results of engagement. In the Renaissance, both were recognised, but as in the present day, medicine was more interested in the illness effects.

[1]Kirkman Gray B. A History of English Philanthropy. London: P. S. King and Son, 1905; 15.
[2]Isaacs A, ed. Thomas Linacre. In: Macmillan Encyclopedia. London: Macmillan, 1990; 725.
[3]Harvey P, ed. The Oxford Companion to English Literature. 4th edition. Oxford: Clarendon Press, 1967; 479.
[4]Porter R. Disease, Medicine and Society in England 1550-1860. Basingstoke and London: Macmillan Education, 1987.
[5]Porter. Disease, Medicine and Society.
[6]Porter. Disease, Medicine and Society.
[7]Porter. Disease, Medicine and Society.
[8]Porter. Disease, Medicine and Society.
[9]Porter. Disease, Medicine and Society…; 13-17.
[10]Porter R. The Greatest Benefit to Mankind: A Medical History of Humanity from

Antiquity to the Present. Harper Collins (first published 1997). Paper back edition 1999; 126-128.

[11]Macdonald EM. World-Wide Conquests of Disabilities: The History, Development and Present Functions of the Remedial Services. London: Baillieie Tindall, 1981.

[12]Macdonald. World-Wide Conquests of Disabilities.

[13]Isaacs. Macmillan Encyclopedia…; 1264.

[14]Girling DA, ed. New Age Encyclopaedia. 7th edition. Sydney & London: Bay Books, 1983.

[15]Macdonald. World-Wide Conquests of Disabilities…; 62.

[16]Macdonald. World-Wide Conquests of Disabilities…; 64.

[17]Blundell JWF. The Muscles and their Story from the Earliest Times (an Adaptation of the 'Ars Gymnastica') including the Whole Text of Mercurialis, and the Opinions of other Writers Ancient and Modern on Mental and Bodily Development. London: Chapman & Hall, 1864; 34-36.

[18]Georgii A, ed. Ling's Educational and Curative Exercises. London: Renshaw, 1875; 12.

[19]Marti-Ibañez F, ed. Henry E. Sigerist on the History of Medicine. New York: MD Publications, Inc., 1960; 49-51.

[20]Macdonald. World-Wide Conquests of Disabilities…; 67-68.

[21]Kirkman Gray. A History of English Philanthropy.

[22]Kersler GD, Glyn G. The History of the Royal National Hospital for Rheumatic Diseases Bath. Bath: Friends of the Royal National Hospital, 1965; 4.

[23]Macdonald. World-Wide Conquests of Disabilities…; 67-68.

[24]Porter. Disease, Medicine and Society in England.

[25]Kaske CV, Clark JR, eds. Marsilio Ficino. On a long life. In: Three Books on Life: A Critical Edition and Translation with Introduction and Notes. Binghamton: Centre for Medieval and Early Renaissance Studies, 1989.

[26]Kaske & Clark. Marsilio Ficino. On a long life…; 131.

[27]Marti-Ibañez. Henry E. Sigerist on the History of Medicine…; 49.

[28]Ulrich Ellenbog. Von den Gifftigen Besen Tempffen und Reuchen, 1473. Eine gewerbehygienische Schrift des XV. Jahrhunderts, herausgegeben von Franz Koelsch und Friedrich Zoepfl, Munich, 1927 (Reprint). In: Marti-Ibañez. Henry E. Sigerist on the History of Medicine…; 49.

[29]Isaacs. Macmillan Encyclopedia…; 924.

[30]Girling. New Age Encyclopaedia.

[31]Marti-Ibañez. Henry E. Sigerist on the History of Medicine…; 49-50.

[32]Macdonald. World-Wide Conquests of Disabilities…; 61.

[33]Girling. New Age Encyclopaedia.

[34]Isaacs. Macmillan Encyclopedia…; 19.

[35]Agricola G. De Re Metallica, translated from the first Latin edition of 1556 by H. C. Hoover and L. H. Hoover, London, 1912.

[36]Agricola. De Re Metallia.

[37]Cited in: Marti-Ibañez. Henry E. Sigerist on the History of Medicine…; 50.

[38]Marti-Ibañez. Henry E. Sigerist on the History of Medicine…; 51.

[39]Ramazzini B. Of the diseases of tradesmen. In: Health Preserved in 2 Treatises. 2nd edition. London: J Whiston, 1750; Foreword.

[40]Marti-Ibañez. Henry E. Sigerist on the History of Medicine…; 51.

[41]Ramazzini B. A Treatise Of The Diseases Of Tradesmen, Shewing The Various Influence Of Particular Trades Upon The State Of Health; With The Best Methods To Avoid Or Correct It, And Useful Hints Proper To Be Minded In Regulaing The Cure Of All Diseases Incident To Tradesmen. London: Printed for Andrew Bell, Ralph Smith, Danial Midwinter, Will. Hawes, Will. Davies, Geo. Straghan, Bern. Linot, Ja. Round, and

Jeff. Wale. 1705; 1-2.

[42]Ramazzini B. Diseases of Workers revised. The Latin text of 1713 Translated by Wilmer Cave Wright, Chicago; University of Chicago Press 1940. New York: Hafner Publishing, 1964; 87

[43]Ramazzini. Diseases of Workers…; 89.

[44]Ramazzini. A Treatise of the Diseases of Tradesmen 1705…; 29-30.

[45]Ramazzini. Diseases of Workers…; 57.

[46]Ramazzini. A Treatise of the Diseases of Tradesmen 1705…; 32-34.

[47]Ramazzini. A Treatise of the Diseases of Tradesmen 1705…; 33.

[48]Ramazzini. A Treatise of the Diseases of Tradesmen 1705…; 54.

[49]Ramazzini. A Treatise of the Diseases of Tradesmen 1705…; 55.

[50]Ramazzini. A Treatise of the Diseases of Tradesmen 1705…; 169-170.

[51]Ramazzini. A Treatise of the Diseases of Tradesmen 1705…; 66.

[52]Ramazzini. A Treatise of the Diseases of Tradesmen 1705…; 189.

[53]Ramazzini. A Treatise of the Diseases of Tradesmen 1705…; 192.

[54]Ramazzini. A Treatise of the Diseases of Tradesmen 1705…; 203, 204

[55]Ramazzini. Diseases of Workers…; 283.

[56]Ramazzini. A Treatise of the Diseases of Tradesmen 1705…; 189-190.

[57]Ramazzini. A Treatise of the Diseases of Tradesmen 1705…; 193.

[58]Ramazzini. A Treatise of the Diseases of Tradesmen 1705…; 193-4.

[59]Ramazzini. A Treatise of the Diseases of Tradesmen 1705…; 194-5.

[60]Ramazzini. A Treatise of the Diseases of Tradesmen 1705…; 247-249

[61]Ramazzini. A Treatise of the Diseases of Tradesmen 1705…; 273.

[62]Ramazzini. A Treatise of the Diseases of Tradesmen 1705…; 195.

[63]Ramazzini. Diseases of Workers…; 401.

[64]Ramazzini. A Treatise of the Diseases of Tradesmen 1705…; 205.

[65]Ramazzini. Diseases of Workers …; 327.

[66]Ramazzini. Diseases of Workers …; 406.

[67]Ramazzini. Diseases of Workers …; 210.

[68]Ramazzini. Diseases of Workers …; 211.

[69]Paynell T. Introduction to Regimen Sanitatis Salerni. England: 1528.

[70]Clendenning L. Source Book of Medical History. (with notes). Dover: 1960, (an unabridged and unaltered republication of the work originally published in 1942 by Constable and Company, Ltd., 10 Orange Street, London W.C. 2.).
Girolamo Fracastoro Translations: The "Syphilis" has several times been translated into English:
(1) First in 1685, by Nahum Tate (1652-1692), poet laureate (partially reprinted in Major's "Classic Descriptions of Disease").
(2) Philmar Company, St. Louis, Mo., 1 9 1 1, prose.
(3) Dr. William van Wych, "The Sinister Shepherd," Primavera Press, Los Angeles, Calif., 1934, in rhymed quatrains.
(4) Heneage Wynn Finch, "Fracastor — Syphilis or the French Disease," London, William Heinemann, 1935

[71]Clendenning. Source Book of Medical History…; 116.

[72]Macdonald. World-Wide Conquests of Disabilities…; 62.

[73]Sydenham T. Observationes Medicae. London: 1676.

[74]Macdonald. World-Wide Conquests of Disabilities…; 70.

[75]Macdonald. World-Wide Conquests of Disabilities…; 58-72.

[76]Isaacs. Macmillan Encyclopedia…; 926.

[77]Macdonald. World-Wide Conquests of Disabilities…; 66.

[78]Paré A. The Author's dedication to Henry the third, the most Christian King of France

and Poland. 1579. In: Johnson T. The Workes of that Famous Chirurgion Ambrose Parey Translated out of Latin and Compared with the French. Printed by Th Cotesand R Young, 1634.

[79]Johnson. The Workes of that Famous Chirurgion Ambrose Parey…; 34.

[80]Johnson. The Workes of that Famous Chirurgion Ambrose Parey…; 35.

[81]Johnson. The Workes of that Famous Chirurgion Ambrose Parey…; 34-35.

[82]Johnson. The Workes of that Famous Chirurgion Ambrose Parey…; 34-35.

[83]Johnson. The Workes of that Famous Chirurgion Ambrose Parey…; 34-35.

[84]Johnson. The Workes of that Famous Chirurgion Ambrose Parey…; 35-36.

[85]Macdonald. World-Wide Conquests of Disabilities…; 66.

[86]Johnson. The Workes of that Famous Chirurgion Ambrose Parey…; 878.

[87]Johnson. The Workes of that Famous Chirurgion Ambrose Parey…; 878.

[88]Johnson. The Workes of that Famous Chirurgion Ambrose Parey…; 878.

[89]Johnson. The Workes of that Famous Chirurgion Ambrose Parey…; 879.

[90]Cornaro LA. A treatise on a sober life. In: Sinclair, Sir J. Code of Health & Longevity. Edinburgh: Arch Constable & Co., 1806; 50-52.

[91]Cornaro. A treatise on a sober life…; 73-74 .

[92]Cornaro. A treatise on a sober life…; 74-76.

[93]Cornaro. A treatise on a sober life…; 77.

[94]Cornaro. A treatise on a sober life…; 78-79.

[95]Cornaro. A treatise on a sober life…; 78.

[96]Cornaro. A treatise on a sober life…; 52.

[97]Sinclair J. The Code of Health and Longevity. Volume III. Edinburgh; Printed for Arch. Constable and Co.; and T. Cadell and W. Davies, and J. Murray, London, 1806; 121.

[98]Sinclair. The Code of Health and Longevity…; 117.

[99]Girling. New Age Encyclopaedia…; vol 25: 202.

[100]Sanctorius Sanctorius. Medicina Statica. In: Sinclair. Code of Health and Longevity.

[101]Sinclair. Code of Health and Longevity…; 175-178.

[102]Sinclair. Code of Health and Longevity…; 176-178.

[103]Sinclair. Code of Health and Longevity…; 189.

[104]Cameron Gillies H. Regimen Sanitatis: The Rule of Health: A Gaelic Medical Manuscript of the Early Sixteenth Century or Perhaps Older. Glasgow: Printed for the author by Robert Maclehose & Co. Ltd., University Press, 1911; Introduction.

[105]Cameron Gillies. Regimen Sanitatis.

[106]Cameron Gillies. Regimen Sanitatis.

[107]Cameron Gillies. Regimen Sanitatis…; 51.

[108]Cameron Gillies. Regimen Sanitatis…; 52.

[109]Cameron Gillies. Regimen Sanitatis…; 52.

[110]Cameron Gillies. Regimen Sanitatis…; 52.

[111]Covey HC. Social Perceptions of People with Disabilities in History. Springfield, Illinois; Charles C. Thomas, 1998; 46.

[112]Johnson. The Workes of that Famous Chirurgion Ambrose Parey…; 884.

[113]Covey. Social Perceptions of People with Disabilities in History…; 49.

Part 3

Enlightened Times

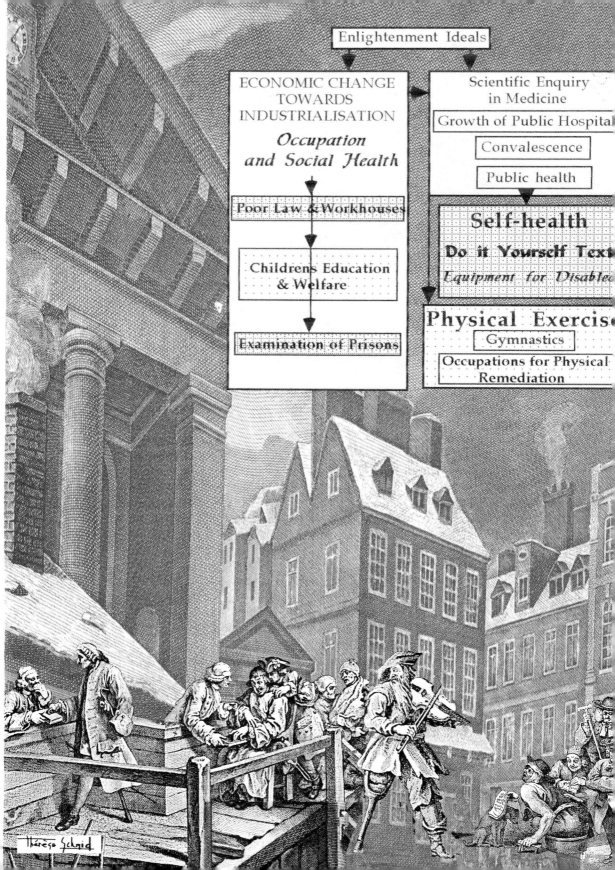

Enlightenment Ideals

ECONOMIC CHANGE TOWARDS INDUSTRIALISATION

Occupation and Social Health

Poor Law & Workhouses

Childrens Education & Welfare

Examination of Prisons

Scientific Enquiry in Medicine

Growth of Public Hospital

Convalescence

Public health

Self-health

Do it Yourself Text

Equipment for Disabled

Physical Exercise

Gymnastics

Occupations for Physical Remediation

Thérèse Schnid

Chapter 7

Occupation for Social and Physical Health in Enlightened Times

Contents

It can be said that modern medicine rests on the heritage of Aesculapius, Hippocrates and Galen. It has also grown from more recent scholarship such as the landmark publication of Vesalius' major work on anatomy (1543) and William Harveys' discovery of the circulation of blood (1628). It was not until the Enlightenment, the so-called Age of Reason, however, that orthodox authoritarian beliefs were replaced with rational scientific inquiry.

Armed with that thought, in this section of the history the foundations of modern occupational therapy will be explored. This, too, grew from the heritage of earlier ideas that can be linked with Hippocrates' and Galens' regimens for a Healthy Life and, in the same vein, with Hygiea rather than the heroic traditions of Aesclepius. The health promotion and illness prevention concept did not get lost in the Middle Ages but, in the context of that time, became largely subservient to a spiritual view of the relationship between occupation and health. It grew again, in a relatively modern sense, as the written word carried the ideas further afield so that they reached more people. Additionally, as Enlightenment thinkers espoused liberty and individuality along with scientific discovery and industrial capitalism, occupation was viewed as a necessity for the remediation of social ill health. That was, in large part, due to the way industriousness was deemed to be of inestimable worth.

During the eighteenth century, three occupationally based social health issues demanded attention. The first was unemployment, often for people with mental or physical ill health or disability, the aged, the young and the socially disempowered. The second was lack of education and vocational training for pauper young. The third was the appalling conditions in places of detention like gaols and Bridewells. These issues were largely tackled at a population level, which perhaps points to a different way forward for occupational therapists in the 21st century as they encounter and address problems of occupational deprivation and occupational injustice.

Despite the modern day World Health Organisation recognising social as well as physical and mental well-being as a component of good health, and its having been addressed in the eighteenth century, it was largely overlooked in the twentieth by medically based practitioners. That has been unfortunate for occupational therapists because occupation is an entity that interlinks social and medical domains and provides scope for practice that has been largely unexplored. Despite that, occupation for social health has been found to be effective across physical health domains. For example, there is plentiful research evidence that unemployment is related to an increase in most types of morbidity and some mortality,[1] and that lack of meaning in employment can be as detrimental to health as unemployment.[2] There is also evidence that there are significant benefits for the independent elderly in preventive occupation programs across health, function, and quality of life domains;[3] and even that social and productive occupations do not have to have apparent physical "exercise" benefits to lower the risk of all cause mortality.[4] Occupational therapy, as it becomes a force for health from its own perspective and in its own right will, hopefully, take on a more dominant role in social health issues as the next century progresses along with an illness preventive and health promotive approach.

The Enlightenment was the time when a belief in an individual's right to moral autonomy and self-realisation began to surface.[5] As those ideas are central to the modern discipline of occupational therapy it is important to explore, albeit briefly, their development, and the people who espoused them, in order to understand their place in health care and their influence in the present. The chapter also contains a brief discussion about the social context of the age largely from an occupational perspective, and informative extracts from contemporary sources about occupational initiatives taken to address social health issues typified by what happened in charity schools, workhouses and gaols.

An understanding of the social background sets the scene for the inquiry into physical health through occupation, which is advanced later in the chapter. To capture that story, issues explored range through the growth of hospitals and organisation of medical services, lay practitioners and self health. The latter became particularly important as during that period greater literacy led to a proliferation of published works, some of which included notions of the relationship of occupation with maintaining health. That is followed by discussion of new theories with potential occupational therapy ramifications. The place to start, though, is with an overview of the social context of the times and, here, the medico-historical works of Porter have proved an invaluable source.

The Enlightenment

The Enlightenment, an eighteenth century intellectual movement, was unmistakably influenced by the advent of modern science as well as the religious conflict that followed the Reformation. It continued the work of great 17th century thinkers such as Galileo and Descartes, and English empiricists like Francis Bacon, Isaac Newton and John Locke. Those trailblazers had developed methods of rational inquiry which demonstrated the possibility of applying scientific discovery and related ideas to benefit people and the world in which they lived. Enlightenment thinkers such as Denis Diderot, David Hume, Immanuel Kant, and Pierre Voltaire advocated for an enlightened, and largely materialistic, conception of human nature emphasising self-expression and fulfilment as part of a philosophical rationalism based on science and nature. This they envisaged would replace religion as the means of knowing about the destiny of humanity. They also advocated for equality and justice, and for liberating people from restrictive political and religious systems, thus paving the way for American and French Revolutions. In this they were assisted by the French Encyclopedistes such as Jean-Jacques Rousseau (1712-78), who attributed evil to society rather than individual sin, and Utilitarians, like Jeremy Bentham (1748-1832), best known for his theory that the measure of right and wrong is according to the greatest happiness of the greatest number of people.[6] Bentham's Utilitarianism, which was saluted by social and occupational health activists of the next century, appears to have some concepts in common with occupational therapy which links how people feel with what they do, and with individual and community well-being and physical health.

During the eighteenth century in England, not only the pursuit of and right to happiness but also personal fulfilment was a theme of social essayists. That encouraged the population generally, within the bounds of the social conventions of the day, to maximise pleasures and avoid pain as they sought to achieve their own ends.[7] That appeared to be epitomised in two main ways. Either people sought to enhance individual potential through engagement in occupations with personal meaning, or to maximise wealth in the belief that material gains paved the way to happiness. In this regard Erasmus Darwin (1731-1802),[8] an unconventional and freethinking physician, poet, naturalist and botanist who anticipated aspects of his famous grandson's evolutionary theory, advocated that 'one must do something … otherwise one grows weary of life and becomes a prey to ennui.' According to Darwin, work was a means of staving off the nihility of all things, as well as an ongoing source of pleasurable activities. Work was also advocated as a means to maximise wealth and the government of the day, just as in the present, put the economic wealth of the state ahead of steps to enhance individual's personal potential.

Such ideas coincided with the passing of pre-industrial society in England.[9] They probably applied more to the upper and middle echelons of society who, on the whole, were enjoying increasing prosperity as the country's capitalist economy began to experience sustained and accelerating growth with the advance of industrialisation, in contrast to most other European countries. Alongside that the population of farmers, merchants, tradesmen, artisans, shopkeepers, clerks, and the like, also expanded. More people had money to spend on items formerly available only to the rich. Porter reports that, according to account books of the period, many spent their earnings on services like libraries, hairdressers, music lessons, educating children, and medical practitioners. Indeed, they were able to make choices about the kind of health care they wanted or could afford. As well, many traditional occupations of daily life like making clothes changed from functions undertaken within a household to being bought from outside. Just as in the present day people are more and more choosing to eat out than prepare food at home, then the change involved the demise of domestic occupations like making soap, starch, and furnishings in favour of purchasing these commodities.[10]

It was a progressive period during which agricultural, commercial, and manufacturing sectors thrived, leading to an ethos which celebrated industrious, energetic, and practical individualism and denigrated failure. The latter was punished by disgrace, destitution, becoming dependent on the Poor Law or possibly incarceration in a debtors' prison, and in many cases could result in physical or mental illness as well. Whilst help from extended families, kinship networks, friends and communities was possibly more prevalent than nowadays, family units were nuclear, and social as well as mental and physical well-being was ultimately the responsibility of self or immediate family. There was no Welfare State or Church to draw upon.[11]

The amount of poverty differed from time to time, with the degree of distress coinciding more or less with the rise or fall of corn prices, combined with low wages for labour, as Cary of the Bristol workhouse found through his ongoing contact with the inmates. When prices were high not even a man in regular employment could subsist.[12] Apart from some general understanding that there could be many causes of poverty, the most commonly held view was that profligacy and idleness were the main ones:

> ... *let everyone wipe his eyes, and make use of his head, and his hands to preserve or recover himself out of the quagmire of want: It being certain that still everyman in health and strength may forge himself out a fortune by industry and frugality, and obtain a comfortable subsistence.*[13]

The Reverend Townsend, an adherent of that doctrine argued that the fear of hunger should be accentuated to goad the poor to work. He propounded this view even though, if it was too successful, he was fearful that there would be no one left to do the most servile, sordid, and ignoble jobs required in any community.[14]

In many respects similar to recent times, it was a period in which there was a clear division between the "haves and have-nots" and also of worrying recessions. Particularly in country districts, whole families including very young children were forced to labour by 'extreme poverty and ignorance ... in a far greater degree than is popularly supposed'. Frederick Watson, the son-in-law of the pioneer of recuperative workshops, Sir Robert Jones, in his 1930 text *Civilization and the Cripple*, argued that, especially for children, such labour contributed to a 'fair share of lives crippled in mind and limb'. He pointed to cottage crafts such as the production of Buckinghamshire laces, which have a romantic image, as leading to '"almost universal" distortion of children's spines, premature blindness, chronic ill health and maternity fatalities through malformations'.[15] He cited Ivy Pinchbeck's *Women Workers and the Industrial Revolution, 1750-1850*. In it she told of 3-4 year olds being taught to handle lace bobbins and working regular hours in "lace school" at 5 years of age; of children in the straw plaiting cottage industry 'sorting straws at 4, plaiting at 5 and earning a regular wage at 6; and in glove- and button-making, knitting and embroidery, they were regularly at work at 6 and 7'. Children's hours of labour could be twelve or more hours each day, giving them little chance to play.[16] As well and apart from children, the physical sufferings were immense for large sectors of the work force engaged as muscle power in a manufacturing industry far from automated.[17]

So whilst the plebeian culture of the early eighteenth century exhibited many new trends and traditional features and expectations, deteriorating economic conditions for the masses possibly influenced the surge of interest in humanitarian values which occurred across Europe. Porter suggests that there arose:

> ... *a new recognition on behalf of opinion-makers that the health of the people mattered. Piety and humanity demanded compassion for the sick; utility taught*

that neglecting disease ran counter to enlightened self-interest: for diseases readily spread from the poor to the better off, and sick and disabled labourers made inefficient employees.[18]

An example of that interest was a text by Robert Nelson, published in 1715. It was entitled *An Address to Persons of Quality and Estate, Ways and Methods of Doing Good,* and was aimed at persuading the rich towards charitable impulses and to demonstrate methods by which 'the inferior part of mankind' could be helped. Nelson suggested that more support for churches and charity schools was required and that superior school teachers should be trained. He also suggested that support was needed for widows and orphans of the clergy, distressed housekeepers, "decayed" tradesmen, poor prisoners, and existing hospitals. As well, Nelson identified a need to establish other hospitals for many types of illnesses, for foundlings, "young women convinced of their folly", "converts from popery", and "decayed" gentlefolk, as well as initiatives to place "the poor in a way of industry".[19]

Kirkman Gray argued that the charitable notions of the day were far from selfless, despite Nelson's reminder of the common, but maybe largely unspoken understanding 'that those who have this world's goods should share with those who have them not ... "God only requires from us superfluities"[20,21] The inducement was both 'in this world and the next' for as well as charity providing immediate profit in some cases, it was also a way of procuring a place in heaven by investing in 'spiritual banks ... where profit is as durable as their souls' enabling rich men to 'cover their sins, escape oblivion, and gain immortality'.[22]

That text was far from unique. Throughout Europe, enlightened men of letters became interested in popular education, promoting and producing many dictionaries, handbooks, and encyclopaedias to set forth and popularise a more reasonable view of life among the people of their time. Additionally, growing literacy and geographic mobility added to the impact of social labour becoming increasingly free of traditional controls, which, for centuries, had been provided by gentry, church, and parish.[23] The spoken word had always been their principal means of control. It had also been the means for transmitting ideas from generation to generation and providing apprenticeship into adult skills and mature occupations such as domestic duties, child rearing, farm work, trades, mining and manufacturing.

The literary explosion expanded into the promulgation of the centuries old ideas espoused in the *Regimen Sanitatis* about the maintenance of health through lifestyle factors such as diet, environment, activity and rest, as well as remedies to alleviate ill health. While applicable to all, however, they were probably only available from choice for the more affluent.

Social health: The parish, Poor Law, workhouses and charity schools

In terms of this history the parish, workhouses and charity schools were the antecedents of many of the hospitals and special homes and institutions in which occupational therapists worked during the twentieth century. Although very different to those of the modern day, all were imbued with an occupational philosophy that dominated the day to day lives of residents.

The parish was, traditionally, the smallest organisational entity of the Church of England. From the sixteenth century, parishes began to acquire secular functions, and most importantly, from 1601 the provision and local administration of poor relief.[24] The parish system provided a last resort for those without any means of support: the out of work or those not capable of working, the very old and very young paupers, the sick or disabled, and the orphaned. Before the workhouse system was universally implemented in 1834, the old Poor Law was usually humane and often generous, with parishes providing financial support for food, shelter, fuel, clothing, and medical care. Such generosity was prompted by enlightened self-interest in the belief that early intervention might reduce or negate ongoing or more expensive ones later on. Even so, many of the poor battled on without help in preference to accepting it from the parish and the stigma that went with its charity.[25] Downing, for example, noted that before the establishment of the workhouse and school in Mile-End, Stepney, there were upwards of 70 poor who received pensions. All of them, except 6 women, chose to subsist by their own industry, rather than enter the workhouse when it was founded.[26]

Workhouses, as part of poor relief, are relevant to this history because, in a way, they were the forerunners of many modern institutions where occupational therapists work such as nursing homes for the aged and establishments for the permanently incapacitated. It is appreciated that this was not always the case for, whilst some workhouses only admitted the impotent, in others the sick were excluded and the house was largely used as a "terror to the idle".[27] Workhouses also encapsulate a concept which is integral to occupational therapy: that occupation provides meaning within every person's life and that it may need to be introduced to overcome deprivation, whether the cause of its lack be physical, mental or social. Unfortunately that was overlaid with judgemental and pecuniary ideas which nowadays would be viewed as far from health giving. According to the tenets of the time, industry itself was lauded, without any understanding of the need for meaning in occupations before they could be thought to have remedial purpose.

A few workhouses had been established in the 17th century at, for example, Blackfriars, Minories, Reading, and Bristol. They were usually founded as a result of private, often Anglican, philanthropy, especially for children. Most often these workhouses had education as well as work skills in mind, but with an industrial rather than a religious purpose as the driving force. As well as children, the early inmates were, as a rule, old people, and some of the founders experienced great pleasure in 'watching decrepit men and babies industrious at their wheels or diligent at their books, or devoutly praising God for his signal mercies towards them'.[28] The occupations used within them were mainly of a simple, and often domesticated nature, included weaving, spinning, knitting, carding, straw plaiting, stocking, lace, and hop-bag making, hop picking, and domestic work. However, on the whole they failed to provide 'dignified work for competent men under honourable conditions', although this had been a feature of some early experiments. One such was at Reading where a genuine dyeing and cloth making industry had been carried on until halted by the Civil War, and never resumed. Over time workhouses became less and less centres of occupation and more and more refuges "for profligates".[29] People like William Bailey attempted to remedy the situation, to ensure that workhouses met an objective of producing health and happiness for the poor, but they were largely unsuccessful.[30]

Figure 1.7 1: **A workhouse scene in 1720. Sketch from an illustrated playing card.**

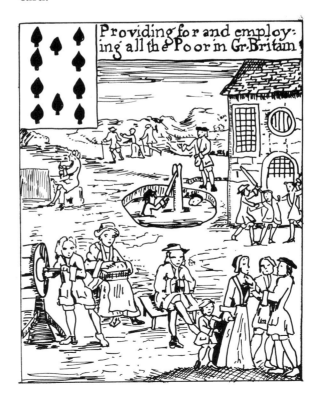

Early in the piece, though, there was a general feeling in the community of the Enlightenment period that the idea of workhouses was the "right one". It fitted with the notions of the time about practical solutions being the best, and the moral values of industry and energy, and was one of its most popular philanthropic expedients. Such feeling was attested to by Thomas Cooke who preached a sermon entitled *Work-houses the Best Charity* at the Cathedral Church of Worcester in February, 1702. So much was the sermon admired that the Mayor and Aldermen requested it be published. Extracts of his response to their request demonstrate not only the Reverend Cooke's gratification but also provide some idea of the local and national interest:

> *To the Right Worshipful Henry Gyles Esq; Mayor of the City of Worcester, and the Worshipful the Aldermen his Brethren.*
>
> *Gentlemen,*
>
> *YOUR earnest request to have this Sermon Published, is a convincing Argument of your great Zeal towards such kinds of Charity: And the Conferences I have had with some of you about a means to procure such a Provision for your own Poor, gives me assurance that nothing will be wanting in your Endeavours that may Contribute thereunto. It is a Duty recommended as a National care by the truest Father of his Country we could ever yet boast of; but it is not in the Power of the wisest Senate in the World, to compleat so suitable a Provision by one universal Law, as (by leave of their Authority) may be form'd for each single Country; by adapting that Provision to their proper Circumstances …*
>
> *You have promises of great Contributions and prospects of more; the Parliament are now sitting, and your representatives both for the City and County are Gentlemen of great Estates and Interests, and have been always forward to serve their country. All these Occurrances look Auspiciously on your design, to which only let me add this further Motive, that there is no one Act the Wisdom of Man can invent, that will more contribute to (what the Nation seems industriously at this time to Aim at, viz.) a general Reformation of Manners, than this will do.*[31]

The sermon itself was taken from the *Second Epistle of Paul the Apostle to the Thessalonians*, chapter 3, verse 10: 'For even when we are with you this we Commanded you; That if any would not work, neither should he Eat.' In it Cooke rails against 'Sloth and Idleness, which are so destructive of all Religion, and foster the Seeds of every kind of Vice' saying:

> *… so displeasing is this Sin to God, so detestable to all good Men, so Scandalous in it self, and so fatal in its Consequences, that the Apostle here Condemns it, and that beyond the extent even of Charity it self to Pardon; no Pity, no Commiseration, no Relief, must be extended to the Lazy Begger; But if any will not Work, neither shall he Eat.*[32]

Cooke proposed that the words of the text inferred several advantages. These included that people who provided for their needs solely by their own endeavours were more diligent than others as they went about their regular occupations; and that the country was advantaged by diligent workers. They also inferred that "inconvenience" and "damage" accrued when that did not occur and that "a cure" for the latter were workhouses to make every such "particular person" and "public State" happy. Going on to address the first of those points, he stated 'it is their peculiar care, whose whole Support is from their Hands, to bestowe their utmost diligence in their particular Callings, that they may earn their own Bread, the pleasing product of their proper Labours'.[33] Cooke called upon material from 'Nature, Reason, Law, Scripture and Religion', the first of which is offered below:

> *First from Nature: And truly he would hardly seem to be of natural Composition that wants to have this Motive urged: Let him survey the whole frame of Nature and tell me what part of the Creation is Unimploy'd; … to indulge our Avarice, and support our Health: Or lastly, to limit his Inquiry to a nearer Speculation, let him look no further then to his own Structure, and in the little World of his own Anatomy, convince me which of the most idle Members (ceasing its imploy,) would not be mist. In the politick structure of the human Body, Labour is indeed reduced to perfect Harmony, in which the Sphears are not boasted more regular nor exact; insomuch that the least disorder of its course, or irregular circulation of its Blood, would make as formidable a change in the Countenance, as in the languid Face of Nature, when the luster of the Sun were in Eclipse.*
>
> *In short, each product of Nature seems industrious by a self conscious Law, and the Labour of each Part is mutual from the expectation of a Reciprical return; so that Nature seems to abhor Idleness, for the same reason that she fears a Dissolution; and the same natural Motive that perswades us to self Preservation, will be sure to instruct our Heads to Project, and our Hands to execute the bussiness of our several Callings, that there may be no Scism in the Body thro' any negligence of its Members, but each performing its proper Office, the whole may be supported after the wise design of Nature.[34]*

In considering Cooke's message, it is interesting to note the health maintaining and remedial nature of part of his theme, which obviously struck a chord within the congregation. It should also strike a chord within occupational therapists reading it, as it provides an 18th century view of the place of occupation in the provision of health. In short, he stated that every aspect and law of Nature appears to incorporate occupation (labour, work) and that these are all interdependent. Further, he believed, Nature, including humans cannot exist without occupation and that all parts of the body and mind work together as part of our various callings, motivated by self preservation and health so that 'the whole may be supported after the wise design of Nature'. Cooke went on to argue that those and other parts of his sermon led to his conclusion that workhouses, combined with hospitals, were essential:

> *We must betake our selves to this only Cure for all this, because hereby the Aged and the Impotent will be sufficiently discriminated from the lazy idle Beggar, and both will be taken care of as the Law directs.*
>
> *For truely as matters now stand, the Aged and the Impotent suffer for the*

Lazy and the Idle: If there be an Aged person or a Cripple in the Family or one that is able to Work and will not; the very consideration of his Idleness is a Barr against the Charity intended, because they know the Impotent shall have the least share of it: Whereas in a Publick Work-house the proper circumstances of every Person is considered: For I would have no Work-house that should not also be an hospital; and as it contains a Bridewel to compel the Lazy, so should it have proper receptacles to succour the distressed: Aged and Impotent Persons there will be among us as long as the World endureth, and God forbid but they should be taken care of.

These are the Poor which Moses tells us will never fail, and these the only ones for which all our charitable Laws were e'er intended.[35]

A punitive view of the workhouses' purpose was apparent in some quarters, probably based on an economic rather than humanitarian or rehabilitative ideology that was to prevail into the next century. Jacob Vanderlint, for example, in an essay published in London in 1734, argued:

… for extirpating idleness, debauchery and excess, promoting a spirit of industry, lowering the price of labour in our manufactures and easing the land of the heavy burden of poor rate, we suggest the device of shutting up such labourers as become dependent on public support - in a word, paupers - in "an ideal workhouse", such ideal workhouse to be made a House of Terror and not an asylum for the poor. In this House of Terror, this "ideal workhouse", the poor shall work fourteen hours in a day, allowing proper time for meals, in such manner that there shall remain twelve hours of neat labour.[36]

Indeed, various changes were enacted to the Poor Law legislation during the 18th century towards those less charitable ends. In 1723 the Workhouse Test Act authorised parishes to withhold relief from those who refused to enter workhouses. Some sixty years later, in 1782, because the sick, aged, and able-bodied were herded indiscriminately into workhouses a further change of the Act forbade the admission of able-bodied unemployed into workhouses. Instead it charged parishes to find them work or, if this was impossible, to provide outdoor relief (support in kind without being admitted to a workhouse). That Act also provided parishes with the power to unite which they did Berkshire in 1795 when the justices adopted the Speenhamland system to subsidise agricultural worker wages out of the poor rates to bring them to subsistence levels after a rise in the price of wheat.[37]

The first relevant Act for poor relief in Ireland where masses of destitute poor had long been unaided[38] was passed by the Irish Parliament in 1703. That provided for the erection of a "House of Industry" in Dublin 'for the employing and maintaining the poor thereof', and in the main catering for "sturdy beggars", "disorderly women", the old and infirm, and orphan children.[39] Vagrants and sturdy beggars were "to be employed" and to work "voluntarily" or were liable to be flogged, imprisoned, receive "severe usage" or be treated with proportionate vigour.[40] 'Any poor child or children found or taken up within the said city or liberties above five years of age' were to be apprenticed out to any "honest person" until the age of twenty-four if male, and twenty-one if female. Alternatively, they could be kept in the service of the corporation until the age of sixteen.[41] Up to five years of age homeless children were the responsibility of parish authorities.[42]

The ongoing modification of the Poor Laws thus showed a general tendency towards greater rigidity, with the conditions of relief becoming more strictly defined as time passed. There was, obviously, concern about the children and youths dependent on the system, particularly as the cost of Poor Law relief fell substantially during the first fifty years of the century, which would have meant that the amount of help and support decreased during that time.[43]

Joseph Downing, in 1725, provided an account of several workhouses for employing and maintaining the poor, substantial extracts of which are provided below to illustrate how occupational deprivation was addressed in the institutions set up to remediate social health problems of Enlightenment times:

> The House is divided into Two Parts, one Part is called the Steward's Side, where poor Children are taken in from Benefactors giving 50/- or 70/- as before mentioned, and these Children are by that Means, and their Labour, rather a Profit than Charge to the House; and on this side are also taken in such Children as are a Charge to the several Parishes of this City and Liberties to which they belong. And all these Children are religiously Educated according to the Church of England, and are employ'd in Spinning Wool, Flax, Sewing, or Knitting; they are Dieted and Cloath'd, and duly taken Care of in Sickness. They are taught to Read, Write and Cost-Account, whereby they are qualified for Services and honest ways of Livelihood, and at their going out they have a Suit of Cloaths, or 20s. But Freemens Children have a larger Allowance out of a Benefaction directed to be appropriated to that purpose.
>
> And the other Part of the Work-House is called the Keeper's Side, where Vagabonds, Beggars, Pilfering and other Vagrants, Lewd, Idle, and Disorderly Persons, (duly Committed have such Relief as is proper for them), and are employ'd in Beating Hemp, Picking Oakum, or washing Linen. And these Vagrants and Beggars, etc after they have been some Time confined to hard Labour, and have been taught therby how to maintain themselves honestly, are sent to their respective Settlements as the Law directs; so that from Easter 1700, to Easter 1713 the Number of Vagrants, Beggars, etc discharged is 5555, during which Time there died 54 and at Easter last there remained 40.
>
> The Number of Children put out Apprentices during the same Time, is 1243 during which Time there died 118 and at Easter 1713 there remained 279.
>
> The children, and all others in the Work-House, are required to attend Divine Service Morning and Evening, which is regularly and duly performed in a convenient Place of the House, set apart for that purpose. But it would take up more room than can be spared in a brief Account to set down particularly the

Orders relating to the Christian Education of the Children, and how they are Cloathed, Fed, and Taught, and brought up to Write.[44]

In his account, Downing provided material from reports of several committees appointed by the Common Council, which are of interest. The first indicates that examination of what occurred within the workhouses was part of the system just as external reviews of service institutions are today. 'The Committee say, They have view'd the several Appartments, and the Method used in Employing the Children and others Committed there to Work, according to their several Capacities and Abilities, and do well approve of the same.'[45] Probably, but disappointingly, the economic aspects of the system appear to have been a driving force in the choice of occupations used, rather than those likely to develop the particular skills and interests of those engaged. In the following report, the Trustees, in fact, looked for occupations that demanded little strength or skill having taken a negative outlook on what was possible. The fact that workhouse residents were very old, very young, or infirm was regarded as a disadvantage rather than a challenge that was central to the charitable impulse of the workhouse concept. Such attitudes may have resulted in the systems ultimate failure:

> *Though much Profit could not be expected from the Labour of People, old or infirm, or under Age, and who were all to learn the Business they were to be imploy'd in; they Trustees took into Consideration how to set them to work in some easy Business, consistent with their Strength and Unskilfulness; and resolv'd, that they should work for nothing, for anybody that would instruct them to work till their Hands were in. Upon which a Weaver in the Neighbourhood provided them with Hempen Thread, call'ed Ruffia Yarn, to wind upon Rills for the Use of Sack-cloth and Sail-cloth Weavers.*
>
> *So many People work at this, as wind off about 60 pound weight in a Day.*
>
> *The same Gentleman finds Junk (Pieces of old Cable) to imploy others in picking Oakum; about 12 work at this, and pick about 1000 Weight in a Week.*
>
> *The Children are imploy'd in learning to read, and picking Oakum: and the rest in making the Beds, and keeping the House clean.*[46]

Picking oakum, or beating kemp, were occupations which were constantly chosen for remedial purposes across the centuries whether for pauper children or adults, the elderly and decayed or decrepit, the physically or mentally handicapped, or prisoners in gaols. Unlike riding which was selected for particular features valued as assisting the normalising of humoural physiology, picking oakum had little to recommend it except simplicity and repetitiveness. Oakum was a fibrous matter that was used for caulking boats, obtained from picking at old ropes. It can be viewed as analogous to the simple repetitive tasks that occupational therapists have used from time to time when other occupations appear too difficult or time demanding to encourage, or when physiological requirements from other ideologies dominate, submerging the concept of meaningful occupation.

Figure 1.7.2: Harlots Progress. Plate 4. Moll Hackabout in Bridewell beating hemp, by William Hogarth (1697-1764).
(The Wellcome Library)

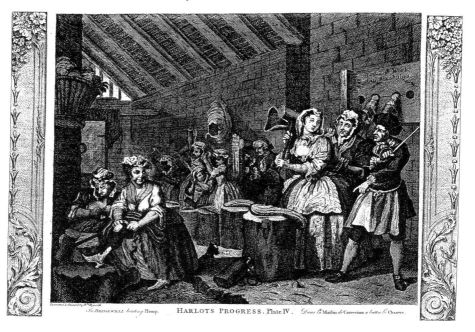

The reports went on to discuss further some of the feelings that appear to have been commonly expressed which relate to the benefits of workhouses for pauper children:

> *... if this part of the Design be so necessary and useful, how much more Useful and Beneficial ... (is the) ... due Provision of Relief and Employment of Poor Children, and to prevent their perishing for Want. Add to this, the inestimable Benefit of their being Nutured and brought up in a Religious Education, and taught to Work as soon as they are able, whereby they at present help to Support themelves, and wherby they are fitted for honest Trades and Services, and are not only kept from Perishing for Want, but from Pilfering, and turning Vagabonds, and incorrigible Rogues, and made useful Members of the Community; and great must needs have been the Advantage of having above 1200 poor necessitous Children so brought up and put out into the World. And suppose they had been otherwise kept from perishing for Want, yet great would have been the Loss of their honest Labour and Industry, at least to themselves; and greater would have been the Evil, if they had follow'd the wicked Practices their miserable Condition expos'd them to.[47]*

In the 1725 Report of the workhouse at Mile-End, Old Town Hamlet, Stepney which had been converted from a 'Musick-House of no good Repute', we learn that it housed 6 Women, 12 Boys, and 5 Girls. All were employed at picking oakum, 'under the care of a poor Man and his Wife, who are allow'd 5s. per week with their Lodging and Maintenance in the House'. Six trustees, each of whom had charge of the House on a monthly rotation, governed it. Inmates had milk, bread, cheese and butter for breakfast and supper, and meat three times a week. As well there was a charity school for 21 boys and 10 girls in the lower part of the house, looked after by the mistress of the girls who had an apartment. There, 'such of the children as are parish orphans, are set to work, as well as taught to read and write'.[48]

The 1725 report introduced the notions of charity schools for the poor. These had a similar mission to workhouses, relating to the importance of work and domestic occupations in the preparation of children for later independence. Downing provided an account of two of the schools. First, the Grey-Coat Hospital in Westminster:

> A proposal being made to the Vestry at St Margaret's Westminster, about the Year 1701, they agreed to let the Trustees of the Grey-Coat-School have a large House belonging to the Parish Rent-free for Seven Years; which Grant has been renew'd from time to time ever since, for the Reception of as many of the Parish-Children (with the usual pensions given to their Nurses) as the Trustees would undertake to maintain and imploy with Work.
>
> At first the Trustees took in the 50 Boys belonging to the Charity-School, and at several Times afterwards so many Boys and Girls as have sometimes increas'd the Number of Children to above 130, which is the Number of them at present, including those on the Parish Account, and have set them all to Work; some upon spinning of Wool, others upon Housewifry, sewing, knitting, etc. And the Incomes of the Charity, with their Earnings, are appointed towards finding them in Diet, Lodging, and other Necessaries: The Management whereof succeeded so well, that, in order to lay a more solid Foundation for its Support and Maintenance, Her Late Majesty was pleas'd, in the 5th Year of her Reign, to incorporate the said School, and to make the trustees One Body Politick, by the Name of The Govenours of the Grey-Coat-Hospital in Tothil-Fields, of the Royal Foundation of Queen ANNE. [49]

Second, a girls school at Greenwich:

> In the Year 1700, several Charitable Ladies of this Town, join'd their Subscriptions for setting up a School for Teaching and Cloathing 30 Girls. Some Time after a Proposal was made to the said Gentlewomen, that if they pleas'd to allow the Charge that was usually allowed for Cloathing the Children, to be laid out in Materials for setting them to Work, the Mistress might teach the Children to make their own Cloathes; which would have this Advantage in it, that tho' nothing might be sav'd in the Charge, yet the Children, by being inur'd to Labour, would be better prepar'd for Services in the Families where they might afterwards be plac'd. A Tryal of this Proposal for one Year was soon resolv'd on, and the Success was such, that it has been continu'd, with some Improvements, ever since[50]

Despite the hope that Enlightened views of humanity may have led to a clear understanding of the social health needs for meaningful occupation, the history of workhouses and elementary education of pauper children during the eighteenth century is bound up in many ways with employing cheap child labour. Thomas Firmin's spinning school, which was started in 1775, is an example, although his interest in the poor was strong. His establishment in Little Britain, supported by many charitable donors, was part school, part factory to which children aged three were admitted. For the first year they had a literary education, and then their technical instruction began with only an interval for reading each day. At five or six they could earn 2d a day, and later 3d, until they were old enough to be apprenticed. Their labour paid, in large part for their instruction, which was provided by a woman, employed at 5 shillings a week, to teach spinning and reading.[51]

Charity schools differed from Firmin's in that they were the outcome of a large number of associations, usually started by members of the Church of England, rather than the work of one man. By the year 1734 there were 132 such schools in London, and 1,329 in the country, with over 24,000 students attending them. They usually had a religious bent and were sometimes founded to prevent children's attendance at a school provided by other religious groups such as Quakers, Papists, Dissenters, or Infidels. In the schools, to fit the boys for apprenticeships and the girls for domestic service, children were taught:

… civility and good manners, and reading, and catechizing: in some of them the boys learn writing and arithmetick, and navigation; and the girls are taught to knit and sew, and mark, and spin, and card, and mend and make their own cloathes[52]

From an early period some of the schools also acted like workhouses, having the children work at commercial projects as well as receiving an education and deriving a profit from the undertaking. That became more so as time went on. There was parental opposition to that, which was met in one school where children were allowed every other day to be employed in servile labour for their parents. There was also industrial criticism especially about the revolutionary effects that learning could produce.[53]

Despite such initiatives, children of the lower classes were often the victims of brutality and neglect. If they survived at all, they could not expect to have any encouragement to use whatever skills they had in other than ways concerned with survival at its most fundamental and degrading. That was occupational deprivation and social ill health at its worst. Many of the Poor Laws' charitable foundations had broken down, partly because of changes in public sentiment from time to time, and perhaps as a result of the South-sea speculations. Some concerned citizens, such as Joseph Addison (1672-1719), a poet, dramatist, and politician who foreshadowed modern journalism, sought to answer at least some of the problems. In the *Guardian* (No. 105) in 1713, the year of the paper's foundation, he advocated the establishment of a foundling hospital:

> *Since I am upon this subject, I shall mention a piece of charity which has not yet been exerted among us, and which deserves our attention the more, because it is practised by most of the nations about us. I mean a provision for foundlings, or for those children who, through want of such a provision are exposed to the barbarity of cruel and unnatural parents.*[54]

Figure 1.7.3:   **Thomas Coram**
(The Wellcome Library)

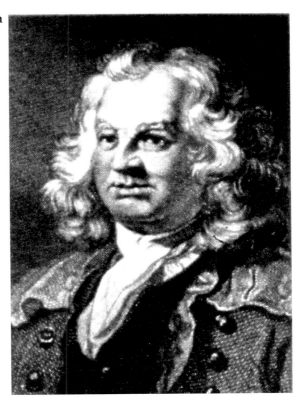

The establishment of a foundling hospital in London took some thirty or more years from Addison's call. It came because an elderly philanthropic sea captain, Thomas Coram (1668-1751), pictured in figure 1.7.1, saw newborn infants left to die on dunghills in and around London and abandoned by the wayside on his journey to and from the capital from Rotherhithe where he lived. The terrible waste of human life both shocked and angered him, especially as he had just returned from the New World where human labour was the greatest need. He determined to establish a foundling hospital similar to institutions known to exist on the continent. It opened, with a Royal Charter, on March 25, 1740. A shield especially designed by Hogarth for the use of the Hospital was set over the door of the premises in Hatton Garden, and the first 60 children admitted. During the first year 136 children were received of whom 56 died.

Figure 1.7.4 **"Captain Coram and children carrying implements of work".**
Engraving by T. Cook, 1809, after W. Hogarth, 1739
(The Wellcome Library)

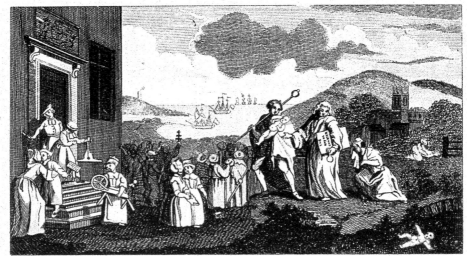

SEVERAL CHILDREN OF THE FOUNDLING HOSPITAL.

Published by Longman, Hurst, Rees, & Orme, July 1st 1809.

THE **ROYAL CHARTER** *Establishing an* **HOSPITAL** FOR THE **Maintenance and Education** *Of exposed and deserted* **YOUNG CHILDREN.**
George the Second, by the Grace of God, and so forth, to whom these Presents shall come, Greeting.

WHEREAS Our Truly and Well-beloved Subject, Thomas Coram, Gentleman, in behalf of great Numbers of helpless infants, daily exposed to destruction, has by his Petition, humbly represented unto Us, that many Persons of Quality and Distinction, as well as others, of both Sexes (being sensible of the frequent Murders committed on poor miserable Infants by their Parents to hide their Shame, and the inhuman Custom of exposing new-born Children to perish in the Streets, or Training them up in Idleness, Beggary, and Theft) have, by Instruments in Writing, declared their Intentions to contribute liberally towards the erecting of an Hospital, after the Example of other Christian Countries, and for supporting the same, for the Reception, Maintenance, and proper Education of such helpless Infants, as soon as We should be graciously pleased to grant Our Letters Patent for that good Purpose: That several Legacies having been bequeathed for the same, to be paid by Executors, when any such Hospital shall be properly established here; the Petitioner therefore hath humbly prayed Us, that We would be graciously pleased to grant Our Royal Charter for incorporating such Persons, as We shall think fit, for receiving and disposing of Charities for erecting and supporting an Hospital for the Reception, Maintenance, and proper Education of such exposed and cast-off Children as may be brought to it, under such Rules and Regulations, as to Us may seem met.[55]

In 1748 it had been publicly announced that the boys were intended for sea service and husbandry but whilst resident in the Hospital would engage in open-air work. Sheds for that purpose were built alongside the walls that enclosed the grounds and offers for the children's employment were invited. These led to proposals that the boys should undertake oakum picking and net knitting and the girls be occupied at silk winding, domestic work, "sowing", and spinning. Not long after the Hospital was established there appears to have been some need for measures to be taken that would improve the children's physical health. Bathing in the sea at Brighthelmstone (Brighton) was the chosen health enhancing occupation, however that appeared too expensive. In its place "Dr. Mead" advocated that 'Drinking the said Sea Water here would answer the same purpose'. A few years later a "Cold Bath" was constructed in the hospital, 16 feet by 10 feet, and "lined with stucco" where, presumably, communal bathing took place.[56]

Social health: Prisons

Although not a large part of practice, occupational therapy has been used in prisons during the twentieth century. It has been thought to have a number of uses, such as assisting in the social rehabilitation process, and reducing the boredom that results from occupational deprivation and can lead to ill health or to unacceptable behaviour. Prisoners in 18th century gaols were also subject to occupational deprivation and boredom and concomitant disorders. That appears to have been understood by John Howard, a trailblazer in terms of prison reform.

John Howard (1726-90), the well known philanthropist, pictured in figure 1.7.5, had his interest in prisons aroused when he was captured and imprisoned by the French whilst attempting to go to the relief of survivors of the 1755 Lisbon earthquake.[57] Later, when he became High Sheriff of Bedfordshire, he began an investigation of gaols when he discovered that many prisoners in his county only remained there because they could not pay the gaoler's fees after their original sentence was completed. He travelled widely visiting prisons and hospitals throughout Britain and Europe, insisting on penetrating their darkest and most miserable conditions. Indeed 'his clothes became so impregnated with the gaol smell that he found it necessary to travel on horseback; his notebooks had to be treated by fire before he could use them'.[58] He published two works, *The State of Prisons, in England and Wales, with an Account of some Foreign Prisons* in 1777, and *An Account of the Principal Lazarettos in Europe* in 1789. His style was unemotional. He compiled the facts without picturesque detail, and his works were the more powerful for it, presenting as an 'accumulative, a monotonous repetition of horrors prosaically stated as though they were entirely commonplace and normal'.[59] Halle, the French health encyclopaedist, argued that 'the system of prisons is still more remote from perfection than that of hospitals' and praised Howard as 'one of the most celebrated friends of humanity'. Howard's talent, said Halle, was to place before men's eyes the calamities of their fellow creatures whilst also pointing out 'the measures which they ought to have adopted for the purpose of increasing their happiness'.[60]

Figure 1.7.5:   **John Howard. Line engraving by M. Davis, 1787**
(The Wellcome Library)

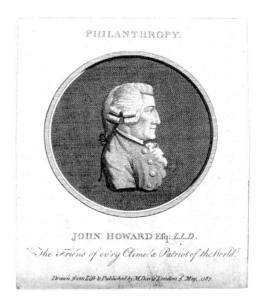

Whilst Howard did not personally aim at rectifying the abuses, he determined to alert the community as a whole about them so that collective effort was aroused. He was successful in forcing the Government to become responsible for the state of prisons and for many reforms that were instigated from that time.[61] He also provided some insight about his requirements for a "model" gaol when he made suggestions for a proposed prison at Islington:

> *The penitentiary house for female convicts, and its inhabitants … with respect to healthiness.* (Note here reads:) *In respect to healthiness the situation at Islington is much more eligible than any of the populous parts of the city - so that by providing airy apartments, free ventilation, plenty of water; and by promoting cleanliness, accompanied by wholesome food, and **a proper degree of labour;** the convicts may there **enjoy better health** than falls to the lot of many thousands of reputable tradesmen and mechanics.[62]*

Figure 1.7.6: **John Howard (?)**
visiting a prisoner.
Etching after
Armitage
(The Wellcome Library)

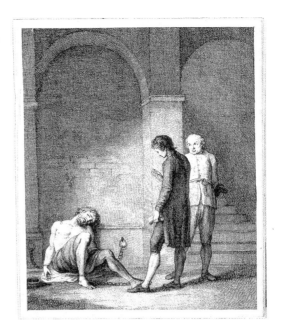

With that reference to the place of labour or occupation in regard to the health of the prisoners firmly in mind, some excerpts have been selected from Howard's reports that comment on matters that will be of interest to occupational therapists. For example, of New Ludgate prison he wrote: 'Here are several improvements … In the large workroom I always found either chair-makers, basket-makers, or coopers at work.' At the New Prison, Clerkenwell, he found 'no sick ward for women: no bedding. The bath never used: no water in that pump for two years. Chapel badly contrived: not white-washed. Men and women separated; but all sorts of prisoners associate together, playing cards &c.' Of the Manchester gaol he said: 'The women's side is very clean. Employment, winding, spinning and picking cotton. The prisoners have their earnings as there is no allowance except two-pence a day to the sick.' At the county Gaol in Chester Castle Howard found 'here at both my visits, a prisoner, who had been reprieved, employed in the instruction of nine young prisoners, whom he had taught to read'.[63]

Howard's thorough analysis of the prisons also included what happened in the Hulks. This was a "temporary" expedient of confining prisoners in old warships which was adopted in 1776 to hold felons sentenced to transportation to the colonies, which lasted for 82 years.[64] It can be imagined how terrible conditions may have been, so it comes as no surprise that Howard expressed general disquiet about them. 'I think it will be admitted that the mode of confinement and labour in the hulks is too severe for the far greater number of those who are confined in them.'[65]

He gave some detail in occupational terms. On the Plymouth Hulk 'the prisoners were all in total idleness, except six or seven who were making a boat for the captain. One ingenious man had made a small ink-stand (which I have by me) out of the bone of his meat; but his knife was taken from him.' In contrast on the Portsmouth Hulks: 'All Saturdays be spent on cleanliness … viz. bathing, washing and mending their clothes, shaving, cleaning themselves and every part of the ships, and beating and airing their bedding' and 'on other days none who are able should be excused from work'. Some were even employed on shore in public works.[66]

Foreshadowing occupation as rehabilitation during prison confinement, of penitentiary houses Howard said:

> The act for establishing penitentiary houses, drawn up by two of the wisest men this kingdom has produced, was "a work of long and continued labour and inquiry," and the legislature fully expressed their wise and humane sentiments in the following terms; "that if many offenders convicted of crimes for which transportation had been usually inflicted, were ordered to solitary imprisonment, accompanied by **well regulated labour**, and religious instruction, it might be the means, under providence, not only of deterring others from the commission of the like crimes, but also of **reforming the individuals, and inuring them to habits of industry**".[67]

Indeed, reminding the reader of the old cartoon about the patients building their own occupational therapy department under the National Health Service, Howard suggested that the prisoners in his time should build their own gaol:

> The penitentiary houses I would have built, in great measure by the convicts. … Let one or two hundred men, with their proper keepers, and under the directions of the builder, be employed in levelling the ground, digging out the foundation, serving the masons, sawing the timber and stone: and as I have found several convicts who were carpenters, masons, and smiths, these may be employed in their own branches of trade; since such work is necessary and proper as any other in which they can be engaged. …. By this method, they may be kept most usefully employed; and at the same time, by regular labour, some degree of separation, and proper conduct of their overseers to them, they may perhaps be a little reformed … Many have been reclaimed and made useful members of society, in foreign houses of correction, and have thanked God for their confinement in them.[68]

He proposed that some general regulations needed to be established within all types of correctional institutions. Within those Howard recommended occupations to ensure cleanliness of themselves, their clothes and bedding and the "House" as necessary to the ongoing health of inhabitants. As well he proposed that occupations be "proportioned to strength" and "to the degree of criminality". He considered the hours and kinds of occupations; whether they should be within doors or without; the numbers who should work together; whether occupations should include "mere labour" or "ingenuity"; and the saleability of the products. He also argued that the labour of each should be distinguished from that of others and that, when appropriate, prisoners should work at their own trades, supplying the needs of the prison with a proportion of the profit being allowed to the prisoners. He also argued that the occupations should be wholesome; and that it should be ensured that the tools used were not dangerous and were returned at night.[69]

In an earlier chapter the origin of Bridewell Hospital was discussed. Pennent, writing in 1790 described the institution as 'not only a prison for the dissolute, but a hospital for the education of the industrious youth'. However, as the years went by the original idea of it being a place where the needs of the occupationally deprived could be met was largely lost in favour of its other purpose to house the occupationally depraved. The former purpose was subsumed into the educational notion of "schools", the latter lost its remedial focus, and as other bridewells were established, unfortunately, the name became synonymous with gaol.

John Howard visited the original and new bridewells. He reported that in the original establishment there were, in 1783 as many as 1,597 vagrants and others committed to "this prison". A year later the figure rose to nearly 3,000 then fell dramatically to 612, followed by 716. Twenty-six men and 25 women were in residence in 1787 and in the following year, 19 men and 10 women. He commented on occupations and conditions:

> *Each sex has a workroom and a nightroom ... Some were picking oakum, and others were making ropes, which is a new and proper employment. Mr Hardwick, a hemp dresser, has their labour, and a salary of twenty guineas a year. - Allowance a penny loaf each, and four days in the week ten ounces of beef without bone etc. The allowance for persons constantly employed, is not too much; but would it not be better if they had less meat, and more bread? The prison wants white-washing, and the men's night room more light and air. At my first visit two were in the infirmary; at my last, only one.*
>
> *There are very properly solitary cells for the Bridewell boys, in which one was confined and employed in beating hemp.*[70]

The Lincoln City Bridewell, however, appears to have kept closer to the original concept of remediating occupational need, which was perhaps facilitated by it being endowed and housed in 'two rooms adjoining spinning school. Allowance, a shilling a week and half the earnings. No water. The master of the school is keeper.' A note reads:

> *The spinning school is supported by a legacy of 700 pounds left in 1686. The master has a salary of 30 pounds to teach the children of the poor in this city to spin. There were about twelve spinning worsted in a large room. Mrs. Yorke, the present Bishop of Ely's lady, when she resided in Lincoln, frequently visited this school; and by her attention, and encouragements to the most cleanly and industrious children, it was then in a flourishing condition.*[71]

Howard's reports warrant further investigation as the original brief of Bridewell was a very exciting concept in terms of this history. At the beginning of the period, during Queen Anne's reign, Bridewell's charitable role was in overcoming occupational deprivation by enabling the young to find an outlet for their capacities and talents and thereby to experience some enjoyment. This intent was still evident in, for example, the annual spectacle of the children from the two Royal hospitals in 'great cavalcade' through the streets, with 'colours and streamers'. 'The procession of these and the children of Christ's Hospital on Easter Monday and Tuesday affords to the human mind the most pleasing spectacle, as it excites the reflection of the multitudes thus rescued from want, profligacy, and perdition.'[72] In later years this 'was no more to be seen'.[73] Another source of excitement for the apprentices of Bridewell, who wore a distinctive blue dress and white hat, was the tradition of attending fires with an engine that belonged to the hospital.

> *Whenever intelligence of a fire breaking out (and it always was conveyed), whether at Wapping or Westminster, arrived at the Hospital, the beadle at the gate immediately rang the fire bell in the courtyard. If it was in the daytime, the apprentices immediately rushed from their work. If it happened in the night, those who were first come down went round knocking at the Art Masters' doors till all the inhabitants were awakened and the boys called out.*[74]

The service was discontinued in 1735 because although the boys were "active" and "serviceable", there were concerns about them being thrown amongst 'profligates which are collected in the streets', the master's loss of a day's work, and because many boys got hurt or "disabled from work" for a long time. In the previous extract the term "Art Masters" occurs, which is defined below:

> *Here* (Bridewell) *many Arts Masters (as they are styled), consisting of decayed tradesmen, such as shoemakers, taylors, flax dressers, and weavers, have houses and receive apprentices who are instructed in several trades, the masters receiving the profits of their labours. After the boys have served their time with credit, they are paid ten pounds to begin the world with, and are entitled to the freedom of the city.*[75]

However, apparently all was not going well. Various reforms were undertaken during the 18th century, with new and stricter regulations being tried out, but by 1798 there was still general dissatisfaction at the way in which the affairs of Bridewell were administered. A select committee was appointed to inquire whether and by what means the estates and revenues of the Hospital could be used with better effect to benefit the original objectives according to the intention of the royal founder. The situation apparently did not improve as some twenty years later, in the nineteen century, a Committee of the House of Commons was appointed to inquire into the prisons of the metropolis, including Bridewell. That Committee's report condemned the state of affairs and the arrangements in force at the Hospital.[76] The training of apprentices eventually was developed into King Edwards School, now at Witley in Surrey.

Figure 1.7.7:   Bridewell Hospital: An aerial view. J. Stowe, Survey of
London, 1754-57
(The Wellcome Library)

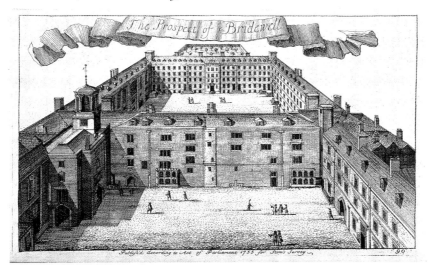

In Summary:
The enlightened use of occupation for social health

The Enlightenment proved to be a period in history during which occupation, particularly in the sense of work or labour, was valued as a way towards liberty, independence, individuality, and self realisation, which Enlightenment thinkers and modern occupational therapists both espouse. Then, the leaders of society applauded energy and industry, and idleness regarded as one of the greatest illnesses necessitating remedial action. Philanthropic, charitable, and religious endeavours combined with government legislation led to many occupation based initiatives in new and old institutions such as charity schools, workhouses, hospitals and gaols. Here, it would seem, was one foundation of an occupational appreciation of health. Present day practitioners should not neglect what can be learnt from occupation-based programmes at workhouses, nor reject them, as they are an obvious precursor to current ideas.

Occupation as a holistic concept was not appreciated at the time, and one aspect, namely labour, was picked out as more important than others, as it still is. Then, industrial capitalism was emerging with a demand for "manpower" which had little to do with meaning, self realisation, or well-being, but more with economic gains for industrial leaders, and celebration of a few human's ingeniousness. In the process of realising the wealth of a few, and the upward mobility of the middle classes, remediation of the health and happiness of the suffering masses was relegated to institutions. These could have, but did not, meet their occupational needs, or even their economic ones, whilst being promoted as doing both. Whilst such institutions have to be a source of embarrassment to an occupationally based profession, at least they were wide spread and generally regarded as necessary. That suggests that new schemes addressing the occupational aspects of social health could be possible, if done with people's occupational health needs in mind rather than economic and materialistic goals.

Occupational regimes towards physical health

In the next section of the chapter a view of eighteenth century regimes aimed at maintaining and restoring physical health will be considered through the lens of occupational therapy. At this time of change from long held agricultural traditions of employment and concomitant social ideologies and personal aspirations, one would expect to find concurrent developments in the provision of health care for the treatment of physical disorders. And, indeed, the time of the Enlightenment was one of expansion of medical ideas and discoveries, as well as political, economic, social and scientific developments that were embraced across nations. Both positively and negatively influenced by a thriving market economy and by exemption from censorship of information, Enlightenment ideals were realised in England in practical terms. 'Economic growth, social change and the march of mind in turn played their parts in shaping responses to the threats to health, livelihood and even life itself posed by rampant disease.'[77]

Porter and Porter describe how in the eighteenth century, as in earlier times, disease, sickness and suffering was something all people expected to some degree or other, and in many cases nothing could be done to save life. Not all resulted in death, but caused pain and suffering to the extent that people were unable to go about their everyday lives or maintain employment, permanently or temporarily, whilst experiencing little pleasure, well-being or peace of mind. Many diseases were caused by lack of food or knowledge, poverty or overwork, accidents or unhygienic practices, which are now things of the past or easily fixed.[78] There would have been widespread agreement with the resignation expressed by Elizabeth Montagu, one of the leaders of "blue stocking" circles, a beauty and a wit, who, in 1739, when she would have been all of 19 years old, proclaimed:

> I have swallowed the weight of an Apothecary in medicine, and what I am
> better for it, except more patient and less credulous, I know not. I have learnt to
> bear my infirmities and not to trust to the skill of physicians for curing them. I
> endeavour to drink deeply of philosophy, and to be wise when I cannot be merry,
> easy when I cannot be glad, content with what cannot be mended, and patient

where there can be no redress. The mighty can do no more, and the wise seldom do as much.[79]

If such sentiments were the lot of many, it is somewhat heartening to find that increasing humanitarian beliefs, mixed with liberal doses of self interest, led to the establishment of institutions for the relief of those suffering physical illness and disability. Helpful, too, was the proliferation of do-it-yourself "health" books, which sustained the "self-healthers". Alongside that, a free market approach led to increased opportunities opening up for lay health practitioners. At the same time there was a birth of new theories and initiatives that came to be important in the eventual advancement of occupational therapy and related disciplines.[80]

Growth of hospitals and medical services

With the rise of capitalism the economic possibilities of the medical profession began to be recognised. This led, more and more, to physicians recruiting themselves from the middle classes, many with the hope that they might become physicians to a person of high rank, which would give them an assured income. For those inclined towards altruistic work, such positions often provided the opportunity to devote some time to charity if they felt so inclined.[81] At that time it became common practice for parishes to contract a particular physician to care for its poor for an annual fixed sum. It is worthy of note that as pauper hospitals were few and far between 'charity and Poor Law relief combined to offer at least some medical attention to the lower orders'.[82]

Prior to the 1750s there was but faint resemblance to the current organisation of medical services, although as has been discussed earlier, practitioners fell into three main divisions not dissimilar to today; physicians, surgeons, and apothecaries and, at least in the country, often combined those roles. Physicians, with a university degree, continued to treat internal disorders following observation and the taking of a detailed history. Surgeons treated external disorders by manual procedures and, for the first half of the century still retained their traditional link with barbers. Apothecaries continued to dispense the prescriptions of physicians, but also "treated" over the counter and sometimes in homes. Despite the division of labour between them there was constant tension and rivalry for clients, power and status. In 1704, for example, The College of Physicians lost its monopoly, in London, on the prescription of medicines. From that time the College, which was in effect an exclusive club whose fellowship was reserved for gentleman graduates of "Oxbridge" and members of the Church of England, had to share prescribing rights with apothecaries on the proviso that they did not charge for advice.[83]

Medical historians have noted that, despite this division and tension, medical care grew rapidly in England in the eighteenth century whilst not necessarily improving or reducing the experience of morbidity or mortality of patients.[84] Watson suggested, for example, that there was a considerable advance in the study of orthopaedics, but that it could only be described as experimental. Francis Glisson (1597-1677) had pioneered the subject of infantile rickets in the previous century, Nicholas Andre (1658-1742) the case of crippled children, and Percival Pott (1714-1788) and John Hunter (1728-1793) laid the foundations of joint surgery.[85] Hunter had also been supportive of Pugh's work towards developing remedial movement of muscles for contractions of joints, paralytic weakness, and other affections. Pugh's book on the science of muscular action was published, in 1794, after Hunter's death.[86] Pott, of St Bartholomew's Hospital, mainly concentrated on industrial pathology, but is remembered for his description of what is now known as "Pott's Disease" and "Pott's Fracture", the latter being based on personal experience of a fractured ankle when he fell from his horse.[87] In addition to orthopaedics, neuro-physiological research began to gain momentum during the eighteenth century. Swiss, Albrecht von Haller (1708-1777), for example, worked on muscle fibres and their contraction relating to movement and William Cullen (1710-1790) a professor of medicine at both Glasgow and Edinburgh Universities outlined the production of movement through stimulation of the nervous system.[88] Studies also advanced in paediatric care. William Cadogan, for example, wrote *An Essay upon Nursing and Management of Small Children,* and George Armstrong set up a clinic specifically to treat children. Such advances as those led, gradually, towards a time when occupation would be recognised, for its physiological attributes, in the treatment of many types of disorder for people of all age groups.

It is clear that physical medicine, and medical men, profited from the secular nature of the Enlightenment's thriving consumer economy, when bodily needs eclipsed those of the soul. During this period, medical practices accelerated, incomes rose, "sidelines" emerged such as Poor Law contracts, hospital posts, and smallpox inoculations, and doctors began to occupy diverse and increasingly prestigious niches in scholarly fields and community service as well as of a professional nature.[89]

Extensive changes within the medical establishment continued to occur throughout the 18th century. For example, the apprenticeship and growth of man-midwives (current day obstetricians) from the 1730s on led ultimately to the medicalisation of childbirth.[90] The surgeons severed their links with barbers when the Company of Surgeons was established in 1745, and Loudon suggests that within the medical hierarchy even the 'traditional superiority of the physician' was diminished substantially. This was 'due in part to the advances in anatomy and surgery as academic disciplines and in part to the rise of the voluntary hospitals' both of which led to the 'spectacular rise in surgery'.[91]

At the start of this period, 1700, there were still only two endowed medical hospitals in Britain, St Bartholomew's and St Thomas's, in London.[92] A forward thinking pamphlet of the time argued for the provision of localised institutions for a whole range of "defectives and unfortunates", inclusive of those with physical, mental or social disorders. It stated:

> *There should be one General Hospital erected in each County … for the Reception and Maintenance of all poor Lunaticks, Ideots, Blind Persons, Maim'd Soldiers and Seamen, Cripples uncapable of relieving themselves by any Manufacture or Labour, and Bed ridden Persons beyond a prospect of Cure, that are or shall be Inhabitants of that County. Such hospitals should be charged to the rates and overseen by parliamentary visitors.*[93]

The pamphlet was indicative of a changed perception amongst policy makers that maintaining people's health was important, and sickness worthy of compassion. Enlightenment thinking, which refocussed philanthropic action towards humanitarian and secular rather than religious charities, resulted in quite unprecedented largesse directed at the establishment of institutions for the succour of the sick poor without charge to them, although this did not include Poor Law paupers.[94] Sickness often posed a threat to those more affluent because infection could spread and, then, there was little available to halt it. Another reason for the change of view which also appeared common sense was that as industry was emerging as the basis of future economic growth, people could increasingly become the victims of occupational disease as toxic chemicals and dangerous machinery were being used more and more. Bearing this in mind it is not difficult to recognise, as was the case then, those workers who were sick or handicapped decreased productivity and profits. Many employers made contributions to hospital charities that entitled their workers to treatment and care. Others, such as Josiah Wedgwood, of pottery fame, established insurance schemes into which employees made compulsory payments in return for treatment and sick pay should the need arise.[95]

Whether prompted by more humanitarian views of the Enlightenment, self-interest, or pamphlets, in the first half of the century voluntary general hospitals were built in over thirty ancient towns and cities as well as in new centres of industry such as Manchester and Birmingham. They included Westminster (1720), Guy's (1724), The Edinburgh Royal (1729), St George's (1733), Winchester and Bristol (1736-7), The London and York (1740), Exeter (1741), Bath (1742), Northampton (1743), and The Middlesex (1745).[96] Specialist hospitals, too, were opened, some of which bespeak the decline of older religious judgments which still lingered, that some diseases were punishments to be borne. Exemplifying that suggestion are the hospitals that were established for those with venereal disease; for the "lying in" of maternity cases; as well as those mentioned earlier in the chapter for foundlings where unwanted children were brought up, educated and taught a trade; and for penitent prostitutes where they also could learn a new trade and prepare for a different way of life.[97,98,99]

Kersley and Cosh suggest in their history of the Royal National Hospital for Rheumatic Diseases at Bath that 'the eighteenth century has been called the "age of hospitals"' because of the number established during that period.[100] Indeed the establishment of voluntary institutions was largely a lay enterprise. In turn, hospitals provided benefits to members of the medical profession, many of whom recognised an opening of opportunity which, incidentally, led eventually to their almost unassailable position in the present time. In the main, though, physicians did not undertake the management of those hospitals at their genesis. Rather, lay philanthropists who gave generous donations to their continuance as well as their establishment, as a reward, were given voting rights on boards of management.[101] So it can be said that it was the thriving consumer economy of the eighteenth century which encouraged philanthropists and humanitarians from many walks of life, inspired by Enlightenment philosophies, to support medical charities and found hospitals for the poor.

Lady Elizabeth Hastings provides us with an example. It was she who proposed in 1716 that a hospital for the sick poor from anywhere around the country should be established in Bath. She gathered together a group of like-minded collaborators including Henry Hoare a banker and a founder of the Westminster Hospital during the same year, Doctors Cheyne, Bave and Quinton, and Richard (Beau) Nash who was a dandy and gambler as well as a leading socialite of the town. The latter was a generous backer of the hospital for the rest of his life, canvassing financial support from the nobility and gentry with whom he associated.

Although there were already three hospitals in the town there was an urgent need for another. Those in existence were St John's, founded in 1180 as part of a religious institution and by then a secular home for the poor and needy, along with a small medieval leper hospital, and Bellott's Hospital founded in 1609 for twelve poor strangers in need of taking the waters. The Act of 1597, which permitted the diseased and impotent poor of England to free use of Bath's waters, had resulted in a tripling of the entire population and a very large community of beggars seeking alms. The Act was repealed in 1714, probably 'to the relief of the gentry then beginning to patronise the city'. Patients of the 150-bed hospital, though, were entitled to 'free use of the Hot Bath and the Old pump', when the plans came to fruition and the hospital, known as the *Royal Mineral Water Hospital* opened in 1742. The main treatment, not surprisingly, was taking the waters, either internally, under a douche according to a prescribed number of pump strokes, or as a bath. In addition to those remedial occupations, ambulant patients were required to assist with the care of those more disabled and with the cleaning.[102]

Spa physicians, George Cheyne and William Oliver, who practised in London or other parts of the country when it was not the season "to take the waters" often concentrated on rheumatology, particularly arthritis and gout, and wrote about the topic. Despite only about 26% of patients at the *Royal Mineral Water Hospital* being recorded as having rheumatism, Cheyne and Oliver must have also had plenty of patients from amongst the nobility and gentry who frequented the fashionable resort town. Buxton, in Derbyshire, was a less exalted spa resort that offered treatment 'restricted to patients from beyond a seven-mile radius'. Formerly also a Roman baths, it was opened in the 16th century under the patronage of the Earl of Shrewsbury in association with the Buxton Bath Charity which was founded in 1572.[103]

As well as hospitals and spas, lay philanthropists also had a hand in the establishment of dispensaries, which by 1800 treated up to 50,000 cases a year. These provided advice, free medicine and 'domiciliary visits by eminent physicians' to 'the sick poor for whom there was no room in hospitals or whose complaints were unsuitable for hospitalisation'. Such visits provided first-hand experience of the life styles of the poor, and gave impetus towards public health initiatives for improved housing, sanitation and health education.[104,105]

John Howard, in his observations of European and British lazarettos, prisons and other hospitals summed up his view of the London hospitals in the late eighteenth century.

> *The securities and fees required at admission into many of the hospitals bear hard upon the poor, and absolutely exclude many of those who have the greatest occasion for charitable relief. The nurses fees in particular open a door to many impositions.*
>
> *The visits of governors are too often only a matter of form, the visitor hurrying out of an offensive room, and readily acquiescing in the reports of nurses &c. Hence I apprehend, many instances of neglect in surgeons and their dressers, as well as other officers, go unnoticed.*
>
> *I have never found any clergyman administering consolation and admonition to the sick; and prayers are usually attended by very few.*
>
> *White-washing the wards is seldom or never practised; and injurious prejudices against washing floors, and admitting fresh air, are suffered to operate.*
>
> *Bathing, either hot or cold, is scarcely ever used; I suppose, because it would give trouble to the attendants.*
>
> *The admission of great quantities of beer for the patients, from ale houses, by alleged, or pretended orders from the faculty, is a great and growing evil. Every proper article of diet should be provided by the hospital, and no other, on any account, be admitted.*

With remarkable foresight, Howard noted, possibly for the first time, that acute hospitals had a need for occupational regimes aimed at "daily life" skills. He also identified the need for suitable environments for their implementation when he observed that 'there are no convalescent wards or sitting rooms, so that patients are often turned out very unfit to work, or the common mode of living'.[106] In his recommendations he suggested the requirement of 'airy rooms and refectories for convalescent patients' as well as 'a piazza and spacious walk to induce patients to take air and exercise'. He added 'it is a pity that for want of attention to these circumstances, such noble intentions should be rendered of much less public utility, than was intended by their generous founders and supporters'.[107]

Of *The Royal Hospital* at Hasler, near Gosport, Howard reported that 'all the nurses here, and in the hospital at Plymouth, are women, which is very proper, as they are more cleanly and tender; and they more easily pacify the patients, who are seafaring men'. He noted that 'the staircases are spacious but they are of wood: the rises are too high; and there is no handrail on the wall',[108] and that the regulations stated:

> XIV. That no cards, or gaming of any kind, be permitted in the hospital.
>
> XV. ... that the nurses take care, that such patients as are able to attend divine service whenever it is performed; and report to the physician or surgeon, such persons who neglect going there.[109]

As hospitals for the masses, rather than the few, were a relatively new facility in the eighteenth century it was perceptive that anyone at that time recognised the part occupation could play in recovery and rehabilitation processes, and to comment on its absence. Few between then and the twentieth century made that connection within hospitals for the treatment of physical disorders, although they certainly did so for hospitals offering intervention to address mental or social disorders and difficulties. Also surprising is his observation about the absence of rails and the height of the steps on the hospital staircase. Howard's perceptiveness might have resulted from his all-encompassing research during which he visited and evaluated most of the facilities in Europe. In these he must have become aware of the possible devastating effects of lack of occupation, which in turn triggered an understanding of the need for its inclusion along with subsequent environmental additions to the buildings.

Convalescence

It was towards the end of the eighteenth century that the necessity for convalescence after acute hospitalisation became realised. That idea was an antecedent to the later notion of rehabilitation. Some might regard it as the antithesis, because, in the minds of many, convalescence suggests a picture of rest and inactivity, whilst allowing the body or mind to recoup. Rehabilitation, in contrast, is an active process towards recovery. What they have in common is an understanding that an extension of time and support is required following a period of acute hospitalisation, to enable return to a previous way of life, or an adapted one. Neither are currently in vogue to the extent they were previously, with fewer facilities being provided by the State for those specific purposes and many people being expected to convalesce or rehabilitate according to their own resources.

Kirkman Gray tells the story of the beginning of the realisation that acute care was not enough:

> As is so frequently the case this further development of care for the diseased owes its origin to a particular case of hardship. It happened that one day in 1791 a gentleman met in the Uxbridge Road a man of decent appearance sitting on the bank with a pair of crutches by his side. The cripple, in response to enquiries, gave this account of himself: "That he was a Gloucestershire manufacturer; that he had been a short time in London, where he had the misfortune to break his leg, and had been admitted a patient into an hospital; that his leg had been very well set, and all proper care had been taken of him; and upon his discharge that morning, some gentleman had kindly given him a shilling." Oh, useless shillings! He could not ride into Gloucestershire. What remains reflects the narrator, but to beg, to steal, or to perish. The story was not related in vain. The Samaritan Society was formed in connection with the London Hospital.[110]

The convalescent scheme took some years to evolve and was to become an important part of treatment regimes during the next century. However it is worth noting its genesis was at this earlier time. It grew alongside a developing appreciation that, following hospitalisation, many would not have the resources to even be certain of where they would live. Apart from that some would need time to overcome such handicaps as lameness, blindness, or depression, or to reconcile future lifestyles with an incurable condition. The "Friends" of every hospital were urged to establish societies similar to the Samaritan. Of similar timing, but slightly different origin was another convalescent type hospital. The Royal Sea Bathing Hospital at Margate was founded in 1796, and in the first year had 16 patients which number rose to 86 by the turn of the century. They were required to pay 5 shillings a week for board, and were transported cheaply, from London, by ship down the Thames.[111]

Prescription of occupations–equitation, travel etc.

Apart from hospitals, and despite a growing tendency towards increased use of drugs, the wider view of interventions towards good health still included medical recommendations to change lifestyles towards healthy regimes. Backing up pharmaceutical recommendations, the *Regimen Sanitatis* remained in force, with riding apparently still being the most popular occupation prescribed. It will be recalled that horse riding was considered healthful and often prescribed or used in Classical times. Xenophon, who was a friend and disciple of Socrates, wrote in *Oeconomicus* that Socrates highly approved of riding as a mode of exercise which he said, 'gives you at the same time both health and strength of body'.[112] Some hundred years later Oribasius provided, possibly, the first directions relative to exercise on horseback, and Galen even later described it as a 'mixed kind of exercise', combining active exercise in which the body moves itself and passive exercise in which the body is moved by an external force. The Greeks did not use stirrups so the occupation provided different and more fatiguing exercise than later.[113]

Physician, Erasmus Darwin (1731-1802), in *Zoonomia* provided a case study of himself illustrating the efficacy of equitation (riding):

Currie was in this way cured in early manhood of phthisis; and the writer of this article was in this way cured, also in his early manhood, of agrypnia, a painful and distressing want of sleep, which continued for nearly a year. The case is an interesting one, and may be worth recording. He had gone to Edinburgh for his last medical session. He was a clinical clerk at the Infirmary; and was an active president of the Royal Physical Society; and he had to prepare for his examination, for which purpose he was a pupil of excellent Fletcher. He was lodging in that unamiable street known as "College Street". During an intensely cold night, he was summoned from his bed by his landlady to see the maid of all work, who had been suddenly taken ill. He saw her in the homely kitchen of the second flat, and he had, in consequence of exposure in a bitter cold night in the mid-passage of that villainous flat, a severe attack of meningitis.

He was in those days a hard student; his brain had been taxed to the full, by reading, and lectures, and hospital practice, for he had to prepare the notes for the clinical lectures, besides his other kinds of necessary work. Inability to read, or sleep, or think; a quick wiry pulse, headache, and other such symptoms, took the pluck out of him - at that time he had more than enough of it. He went to his masters at the Infirmary, to the dons of the University - they all scouted the idea of there being inflammation of the brain. "You have worked too hard; live generously, shut up your books, drink wine, and work no more for the present." In the sense of reading, he could work no more; but he had himself bled once and again. He was not plucked; and at the close of that year he went to British Guiana, six degrees from the Equator. For nearly twelve months he did not sleep more than two hours in the twenty-four; sometimes not more than one hour; sometimes not at all. After trying everything he could think of, he bethought him of horse exercise, and pursued it steadily, riding for very many hours every day, and gradually his sleep returned to him; from that time to this he has slept like a top.

Physician, William Brownrigg's eighteenth century Casebook provides a number of recommendations for horse riding as treatment. He prescribed it for a variety of complaints, and Mrs Waters, a gentlewomen aged 49 with asthma, apparently found it both enjoyable and refreshing. Mr Boodle, a ship's captain in his fifties, was advised to 'indulge in horse-riding' for violent headaches, sickness, breathlessness and coughs and, in 1739, a Mrs Harriman of Workington, when experiencing pulmonary congestion was given a prescription to 'take frequent exercise' especially 'diligently by riding'. Brownrigg recommended exercise particularly on horseback as well as 'rubbing' to be of benefit for skin disorders, while for a studious 19 year old man with rickets a good deal of exercise but no mention of horses was advised. In a letter dated 1742, to J. Christian Esq., at Unerigg, Brownrigg prescribed a great deal of exercise by walking, in a chaise, and riding, along with reasonable hours of sleep, a moderate application to business, and abstinence from working at night, and from too much study. Christian apparently suffered from heaviness all over the body and his speech was affected from a disorder of 'slight resolution of certain nerves'.[114]

Probably the other most common occupational pursuit recommended was travel to a different clime, for those who could afford it. Porter provides the case of Lady Duncannon as illustrative of such intervention. In 1790 she was "spitting blood" and had an "abominable cough", 'her legs were so weak, she was on crutches. Everyone presumably thought it was consumption, although the term was not used.' Her family chose to consult the physician, Sir Richard Warren. 'He was in no doubt: she must winter in the South of France; in fact she remained there three years.'[115]

Public health, health promotion and occupational health

During the eighteenth century some improvement in hygiene occurred which Sigerist described as 'hygiene from below' suggesting that it was influenced by many publications designed to teach self health, as well as more general literary works of the period. In Rousseau's writings, for example, he argued that people must be enlightened about everything concerning health and disease so they could help themselves. That flowed on from his opposition to absolutist governments and belief that all people are good by nature, but unhappy because unenlightened and ill because ignorant.[116]

Another text worthy of note is the 1789 French *Encyclopedie Methodique*. Within that, Halle published a treatise on Hygiene that included a history of preventive and health promotive methods in the tradition of the *Regimen Sanitatis Salerno*. However it was much more inclusive of ideas other than about diet.[117]

Halle explained that medicine is concerned with two important issues, the state of health and the state of disease, an issue which is often mixed up in the present day when "health-care" is used to describe intervention for states of ill health. The central issue of the first of these, he said, was Hygiene–used in its broadest sense, and of the latter was therapeutics–the art of healing. Hygiene was the name given to what would now be known as public health. He defined it as 'that department of medicine, the object of which is the preservation of health'.

Halle suggested that government in the classical world made an important distinction between *public* and *private hygiene* which 'legislators of modern times have neglected'. In the public sphere people were considered collectively, or in society, and in the private in an individual capacity. The Ancients recognised, he said, 'the mutual dependence between the physical and moral virtues', and their wise regulations ensured health and vigour.[118] It was in public hygiene, Halle wrote, that 'the philosophical physician becomes the legislator's soul and adviser'.[119]

From his appreciation of the Classical viewpoint he explained that hygiene has three major objects. Firstly, 'the various conditions which a healthy man may experience in respect to the influences to which he is exposed; this is the study of temperaments and constitutions' and 'his wants and faculties'. Second, 'the causes, the nature, and the effects of these influences; this is what has been very preposterously termed the non-naturals', including 'the knowledge of the things which he uses and enjoys, and of their effects upon his constitution and organs'. Thirdly, 'the laws deduced from these sources of knowledge, and determines the bounds within which his enjoyments must be limited, if he would wish to enjoy a confirmed state of health' and 'the method of regulating or modifying these influences, so as to render them conducive to the preservation of health; this department of the subject has been properly denominated regimen or dietetic'.[120]

Following his history of the topic, Halle provided his own detailed plan of Hygiene as a department of medicine. He finalised his "complete treatise" with an "important inquiry", namely 'the consideration of the light which hygiene reflects on the art of healing'. His extensive plan is provided below, in which many of the topics and issues of concern are of interest to occupational therapists.

HYGIENE

PART FIRST

Subject of Hygiene:
Or the knowledge of Man, in a sound state of Health, in his Relations, and in his differences; that is to say, *in society, or in his individual capacity.*

PART SECOND

Matter of Hygiene:
Or the knowledge of those things which Man uses or enjoys, improperly denominated *Non-naturals*, and of their Influence upon our Constitution and our Organs.

PART THIRD

Means or Rules of Hygiene:
Or Rules which determine the measure within which the use of the things

called *Non-naturals* ought to be restrained for the preservation of Man; considered either *as a member of society*, or in his collective capacity, or as an individual.

PART FIRST
Subject of *Hygiene*

Division of the First Part into Two Sections

SECT. I.
Knowledge of Man in a sound State of Health, considered in Society or in his relative Capacity.

1, Relations resulting from *Climates* and *Situations.*

2,   '   '   from Associations in common Habitations or Places of Abode.

3,   '   '   from Uniformity in the Mode of Living with regard to Occupations, with regard to the common use of Air, of Food, &c.

4,   '   '   from Uniformity in *Customs* and *Manners*, Laws, Governments, etc.

SECT. II.
Knowledge of Man, considered individually, or in his Peculiarities.

1, Peculiarities relative to different Periods of Life.

2,   '   '   to the Sexes.

3,   '   '   to Temperaments.

4,   '   '   to Habits.

5,   '   '   to Professions.

6,   '   '   to different Circumstances of Life; Poverty, Convalescence, Travels, &c.

PART SECOND
Matter of *Hygiene*

CLASS

I. *Circumsusa:*	Or things with which we are surrounded.
II. *Applicata:*	Or things applied to the Surface of the Body.
III. *Ingesta:*	Or things destined to be introduced into the Body by the primary Passages.
IV. *Excreta,* Excretions:	Or things destined to be expelled from the Body.
V. *Gesta,* Actions:	Or functions which are exercised by the voluntary Motion of the Muscles and Organs.
VI. *Percepta:*	Perceptions: Or Functions and Impressions which depend upon the Sensibility and Organisation of the Nerves.

CLASS V
Gesta, Divided into Four Orders

ORDER I. *Watching*

ORDER II. *Sleep*

ORDER III. *Motion and Locomotion*
1, General Motion, impressed, spontaneous, mixed.
2, Partial; of the Limbs, of the Organs of the Voice, of Speech, etc.

ORDER IV. *Rest*
1, Absolute, or Inaction.
2, With active Disposition, without Locomotion; Position; Station, Efforts.

CLASS VI
Percepta, Divided Into Four Orders

ORDER I. *Sensations*
1, The external Senses.
2, Hunger, Thirst; and the Sensation of all our physical, moral, intellectual, and habitual Wants.
3, Physical Love.
4, Sympathy and Antipathy.

ORDER II. *Functions of the Soul.*
1, Passive Affections; agreeable, painful.
2, Active Affections; Attachment, Aversion.

ORDER III. *Functions of Mind.*
1, Intelligence.
2, Imagination.
3, Memory.

ORDER IV. *Debility, or Privation of Perceptions.*
1, Of the Senses; Apathy.
2, Of the Soul; Indifference.
3, Of the Mind; Inactivity.
4, Ennui; *Restlessness, Uneasiness of Mind.*

PART THIRD
Means of Hygiene

DIVISION I. *Public Hygiene:* Or Rules for the Preservation of Man, considered as a Member of Society, or in his collective Capacity.

DIVISION II. *Private Hygiene:* Or Rules for the Preservation of Man, considered as an Individual.

DIVISION I

Public Hygiene, arranged into Four Sections

SECT. I. *Rules of Public Hygiene* relative To Climates and Situations.
II. ' ' ' To common Places of Abode or Habitations.
III. ' ' ' To the common Mode of Living; in respect
to common Occupations, to the common
Use of Air, of Aliments, etc.
IV. ' ' ' To Customs, to Manners, to Laws, etc.

DIVISION II

Private Hygiene, in Three Sections.

SECTION III

Particularities of Regimen: Divided into Six Orders

ORD.`1, Regimen in different Periods of Life.
    2, ' of Sexes
    3, ' of Temperaments.
    4, ' relative to Habits.
    5, ' relative to Professions.
    6, ' relative to Circumstances of Life, Poverty, Travels,
Convalescence etc.

CONSEQUENCES OF *HYGIENE*, OR ITS CONNECTIONS WITH THE ART
OF HEALING

I. SPECIES OF CONNECTIONS: *Concerning the Differences* of Man in a sound
State of Health, with the predisposing *Causes* to Diseases.
    1, Of Man in his social Capacity; epidemical and endemial Dispositions.
    2, Of Man considered as an Individual: individual Dispositions to
Diseases, according to the Period of Life, Sex, Temperament, etc.
II. SPECIES OF CONNECTIONS, *concerning the Knowledge of the things called
Non-naturals,* with *the occasional Causes* of Diseases dependent on the
State of the Air, etc.
III. SPECIES OF CONNECTIONS, *concerning the prophylactic Rules of Hygiene,*
with *preservative and curative Precepts.*
    1, Of epidemic and endemial Diseases.
    2, Of sporadic Diseases.[121]

Halle provided a useful overview of his explorations and analyses. 'In truth,'
he wrote:

> ... *the different shades of the state of health conduct us to the different
> dispositions which render us obnoxious to disease. The varied effects which the
> things that man uses and enjoys produce upon his constitution, lead us to the
> causes which derange and disturb his health; and the difference of the measures*

within which his enjoyments ought to be confined, according to the diversities of his constitution, places us in the immediate vicinity of the variations of regimen, suited to the different conditions of the man who labours under disease.[122]

Within the public sphere, attention to occupational health matters was beginning to increase with Denis Diderot (1713-1784), the French encyclopaedist, providing comment on the forms of occupations in factories and other work centres.[123] Interest was also advancing within medical ranks, perhaps inspired in part by Ramazzini's text, discussed in a previous chapter, which was published at the beginning of the century. Like that famous predecessor, Antoine Lavoisier (1743-1794), a French chemist, concerned himself with analysis of movement aspects of manual work but, a sign of the times, concentrated on those in industry. He also gave attention to other physical problems such as unsuitable lighting, ventilation, food and water supplies, drainage, and insanitary workshops. A man of many interests, he proposed savings and superannuation funds for workers and, on a different tack, education and prison reform.[124]

Both Percival Pott, in 1775 and Benjamin Bell in 1794 noted the high incidence of testicular and scrotum cancer in trades associated with soot, such as chimney sweeping. Consumption was described amongst Redditch needle pointers, Sheffield cutlery grinders, and Edinburgh stonemasons.[125] In the armed services, Sir John Pringle observed and wrote about diseases apparent in the army,[126] and Gilbert Blane published a text on diseases of seamen[127] James Lind (1716-94), a Scottish surgeon, also had a particular interest in the health of sailors, having served as naval surgeon for 34 years. He investigated the causes of scurvy from which many sailors suffered, publishing his classical *Treatise of the Scurvy* in 1753. In that year he urged the issue of lemon juice to sailors as a preventive measure and, surprisingly, seems to have been heard. Eventually scurvy was eradicated especially as well-known explorers of the ilk of James Cook, heeded his advice. Four years later Lind published *An Essay on the Most Effectual Means of Preserving the Health of Seamen*[128] which dealt with the appalling conditions in which sailors lived when on board ship, and measures to improve them.[129]

The growing awareness of the hazards of industrialisation resulted in the establishment of societies that provided free surgical appliances to those threatened by ruptures as a result of heavy labouring jobs. Similarly, concern for other types of accident resulted in specialised charities being founded, such as the Royal Humane Society in 1773. That aimed to teach resuscitation to those rescued from drowning, which seemed to have been on the increase as economic expansion led to greater density of work around ports, rivers and canals.

Lay health care

Loudon, the medical historian, argues that with the growth of formalised medicine in the eighteenth century it would be easy to assume that this would be at the expense of the lay practice of the past. Yet, he describes how people in all walks of life continued to practice health care and describe themselves as medical practitioners.[130] George Winter, a practical farmer, was a case in point. He 'practised physic on his servants, and the poor of the neighbourhood' after coming into possession of his, physician, uncle's books.[131]

Members of the clergy and the gentry, men and women, frequently took on a doctoring role, actively physicking servants, employees, and villagers. Sometimes, like the Reverend George Woodward, they treated numerous servants and labourers, pets and livestock, and like the Duke of Montagu, who ran a hospital for old cows and broken-winded horses, they combined the roles of physician and veterinarian. Such role appropriation could result in a potentially lucrative practice and status. Indeed, clergyman Richard Wilkes (1690-1760) of Willenhall, Staffordshire, with an MA from St John's College in Cambridge proved that it was possible for people untrained in medicine, surgery, midwifery, or pharmacy to become fashionable physicians.[132]

Home treatment, and care of others in the community by those with aptitude and interest in doing so, was extensive. This was because of the common experience of ill health and early death, along with the scarcity of people trained in medical matters, the lack of success of many of their treatments, and their cost. Whilst it is probable that the place of the "wise woman" in health care became a dying tradition, as can be seen, great diversity in providers of "medicine" remained an integral part of society.[133] It remained a free market so vendors of patent medicines and quacks flourished as the incidence and prevalence of diseases such as rickets, tuberculosis, and typhoid increased with the growth of more urban populations living in crowded, squalid conditions. The main difference between quacks and trained physicians was the merchandising style. Whilst the academically trained physician recognised that illness was a disorder symptomatic of the whole system, in the way of Classical Greek Medicine, quacks treated "symptoms" with "potions".[134] They could run lucrative businesses with 20th century-like entrepreneurial flair making big promises, offering money-back guarantees, special deals, free gifts, seductive packaging and names, and "mail order" patent medicines for country readers. Saturation advertising on the streets and in the newspapers became commonplace.[135] In what was described by Porter as the first consumer revolution, practitioners targeted deeply ingrained self health traditions, advocating Nature rather than physicians, and prevention before cure.[136]

Figure 1.7.8: Doctor Bossy, an imfamous medicine vendor selling his wares to a crowd of sick and crippled people at Covent Garden. Etching 1795, after A.van Assen.
(The Wellcome Library)

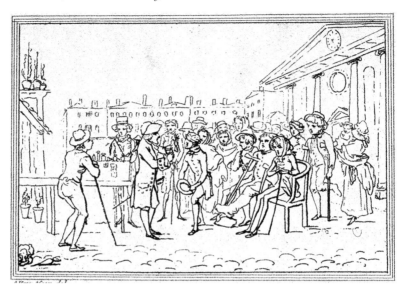

Self as occupational and health practitioners

Just as in the present day there are some illnesses that people self diagnose and treat, like the common cold, headache, or rheumatic twinges, so in the eighteenth century did people act as their own health practitioner. They made use of religious, philosophical, moral and personal strategies, particularly valuing practical activity to prevent and counter illness and cope with death. Self-diagnosis and prescription were even more common than now, and ranged over more types of disorder. The patriarch of a house assumed responsibility for its health as well as its morals, and a "good housewife" was expected to practice family or "kitchen" physic just as they cooked, brewed, and sewed. Health care and medicine were constant subjects of discussion amongst the educated, but more than that, could have been a form of occupational therapy for often distressed family members as they sought feelings of competence. 'Caroline Fox, for example, suggested to her sister, the Marchioness of Kildare, when her husband was sick: "Don't you as a physician think bathing in the sea would do him good?"'[137]

James Boswell's London Journal, 1762-1763 provides an example of how he self diagnosed and treated gonorrhoea. Boswell (1740-1795), pictured in figure

1.7.9, the son of Scottish judge Lord Archinlech, was a biographer most famous for his friendship with, and biography of Dr Samuel Johnson.

Figure 1.7.9: **James Boswell,**
pencil sketch by
Thomas Lawrence
(National Portrait
Gallery)

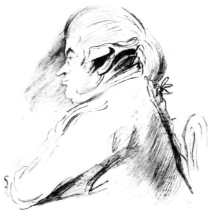

The extract from his journal, below, tells of his illness which followed a couple of previous bouts, how he discussed it with colleagues, and that he recognised how it would curtail many of his usual "health giving" activities for some little time. It also identifies how he included different occupations in his daily life to lessen the effects of the disease and increase his experience of well-being:

THURSDAY 20 JANUARY. I rose very disconsolate, having rested very ill by the poisonous infection raging in my veins and anxiety and vexation boiling in my breast. I could scarcely credit my own senses. What! thought I, can this beautiful, this sensible, and this agreeable woman be so sadly defiled? Can corruption lodge beneath so fair a form? Can she who professed delicacy of sentiment and sincere regard for me, use me so very basely and so very cruelly? No, it is impossible. I have just got a gleet by irritating the parts too much with excessive venery. And yet these damned twinges, that scalding heat, and that deep-tinged loathsome matter are the strongest proofs of an infection. ... Am I now to be laid up for many weeks to suffer extreme pain and full confinement, and to be debarred all the comforts and pleasures of life? And then must I have my poor pocket drained by the unavoidable expense of it? And shall I no more (for a long time at least) take my walk, healthful and spirited, round the Park before breakfast, view the brilliant Guards on the Parade, and enjoy all my pleasing amusements? And then am I prevented from making love to Lady Mirabel, or any other woman of fashion? O dear, O dear! What a cursed thing this is! What a miserable creature am I!

In this woeful manner did I melancholy ruminate. I thought of applying to a quack who would cure me quickly and cheaply. But then the horrors of being imperfectly cured and having the distemper thrown into my blood terrified me exceedingly. I therefore pursued my resolution of last night to go to my friend Douglas, whom I knew to be skilful and careful; and although it should cost me more, yet to get sound health was a matter of great importance, and I might save upon other articles.[138]

SATURDAY 22 JANUARY. Calmly and considerately did I sit down in my arm-chair this morning and endeavour to call up all the philosophy that I could. A distemper of this kind is more dreadful to me than most people. I am of a warm constitution: a complexion, as physicians say, exceedingly amorous, and therefore suck in the poison more deeply. I have had two visitations of this calamity. The first lasted ten weeks. The second four months. How severe a reflection is it! And, O, how severe a prospect! Yet let me take courage. Perhaps this is not a very bad infection, and as I shall be scrupulously careful of myself, I may get rid of it in a short time.[139]

WEDNESDAY 9 FEBRUARY. I got up excellently well. My present life is most curious, and very fortunately is become agreeable. My affairs are conducted with the greatest regularity and exactness. I move like very clock-work. At eight in the morning Molly lights the fire, sweeps and dresses my dining-room. Then she calls me up and lets me know what o'clock it is. I lie some time in bed indulging indolence, which in that way, when the mind is easy and cheerful, is most pleasing. I then slip on my clothes loosely, easily, and quickly, and come into my dining-room. I pull my bell. The maid lays a milk-white napkin upon the table and sets the things for breakfast. I then take some light amusing book and breakfast and read for an hour or more, gently pleasing both my palate and my mental taste. Breakfast over, I feel myself gay and lively. I go to the window, and am entertained with the people passing by, all intent on different schemes. To go regularly through the day would be too formal for this my journal. Besides, every day cannot be passed exactly the same way in every particular. My day is in general diversified with reading of different kinds, playing on the violin, writing, chatting with my friends. Even the taking of medicines serves to make time go on with less heaviness. I have a sort of genius for physic and always had great entertainment in observing the changes of the human body and the effects produced by diet, labour, rest, and physical operations.[140]

Boswell's sexually transmitted disease was not a disorder considered shameful or necessary to hide. Sex, at least among the higher social strata, and for both men and women, was regarded with an earthy matter-of-factness, openness and bawdiness far different from the next century. Erasmus Darwin described sex as the 'chef d'oeuvre, the masterpiece of nature', 'the purest source of human felicity, the cordial drop in the otherwise vapid cup of life'. His attitudes were not surprising in a medical man as sexual activity was prescribed for medical and psychological reasons, especially as retention of semen was believed to be harmful, and sexually deprived women frustrated and ill-tempered.[141]

The sexual freedom of the time was one aspect of the Enlightenment championing of liberty, individuality, and the right to personal fulfilment, which was critical of blind traditionalism and moral judgements of Catholic or reformed churches alike. The pursuit of, and right to, happiness in combination with the idea that it was fitting to seek after worldly well-being led people to be more indulgently reflective about their own psychological needs in diaries and auto-biographies. Boswell for example, in expansive tone wrote: 'I felt a completion of happiness. I just sat and hugged myself in my own mind.'[142]

Self-help practitioners not only drew upon theories and practices derived from personal and other's experiences but they also had access to the many written texts mentioned earlier.

Self health texts

Analogous to the growth of computer literacy in the present day, during the 18th century there was a growing level of literacy prompted and encouraged by a wide range of information in books, innumerable pamphlets, almanacs, primers, newspapers, and magazines. Many were about health and illness, or partly so. The *Gentleman's Magazine,* for example, provided opportunity for educated readers and medical practitioners to communicate through the correspondence columns about health issues. Recognising their potential for good, or perhaps with less charitable thoughts, for advertisement, respected medical men were often the authors of texts aimed at self and lay health practitioners.[143]

Quite a number of the books were devoted to advice about health promotion and disease prevention in the tradition of the *Regimen Sanitatis.* In *Every Man His Own Doctor* John Archer outlines both prevention and cure:

> How every one may know his own Constitution and Complection, by certain Signs. Also the Nature and Facilities of all Food as well Meats, as drinks. Whereby every Man and Woman may understand what is good or hurtful to them. Treating also, of Air, Passions of Mind, Exercise of Body, Sleep, Venery and Tobacco etc. The Second part shews the full knowledge and Cure of the Pox, and Running of the Reins, Gout, Dropsie, Scurvy, Consumptions, and Obstructions, Agues. Shewing their causes and Signs, and what danger any are in, little or much and perfect Cure with small cost and no danger of Reputation.[144]

George Cheyne's *Essay of Health and Long Life* (1724) was an early offering along the lines of the *Regimen Sanitatis* providing timely advice about healthy and moderate lifestyles. Cheyne was, obviously, a diplomat, because by his moderate rather than severe approach his work proved to be a firm favourite throughout the century, especially with the upper classes. Like earlier texts and others of the kind, it concentrated on the non-naturals recommending the avoidance or reduction of eating or drinking too much, late nights, and sedentary occupations.

> It is a common saying, that every man past forty is either a fool or a physician: … for as the world goes at present, there is not anything that the generality of the better sort of mankind so lavishly and so unconcernedly throw away as health, except eternal felicity. Most men know when they are ill, but very few when they

Figure 1.7.10: George Cheyne
(*The Wellcome Library*)

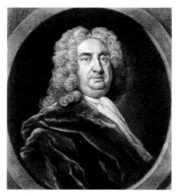

are well. And yet it is most certain, that it is easier to preserve health than to recover it, and to prevent diseases than to cure them. Towards the first, the means are mostly in our own power.[145]

As he went on to discuss the six non-naturals, he provided the following rationale for the inclusion of active and passive occupations:

To restore this decay and wasting of animal bodies, nature has wisely made alternate periods of labour and rest, sleeping and watching, necessary to our being; the one for the active employments of life, to provide for and take in the materials of our nourishment; the other to apply those materials to the proper wasted parts, and to supply the expenses of living.[146]

With something of the concern of a present day occupational scientist Cheyne obviously studied the nature of occupation and its effects upon productivity, health, and freedom from stress. His observations on the timing of occupation to best effect would provide worthwhile current day research topics as the answers would be valuable, not only to scholars but, to students and rehabilitees. In common with experience recounted by many modern writers he observed that most people are able to engage most fruitfully in intellectual occupations after a nights sleep, and so he recommended that this should be borne in mind and acted upon. Cheyne introduces the idea as a well-known fact:

All the nations and ages have agreed that the morning season is the proper time for speculative studies, and those employments that require the faculties of the mind. For then the stock of the spirits is undiminished, and in its greatest plenty; the head is clear and serene, the passions are quieted and forgot; the anxiety and inquietude that the digestions beget in the nervous system, in most tender constitutions, and the hurry the spirits are under after the great meal, are settled and wrought off. I should advise, therefore, those who are of a weak relaxed state of nerves, who are subject to hypochondriacal or hysterical disorders, whose professions lead them to much use of their intellectual faculties, or who would indulge in speculative studies, to go early to bed, and to rise betimes; to employ their morning hours in these exercises till eleven o'clock, then to take some agreeable breakfast of vegetable food; to go on with their studies and professions and then to take all the rest of the day off all study and thought, divert themselves agreeably in some innocent amusement, with some gentle bodily exercise; and as soon as the digestion is over, to retire and provide for going to bed, without any further supplies, except it be a glass of fair water, or warm sack-whey. But the aged and sickly must go sooner to bed and lie longer, because age and sickness break rest, and the stiffened and hardened limbs of the ancient become more pliant and relaxed by much sleep, a supine posture, and the warmth of the bed.[147]

As well as balancing time between physical and intellectual occupations, Cheyne referred to occupational balance in terms of energy and restfulness. He considered in some detail how he saw the relationship between what people "did" and their physiological processes, so supporting his argument that occupation is 'almost as necessary to health and long life, as food itself'. A very similar statement was made by Dunton, an American occupational therapy pioneer, early in the twentieth century, the major difference being that Dunton did not include the "almost". Cheyne, in the spirit of his time, used the biblical story of Genesis rather than scientific proof to support his observations.

We proceed in the next place, to the consideration of exercise and quiet, the due regulation of which is almost as necessary to health and long life, as food itself. Whether we were so made before the fall, as to live in intire health, in a rigidly sedentary and contemplative life, is a speculation of no great consequence, nor easily determined in our present situation; for there is no certain analogy between things as they now are, and as they might have been then. As there happen'd an intire revolution in the complexion and qualities of the minds of the first pair; so, to me, there appear, to be evident indications of a designed change and alteration of the material world, and the nature of the animals and vegetables which subsist on this globe, from what they were when God pronounced every thing good that he had made. Nor seem the celestial bodies to have escaped, so far as they regard us. Whatever be in this, the passage where God tells Adam, "That in the sweat of his brow he shall eat bread" (Gen. iii. v. 19), seems to be the injunction of a salutary penance; that is, not merely a punishment, but also a remedy against the disorders his body would be liable to in this new state of the creation, and against the poisonous effects of the forbidden tree he had eaten the fruit of. I am the more confirmed in this belief, that I observe, the absolute necessity of labour and exercise, to preserve the body any time in due plight, to maintain health, and lengthen out life. For let whatsoever diet be pursued, however adjusted in both in quantity and quality, let whatever evacuations be used to lessen the malady, or any succedaneum (equivalent) be proposed, to prevent the ill effects, our bodies are so made, and the animal oeconomy now so contrived, that without due labour and exercise, the juices will thicken, the joints will stiffen, the nerves will relax, and on these disorders, chronical distempers, and a crazy old age must ensue. Nor is this necessary only in the colder climates, and where the food is gross, but even in the warmest climates, and where the food is lightest. For though the warmth of the air may keep the perspiration free and open, or rather, where it is very great, promote sweating; yet, at the same time, and by consequence, it will thicken the fluids, and relax the fibres; to prevent both which, exercise is absolutely necessary: but in such a climate it ought to be gone about in the cool of the day. And tho' light food may, in great measure, prevent the thickening of the fluids, yet it cannot do it sufficiently without exercise; nor can it at all keep the fibres in due tension; for to that purpose exercise is absolutely necessary. Nay, the joint power of warm air and light food cannot supply the place of exercise in keeping the joints pliant and moveable, and preserving them from growing resty and stiff.[148]

In turning from theory to practice Cheyne discussed the occupations he considered of particular use, both in terms of sick and well, young and old. As in many similar recommendations throughout the centuries he pointed to riding and walking, as others before him had, as most useful occupations for many purposes. Horseback riding was, for example, much in favour as a form of rest. For example Benjamin Marten, in a book on consumption published in the previous century, had recommended riding because it entertained patients in a restful manner, in contrast to the physical and mental fretfulness resulting from prolonged residence in dark, smelly, and stuffy bedrooms.[149] Both riding and walking may also have been considered particularly useful because the circulation and elimination of fluids was considered vitally important within the "humoural" theories of health. Cheyne wrote:

Of all the exercises that are or may be used for health (such as walking, riding a horseback or in a coach, fencing, dancing, playing at billiards, bowls or tennis, digging, working at a pump, ringing a dumb bell, etc) walking is the most natural, as it would not spend too much of the spirits of the weakly. Riding is certainly the most manly, the most healthy, and the least laborious, and expensive of spirits, of any; shaking the whole machine, promoting an universal perspiration and secretion of all the fluids (to which may be added, the various changes of the air, thro' which they so quickly pass, every alteration of which, becomes, as it were, a new bath) and thereby, variously twitching the nervous fibres, to brace and contract them as new scenes amuse the mind. Those who cannot ride, must be carried in a coach or litter, which is the best exercise for the lame and crazy, and the only one proper for old and decrepid persons, as well as those that are so young, that they are not able to manage their own exercise. The home exercise, such as playing tennis and billiards, dancing, fencing, and the like, ought to be follow'd only when the season forbids them being abroad; for being in the air, contributes much towards the benefit of exercise. 'Tis beautiful to observe that ernest desire planted by nature, in young persons, to romp, jump, wrestle and run, and constantly be pursuing exercises and bodily diversions, that require labour, even till they are ready to drop down; especially the healthier sort of them: so that sitting or being confined, seems to be the greatest punishment they can suffer, and imprisoning them for some time, will much more readily correct them than whipping. This is a wise contrivance of Nature; for thereby, their joints are render'd pliable and strong; their blood continues sweet, and proper for a full circulation; their perspiration is free, and their organs stretched out, by due degrees, to their proper extension.[150]

Occupation was recognised by Cheyne as the mechanism by which bodily organs were maintained as Nature intended they should. He, tactfully, suggested that the occupations of "working men" were more healthful than those of the wealthy who devoured his opinions:

> It is also very agreeable to observe, how the several different organs of labouring men are strengthen'd and render'd brawny and nervous, as they happen to be most employed in their several vocations, let them be otherwise ever so small or weakly. The legs, thighs and feet of chairmen; the arms and hands of watermen; the backs and shoulders of porters, grow thick, strong and brawny by time ... And if due pains were taken by the labour proper to them, the organs of all the functions of the animal oeconomy might be strengthen'd and kept in due plight.[151]

As a proto-occupational therapist he made recommendations about what type of occupations should be recommended for particular cases with cure in mind:

> ... to the asthmatick, and those with weak lungs, I should recommend talking much and loud, even by themselves, walking up an easy ascent, and when any degree of weariness warns them, to sit and rest, till they are easy, and then return to their walking again, and so to increase it every day, till they are able to walk a reasonable distance, in a reasonable time. To those who have weak nerves and digestion, and to those who are much troubled by head-aches (most of which arise from the ill state of the stomach and bowels) I should recommend riding on horseback as much as possibly they could, in the clearest and driest air, and to change the air daily, if possible. To those who are troubled with the stone or gravel, to ride much over rough causeways in a coach. To those that have rheumatick pains, to play at Billiards, tennis or cricket, till they sweat plentifully, and then go immediately into a warm bed, and drink liberally of some warm thin liquor, with ten drops of Spirit of Sal Armoniac or Harts-horn in each draught, to encourage the sweating. To those who have weak arms or hams, playing two or three hours at tennis, or at football every day. To those who have weak backs or breast, ringing a bell, or working at a pump. Walking thro' rough roads, even to lassitude, will soonest recover the use of their limbs to the gouty; tho' riding on horseback or in a coach will best prevent the distemper. But the studious and contemplative, the valetudinary, and those of weak nerves, if they aim at health and long life, must make exercise a part of their religion, as it is among some of the Eastern nations, with whom pilgrimages, at stated times, are an indispensible duty, and where mechanical trades are learned and practiced by men of all ranks. Those who have their time in their own hands, ought to have stated seasons for riding or walking in a good air, as indispensible, as those for going to dinner, to bed, or to church. Three hours for riding, or two for walking, the one half before the great meal, and the other before going to bed, is the least that can be dispensed with.[152]

Cheyne also considered associated conditions that were advisable when undertaking remedial occupation:

> There are three conditions of exercise to make it the most beneficial that may be. First, that it be upon an empty stomach (as, indeed, that is the time for all

medicinal evacuations) for thereby, the now concocted crudities, or those superfluities Nature would be rid of, and has fitted, by going through the proper secretions, for being ejected, but cannot throw off without foreign assistance, will be readiest discharged. For on a full stomach exercise would be too tumultuous, precipitate the secretions, and throw off the found juices with the corrupted humours. Secondly, that it be not continued to down-right lassitude, depression of spirits, or a melting sweat. The first will wear out the organs, the second spend the strength, and the third will only do violence to the natural functions. Thirdly, due care is to be had after exercise, to retreat to a warm room and proper shelter from the injuries of the weather, left sucking into the wasted body the nitreous particles of the circumambient air, they should imflame the blood, and produce a rheumatism, fever or cold. I might add a fourth condition, joining temperance to exercise, otherwise the evil will be as broad one way, as 'tis long the other. For since exercise will create a greater appetite, if it is indulg'd to the full, the concoctive powers will be as unequal to the load, as they were before.[153]

Apart from Cheyne, others provided similar therapeutic advice in self health texts. William Buchan, a medical practitioner trained in Edinburgh, provided the middle class with a style of advice that they appreciated. *Domestic Medicine* which was aimed at self-healthers rather than his own profession, appeared in 1769 and this, like Cheyne's text, offered simple preventive advice on how to care for health by taking control over life-styles and environments. He set out the rules of health according to the headings of the non-naturals, as well as some simple remedies of a practical nature.[154] Porter suggests that Buchan 'struck a chord with thousands of sturdy, independent-minded self-help readers - his followers were dubbed "Buchaneers"–anxious to maintain and maximise control, wherever possible, over the fate of their own bodies'.[155] From the point of view of this history it is worth noting that Buchan stressed the advisability of men 'learning some mechanical employment' which netted successful results as a health measure to counter the frustrating effects of inactivity.[156]

John Wesley's (1703-91) book *Primitive Physick* was published in 1747. It was also a favourite, but was concerned with cures rather than health maintenance, although he cited Cheyne's general health advice. An upholder of self-healing as well as being the founder of the Methodist faith, Wesley put trust in Nature whilst offering simple instructions using common ingredients and traditional knowledge in preference to quack remedies. In essence his publication was a recipe book to help, particular the poor, in times of sickness because in most instances they could not afford to take time off work.[157]

In a slightly different mode, and reminiscent of the popular verse of the medieval Regimen, John Armstrong (1709-79), a physician and poet, and brother of paediatric physician, George, published a poetic account of *The Art of Preserving Health* in 1744.[158] True to type, it includes reference to the value of air, warm ablutions, and appropriate diet as well as to exercises, graded walking, work, and the pleasurable and health giving effects of fishing and gardening in what Harvey, the editor of *The Oxford Companion to English Literature*, describes as a surprisingly pleasant poem in spite of its unattractive title.[159]

According to their sales, health-care books were popular, and from contemporary diaries and letters it seems clear that they were not only purchased but also well used.

Occupation for health: New theories and initiatives

As modern day occupational therapists are deeply interested in physical mobility and aids to occupations of daily life, the first part of this section considers their development during the Enlightenment.

Physical mobility and aids to daily occupations

As Bath was a place where many people with disability could be found taking, or bathing in, the mineral waters it is an appropriate place to consider what was available to assist them. In fact, the patients of the voluntary hospital had to walk through the streets to the site of their "hot spring" treatment. Sedan chairs and chairmen were provided for those who couldn't walk. Although their diagnoses were varied, there would have been quite a few who experienced difficulties, for many were described as suffering rheumatism, and palsy (which was often due to lead paint), as well as fever, and leprosy which diagnosis possibly also referred to other types of skin disorders. Men and women were segregated, with women attending the baths on Mondays, Wednesdays and Fridays, and men on the other days.[160]

Furniture makers at this time began to create chairs that incorporated wheels in their designs. These became known as Bath chairs because they were most commonly found there, despite the fact that many requiring assistance got around in a sedan or less formal and comfortable litter. British cartoonist, Thomas Rowlandson (1756-1827) featured litters in his satirical cartoons. One called *Bath Races* is shown in figure 1.7.11. Originally Bath chairs were made of wood, and were quite heavy and cumbersome, requiring at least one assistant to propel them. Later they where made so that people could use them by self-propulsion.[161]

Figure 1.7.11: Bath races: Coloured Etching by Thomas Rowlandson 1756-1827.
(The Wellcome Library)

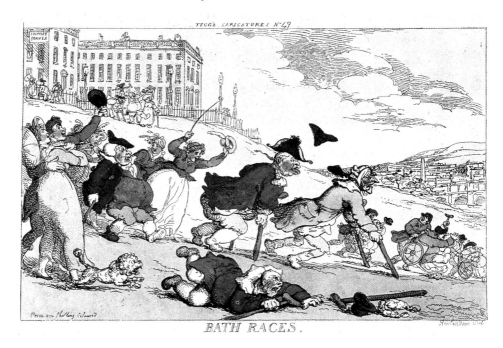

The Enlightenment saw private enterprise making a profit from specially devised furniture to aid people with disability. The story of John Joseph Merlin, an inventor of such furniture, is worthy of a little scrutiny as it provides some clues about the need for entrepreneurial flair in getting such messages across. Merlin was born in 1735 in Belgium, possibly from a family of inventors or mechanics. When he was about 19 years old he lived in Paris for a number of years with, perhaps, the encouragement of the Academie des Sciences. Here he began to make his mark in "mechanical" circles. In 1760 he moved to England under the patronage of a Spanish nobleman, the Conde de Fuentes, who was appointed Ambassador Extraordinary. Merlin was accepted by English society, apart from his skill, because of his eccentricity, which was probably deliberately cultivated, and his appearance of a gentleman rather than a tradesman. He established Merlin's Mechanical Museum in Princes Street, Hanover Square, a fashionable address, which opened its doors to the public somewhere between 1783 and 1788 and became one of the "entertainments" of late eighteenth century London. He died in 1803 but his museum possibly remained open another five years. Some items from his catalogue are described below.[162]

Morning Amusement
M E R L I N' S

Mechanical Exhibition
C A T A L O G U E
of the
DIFFERENT PIECES
of
M E C H A N I S M
Exhibited
At his GREAT ROOM
No. 11 Princes Street, Hanover Square
Which is open every day (Sundays excepted)
from Eleven 'till Three o'Clock
ADMITTANCE 2s. 6d.
N.B. Such persons as visit this Exhibition will have
the liberty of using not only the Hygaeian chair but also the Escarpolets

VI.   A portable Hygaeian chair, by which Persons may swing themselves with perfect Safety, and so as to afford an easy Motion, and uncommonly pleasing Exercise.
For the peculiar Advantages of this to Health, the Reader is referred to Dr. Carmichael Smith's excellent Pamphlet on the Utility of Swinging in Pulmonary Consumptions and other Disorders.

VII.   *Morpheus's Chair,* made to fall back at Pleasure, and form a Bed for Repose of the Infirm. It has curtains and a Calash over the Head, with a Cradle for the Legs, and also wheels about at Pleasure. Price 40 Guineas.

VIII.   A new-invented Mechanical Table, which may be raised to different Heights with great Ease, and will serve for reading, writing or Music for six performers, with four Candles, three Drawers, and two Tablets. It also makes a compleat Breakfast or occasional Dining Table, and takes up no more Room than a Pembroke Table. Price from 10 guineas to 20.

IX.   A curious new-invented *Tea Table,* by which any lady can fill twelve Cups of Tea and shift them round by the Pressure of the Foot, without the Assistance of her hands.

XII.   *Mechanical Easy Chairs* for the Gouty and Infirm to wheel themselves about, with Curtains and a Cradle to rest the Legs upon. Price from 14 to 20 Guineas.

XIV.   An *Escarpolet*, by which two Persons may swing themselves, sitting in a double Hygaeian Chair, with perfect Safety, for similar Purposes with No. VI.

XXII.   A new invented Oscillatory Machine by which Persons may swing themselves sitting in an Hygaeian Chair, or lying on a Sopha.

It is possible that Merlin based some of his designs on similar ones that he had seen earlier in France, imported to England and developed. One such was his invalid or gouty chair which had an almost identical mechanical arrangement to the 'fauteuil … pour ceux qui ont la goute au jambes', built by the master cabinet maker Jean Francois Oeben for the Duc de Borgogne, as well as the invalid chair catalogued by *Grollier de Serviere* in 1751:

> **B19. Recueil d'Ouvrages Curiex de Mathematique et de Mechanique (ou Description du Cabinet)** *2nd edition, Paris, 1751. Grollier de Serviere*
> *Amongst his descriptions of fantastic mechanical devices, Grollier de Serviere includes this eminently practicable design for an invalid chair. Whereas some of his schemes may be traced back as far as two hundred years in earlier collections there is no known precedent for this design. In essence this is Merlin's "gouty chair" and one must suppose that Merlin either saw this book or an actual example, probably when he was in Paris from 1754-1760.*[164]

Interest in many other aspects of daily living emerged at this time. Macdonald reported that Dr Thomas Percival (1740-1804) was concerned with appropriate dwellings and social conditions for the working class, that Johann Frank (1745-1821) gave consideration to suitable clothing.[165]

Occupation for curative or rehabilitative purposes

The Enlightenment proved to be a period in history when occupations that provided physical exercise became clearly recognised as health maintaining. As in earlier times this was linked with a very broad notion of gymnastics, which appeared to cover a range of therapeutic interventions that were later separated into physiotherapy, remedial gymnastics and occupational therapy. In considering reports that tell of those therapeutic practices, the ones of an occupational nature will be selected.

Halle argued that 'with regard to established institutions, to practices, and to customs, we find nothing among modern states which corresponds to the gymnastic schools of the ancients'. They, readers will recall from an earlier chapter, were places of learning and music as well as exercise, where the mind, body and spirit could flourish in social and individual pursuits. Halle went on to suggest that the games used in educational institutions might be considered for the same purposes:

> *It were nevertheless an injustice to exclude from the number of gymnastic practices, the games common in our colleges. Those of hand-ball, of tennis, of the football, of prison bars, and many others, as they stimulate self-love, by the honour of a victory due at once, to strength, to agility, and to adroitness, were invented with perfect propriety for the purpose of developing the whole muscular power of the body, of perfecting the external senses, by increasing their accuracy and precision, and of unfolding in the youth the germs of more than one sort of useful industry. The tennis resembles in many respects the game which Galen so much extols under the name of the small ball.*[166]

One worker in the field, Clement Joseph Tissot (1750-1826), in *Gymnastique Medicinale et Chirugicale* began to classify the exercise elements of occupation as active, passive, or mixed, and identified some he considered of particular value for health purposes. These ranged widely across manual and domestic occupations such as sewing, sawing, hammering, sweeping, and wood chopping, to others of recreational character like billiards or tennis. Tissot also identified occupations of a communal nature like bellringing and those with creative appeal such as violin playing. In the following quotation, Tissot's concern about the lack of knowledge regarding how best to use movements emanating from occupations pre-empts parallel concerns of early 20th century occupational therapists:

> *It has been demonstrated that to prevent and remedy rigidity of muscles and ligaments, motion is necessary, but this knowledge is not sufficient, we must know at what period in the disease to begin, how and to what extent we should use it.*
>
> *Motion should not begin until pain, inflammation and swelling have subsided. It would be dangerous to move joints while these are still present since they might be aggravated. We have seen persistent swelling, inflammation, pain and convulsions in cases where motion was begun too early.*
>
> *When we are convinced that the synovia is attenuated and softened enough to be resorbed by motion and that the part can be exposed without danger to the effects of the exercises suited to reestablish its former status we should choose exercises according to their immediate and particular action on the involved part. We should begin with moderate exercises and avoid stenuous motions in patients who have not recovered their strength.*[167]

Tissot's recommendations for the correct timing of therapy relate to the progress of symptoms, and depend on close monitoring of the injured body part. Starting with injuries to the upper limb, he provided advice about the appropriate choice of occupation for best effect. The first example referred to humero-scapular movements:

> *... if the arms are atrophied and weak or still show the effects of paralysis, there is nothing that will absorb the synovia, re-establish play in the joint and return strength to the arms better than turning the wheel of a printing press by*

*its handle, of cutting wood, filing, using the wimble, throwing stones with a
sling, making stones ricochet on the surface of the water, and all other directions
in its socket. More than once we have seen workers who use the file, the saw and
the lathe recover motion of their stiff or paralysed arms as soon as they were
strong enough to return to their shops.*[168]

In a second example, Tissot considered movements of the elbow and forearm:

*If the movements of articulation of the humerus with the ulna and those of the
ulna with the radius are still difficult and there is ankylosis as a result of disuse;
if the muscles and ligaments of the joints are stiff to such an extent that flexion
and extension of the arm are virtually impossible (as well as pronation and
supination) and if the articulation of these same bones with the metacarpus is
equally involved - what could be more fitting in filling the remedial objectives
than the act of making holes in wood with a drill, of using a small or large
carpenter's plane, or playing the violin or fencing. What exercises more pleasant
and moderate than billiards, quoits, ninepins, etc. But even more effective for
ankylosis or stiffness of the elbow would be the action of bell ringing, drawing
water from a well, climbing a tree, ... Let us repeat that the act of carrying a
lightweight in the arm extended also helps to gain the objective.*[169]

Tissot went on to suggest that the use of occupation could be graded
according to remedial demands in order to progress recovery:

*Shuttlecock and tennis move all the joints of the arm and forearm and call
forth even greater activity and speed than the preceding, and fulfil perfectly all
the remedial requirements. The inflated ball which requires more strength and
nerve to throw would complete the cure which was begun by the other activities.*[170]

Tissot's third example of a remedial occupation programme is in respect of
hand therapy from wrist to fingers. Of particular interest is that he obviously
favours occupations with purpose and meaning ahead of those which exercise
without a particular purpose:

*If it is the wrist or fingers which require re-establishement of their motion,
exercises which place the entire hand in motion as playing the violin, the cithern,
fingering the harpsichord, etc., etc., all satisfy the indications for re-establishing the
agility of these parts and of relieving the stiffness of the flexor and extensor muscles.*

*If these exercises are not available, we can offer others such as squeezing sand
in the fist, turning a box in the hand, kneading and moulding wax, bending and
stretching sheets of lead, etc. We have frequently employed such exercises with
success in breaking up the tophaceous humors which are found in the joints of the
fingers following attacks of gout which have produced a sort of ankylosis.*[171]

The last paragraph is reminiscent of occupational therapy treatment that
became particularly popular in the 1970s and 80s, such as kneading exercise
putty and finding objects in rice or sand. Tissot concluded by encouraging
others to consider different conditions of upper limbs that could be helped by
similar occupational treatment, adding that 'there are probably other surgical
conditions of the upper extremities to which such methods can be applied'. He

then progressed 'to the treatment of these same diseases in the lower extremities':

When these diseases have affected the lower extremities, we should use those exercises which place these parts in motion with respect to the duration of the disease, beginning with the most moderate such as walking, climbing and descending ladders or an inclined plane; billiards, quoits, swimming etc., the effects of which are to make the head of the femur move moderately in its socket at the same time as the joints of the knee and foot.

The pleasure which is associated with most of these exercises is capable of encouraging patients to participate without realising they are performing movements suited to stimulate circulation in these parts and return better activity to the muscles, to break up the thickened synovia in the joints and to loosen them; to elongate stiffened shortened muscles; finally to gain enough strength and vigour of the extremities to permit the earlier return of a condition to support more active and strenuous movements.

For this purpose we recommend shuttlecock, tennis, mall, football, dancing which requires rapid walking and nimble running; hunting which requires walking on sandy, stony paths or on heavy broken ground and necessitates climbing, descending, running, jumping over ditches, scaling heights; the game of barriers which frequently requires running on all fours. It is in these ways, I say, that all these exercises by setting in motion all the joints of the hips, knees and feet will contribute greatly to the relief of the sequelae of all these chronic diseases and achieve their cure by moderate exercise.[172]

Of particular interest in the last quotation is Tissot's reference to the often "unconscious" nature of "occupational" therapy, which has been both applauded and regretted during the twentieth century. The regret, one has to remark, is often on the side of the therapist who would like recognition for the part played in the treatment programme, but who, because of the often unrecognised benefits of occupation, feels that both therapist and occupational treatment is unappreciated.

In the United Kingdom, Francis Fuller MA, the Younger, published a work on the subject *Medicina Gymnastica* in 1707. This proved so popular that it was republished many times. In the preface, by way of introduction to the topic, he complained of the narrow confines of medicine, and the small notice given to exercise as a remedial measure despite its many positive effects, which if ascribed to a more expected type of medicine would be held in high esteem:

The generality of men, have for a long time had too narrow thoughts of physick, as if it were in a manner confin'd to little more than internals, without allowing themselves the liberty of common reasoning, by which they easily might have found that the humane body is liable to, and requires several administrations of a very different Nature, and that it is very unreasonable to suppose, that since there are so many ways for diseases to enter upon us, there should be so few for health to return by ...

As for the exercise of the body, which is the subject of this ensuing discourse, if people would not think so superficially of it, if they would but abstract the benefit got by it, from the means by which it is got, they would set a great value upon it: If some of the advantages accruing from exercise, were to be procured by any one medicine, nothing in the world would be more esteem than that medicine would be.[173]

Going on to discuss the acquisition of strength through ongoing occupational habit, Fuller noted the surprisingly slim physique of many people with great strength. He recommended that those who suffered from habitually poor health might discover striking improvement if they were to engage in strength giving exercise over time:

... we see what excessive strength some men gradually acquire by a constant practice of vehement motions, begun when they are young, which growing upon 'em by degrees, they are not so sensible of the encrease of it. This is the case of tumblers, rope dancers, and the like, in whom the nervous and solid parts must be incomparably more wound up, more tense, than in other people; and thus we see the strongest men are often thin and raw-bon'd, as we call it; that is, tho' daily hard labour, and great perspiration carry off a great deal of the grosser fluids of the body, yet are the muscles not flaccid, but tense and firm, capable of greater actions than the muscles of those who seem to have a better habit of body; which plainly indicates, that exercise does communicate some strength to the nervous parts, which cannot be any other way procur'd; and that we may argue from the greater to the less; that if healthy persons may acquire such monstrous strength by use, people that are valetudinary may, by setting themselves upon a resolute and diligent practice of moderate exercise, obtain a proportionable increase of strength.[174]

In the 1777 version of Fuller's book (the ninth edition) he added a new section titled "Everyman his own Physician". In this he described what he meant by curative exercise:

By exercise then I understand all that motion or agitation of the body, of what kind soever, whether voluntary or involuntary, and all methods whatsoever, which without the use of internals may (or without which internals alone may not always) suffice to enable nature to expel the enemy which oppresses her; confining myself to the consideration of it, only as it may prove curative, not as palliative, or barely preservative.

That the use of exercise does conduce very much to the preservation of health, that it promotes the digestion of the humours, raises the spirits, refreshes the mind, and that it strengthens and relieves the whole man, is scarce disputed by any.

In what remains substantially true in the present time, Fuller went on to discuss the difficulty of people's acceptance of it as a health measure, despite exercise producing effects beyond that of medicine alone:

... but that it should prove curative in some particular distempers, and that too when scarce anything else will prevail, seems to obtain little credit with most

people, who, though they will give a physician the hearing, when he recommends the frequent use of riding, or any other sort of exercise; yet at the same time look upon it as a forlorn method, and the effects rather of his inability to relieve them, than of his belief that there is any great matter in what he advises: Thus by a negligent diffidence, they deceive themselves, and let slip the golden opportunities of recovering, by a diligent struggle, what could not be produced by the use of medicine alone.

Fuller wondered at the variation of attitudes in different places, perceiving that those in more southern climes accepted exercise. However, most people in the eighteenth century, he believed, seemed to prefer internal medicine, which they accepted as a "quick fix" requiring no time or effort on their part:

Whether this proceeds from the custom of these northern nations, so different from those of more southern countries, who seem to have placed almost as much in their methods of exercise, as in the internal physic; or whether from the narrow notions most people have conceived of the art of physic, as if it implied little more than internals only, without considering that external, mechanical, and all other means whatsoever that give relief, properly belong to it; this I shall not pretend to determine: But this, I think, I may venture to affirm, that most men indulge themselves in the expectation of more sudden relief, than the nature of the case will admit of; as if they thought medicine was always to take like a charm, without putting them to the expence of much time or pains. They do not consider the wonderful variety of the disorders of nature, and the stubborness of some cases, which will not permit the sick to be wholly passive, but indispensably oblige him to conspire with his physician, and strive indefatigably to exalt his constitution to a degree requisite to supply the defect of internal physic; which industrious striving on the part of the sick, being what is here meant by exercise, and which it is my purpose to represent as more efficacious than it is generally believed to be.

Riding, which has already been observed as a favoured occupation for physicians and self health practitioners, remained the case for therapeutic gymnasts. Fuller devoted a whole chapter to the topic, and explained:

... upon several accounts, this may be esteemed the best and noblest of all exercises for a chronic and sick person, whether we consider it with respect to the body or the mind. If we enquire after what manner it affects the body, we shall find that it is a kind of mixed exercise, partly active and partly passive; the lower parts of the body being in some measure employed, while the upper parts are almost wholly remiss, or relaxed: Nay, where a man is easy, is sure of his horse, and rides loose, there is very little action on his part, but he may give himself to be careless almost as if he were seated on a moving chair, so that he may be said to be exercised, rather than to exercise himself; which makes the case widely different from almost all other sorts of exercise, as walking, running, stooping, or the like; all which require some labour, and consequently more strength for their performance; in all which the muscular parts must be put to some stress, and

some of the secretory vessels made to throw off too much, while others throw off too little; whereas riding, the parts being incomparably relaxed, there is better disposition towards an equal secretion of the morbific particles, and a less expence of the animal spirits, the chief agents in all irregular secretions; so that a sick person may by this means be greatly relieved, and not tired; wheras by other more violent ones, it is possible he may be tired, and not relieved.[175]

Fuller finishes by including *Rules for health and a long life written by an eminent physician*. It can be speculated that this may well have been Cheyne, although publishing laws were less stringent at that time and there are many similarities between texts. Perhaps the repetition of the "rules" is attributable to the need for ongoing promulgation of the *Regimen Sanitatis*. In Rule IV, which deals with exercise and quiet, the eminent physician stated that:

Whatever was the original constitution of man, in our present state, a due degree of exercise is indispensibly necessary towards health and long life.

Animal food, and strong liquors, seem not to have been designed for man in his original make and frame; but rather indulged, to shorten the antediluvian length of life, in order to prevent the excessive growth of wickedness.

Walking is the most natural and effective exercise, did it not spend the spirits of the tender too much. Riding a horseback is less laborious, and more effectual for such. Riding in a coach is only for the infirm, and young children. House exercises are never to be allow'd, but when the weather or some bodily infirmity will not permit going abroad; for air contributes mightily to the benefit of exercise, which wonderfully promotes their health, increases their strength, and stretches out their organs.

The organs of the body that are most used, always become strongest, and therefore we may strengthen any weak organ by exercise.

Etc.[176]

Goodbody, in the *Illustrated History of Gymnastics* gives the credit of developing a "system" of health maintaining exercise to Johann Frederich Guts Muths, a German. Much of his teaching was based on ideas of the ancients, that gymnastics could be used to raise the fitness level of the ordinary population. To the Greek's range of physical exercises he added climbing, balance movements, marching, and military drills, but also recommended 'exercises for the senses, as well as reading aloud and recitation' and 'stressed the importance of handicrafts and gardening.' Muths sought to attract young people to gymnastics, writing *The Games for the Exercise and Recreation of Body and Mind* as well as his seminal work *Gynmastik fur die Jugend* (Gymnastics for the Young) in 1793, which was translated into French, English, Swedish and Danish.

Farther south, in Pavia, an ancient Italian University town, Simon Tisset (1728-1797), who was an instructor of clinical medicine, also became interested in physical exercise. Along with Johann Frank, a medical practitioner, he encouraged young people to undertake gymnastic exercises. In a snowballing effect, Franz Nachte Gall, a Danishman, influenced by Tisset and also by Muths' text, established a gymnasium in Denmark encouraged by the Crown Prince (later King, Frederick VI) who was interested in it as military training. Pehr Henrik Ling (1766-1839) of Sweden, who was to become one of the best known advocates for medical gymnastics, was one of his pupils. Ling studied medicine and then used gymnastics in promoting health and remediating disease, stressing the need to gain the interest and cooperation of those undertaking such treatment. From being a gymnastic and fencing instructor at Lind University, he went on to found the Central Institute of Gymnastics in Stockholm which is discussed further in chapter 10. Another of the influential Northern European leaders was Johann Friedrich Jahn (1778-1852) of Germany and yet another was Jacques Delpech, a contemporary of Ling, who founded an orthopaedic institution between Montpellier and Toulouse, with a winter and summer gymnasium and bath. His particular health interest was in using gymnastics to correct deformities. Indeed, the interest continued expanding into various parts of Europe from both northern Europe and further south.[177][178]

The popularity of physical occupations such as gymnastics as a way to maintain and improve health had been advanced in writings of learned Renaissance men such as Montaigne and Locke, who stressed the need for healthy bodies as a prerequisite to healthy minds. Montaigne, the French essayist, had recommended exercise in *Of the Education of Children*. British philosopher John Locke in *Thoughts Concerning Education,* along with the later "enlightened" Jean-Jacques Rousseau in *Emile,* were both enthusiastic about physical training for young men. Rousseau wrote: 'Exercise his body continually; make him strong and healthy that you may make him wise and reasonable.' Such sentiments were influential.

Johann Heinrich Pestalozzi (1746-1827) the Swiss educationist put Rousseau's theories about physical development according to Nature into practice. He based his own child's education on Rousseau's *Emile*, and went on to try out his adaptation of the theory, first on a group of destitute children, and then in an orphanage. After that he founded his own institution to which many foreign educationalists came for inspiration.[179] In a later chapter it can be seen that a link began to emerge between the ideas of the enmeshing of physical and mental occupation made at that time, to modern-day occupational therapy. The mother of Octavia Hill who was influential in the development of British 20th century occupational therapy, was a Pestalozzian teacher and taught her children along those lines.

The development of schools for the blind

Typically, since their inception, schools for the blind have used occupation to improve well-being, as well as aiming towards some degree of self sufficiency and independence of those affected. In a historical sketch of organisations that developed for the education of the blind, Richie described the Paris School as the first. Its founder was Valentin Hauy who was born in Picardy in I745. He worked as a junior official in the Foreign Office in Paris, and an incident on one of the City's Boulevards which revolted his sensibilities turned his thoughts in the direction of what was to become his life's work. 'A dozen blind men grotesquely attired and with pasteboard spectacles on their noses' delighted the audience of a fashionable cafe where people thronged of an evening, by executing a discordant symphony. Later, Hauy took in hand the education of a 17 year old boy, Francois le Sueur, who had lost his sight when he was six weeks old and supplemented the family income by begging at the church door of St Germain des Pres. The experiment was so successful that in six months the boy was able to read, and a couple of years later, had made excellent progress in French, geography, and music.[180]

Early in 1785 Hauy, in company with Francois, read a paper on the education of the blind to the learned assembly of the Academy, which was so well received that some of the members supported a more general experiment which became known as L'Institution Nationale des Jeunes Aveugles. Hauy studied the methods used by blind individuals in their efforts to self educate, and adopted all that seemed useful for his first class, which was made up of a few blind children who received monthly gratuities from a philanthropic society. Richie claimed that 'it was a time when philanthropic enterprises of various kinds became successively fashionable, and for a few years the Institution for Blind Children enjoyed this fickle fortune'. In that vein, in the same year he was summoned to appear, with Francois, before the Court at Versailles.[181]

By 1786 there were thirty lively youngsters in Hauy's institution, but the turmoil of the Revolution was to result in less interest and charity as people grimly went on with matters of vital import to their own survival. Fifteen years later Napoleonic bureaucrats decreed that the pupils should be moved to the Paris Blind Asylum, the hospital des Quinze-Vingts. However good the intent, this was disastrous for the pupils whose education languished in the new environment, especially as Hauy was thanked for his past services and turned out of office.[182]

By the end of the eighteenth century, four British institutions had followed in the footsteps of L'Institution des Jeunes Aveugles. The first, in I791, was established in Liverpool by Edward Rushton, who was a man of forceful personality, said to be unselfish and courageous. He lost his sight as a youth on board a slave ship, whilst labouring to mitigate the sufferings of the captives during an epidemic of ophthalmia. Rushton partially regained his sight, but his experience stimulated an active desire to lessen the trauma of blindness.[183]

Rushton described his scheme in the *Liverpool Mercury*. He told how in 1790, at a weekly literary discussion group that he regularly attended, he learned how the recently established Marine Board had declined to accept any small donations. It immediately occurred to him that:

> ... *if an institution could be formed in Liverpool, for the relief of the numerous and indigent blind, the small donations thus declined by the Marine Committee, might be brought to flow in a channel, not less benevolent and prove of essential service in the establishment of a fund for the benefit of that unfortunate description of the community.*[184]

Almost immediately the idea was associated with occupation of a musical nature and with "the blind helping the blind". One member of the Literary Society, who enlisted help from several wealthy gentlemen, was a Mr Lowe, a respectable musician who was himself blind. Another musician, who was also blind, John Christie, recommended to Rushton where the blind might receive free instruction on the harpsichord and violin. The practice of the latter was forbidden at the outset, however, for fear the city would be filled with blind fiddlers. The public was informed that the occupations to be tried out at the start would be:

> ... *the winding of Cotton, the spinning of Worsted, the knitting of the Worsted Stockings, the making of Whip-lashes, the winding of Worsted into balls and hanks for the hosiers, the picking of Oakum, the making of Cabbage Nets, Net Caps, etc., the Lining of Hats, Music, etc.*[185]

The Institution, formally constituted in 1793, admitted only "moral" persons between the ages of fourteen and fifty from Lancashire and Cheshire, and had about 25 to 45 attendees who were neither lodged nor fed there, but paid in proportion to their labour. It resembled a factory, but the rooms had good fires, and masters were employed to provide instruction in music and handicrafts.[186]

Two more institutions were founded, in 1793, one in Edinburgh for young people and adults and aimed mainly at industrial training and employment, and one in Bristol which was founded by two members of the Society of Friends. The founder of the Edinburgh Society for the Relief of the Indigent Blind, which soon became the Asylum for the Industrious Blind was David Johnston, an energetic divine of Leith. The Bristol Institution, which began with only four boys and two girls who attended daily, was aimed at training in industrial occupations and employment. Early in the next century it became a residential institution. In 1799, the last British institution to claim birth in the eighteenth century was the School for the Indigent Blind of St George's, Southwark. There, fifteen blind people were to be 'educated, maintained and taught a trade'.[187] The occupations that were found most useful in these early institutions of training were, apart from encouraging literacy, plaiting whips and spinning flax, basketry, mat and mattress making, and making music.

Following the upheavals of the French Revolution and the Napoleonic era (1789-1815) the Enlightenment movement declined, eroded by Nationalism, the growth of a new wealthy educated class of industrialists, and the religious revival of the 1790s and early 1800s.

In summary, the lasting heritage of the Enlightenment has been 'its contribution to the literature of human freedom and some institutions in which its values have been embodied'.[188] Included in the latter are many facets of modern government, education, and philanthropy and, it can be argued, the professional philosophy of occupational therapy which embodies notions of self realisation, moral autonomy and independence, liberty and justice with regards to people's occupational health needs. In the remediation of physical health through occupation there were clearer directions with physiological questions, rationales and practice within the field known then as gymnastics. Along with that was a burgeoning of mobility aids to enable people with disability to live more fulfilled and active lives. Additionally, the advent of literature that assisted self-healthers to follow the advice about occupational aspects of maintaining health, from the ancient authority of the *Regimen Sanitatis* and similar counsel, was probably more advanced than in the present.

---

[1]Smith R. Unemployment and Health: A Disaster and a Challenge. Oxford: Oxford University Press, 1987.

[2]Winefield A, Tiggerman M. A longitudinal study of the psychological effects of unemployment and unsatisfactory employment on young adults. Journal of Applied Psychology 1991; 76(3): 424-431.

[3]Clark F, Azen SP, Zemke R, Jackson J, Carlson M, Mandel D, Hay J, Josephson K, Cherry B, Hessel C, Palmer J, Lipson L. Occupational therapy for independent-living older adults: A randomized control trial. Journal of the American Medical Association 1997 (22 October); 278: 1321-1326.

[4]Glass TA, de Leon CM, Marottoli RA, Berkman LF. Population based study of social and productive activities as predictors of survival among elderly Americans. British Medical Journal 1999; 319: 478-483.

[5]Porter R. English society in the eighteenth century. The Penguin Social History of Britain (revised edition). London: Penguin Books, 1990; 256.

[6]Emerson RL. Enlightenment. Grolier Multimedia Encyclopedia 1995. Grolier Electronic Publishing, Inc. (CD Rom), 1995.

[7]Porter D, Porter R. Patient's Progress: Doctors and Doctoring in 18th Century England. Cambridge: Polity Press, 1989; 9.

[8]Erasmus Darwin, wrote Zoonomia, or the Laws of Organic Life. Dublin: Printed for D. Byrne, and W. Jones, 1794-96, (a Lamarkian interpretation of evolution and the laws of organic life which he considered to be much influenced by environment) [Harvey P, ed. The Oxford Companion to English Literature. Oxford: Clarendon Press, 1967; The Hutchinson Dictionary of Ideas. Oxford: Helicon, 1994; 136; "Darwin, Erasmus" in 1995 Grolier Multimedia Encyclopedia. CD Rom. Grolier Electronic Publishing, Inc. 1995.]

[9]Langford P. The eighteenth century (1688-1789). In: Langford P, Harvie C. The

Eighteenth Century and the Age of Industry. The Oxford History of Britain, Vol. 4. Oxford: Oxford University Press, 1984; 26.

[10]Porter R. Disease, Medicine and Society in England 1550-1860. Basingstoke and London: Macmillan Education, 1987.

[11]Porter & Porter. Patient's Progress: Doctors and Doctoring…; 7-8.

[12]Kirkman Gray B. A History of English Philanthropy. London: P. S. King & Son, 1905; 205-212.

[13]The art of thriving. Cited in: Kirkman Gray B. A History of English Philanthropy…; 208.

[14]Townsend J. Dissertation on the Poor Laws. By a Well-Wisher to Mankind. London: 1786; 34, 85-87.

[15]Watson F. Civilization and the Cripple. London: John Bale, Sons & Danielsson, Ltd., 1930; 7.

[16]Pinchbeck I. Women workers and the industrial revolution, 1750-1850. London: G. Routledge & Sons, 1930. Cited in: Watson. Civilization and the Cripple…; 7-8.

[17]Porter. Disease, Medicine and Society in England 1550-1860.

[18]Porter. Disease, Medicine and Society in England 1550-1860.

[19]Nelson R. An Address to Persons of Quality and Estate, Ways and Methods of Doing Good. 1715; 100, 189, 191, 199, 215.

[20]Nelson. An Address to Persons of Quality…; 241.

[21]Kirkman Gray. A History of English Philanthropy…; 98.

[22]Nelson. An Address to Persons of Quality…; 12, 103-4. In: Kirkman Gray. A History of English Philanthropy…; 98-99.

[23]Thompson EP. Customs in Common. London: Penguin Books, 1993; 7-9.

[24]Girling DA, ed. New Age Encyclopaedia. Volume 22. 7th edition. Sydney & London: Bay Books, 1983; Vol. 22: 114.

[25]Porter & Porter. Patient's Progress: Doctors and Doctoring…; 8-7.

[26]Downing J. An Account of Several Work-Houses for Employing and Maintaining the Poor, Setting Forth the Rules by which they are Governed … As also of Several Charity Schools, for Promoting Work and Labour (An Alphabetical List of Work-Houses etc). London: 1725 (1732); Vol. 2: 15.

[27]Kirkman Gray. A History of English Philanthropy…; 217.

[28]Downing. An Account of Several Workhouses.

[29]Kirkman Gray. A History of English Philanthropy…; 216.

[30]Bailey W. The Better Employment and more Comfortable Support of the Poor. 1758.

[31]Cooke T. Letter to the Mayor and Aldermen, London, 1702. In: Work-houses the Best Charity: A Sermon Preacht at the Cathedral Church of Worcester, February 2d 1702. By Thomas Cooke Master of Arts, and Rector of St Nicholas in the City of Worcester. Published at the Request of the Mayor and Aldermen. London: Printed for John Butler, Bookseller in Worcester, and sold by most Booksellers in London and Westminster, 1702.

[32]Cooke. Work-houses the Best Charity…; 6.

[33]Cooke. Work-houses the Best Charity…; 6.

[34]Cooke. Work-houses the Best Charity…; 7.

[35]Cooke. Work-houses the Best Charity…; 25.

[36]Vanderlint J. Money Answers All Things; or an Essay to Make Money Sufficiently Plentiful amongst all Ranks of People: and Increase our Foreign and Domestic Trade etc. London: 1734.

[37]Girling. New Age Encyclopaedia…; 134.

[38]O'Connor J. The Workhouses of Ireland; The Fate of Ireland's Poor. Dublin: Anvil

Books, 1995; 29.

[39]O'Connor. The Workhouses of Ireland…; 31.

[40]Wodsworth WD. Brief History of the Dublin Foundling Hospital. Dublin, 1876.

[41]O'Connor. The Workhouses of Ireland…; 32.

[42]O'Connor. The Workhouses of Ireland…; 33.

[43]Nichols RH, Wray FA. The History of the Foundling Hospital. London: Oxford University Press, Humphrey Milford, 1935; ch 1, introduction.

[44]Downing. An Account of Several Work-Houses…; vol 1: 8-9.

[45]Downing. An Account of Several Work-Houses…; vol 1: 11.

[46]Downing. An Account of Several Work-Houses…; vol 1: 11.

[47]Downing. An Account of Several Work-Houses…; vol 1: 14.

[48]Downing. An Account of Several Work-Houses…; vol 2: 15.

[49]Downing. An Account of Several Work-Houses…; vol 2; 17.

[50]Downing. An Account of Several Work-Houses…; vol 2; 24.

[51]Firmin T. Some Proposals for the Imployment of the Poor and for the Prevention of Idleness and … Begging … London: Printed by J Groves, 1681.

[52]Kennet W. Bishop of Peterborough Twenty-Five Sermons. London: 1706; 72.

[53]Kirkman Gray. A History of English Philanthropy…; 105-114.

[54]Addison J. Guardian (No. 105), 1713. Cited in: Nichols & Wray. The History of the Foundling Hospital…; Introduction to Ch. 4.

[55]Downing. An Account of Several Work-Houses…; vol 3: A2.

[56]Nichols & Wray. The History of the Foundling Hospital…; 130.

[57]Girling. New Age Encyclopaedia…; 252.

[58]Kirkman Gray. A History of English Philanthropy…; 180.

[59]Kirkman Gray. A History of English Philanthropy…; 181.

[60]Halle R. Treatise: Hygiene. In: Encyclopedie Methodique, Medicine, Tome 7, part 1. Livraison 65. Translated in: Sinclair J. The Code of Health and Longevity, Vol III. Edinburgh: Printed for Arch Constable and Co.; and T Cadell and W Davies, and J Murray, London, 1806; 327-8.

[61]Kirkman Gray. A History of English Philanthropy…; 183.

[62]Howard J. An Account of the Principal Lazarettos in Europe; With Varios Papers Relative to the Plague: Together with further Observations on some Foreign Prisons and Hospitals; And Additional Remarks on the Present State of those in Great Britain and Ireland. Warrington: Printed by William Eyres, MDCC LXXXIX. 1789; 225.

[63]Howard. An Account of the Principal Lazarettos in Europe…; 126, 127, 206, 207.

[64]Girling. New Age Encyclopaedia…; 241.

[65]Howard. An Account of the Principal Lazarettos in Europe…; 219.

[66]Howard. An Account of the Principal Lazarettos in Europe…; 216, 218.

[67]Howard. An Account of the Principal Lazarettos in Europe…; 220.

[68]Howard. An Account of the Principal Lazarettos in Europe…; 221-222.

[69]Howard. An Account of the Principal Lazarettos in Europe…; 228.

[70]Howard. An Account of the Principal Lazarettos in Europe…; 127.

[71]Howard. An Account of the Principal Lazarettos in Europe…; 163.

[72]Pennant 1790. Cited in: A Short History of Bridewell and Bethlem Royal Hospitals. The Bethlem Art and History Collections Trust. 1899; 12.

[73]Nichols & Wray. The History of the Foundling Hospital…; chapter I, intro.

[74]Pennant. In: A Short History of Bridewell and Bethlem Royal Hospitals…; 12.

[75]Pennant. In: A Short History of Bridewell and Bethlem Royal Hospitals…; 12.

[76]A Short History of Bridewell and Bethlem Royal Hospitals.

[77]Porter & Porter. Patient's Progress…; 10.

[78]Porter & Porter. Patient's Progress.

[79]Porter & Porter. Patient's Progress.

[80]Macdonald EM. World-Wide Conquests of Disabilities: The History, Development and Present Functions of the Remedial Services. London: Bailliere Tindall, 1981; 75.

[81]Sigerist HE. A History of Medicine, Volume I: Primitive and Archaic Medicine. New York: Oxford University Press, 1955.

[82]Porter. Disease, Medicine and Society in England 1550-1860...; 22.

[83]Porter. Disease, Medicine and Society in England 1550-1860.

[84]Hamilton B. The medical professions in the eighteenth century. Economic History Review. 2nd series, IV: 1951; 141-69. Though dated, still a valuable account of the structuring of the medical professions. Use together with the work of Lane, Loudon and Waddington.

[85]Watson. Civilization and the Cripple...; 8.

[86]Georgii A, ed. Ling's Educational and Curative Exercises. London: Renshaw, 1873; 14.

[87]Macdonald. World-Wide Conquests of Disabilities...; 75-6.

[88]Cullen W. Treatise on Materia Medica. 1789.

[89]Loudon I. Medical Care and the General Practitioner 1750-1850. Oxford: Oxford University Press, 1986.

[90]Loudon. Medical Care and the General Practitioner...; 3, 18-20, 86.

[91]Loudon. Medical Care and the General Practitioner...; 24.

[92]Porter R. Mind-forg'd Manacles. London: The Athlone Press, 1987; 122.

[93]Porter. Mind-forg'd Manacles...; 121.

[94]Porter. Disease, Medicine and Society in England 1550-1860.

[95]Porter & Porter. Patient's Progress: Doctors and Doctoring.

[96]Cameron HC. Mr Guy's Hospital, 1726-1948. London, New York and Toronto: Longmans Green, 1954. (Highlights the importance of individual philanthropy in the development of the English hospital system). Clark-Kennedy AE. London Pride: The Story of a Voluntary Hospital. London: Hutchinson Benham, 1979. (A well-researched account of the London Hospital, a new voluntary hospital of the Georgian age). Dainton C. The Story of England's Hospitals. London: Museum Press, 1961; Poynter FNL, ed. The Evolution of Hospitals in Britain. London, Pitman, 1964; Woodward J. To Do the Sick No Harm. A Study of the British Voluntary Hospital System to 1875. London and Boston: Routledge & Kegan Paul, 1974. (A history of the voluntary hospital movement).

[97]Porter. Disease, Medicine and Society in England 1550-1860...; 36.

[98]McClure R. Coram's Children. New Haven, Connecticut, and London: Yale University Press, 1981.

[99]Owen D. English Philanthropy 1660-1940. Cambridge, Massachusetts: Belknap Press, 1965.

[100]Kersley GD, Cosh JA. The History of the Royal National Hospital for Rheumatic Diseases: Bath. Bath: Friends of the Royal National Hospital, 1965; 4.

[101]Porter. Disease, Medicine and Society in England 1550-1860.

[102]Kersley & Cosh. The History of the Royal National Hospital...; 4-6.

[103]Kersley GD, Glyn J. A Concise International History of Rheumatology and Rehabilitation. Royal Society of Medical Services, 1991; 3.

[104]Porter. Disease, Medicine and Society in England 1550-1860...; 37.

[105]Loudon IS. The origins and growth of the dispensary movement in England. In: Bulletin of the History of Medicine, IV: 322-42.

[106]Howard. An Account of the Principal Lazarettos in Europe...; 140-142.

[107]Howard. An Account of the Principal Lazarettos in Europe...; 140-142.

[108]Howard. An Account of the Principal Lazarettos in Europe…; 180.

[109]Howard. An Account of the Principal Lazarettos in Europe…; 182.

[110]Glasse Rev. Dr. Report, Society for bettering the condition of the poor. ii., 99. In: Kirkman Gray. A History of English Philanthropy…; 147-8.

[111]Kirkman Gray. A History of English Philanthropy…; 148-9.

[112]Halle. Treatise: Hygiene…; 383; (Xenophon's complete works have been translated by H. G. Dakyns: 1890-94).

[113]Halle. Treatise: Hygiene…; 382.

[114]Ward JE, Yell J. The Medical Casebook of William Brownrigg MD FRS., 1712-1800. London: Wellcome Institute, 1993; 33, 62, 119, 120-121, 153.

[115]Porter & Porter. Patient's Progress: Doctors and Doctoring…; 157-159:

[116]Marti-Ibañez F, ed. Henry E. Sigerist on the History of Medicine. New York: MD Publications, Inc., 1960; 21-22.

[117]Halle. Treatise: Hygiene…; 260-475.

[118]Halle. Treatise: Hygiene…; 275.

[119]Halle. Treatise: Hygiene…; 464.

[120]Halle. Treatise: Hygiene…; 464

[121]Halle. Treatise: Hygiene….; 466-475.

[122]Halle. Treatise: Hygiene…; 465.

[123]Macdonald. World-Wide Conquests of Disabilities…; 83, 90.

[124]Macdonald. World-Wide Conquests of Disabilities…; 83, 90.

[125]Cited in: Meiklejohn A. The Life, Work and Times of Charles Turner Thackrah, Surgeon and Apothecary of Leeds (1795-1833). Edinburgh and London: E & S Livingstone Ltd., 1957; 37-38.

[126]Pringle Sir J. Observations on Diseases of the Army. 1752.

[127]Blane G. Observations on the Diseases Incident to Seamen. 1785.

[128]Lind J. An Essay on the Most Effectual Means of Preserving the Health of Seamen of the Royal Navy … And an Appendix of Observations on the Treatment of Diseases in Hot Climates. London: 1757.

[129]Girling. New Age Encyclopaedia…; 270.

[130]Loudon. Medical Care and the General Practitioner.

[131]Winter G. (M.D.) A New and Compendious System of Husbandry; Containing the Mechanical, Chemical and Philosophical Elements of Agriculture. 2nd edition. London: 1797.

[132]Tildesley NW. Richard Wilkes of Willenhall, Staffs: An eighteenth century doctor. Transactions of the South Staffordshire Archeological and Historical Society 1965-6; 7: 1-10.

[133]Black WG. Folk Medicine: A Chapter in the History of Culture. London: Publications of the Folk-Lore Society, 1883.

[134]Porter. Disease, Medicine and Society in England 1550-1860.

[135]Porter & Porter. Patient's Progress.

[136]Porter & Porter. Patient's Progress.

[137]Porter & Porter. Patient's Progress…; 35.

[138]Boswell J. Boswell's London Journal 1762-1763. Now first published from the original manuscript prepared for the press, with introduction and notes by Frederick A. Pottle. Melbourne, London, Toronto: William Heinnemann Ltd, 1950. Australian edition, 1951; 155-156.

[139]Boswell. Boswell's London Journal 1762-1763…; 164.

[140]Boswell. Boswell's London Journal 1762-1763…; 183-184.

[141]Darwin E. Cited in: Porter. English Society in the Eighteenth Century…; 260.

[142]Porter & Porter. Patient's Progress…; 256.

[143]Porter & Porter. Patient's Progress.

[144]Archer J. Everyman his own doctor. Cited in: Porter & Porter. Patient's Progress…; 200.

[145]Cheyne G. Essay of Health and Long Life. London and Bath: Strahan, 1724; 77.

[146]Cheyne. Essay of Health and Long Life…; 77.

[147]Cheyne. Essay of Health and Long Life…; 85-86.

[148]Cheyne. Essay of Health and Long Life…; 89-91.

[149]Dubos R. Mirage of Health: Utopias, Progress and Biological Change. New York: Harper and Row Publishers, 1959; 142.

[150]Cheyne. Essay of Health and Long Life…; 94-96.

[151]Cheyne. Essay of Health and Long Life…; 96-97.

[152]Cheyne. Essay of Health and Long Life…; 97-99.

[153]Cheyne. Essay of Health and Long Life…; 99-100.

[154]Buchan W. Domestic Medicine. 1769.

[155]Porter & Porter. Patient's Progress…; 199.

[156]Macdonald. World-Wide Conquests of Disabilities …; 90.

[157]Wesley J. Primitive Physick: Or an Easy and Natural Method of Curing Most Diseases. London: 1747.

[158]Armstrong J. The Art of Preserving Health: A Poem. Dublin: J Smith, W Powell, 1744.

[159]Harvey P, ed. The Oxford Companion to English Literature. 4th edition. Oxford: The Clarendon Press, 1967; 41.

[160]Kersley & Cosh. The History of the Royal National Hospital…; 6.

[161]Covey HC. Social Perceptions of People with Disabilities in History. Springfield, Illinois: Charles C Thomas, 1998; 47, 49.

[162]French A. John Joseph Merlin. An Ingenious Mechanick. London: Iveagh Bequest, Kenwood, Greater London Council, 1985; 15.

[163]French. John Joseph Merlin. The Ingenious Mechanick…; 168-139.

[164]French. John Joseph Merlin. The Ingenious Mechanick.

[165]Macdonald. World-Wide Conquests of Disabilities…; 83, 90.

[166]Halle. Treatise: Hygiene…; 310.

[167]Tissot CJ. Gymnastique Medicinale et Chirugicale. (1780). Extracts in: Licht Dr S, trans and ed. Occupational Therapy and Rehabilitation. Baltimore: Williams and Wilkins. In: The Scottish Journal of Occupational Therapy September, 1951; 6: 3-5.

[168]Tissot. Gymnastique Medicinale et Chirugicale.

[169]Tissot. Gymnastique Medicinale et Chirugicale.

[170]Tissot. Gymnastique Medicinale et Chirugicale.

[171]Tissot. Gymnastique Medicinale et Chirugicale.

[172]Tissot. Gymnastique Medicinale et Chirugicale.

[173]Fuller F. Medicina Gymnastica: Or, Everyman his own Physician, A Treatise Concerning the Power of Exercise With Respect to the Animal Oeconomy. The seventh edition improved. To which is added, Rules. London, 1777; preface.

[174]Fuller F. Medicina Gymnastica: or, a Treatise Concerning the Power of Exercise with Respect to the Animal Oeconomy; And the Great Necessity of it in the Cure of Several Distempers. London: Printed by John Matthews for Robert Knaplock, at the Angel and Crown in St Paul's Church-yard, (MDCCV) 1775.

[175]Fuller. Medicina Gymnastica: Or, Everyman his own Physician…; 164-165.

[176]Fuller. Medicina Gymnastica: Or, Everyman his own Physician.

[177]Goodbody J. The Illustrated History of Gymnastics. London: Stanley Paul, 1982; 12-13.

[178]Macdonald. World-Wide Conquests of Disabilities…; 95.

[179]Girling. New Age Encyclopaedia…; vol 22: 227.

[180]Ritchie JM. Concerning the Blind. London: Oliver and Boyd, 1930.

[181]Richie. Concerning the Blind…; 9.
[182]Richie. Concerning the Blind…; 10.
[183]Richie. Concerning the Blind…; 12-13.
[184]Bickerton TH. A Medical History of Liverpool from the Earliest Days to the Year 1920. London: John Murray, 1936; 30.
[185]Bickerton. A Medical History of Liverpool…; 32.
[186]Bickerton. A Medical History of Liverpool…; 31-33.
[187]Richie. Concerning the Blind…; 14-15.
[188]Emerson. Enlightenment. Grolier Multimedia Encyclopedia1995.

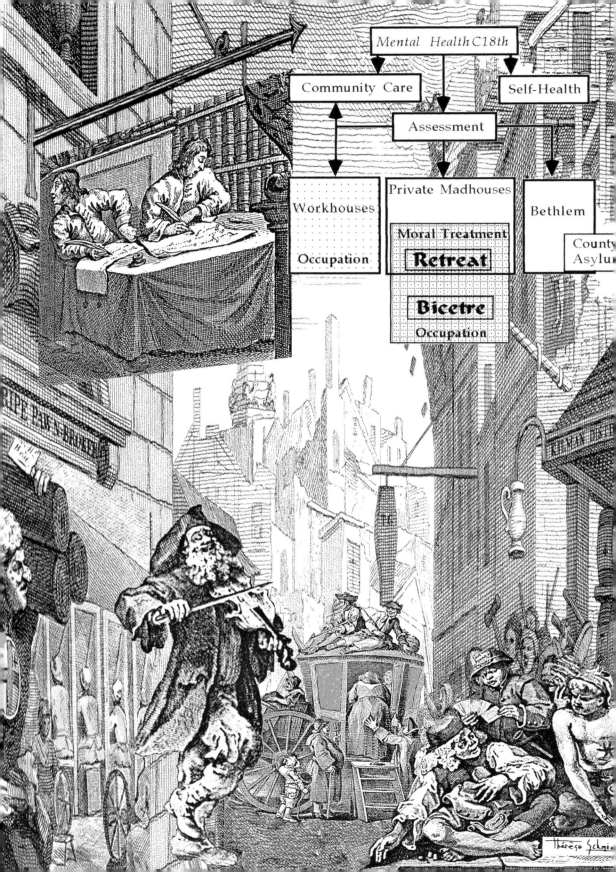

Mental Health C18th

Community Care

Self-Health

Assessment

Workhouses

Occupation

Private Madhouses

Moral Treatment

Retreat

Bicetre

Occupation

Bethlem

County Asylum

Chapter 8

Mental Health and Occupational Regimes in Enlightened Times

Contents

Psychiatry and psychology, like occupational therapy, have been practised throughout time by people of different persuasions and professions. It was not until the eighteenth century, however, with the growth of private and later public asylums and moral treatment that they began to appear as distinct specialities. Such development marked the emergence of occupation as an important aspect of treatment in psychiatry and allows an unbroken link of what could be described as "occupational therapy" to be traced from the 1790s to the present day, in at least one British asylum.

The use of occupation in the care of those with mental disorder though has an even earlier history in the eighteenth century than the start of moral treatment, however important that is. It is therefore relevant to establish, as far as is possible, the extent of occupation's use and to be aware of the changing face of the management of "madness" from the time of the Enlightenment. These changes led to the evolution of public County Asylums in the nineteenth century and eventually, in the twentieth century, to the establishment of occupational therapy as it is now known.

In the last chapter it became clear that with the evolution and wide dispersion of the liberal ideas of Enlightenment thinkers came a gradual reduction of indifference to others less fortunate.[1] This, coupled with a new evangelicalism stressing the brotherhood of man,[2] may have led to more notice being taken of those in need of help for mental health reasons. Subsequently, there was a proliferation of private madhouses in England, an emergence of specialists in the treatment of insanity and, eventually, humane, moral treatment. Added to those humanitarian notions was the need to exclude the voices of irrationality, as religious theories of madness gradually gave way to theories about faulty reasoning of individuals.[3] In an Age of Reason the possibility of retraining thought processes led to the idea that benefits might ensue from institutional and educational confinement to the extent of effecting cure. In Catholic European countries, religious institutions provided the majority of services for those deemed insane, but in England, where such establishments had long since disappeared, there was a void of suitable places. The void provided ample opportunity for free enterprise and no requirement for those who took advantage of the opportunity to be medically qualified.

At the same time the changing face of the economy led others to suppose that those changes were disadvantaging people's mental health. Surprisingly, the middle and upper classes, rather than the poor, were the recognised victims of that perceived disadvantage.[4] King George's very public illness, the seeking out of affluence, luxury and over-indulgence, and rampant individualism, were all blamed for an obvious increase in insanity and particularly for the fashionable, national disease of melancholia.[5] The very growth of madhouses, which were largely populated by more affluent clientele, was seen as evidence. Benjamin Faulkner, an outspoken madhouse proprietor, suggested that the:

> ... truly astonishing ... progress of insanity (and) the rapidity with which the disorder has spread over this country, within the last fifty years, may be attributed, in a great measure, to the increase of luxury, ... inordinate desires, and the indulgence of inordinate passions, not unfrequently subjugate reason, and produce insanity.[6]

William Rowley even blamed a "tolerant" society for the increase:

> The agitations of passions, this liberty of thinking and acting with less restraint than in other nations, force a great quantity of blood to the head, and produce greater varieties of madness in this country, than is observed in others. Religious and civil toleration are productive of political and religious madness.[7]

William Hogarth's final portrayal of A Rake's Progress, published in 1735, (Figure 1.8.1) as he succumbs to madness and is admitted to Bethlem hospital illustrates the commonly held view to which Faulkner and Rowley alluded.

Others, and more particularly with the poor in mind, have blamed the violent social disruption that occurred as the genesis of the industrial revolution altered traditional patterns of occupation and disrupted age old communal structures.[8] In the present day major life changes are seen as potential stressors and causes of mental illness, so it is not hard to imagine that for some people then this may also have been true. Such disruption also had the potential to

Figure 1.8.1:   A Rake's Progress: Chained, raving mad in Bedlam. Engraving by T Bowles, 1735 after W.Hogarth
(The Wellcome Library)

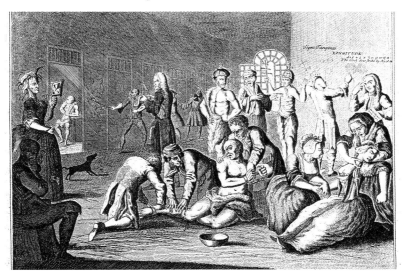

hinder the traditional informal ways that mental illness had been managed and, if that was the case, not surprisingly the numbers of sick appeared to escalate. It is also possible that the increasing availability of services caused the need for more and more of a similar kind as advertising and good marketing made people more aware of the disorder and potential assistance. Indeed, madhouses fostered and nurtured a supply of customers to such effect that need expanded as the number of madhouses grew.[9]

Despite such changes and the apparent increasing incidence of disorder, the treatment of mental health problems and the different types of care available during the early years of the Enlightenment remained similar, in many respects, to care and treatment during the Renaissance. For instance, most people usually remained within their community acting as their own occupation, health, and medical advisers. If this was deemed impossible then supervision, protection or housing within private care in the community, admission to a private madhouse, a workhouse, or Bethlem Hospital were all options. Most of those facilities underwent some form of modification during the century as expertise grew and commercial or moral challenges were taken up. Such modification, by the end of the eighteenth century, saw the genesis of moral treatment and the establishment of County Asylums, institutional care and mental illness as a medical speciality.

The component parts of mental health identified in the conceptual map in the chapter frontispiece provide an outline for the direction taken within this chapter.

In it the history of occupation's use in mental health during the Enlightenment is explored. As, early in the 1700s, the mentally ill were rarely locked up in facilities designed for that purpose, the place to start is with the notion of self-care. Self-care has already been identified as being increasingly significant as the rights and responsibilities of individual people were espoused during the Enlightenment. The mass production of printed texts aimed at the betterment of the human experience included some that addressed issues of mental health.

Self health: Self as occupational therapist

Like physical health and illness, the treatment of mental disorders or the maintenance of mental well-being rested very much in the hands of the ordinary folk rather than experts, who had little to offer and whose services were costly. Indeed, as in earlier times, maintaining mental health and dealing with times of mental distress were part of everyday life for each person and their family and acquaintances, probably many of whom, as part of this process, acted as "occupational therapists" from time to time. Some people wrote in letters or diaries about the experience of themselves or others acting as therapists, or advising about the therapeutic effects and place of occupation for mental health. Such accounts provide evidence of what occupations they considered therapeutic and why. Two of those accounts are provided as examples of self health during the eighteenth century.

The first account concerns the lawyer turned poet, William Cowper (1731-1800), who suffered from what would now be called a bipolar disorder. Following bouts of depression, and at the point of being offered a clerkship at the House of Lords, in 1763 he became manic and attempted suicide. After a spell in Collegium Insanorum at St Albans, a private madhouse set up by Dr Nathaniel Cotton, he retired and went to live in private care with Morley Unwin. After the death of his host he continued to reside with Unwin's widow, Mary, to whom he later became engaged. She continued to care for him when his illness recurred. As soon as Cowper felt able, he worked at carpentry for his own self initiated therapy, and then gardening, which he interspersed with drawing before, some years later, deciding upon poetry. Cowper is best known for his *Olney Hymns* published in 1779, a comic ballad, *John Gilpin's Ride* (1783), and a long discursive poem on rural themes, *The Task* (1785), which he mentions in the letter provided below. Mary Unwin, too, acted as occupational therapist, particularly when she suggested he write satires, eight of which were published in 1782. Following Mary's death he wrote a fine but gloomy poem of despair, *The Castaway,* in her memory, and with probable cathartic effect.[10] When Cowper was 55, he looked back over his illness and told of his self regulated occupation for therapeutic purposes in a letter to Lady Hesketh, his cousin:

TO LADY HESKETH

Jan. 16, 1786

My dearest cousin,

You do not ask me, my dear, for an explanation of what I could mean by anguish of mind and by the perpetual interuptions that I mentioned. Because you do not ask, and because your reason for not asking consists of a delicacy and tenderness peculiar to yourself, for that very cause I will tell you. A wish so suppressed is more irresistible than many wishes plainly uttered. Know then that in the year 73 the same scene that was acted at St Albans, opened upon me again at Olney, only covered with a still deeper shade of melancholy, and ordained to be of much longer duration. I was suddenly reduced from my wonted rate of understanding to an almost childish imbecility. I did not indeed lose my senses, but I lost the power to exercise them. I could return a rational answer even to a difficult question, but a question was necessary, or I never spoke at all. This state of mind was accompanied, as I suppose it to be in most instances of the kind, with misapprehension of things and persons that made me a very untractable patient. I believed that every body hated me, and that Mrs Unwin hated me most of all; was convinced that all my food was poisoned, together with ten thousand megrims of the same stamp. I would not be more circumstantial than is necessary. Dr Cotton was consulted. He replied that he could do no more for me than might be done at Olney, but recommended particular vigilance, lest I should attempt my life - a caution for which there was the greatest occasion. At the same time that I was convinced of Mrs Unwin's aversion to me, I could endure no other companion. The whole management of me consequently devolved upon her, and a terrible task she had; she performed it, however, with a cheerfulness hardly ever equalled on such an occasion; and I have often heard her say, that if ever she praised God in her life it was when she found that she was to have all the labour. She performed it accordingly, but as I hinted once before, very much to the hurt of her own constitution. It will be thirteen years in little more than a week, since this malady seized me. Methinks I hear you ask - your affection for me will, I know, make you wish to do so - Is it removed? I reply, in great measure, but not quite. Occasionally I am much distressed, but that distress becomes continually less frequent, and I think less violent. I find writing, and especially poetry, my best remedy. Perhaps had I understood music, I had never written verse, but had lived upon fiddle-strings instead. It is better however as it is. A poet may, if he pleases, be of a little use in the world, while a musician, the most skilful, can only divert himself and a few others. I have been emerging gradually from this pit. As soon as I became capable of action, I commenced carpenter, made cupboards, boxes, stools. I grew weary of this in about a twelvemonth, and addressed myself to the making of bird cages. To this employment succeeded that of gardening, which I intermingled with that of drawing, but finding that the latter occupation injured my eyes, I renounced it, and commenced poet. I have given you, my dear, a little history in shorthand; I know that it will touch your feelings, but do not let it interest them too much. In the year when I wrote The Task, (for it occupied me about a year) I was very often most supremely unhappy and am under God indebted in good part to that work for not having been much worse. You did not know what a clever fellow I am, and how I can turn my hand to any thing.

William Cowper[11]

The second account concerns that other well known eighteenth century figure discussed in the last chapter, James Boswell, who came from a family with a history of mental illness. Yet, although his brother became a patient in the private madhouse set up by Dr Thomas Arnold, and James was happy with the treatment his brother received, for himself, he engaged in regimens of self-care. In his journal 1762-1763, Boswell wrote about his mental health in relation to occupation, and also about how Samuel Johnson advised him on how to avoid melancholy through constant occupation:

… about the age of seventeen I had a very severe illness. I became very melancholy. I imagined that I was never to get rid of it. I gave myself up as devoted to misery. I entertained a most gloomy and odd way of thinking. I was much hurt at being good for nothing in life … I had been so long accustomed to being out of the world that I could not think of engaging in real life. At last the Guards pleased me. I was opposed in this scheme. This made me fonder of it. I was also an enthusiast with regard to being in London. The charms of poetry also enchanted me.[12]

I complained to Mr. Johnson that I was much afflicted with melancholy, which was hereditary in our family. He said that he himself had been greatly distressed with it and for that reason had been obliged to fly from study and meditation to the dissipating variety of life. He advised me to have constant occupation of mind, to take a great deal of exercise, and to live moderately; especially to shun drinking at night. "Melancholy people," said he, "are apt to fly to intemperance, which gives momentary relief but sinks the soul much lower into misery!" He observed that labouring men who work much and live sparingly are seldom or never troubled with low spirits. It gave me great relief to talk of my disorder with Mr Johnson.[13]

The self-help texts which were published to inform people about what they should do if they experienced mental illness usually followed the tradition of humoral physiology, pathology, and therapeutics often as it was addressed in the *Regimen Sanitatis*. The authors were often general practitioners with an interest in nervous complaints and disordered minds rather than being specialists in "madness". The majority of medical men evinced little interest in mental illness, so, the care of "lunatics" was generally entrusted, if not to the mad person's family, then to a clergymen, jailer, workhouse master or private madhouse keeper who may or may not be a physician.[14] However it was physicians such as George Cheyne,[15] Sir Richard Blackmore,[16] and B. Mandeville[17] who mainly published the texts on helping self or others with mental illness.

In perhaps the best known of those, *The English Malady*, Cheyne recommended a regimen of diet and exercise for nervous distemper. The exercises that he advocated upheld the humoural theories of health in the matter of the mind as well as the body, in fact linked the two as humoural theory did. To that end the exercises recommended labour and occupations which would 'most infallibly strengthen the solids, by promoting and continuing actions and motions'.[18]

> *v. It is of no great consequence of what sort or kind the exercise be, provided it be but bodily exercise and action; certainly riding on horse back is the best of all, because of the almost erect posture, the lesser weariness, and the more universal and natural motion of all the organs, with the constant change of air: and that the lower regions of the body, and the alimentary instruments and hypochondres are thereby not shaken and excited. Next to that is riding in a chaise or chariot. Walking, tho' it will answer the same end and purpose as well as any, and may be more readily and easily used, because it may be equally followed within doors and without, in winter as well as summer, yet it is more laborious and tiresome. Next to these are the active games and sports, such as hunting, shooting, bowls, billiards, shuttlecock, and the like …*
>
> *But certainly the best of all is where amusement or entertainment of the mind is joined with bodily labour and constant change of air … For the entertainment of the mind, and keeping it agreeably diverted from reflecting on its misfortunes or misery, makes exercise infinitely more beneficial, as thoughtfulness, anxiety and concern render it quite useless.*
>
> *vi. It is upon this account that I would earnestly recommend to those afflicted with nervous distempers, always to have some innocent entertaining amusement to employ themselves in for the rest of the day, after they have employed in sufficient time upon exercise, towards the evening, to prepare them for their nights rest.*[19]

Community care and occupation

Whilst in much of Europe centralisation was a key feature of the times, in Britain, local programmes emanated from counties, parishes, squires, justices of the peace and similar authorities following the Restoration of the Monarchy in 1660. That appeared to signal a time of state inertia, community action replacing Parliament or Crown in the provision of social and welfare initiatives. Parochialism and diversity applied across numerous spheres central to this history such as industrial regulations, unemployment, education, public and mental health. Whilst agriculture remained the major form of economy, community initiatives were aided by their smallness and stability.

Most people with mental disorder remained in their parish, cared for and overseen by family and community. People within them knew family histories and individual frailties and what happened in their parish was a matter of interest and concern to them. Those who were unable to adequately care for themselves, or were not the recipient of family care or workhouse relief might be housed with a local cleric or doctor. It was also fairly common practice to board a single lunatic in lodgings with a keeper or willing householder who was compensated for the work by payment from the parish rates.[20] Sometimes such care was supervised, to an extent, by a doctor. Dr Thomas Monro for example, in the latter part of the century supervised J.R. Cozens, the watercolourist. Alternatively, as might be the case in the present, a medical man may be called in to the domestic situation to consult, and it seems that some of them prescribed occupations for remedial purpose. Dr William Pargeter was a case in point. When he was called in to help a young woman with melancholia he recommended not only a change of residence and particular diet, but also exercise and amusements, along with reading and conversation. Soon he was pleased to learn of her complete recovery.[21]

How many individuals with mental illness could be boarded in a house before it was called a madhouse is difficult to establish until later in the century. Early during the Enlightenment, the law, in relation to formal licensing of places of confinement, did not concern itself with "single lunatics" so the practice throve of "boarding houses" within communities. Some of those may well have involved people in occupations as a form of restraint, out of kindness, or for economic reasons. Pinel described one case:

> We are informed by Dr. Gregory, that a farmer, in the North of Scotland, a man of Herculean stature, acquired great fame in that district of the British Empire, by his success in the cure of insanity. The great secret of his practice consisted in giving full employment to the remaining faculties of the lunatic. With that view, he compelled all his patients to work on his farm. He varied their occupations, divided their labour, and assigned to each, the post which he was best qualified to fill. Some were employed as beasts of draught or burden, and others as servants of various orders and provinces. Fear was the operative principle that gave motion and harmony to this rude system. Disobedience and revolt, whenever they appeared in any of its operations, were instantly and severely punished.[22]

Probably many sought to hide disorder. Indeed, Henderson reports that, in Scotland, 'wealthy or well-to-do patients sometimes adopted the most elaborate measures to avoid publicity. Some were confined to restricted quarters in their own homes'.[23]

Assessment of life skills and need for ongoing care

At this period in history, assessment of insanity was not considered physicians' responsibility despite the fact that, from time to time, they had demonstrated an interest in the idea of such disorder as a medical construct. Even assessment for custodial intervention did not require a medical certificate, until 1774, when it became necessary for madhouses to be licensed. A medical certificate was then required to commit people to such places, but there was no rule that determined the qualifications of a medical practitioner.[24] In terms of assessment procedures followed by the few medical men who became involved in the problems associated with lunacy, some, such as Pargeter, took personal and family histories to determine treatment. So too did Thomas Percival. He gathered not only personal details such as age, sex and hereditary constitution, but details of occupation and modes of life as well.[25]

In the main, assessment of whether or not someone was mentally ill or not remained *ad hoc* as before, sometimes involving the judicial system. However the law was, for the most part, also silent on the issue. The mentally ill were dealt with alongside vagrants, according to rulings of local justices of the peace or magistrates.[26] Section 20 of England's 1744 Vagrancy Act allowed any person to detain a vagrant 'who by lunacy or otherwise are so far disordered in their Senses that they may be dangerous to be permitted to go Abroad'. The sanction of two Justices of the Peace was sufficient then to 'cause such Persons to be apprehended and kept safely locked up in some secure place', whilst the assessment of fitness to be released was the responsibility of local magistrates, the keeper, or even the jailer.[27]

An Act was passed in 1714 to realise 'the More Effectual Punishing (of) such Rogues, Vagabonds, Sturdy Beggars, and Vagrants, and Sending them Whither They Ought to be Sent'. This allowed for any person 'furiously mad and dangerous' to be 'safely locked up, in such secure place' so long as 'such lunacy or madness shall continue' following authorisation by any two Justices of the Peace. Whipping was expressly forbidden if the person committed was considered to be a lunatic, and the parish met costs for paupers.[28] A "secure place" for the committal of people with mental disorders was often a workhouse. This may have been because there were a greater number of them than madhouses, and during the century many more were established in parishes across the country following a succession of Acts to that end. Occupation had an important place in workhouses and such as could be engaged would have been.

From medieval times, legal matters to do with property, contracts, estates, heirships, and inheritance had been handled by the justice system, which provided trusteeships for idiots or lunatics. Until the Civil War, the Court of Wards, who appeared to appoint responsible and sympathetic trustees, handled this. To establish whether such intervention was required, or whether the subject was *non compos mentis* (a nincompoop), tests of mental capacity were devised. They were not medical, diagnostic or therapeutic tests but practical ones to establish people's ability to continue to manage their everyday lives. Criteria of competence were elementary such as knowing their name, counting, and recognising key people such as parents. At the time of the Restoration, the Court of Wards was discontinued, and the Chancery assumed responsibility for those functions concerned with the mentally incompetent. Following petition by relatives, the Lord Chancellor issued a writ known as *De Lunatico Inquirendo,* and the case was heard before a jury. If found to be "non compos" the subject's property would be administered by committee under Crown protection.

Public asylums and occupation

Bethlem Hospital

In an earlier chapter, the emergence of Bethlem was traced as the first, and for a very long time, the only hospital for the insane in Britain. It remained the most conspicuous centre for the confinement and treatment of those with mental illness during the eighteenth century, the name Bedlam becoming the epitome of madness itself.

The Hospital was commonly regarded as a place of horror or amusement rather than one that offered the best possible care. Until around 1770 it was partially funded by the pennies dropped into the boxes provided for the many visitors who came to be entertained. Visits to the long gallery day rooms of the imposing Hospital to watch and encourage the bizarre antics of inmates are hard to understand in the present climate. They must have provided people with similar excitement to that experienced today when watching films of scary and freakish behaviours.

Part of the attraction appears to have been the contrast between the grand architecture suited to "my Lord Mayor's Palace"[29] and the crazy, usually poor, inhabitants. Indeed, most of Bethlem's patients came from the ranks of the poor. In retrospect, at least the patient's environment was reasonable during the eighteenth century, particularly when contrasted with some of the conditions endured elsewhere and at other times. In *De Londres Et De Ses Environs* (1788), an unknown French author described what he experienced:

> *I stayed for some time in Bedlam. The poor creatures there are not chained up in dark cellars, stretched on damp ground, nor reclining on cold paving stones ... no bolts, no bars. The doors are open, their rooms wainscoted, and long airy corridors give them a chance of exercise. A cleanliness, hardly conceivable unless seen, reigns in their hospital*[30]

Despite such advantages, and the aim of the governors that the inmates be kept warm and well fed, there are evidences that this was not the case, and stories abound which reflect dissatisfaction with the care received.

As throughout its history, it continued to aim at cure. During this time about 30% of those admitted were said to have been cured, although some of those in that category were re-admitted at a later date. The Records provide some detail of patients discharged as cured. Sarah Carter for example in May 1710:

> ... *appearing in the Judgment of the Committee and Doctor to be restored to her Senses. It is Ordered That she be forthwith discharged from this Hospital.*
>
> ... *And she desiring to goe into Essex where she sayes she has formerly lived It is Ordered that forty shillings be given unto her out of Doctor Tyson's Gift thirty shillings whereof is to be laid out by the Steward of this house for Necessary Apparell & Clothing for her and that the remaining ten shillings be given her to bear her Charges into the Country.*[31]

From 1730 onwards, accommodation was provided for fifty men and fifty women considered to be incurable and who had no families or friends able to give ongoing care.

It seems, however, that Enlightenment thinking failed to penetrate the walls of the establishment, and treatment changed little during the eighteenth century. Physical restraint was employed to control patients and so were traditional medications. In a nepotistic reign, from 1728 to 1853, of four generations of the Monro family as physicians to the Hospital, the principal treatment consisted of "purges, vomits, and blood lettings".[32] Moral management happening in other places was slow to take root in that bastion of insanity.

Yet a few glimmers of embryo moral management emerge from the Hospital's Reports. In 1765 it was recorded, as part of the Matron's duties that she was to ensure that women patients who were 'low spirited or inclinable to be mopish' should be made to get out of bed. Indeed they should not be allowed to slink back to bed and, those who were able, should be employed at needlework. Matrons became, to all intents and purposes, the earliest consultant "occupational therapist" for women patients in many asylums. The case was no different in Bethlem, which can be said to have started the trend. The Report of 1765 records that:

> ... *the Committee further find that the Duty and Office of a Matron has been and is as follows:-*
>
> • *To attend and assist at Bathing and Bleeding the Women*
> • *To look after the maids and see that they do their Duty.*
> • *And we are of opinion that the following regulations and alterations should be made in the office of Matron (that is to say):-*
> • *It is the opinion of this Committee Duty of the Matron (as settled by an Order of Court dated the 6th May, 1736) is only to attend and assist at Bathing and Bleeding the Women and look after the Maids and see that they do their Duty. That the Office of Matron and Nurse on the next Vacancy be united.*
> • *That she shall Distribute the Patients in their proper Cells that each Gallery Maid may have a proper number of such hands, as are fit for work to assist hers and Employ such of the Patients at their needle as are capable when not otherwise Busied rather than let them walk and idle up and down the House Shewing it to Strangers and begging Money.*[33]

It is therefore clear that, in principle at least, occupation for therapeutic purposes was a part of treatment for women with mental health problems, in Bethlem, for the last decades of the eighteenth century. So it is of interest to know the names of those required to initiate and carry out such therapy. There were two Matrons from 1765 to the end of the century: Mary Spencer to January 1793 and Mary White to September 1798.[34]

There were no similar written instructions for occupation to be supplied to male patients, and that of females was restricted to domestic types of work reflecting the pattern of occupations available to poorer women during the Enlightenment. Although there was little opportunity for outdoor occupations because of the city venue, Steward's Accounts and Committee Minutes surviving from earlier in the eighteenth century reveal that, for some patients, work was available throughout its duration. Informally, a very few patients were rewarded with money, alcohol and privileges for engagement in a range of duties such as "cleaning or levelling the yard", "burning the straw" presumably of bedding, screening ash, "trying out the fire engine" and serving provisions. Patients were banned from serving refreshments in 1769, and again in 1785 maybe because of problems caused by jealousy of the privileges. Later in the century medical staff could appoint patients to particular tasks, and in 1796 the resident apothecary, for example, selected a helper to the cook who was allowed a pint of porter a day as a reward.[35]

Other patients obviously found their own means of occupying their time, as can be seen in the Hogarth engraving shown as figure 1.8.1. Apart from various very bizarre activities associated with their disorder, one man is drawing on the wall. In the better known version of this figure one man is playing the violin, and another is, possibly, engaged in a magic trick with a length of string. In terms of more prescribed or organised activities, while not many patients might be engaged in work, a limited number of other occupations were more widely available. The Steward purchased sets of skittles for patient's use in 1773 and more in 1779,[36] and in the patient's sitting rooms, which were gradually added to the wards, newspapers, books and writing material were available. Sophie von la Roche who visited Bethlem in the 1780s reported that she witnessed patients sitting sociably together whilst others sewed, read, or wrote.[37]

Public and County asylums

In answer to an obvious community need, from the beginning of the eighteenth century, there was interest in the establishment of additional institutional facilities for the mentally ill. The anonymous pamphlet dated 1700 calling for the founding of general hospitals in each county described in the last chapter is an example. The pamphlet did not differentiate between people with physical or mental disorder in its appeal for the setting up of institutional care for people who were chronically disabled.[38]

Apart from Bethlem, one very small public asylum had been set up in Norwich by Mrs Mary Chapman in 1713. Another, founded in London in 1751 by public subscription, and necessary because of Bethlem's waiting lists, was St Luke's. St Luke's was called an asylum rather than a hospital or madhouse. Unlike Bethlem, it did not admit the public to be entertained but did admit medical students who learnt about the "trade" under the tutelage of William Battie. Battie, who, like the Monros, also owned a private madhouse was a well respected, energetic and enterprising man who also prognosticated cure as an outcome of his treatment. He asserted that, 'if treated with humanity, lunacy was no less curable than any other disease'.[39] St Luke's does appear to have had some success in this regard. John Wesley recorded:

> *I had the opportunity of looking over the register of St Luke's Hospital; and I was surprised to observe, that three in four, at least, of those admitted receive a cure. I doubt this is the case of any other lunatic hospital, either in Great Britain or Ireland.*[40]

And at least some of the patients there were engaged in occupation. John Howard, already mentioned for the reform of the conditions in prisons, lazarettos and other hospitals reported that:

> *This hospital had two sitting rooms in each gallery, one for the quiet and the other for the turbulent; as well as Large airing grounds for men and women. ... several women were calm and quiet, and at needlework with the matron.*[41]

That report, like the earlier one from Bethlem, identified the Matron as the person responsible for the "occupational regimen" of the women. The key phrase in Howard's report that provides some sense of a therapeutic process is "with the matron". It does not say "for the matron", or "on the instructions of the matron". This, at least, implies encouragement and sharing, as does the use of group or community engaged in the task at hand.

Similar public asylums were established in Manchester in 1766 and Liverpool in 1797, both of which were linked with the General Infirmaries of those cities. John Howard was one key campaigner for the Liverpool establishment along with Dr James Currie. One imagines that at least needlework was used with patients there as the first keeper and matron were both recruited from St Luke's. Other public asylums were established in Newcastle in 1765 and York in 1777, as institutions separate from the care of those with physical illnesses. The Newcastle Lunatic Hospital was privatised within a couple of years by its physician. However York Hospital was started with the fervour of moral idealism and its early years appear to be characterised by enlightened humanity, which was, at a later date, less obvious and the subject of national debate and condemnation.

By the beginning of the nineteenth century, the institutions that would provide asylum and be the basis of treatment of the mentally ill for the next 150 years had slowly begun to emerge from the foundation of enlightened thought.

Few people before then envisaged the notion of asylum as remedy in itself. The managerialism and institutionalisation that arose with industrialisation was yet to supersede the largely individualistic attempts at curing that were part and parcel of small, private madhouses.

Private madhouses and occupation

Although a few philanthropically funded asylums were set up during the eighteenth century, the lack of facilities, in a time that was perceived by some to have witnessed a huge growth in the incidence of lunacy, led to the expansion of private madhouses, (madhouse being the standard eighteenth century term for such institutions). Some of the better known London madhouses included Brooke House at Hackney which was owned by the Monro family, James Newton's house at Clerkenwell, Norman House, a female madhouse in Fulham, and Mrs Wright's at Bethnal Green. In the provinces there was Fonthill Gifford in Wiltshire which was founded in 1718, and Hook Norton in Oxfordshire about 1725. That catered for about a dozen patients, nearly seventy per cent of whom stayed for less than six months. Anthony Addington's madhouse in Reading had between 8 to 10 patients at a time, and the Rev'd John Lord's very small madhouse in Buckinghamshire appears to have specialised in breakdowns occurring at Oxford University. There were at least twenty five madhouses in the county of Edinburgh by the beginning of the nineteenth century.[42] In Dublin, Jonathan Swift founded St Patrick's. Catering for nearly 200, about a quarter of them were paying boarders who found their own bedding. The others were paupers maintained, and supplied with bedding, by charity. They were provided with wooden bedsteads which were in cells 10 feet 8 inches long, 8 feet broad, and 12 feet high with a large window commanding a cheerful view. They opened onto long galleries, which also had windows. The whole establishment was reported to be clean and in good order.[43]

Essentially those madhouses, similar to the many others around the country, were places of confinement, and the growth in their numbers points, not necessarily to an increase in the incidence of mental illness, but certainly to a changing attitude to those deemed insane. In societies which, increasingly, considered that "difference" was not necessarily attributable to "God's purpose" segregation and confinement of those afflicted was a comfortable and convenient option. So, although, as noted in the chapter on the Renaissance, a small but unknown number of people had been placed in custodial care before such opinion became common, by the end of the eighteenth century official figures indicate that around two and a half thousand people were confined in licensed madhouses. The requirement for such licensing was enacted in 1774 and, prior to that date, it is impossible to estimate even the number of madhouses that existed or when they were established. Porter has suggested that probably many householders became madhouse proprietors by default after boarding one or more lunatics for whatever reason, and later choosing to profit from this experience by advertising their establishments as madhouses.[44]

The private madhouses of the eighteenth century were, in many instances, profitable businesses set up by enterprising doctors and keepers from other walks of life in accord with a free market economy. Although there was variation between them, the cost of confinement, in many instances, was expensive even for those who could afford it. Dr Nathaniel Cotton at St Albans, for example, charged each patient three to five guineas a week, which was a similar sum to the wage a female servant earned in a year. The fee for those with "middle incomes" was up to a guinea a week, and about half that price was paid per week to private madhouses by parishes which had no adequate facilities for the custody of the pauper insane who came under their jurisdiction. This was more than the cost of workhouse confinement.

Not surprisingly, the level of accommodation and treatment varied between the social and financial status of the clients. For the right remuneration, proprietors were often willing to provide "special patients" with luxurious accommodation, rooms for servants, favourite foods, or more care, remedies and treatment than the norm. The poor were usually housed in similar style to most servants, apprentices and labourers of the period in detached accommodation such as stables, sleeping on straw mattresses with more than one to a bed, receiving scanty food and limited attention.[45]

But charges and accommodation were not the extent of the diversity between what each madhouse offered. At the simplest level the number housed in them also differed, from a very few, which was more often the case, to over a hundred. William Terry's house at Sutton Coldfield, for example took only eleven new patients in nineteen years from 1793, whilst Hoxton House run by Sir Jonathan Miles at about the same time had over 450. Many were licensed, as part of the 1774 Act, for up to twelve patients. The number housed would, of course, have altered the likelihood of occupation being offered to the inmates.

Some provided only custodial care, whilst others included early forms of remediation. Cure was said to be the aim of most regimes. For example, in the 1779 advertisement for William Finch's establishment, Milford, near Salisbury it is stated that he had:

> ... for many years had great success in curing people disordered in their senses ... the many cures he has performed on Lunatics ... can be attested by the greatest satisfaction he can say, that every person he has had charge of, has, with the blessing of God, been cured and discharged from his house perfectly well'.[46]

There were three principal kinds of remediation which were followed to a lesser or greater extent by the madhouse proprietors or their medical attendants. These were medical in the sense of organic or pharmaceutical "physic", punitive, or moral management. Figure 1.8.2 outlines these approaches and the frequent pairing of "physic" with either punitive or moral management.

Figure 1.8.2: **Mental health: Three types of remediation in the eighteenth century**

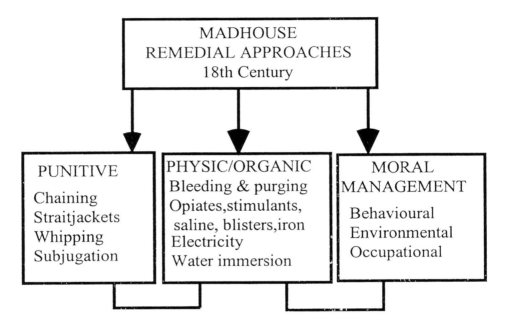

In terms of "physic", physicians had long sought medication for the treatment of disorders of the mind. From the Age of Enlightenment the humoural view of order and disorder had prevailed for ailments of personality as well as those of the body. Different views abounded on what treatment was useful to attain humoural balance and eliminate excesses of blood, choler, phlegm or bile, and madhouse keepers often guarded the secret nostrums of the physicians who attended their patients. To the doses of iron, saline draughts, emetics, valerian, calomel, opiates, and so on, were added physical treatments such as immersion in cold water, electricity and the ubiquitous blood-lettings. None were particularly successful, although as symptoms eased according to nature and time, claims were made that it was the treatment that cured the patient.

Unregulated in any way until licencing became a requirement, and even then in receipt of minimal surveillance, it is not surprising that some madhouses were the scene of improper confinement and neglect. But they also engaged in physical and mental abuse with purpose, using intimidating behavior, restrictive instruments like chains and straitjackets, and physical tools such as whips. This was not frowned upon, as it would be in the present day, as it was, in part, aimed at the elimination of unwanted humours. In addition, such abuse was consistent with the popular stereotype of madness, which still encompassed the notion of demonic possession overcoming the godfearing nature of civilised people. The latter could only be exorcised and therefore "remediated" by severe punishment. Ferriar, an enlightened expert, explained: 'It was formerly supposed that lunatics could only be worked upon by terror; shackles and whips, therefore, became part of medical apparatus.'[47] Not restricted to English madhouses, such practices were widespread across Europe. French physician, Pinel remarked on 'the system of treatment, which is yet adopted in too many hospitals, where the domestics and keepers are permitted to use any violence that the most wanton caprice, or the most sanguinary cruelty may dictate'.[48]

The extent of abuses and brutal punitive therapy is hard to establish as the keepers, knowing that their business depended upon discretion and in some cases secrecy because of a family's wish for anonymity, chose not to keep detailed records. The secrecy makes it difficult to ascertain the regimes of many of the madhouses, so inference has to be drawn from sources such as advertisements and books written on the subject by madhouse proprietors or their medical experts.

From such sources it would seem that harsh treatment was not always the case. Notwithstanding the stereotypes of the age it appears that madhouse keepers could not be sure of success, especially with the affluent, if they marketed their establishments according to those pre-enlightenment views of disorder and treatment. Indeed, some went further. For example Thomas Fallowes, who was, incidentally, probably the first "mad-doctor" to be convicted for illegal confinement, advertised his establishment in Lambeth-Marsh early in the 1700s by criticising 'the rough and cruel Treatment, which is said to be the Method of most of the Pretenders to this cure'. That, he added 'is not only to be abhorr'd, but on the contrary, all the Gentleness and Kindness in the World, is absolutely necessary, even in all the Cases I have seen; I have never us'd any Violence to any Patient'.[49]

Indeed towards the mid-eighteenth century the notion of moral, mental or "mind" management appeared. In many ways moral management was an Enlightenment manifestation of the *Regimen Sanitatis* applied to the treatment of mental disorders. It was also fed by the interest in and following of John Locke's work, an *Essay Concerning Humane Understanding* which grounded knowledge in the senses and the day to day experience of people, as well as the development of personal identity. Madness, in his terms, was more equated with children unable to think straight than of passionate animals who had to be subdued.

As this niche in the health care market began to open up the possibility of prosperity for those of an entrepreneurial nature, proprietors called attention to services that offered all the comforts of home. These services were designed to appeal to families who might not commit a relative to anything less. Fallowes claimed:

> The Conveniences may be easily observ'd upon view; the Situation is in an Air neither too subtle and thin, nor too gross; the Gardens to the House are Commodious, Large and Pleasant, into which the Patients are admitted, in their Intervals, and with a Person to attend them. There is as much Privacy as can be desired, and very good Rooms, and 'tis within such a Distance from the City as any Patient may be visited by their own Physician or Chirurgion, if they think fit; for I shall be ready to admit them.[50]

Responsive to market forces Keepers, as well as advertising facilities and services to meet this requirement, also created new and different ones or re-invented older practices as fresh notions of cure came into being. Joseph Mason Cox's rotating chair was one such innovation. He promoted it as allowing him to subdue his patients because rather than ride in the "whirligig", which caused vertigo and nausea, they acquiesced to his wishes.[51]

The norm, though, during the eighteenth century, saw madhouse advertising proclaiming curative therapy based on fresh air, exercise and diet. Those became part of a moral management approach that included, as well as a comfortable physical environment, at least for those who could pay, a more humane behavioural approach to interaction, and the provision of occupations. It can be questioned whether such advertising was followed to the letter in all cases as "moral treatment" built on the ideals of moral management was not established until the end of the century and its practise appears to have been a revelation to workers in the field.

Occupations as part of the exercise component of the "non-naturals" became a part of treatment within madhouses whose owners based their claims of cure on moral management. In that context the occupations likely to appeal to the well-to-do, the more probable recipients of such interventions, were those most frequently used. Music, embroidery, reading, walking or carriage riding was therefore much in vogue. Fallowes claimed that entertainment was part of the regime he offered and that it was 'such Entertainment as is fit for Persons of any Degree or Quality, in my House, in Lambeth-Marsh'.[52]

In other madhouses occupations were also encouraged that had meaning for the patient. Dr Johnson's very public concerns about the confinement of his fellow-poet Christopher (Kit) Smart because "his infirmities were not noxious to society" and "he did not love clean linen", surely also encompassed a fear that he may not be able to continue with his art. Such was not the case. Smart, particularly remembered for his *Song to David* (1763), spent four years at Potter's madhouse in Bethnal Green. There he was provided with pen and paper, which enabled him to devote time every day to neatly recording the lines that he composed in a document he called *Jubilate Agno*.[53] He also was allowed or encouraged to dig in the garden, play with his cat, read books and magazines, receive and talk with visitors, and from time to time enjoy accompanied freedom. He died in debt, within the rules of the King's bench.[54]

Reading and religious discussion were the occupations sought by William Cowper when he was admitted to the Collegium Insanorum in 1763. This private madhouse, mentioned earlier, was set up around 1740 by Nathaniel Cotton who was well respected for the care he provided. Cowper records:

> I was not only treated with kindness by him when I was ill, and attended with the utmost diligence; but when my reason was restored to me, and I had so much need of a religious friend to converse with, to whom I could open my mind upon the subject without reserve, I could hardly have found a fitter person for the purpose. The doctor was as ready to administer relief to me in this article likewise, and as well qualified to do it, as in that which was more immediately in his province'.[55]

Occupations of a spiritual nature were also part of the regime offered at Fishponds near Bristol. The proprietor, Baptist, George Mason and his family were proud of their humane and homely establishment where they took tea and held prayers with the patients. Not a medical man himself, Mason's successor, Joseph Mason Cox, was and the publicity after Cox became proprietor turned from the simple occupations of home to medical treatment and gadgetry such as the use of his rotating chair mentioned earlier.[56]

Probably the best known of the madhouse proprietors of this period, at least in the present day, was Francis Willis, a Church of England clergyman who had turned to medicine and established a high-class, but small, private asylum at Greatford in Lincolnshire. The Reverend Doctor, who was summoned on 5th December 1788 to cure George the III's "madness", presented himself as a charismatic healer. This allowed him to overrule the King's other physicians and to treat the King man-to-man, in a totally personal, brusque manner, "fixing" him with his "eye", and even having him put into a straitjacket. Despite such subordinating strategies, Willis also encouraged the King to continue his own daily living tasks, to the extent of using a razor for shaving. As well he gave him *King Lear* to read. There must have been a therapeutic purpose behind the use of such an occupation, when one mad king is encouraged to read of the madness of another. Willis took the credit for the King's recovery and received a pension of a £1000 a year by parliamentary vote.[57]

Benjamin Faulkner was another who advocated the use of occupations in his madhouse in Little Chelsea. Faulkner was not a medical man and put forward a case in *Observations on the General and Improper Treatment of Insanity* (1790) that physicians should not be allowed to be proprietors of madhouses. This, he stated, caused a conflict of interest between the need to confine people for as long as possible for the sake of profit versus the need to cure the illness in as short a time as possible. 'It requires no uncommon faith to believe, that the desire of profit and the accumulation of advantages resulting from expensive board and lodging, will, with too many, have more weight than the reputation of an early cure.' It can be wondered whether he believed a doctor should be called at all as the characteristics of the layperson's madhouse of excellence also professed to be curative. His, he claimed provided 'proper objects and amusements to engage and invigorate the mental faculties, proper exercise and proper diet are the grand restoratives in this malady. For the accomplishment of all these my house is peculiarly calculated.'[58]

This claim seems to be of particular relevance to this history as it explicitly captures much of the spirit of modern day occupational therapy as it emerged in the treatment of the mentally ill. Whilst it does not use the term occupation but rather objects and amusements, in the twentieth century also, for much of the time, occupation has not been the word of choice in occupational therapy literature and even common usage. It does point, as early modern texts do, to the therapeutic nature of engagement in "doing" through claims of the restorative and invigorating effects of the occupations provided, linking those with exercise presumably of both mind and body. The clarity of that message from a lay mental health practitioner is also worth noting as it separates occupational regimes from the potions and physical interventions deemed to be the province of medical science. During this period, therefore, there is evidence that both types of experts in mental health, lay and medical, saw the value of occupation as a therapeutic tool.

By the end of the century some of the older established madhouses, such as Fishponds in Bristol, had prestigious standing within the field. Yet few were purpose built. An exception was a new establishment, the Retreat, in York, founded by the Quaker Society for the care of their own members and built in a style reminiscent of a country house. This represented, in large measure, the ideal they envisaged as necessary for enlightened care, and which was to have an enormous impact on the treatment of mentally disturbed people in the future.

Several occupational therapists have linked the origins of moral treatment with the birth of occupational therapy.[59] That makes this story of particular interest in the history. The beginnings of moral treatment and the use made of occupation in York and in Bicêtre, France will be addressed in this chapter. As well, the development of occupation as a treatment method at the Retreat will be discussed further in the next section of the book, within the chapter dealing with mental health in the age of industry.

The Retreat

The genesis of the Retreat will be told in excerpts of the words of Samuel Tuke (1784-1857), the grandson of the founder William Tuke, (1732-1822) who was a Quaker tea merchant and pictured in figure 1.8.3. William Tuke's involvement with the Retreat spanned over thirty formative years, as he remained the manager-in-chief until failing eyesight at the age of 88 caused him to relinquish the post. Such was his prestige within the "lunacy trade" that in that year he was invited by a parliamentary committee concerned with the management of asylums and treatment of the insane to attest to the accuracy of Samuel's 1813 book *Description of the Retreat*. The committee was impressed by the book's account of the Retreat's origins as well the treatment that the patients received. William answered 'I had the revision of it before it went to the press, and I know it to be perfectly correct'.[60] The younger Tuke's account relates how:

> … *the origin of the Institution … has much the appearance of an accident. In the year 1791, a female, of the Society of Friends, was placed at an establishment for insane persons, in the vicinity of the City of York; and her family, residing at a considerable distance, requested some of their acquaintance in the City to visit her. The visits of these Friends were refused, on the ground of the patient not being in a suitable state to be seen by strangers: and, in a few weeks after her admission, death put a period to her sufferings.*
>
> *The circumstance was affecting, and naturally excited reflections on the situation of insane persons, and on the probable improvements which might be adopted in establishments of this nature. In particular, it was conceived that peculiar advantage would be derived to the Society of Friends, by having an Institution of this kind under their care, in which a milder and more appropriate system of treatment, than that usually practised, might be adopted; and where, during lucid intervals, or the state of convalescence, the patient might enjoy the society of those who were of similar habits and opinions …*
>
> *It was believed also, that the general treatment of insane persons was, too frequently, calculated to depress and degrade, rather than to awaken the slumbering reason, or correct its wild hallucinations.*
>
> *In one of the conversations to which the circumstance before-mentioned gave rise, the propriety of attempting to form an Establishment for persons of our own Society, was suggested to William Tuke, whose feelings were already much interested in the subject, and whose persevering mind, rendered him peculiarly eligible to promote such an undertaking. After mature reflection, and several consultations with his most intimate friends on the subject, he was decidedly of opinion, that an Establishment for the insane of our own Society, of every class in accord to property, was both eligible and highly desirable. It was necessary to excite a general interest in the Society on the subject. He therefore, after the close of the Quarterly Meeting at York, in the 3rd Month 1792, requested Friends to allow him to introduce to them a subject, connected with the welfare of the Society … for the care and accommodation of their own Members, labouring under that most afflictive dispensation - the loss of reason'.[61]*

Figure 1.8.3: **William Tuke**
(The Wellcome Library)

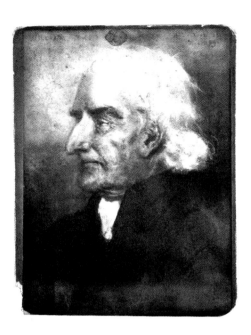

Tuke consulted widely and visited various establishments that treated the mentally ill, including St Lukes. His visits made his commitment to the endeavour stronger as he saw how patients were all too frequently, miserably coerced.[62]

> ... *The Friends with whom the proposal originated, were requested to prepare the outline of a plan, for the consideration of those who might attend the next Quarterly meeting. Several objections, however, on a variety of grounds, soon afterward appeared. ... Some were not sensible that any improvement could be made in the treatment of the insane; supposing that the privations, and severe treatment, to which they were generally exposed, were necessary in their unhappy situation; and others seemed rather averse to the concentration of the instances of this disease amongst us.*

Despite such objections Tuke observed that 'there was a respectable number, who duly appreciated the advantages likely to accrue to the Society from the proposed Establishment, and who cordially engaged in the promotion of the design'.[63]

A firm proposal was put at the next Quarterly meeting, a resolve to establish the institution taken, and subscriptions called for. Some indication of the occupational stance to be followed was apparent in the first of the seven points of that proposal.

> *That, in case proper encouragement be given, Ground be purchased, and a Building be erected, sufficient to accommodate Thirty Patients, in an airy situation, and at as short a distance from York as may be, so as to have the privilege of retirement; and that there be a few acres for keeping cows, and for*

garden ground for the family; which will afford the Patients to take exercise, when that may be prudent and suitable.[64]

Although this only suggests that patients will be encouraged to engage in exercise, use of the word exercise was usually inclusive of occupation during that period. If that was the case it is of interest that such an indication occurred at this early stage and before any formal determinations of the nature of treatment were formulated. In a more recent history of insanity during the Age of Reason, Foucault reminds us of the occupational philosophy underpinning the Quaker faith:

Let us not forget that we are in a Quaker world where God blesses men in the signs of their prosperity. Work comes first in "moral treatment" as practiced at the Retreat. In itself, work possesses a constraining power superior to all forms of physical coercion, in that the regularity of hours, the requirements of attention, the obligation to produce a result detach the sufferer from a liberty of mind that would be fatal and engage him in a system of responsibilities ...

... Through work, man returns to the order of God's commandments; he submits his liberty to laws that are those of both morality and reality, hence mental work is not to be rejected; yet with absolute rigor, all exercises of the imagination must be excluded as being in complicity with the passions, the desires, or all delirious illusions ...

... In the asylum work is deprived of any productive value; it is imposed only as a moral rule; a limitation of liberty, a submission to order, an engagement of responsibility, with the single aim of disalienating the mind lost in the excess of liberty which physical constraint limits only in appearance.[65]

A booklet was published in 1796 that briefly described the work of the Retreat and sought donations and contributions to its establishment. It was titled *State of An Institution near York called the Retreat for Persons Afflicted with Disorders of the Mind 1796*. Within this, too, there is an early indication of the intention to engage patients in occupation to assist their recovery. There is also a suggestion that as some occupations may exacerbate mental illness careful choice must be made to ensure therapeutic effects. As would be expected, in this case, the occupations deemed most suitable were those compatible with the Quaker's religious beliefs:

... on the other hand, when returning reason indicates a restoration of the mental powers, it may greatly tend to advance and establish the patients recovery, to perceive himself under the direction of persons who, whilst they are careful to promote cheerful and salutary amusements, will be concerned, at suitable seasons, to cherish in them the strengthening and consolatory principles of Religion and Virtue, instead of dissipating these impressions, by such diversions as enfeeble the mind, and disqualify it for that solid reflection which leads to substantial peace and comfort.[66]

The details of the Retreat's occupational philosophy of moral treatment, which grew from such small beginnings, were not recorded in detail until

Samuel's landmark book in the next century. It is therefore appropriate that, in this chapter, archival material from the first few years is examined from an occupational perspective. The particulars of occupation within moral treatment are examined in a later chapter, which deals with mental health in the Age of Industry.

The consultations, the gathering in of monies, and the building of the Retreat took a few years:

> Four years had now elapsed since the first Meeting, of the friends to the proposed Establishment; and they felt, as will naturally supposed, a mixture of anxiety and pleasure, in contemplating the progress of their undertaking …
>
> … The house being ready for the reception of patients, according to the expectation given at the last Meeting; and a housekeeper and several servants being provided, the house was opened on the 11th of the 5th month, 1796, and three patients were admitted, early in the following month.[67]

The importance of appropriate staff was recognised and apparently great pains were taken to find those with the right qualities:

> The difficulty of finding suitable persons to have the superintendency of the family, occasioned the Committee no small trouble and anxiety. In the fifth month, however, of the following year, the person who, at present has the management of the female department, was happily engaged; and very shortly afterwards, the present superintendent and apothecary entered on his arduous offices. The conductors and still more the unhappy objects of this Establishment, have great reason to esteem as a blessing, the appointment of these individuals.[68]

The matron, appointed in 1796, was Katherine Allen (1776-1844). She had worked with Edward Long Fox at Fishponds as his female superintendent. In 1806 she married George Jepson (1745-1836) the superintendent appointed in 1797. They remained in charge of the day to day management of the Retreat until 1822. Originally a weaver, Jepson was a self-taught medical practitioner and had been a local counsellor in the West Riding of Yorkshire before his appointment. An indication of their quality is apparent in the following account:

> The female superintendent, who possesses an uncommon share of benevolent activity, and who has the chief management of the female patients, as well as of the domestic department, occasionally gives a general invitation to the patients, to a tea-party. All who attend, dress in their best clothes, and vie with each other in politeness and propriety. The best fare is provided, and the visitors are treated with all the attention of strangers. The evening generally passes in the greatest harmony and enjoyment.[69]

Together the Jepsons seem to have provided the Retreat with an excellent foundation towards developing the helpful, humane and domestic environment that its founders envisaged at the outset. Indeed, in an account of his work in *The Yorkshire Herald* dated July 1892 it is Jepson who is credited with the humane reform for which the Retreat is famous:

> On an occasion soon after his introduction into office, when he had exercised some severity towards a violent patient, he passed a sleepless night in anxious cogitations. He felt satisfied that his mode of treatment in this case had tended to irritate rather than control the patient's diseased feelings, and he determined to try the effect of an opposite system. Following steadily but cautiously the guidance of his judgement and his feelings, he was soon led by observation and experience to abandon the system of terror, and to adopt that which presumed the patient to be generally capable of influence through the kindly affections of the heart, and also in a considerable degree through the medium of the understanding. His system was described by an impartial writer, in an essay on the "Construction and Management of Asylums," published in 1810.[70]

Care was taken in the design of the house and gardens to meet the principles upon which the Retreat was established, including those of an occupational nature, although no room specifically designed for indoor occupations was included:

> The garden is on the north side of the house, and contains about one acre. This furnishes abundance of fruit and vegetables. It also affords an agreeable place for recreation and employment, to many of the patients.[71]

> The superintendent has also endeavoured to furnish a source of amusement, to those patients whose walks are necessarily more circumscribed, by supplying each of the courts with a number of animals; such as rabbits, sea-gulls, hawks, and poultry. These creatures are generally very familiar with the patients: and it is believed they are not only the means of innocent pleasure; but that the intercourse with them, sometimes tends to awaken the social and benevolent feelings.[72]

Even without a designated space for indoor occupation a report brought to the General meeting by the Retreat Committee in June 1797 records the use of therapeutic employment:

> In describing the particular benefits of this undertaking, it seems proper to mention that of occasionally using the patients to such employment as may be suitable and proper for them, in order to relieve the languor of idleness, and prevent the indulgence of gloomy sensations.[73]

Further proof of occupation's use during the founding years of the eighteenth century comes within a letter from Dr Delarive of Geneva to the British Library following a visit to the Retreat in 1798. The Doctor who had examined a large number of public and private institutions for the insane was very impressed with what he saw at the Retreat:

> A new system of education must be adopted to give a fresh course to their (the patients) ideas. Subject them at first (Samuel Tuke who reports this letter does not believe that subjection ever occurred); encourage them afterwards, employ them, and render their employment agreeable by attractive means.[74]

Some of the sparse, hand written case notes from 1796 also reveal the use of occupation with patients. It was reported, for example, that Elizabeth Thompson 'wrote verses of some merit'. She was described as deranged and melancholy, but was discharged much recovered in 1800. Examples of two of the full case notes are provided below.

Case 1:

1796

6. 23   Rachel Row of Reeth single woman Aged abt. 49 years. She has been deranged upwards of two years; maniscal; her Ideas often very wild. Has been much at liberty to walk out though mostly under care of a Keeper for many months past. Her health good.

1823

1. 19   She died this morning at haft past 9 o'clock. She has evidently been growing weaker for nearly all the last year. Aged about 84 years. Very imaginative, described various figures in the clouds & fire - of persons speaking to her etc. Constantly employed in domestic matters about the house. Very fond of doctoring and prescribing strange remedies - of a kind disposition.

Case 13:

1796

11.28   Thos. Ellin of Leeds Aged about 39 years - Has been more or less affected with Religious Melancholy for 5 or 6 year, and had shewn a propensity to injure himself, but seem disposed to guard against it. Little or no medical means have been used for his recovery. Supposed to be a Family disorder.

1800

5.31   Having gradually amended under gentle treatment and employment he was so far recovered as to render it eligible to try him with liberty and he was accordingly sent home this day.

Remark

3mo 6 1807 He followed his business of wool sorting at Leeds for about 2 years regularly and diligently and at last died of a decline.[75]

It is obvious from these excerpts that, at least, some of the patients remained in the Retreat for a long time. In the 1798 report it is observed:

… that out of twenty three cases now in the house, all of them, except two or three, were, at their admission, of so long standing as to be considered incurable. Most of the patients appear much improved, and some of them may be considered in a state of recovery; but from their liability to relapse, and their remote situation from home, their friends wait for further confirmation previously to their removal.[76]

The Retreat, in these early days had only small numbers of patients. By 1801 there were only 40 patients in the House. The report of the State of the Retreat in 1801 recorded:

There have been thirteen patients admitted since the last year. Seven have been discharged in a state of recovery; and two have died. The number now in the house is 40, viz. 24 women and 16 men. Besides the persons recovered, the condition of several others has been so much meliorated, as to afford additional encouragement to those who have interested themselves in this institution.[77]

Tuke makes a point in an explanation of his statistics that patients who appeared to recover and then returned to the Retreat following a relapse were not considered to be "recovered".[78]

Further details of the use of occupation as part of moral treatment at the Retreat will be discussed in Chapter 11. The other giant in the establishment of moral treatment at the same time as the Tukes at the Retreat was Pinel at Bicêtre. Because his text explaining it was first published in 1801 it is included in this chapter as it reports on developments in moral treatment at the close of the eighteenth century.

Pinel, Bicêtre, moral treatment and occupation

In the second year of the French Republic which was declared in 1792, Philippe Pinel (1745-1826) was appointed physician to a "lunatic infirmary" within Bicêtre, a hospital in Paris. There he found patients chained up in dirty cells, and treated as animals. Pinel is renowned for striking off their chains. Metaphorically true, this famous myth followed permission, which he obtained in 1798 from the National Assembly to remove the patient's fetters and permit them reasonable liberty along with other humanitarian treatment and an improved environment. Couthon, a warder, reputedly said to Pinel on that occasion: 'Citizen, are not you yourself crazy that you would unchain these wild beasts', a supposition which was discovered to be unfounded.

Figure 1.8.4: **Philippe Pinel, Lithograph by P.R. Vigneron**
(The Wellcome Library)

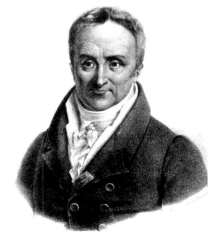

Pictured in figure 1.8.4, Pinel, who had qualified at Montpellier, and written a treatise on manic conditions prior to his appointment to Bicêtre, was known among his colleagues for his acumen in diagnosis. His attention to detail and acute observation which formed the basis for their evaluation of his work is evident in *Traité sur L'Aliénation Mentale,* published in France in 1801, and in English in 1806 as *A Treatise on Insanity.* Excerpts given below from this work record the story of his account of the place of occupation within moral treatment. The excerpts also demonstrate his superior knowledge in the field as he based his work and the ideologies that shaped it on observation and empirical knowledge gained as he worked amongst the afflicted.

He pointed out the difficulties to be overcome in asylums at that time:
Frequent attendance upon lunatic institutions can alone give an adequate idea of the difficulties of the service. New aversions or offences to encounter, dangers unforeseen to incur, perpetual clamours or insulting vociferations to listen to, and violence frequently to repel, are the leading characters of the scene that is daily presented at these melancholy habitations.[79]

As in all good scientific theses, he explained his methods of collecting data and making inferences:
Of the knowledge to be derived from books on the treatment of insanity, I felt the extreme insufficiency. Desirous of better information, I resolved to examine for myself the facts that were presented to my attention; and forgetting the empty honours of my titular distinction as a physician, I viewed the scene that was opened to me with the eye of common sense and unprejudiced observation. I saw a great number of maniacs assembled together, and submitted to a regular system of discipline. Their disorders presented an endless variety of character: but their discordant movements were regulated on the part of the governor by the greatest possible skill, and even extravagance and disorder were marshalled into order and harmony. I then discovered, that insanity was curable in many instances, by mildness of treatment and attention to the state of the mind exclusively, and when coercion was indispensable, that it might be very effectually applied without corporal indignity. To give all their value to the facts which I had the opportunity of observing, I made it an object of interest to trace their alliance with the functions of the understanding. To assist me in this enquiry, I attentively perused the best writers upon modern pneumatology, as well as those authors who have written on the influence of the passions upon the pathology of the human mind. The laws of the human economy considered in reference to insanity as well as to other diseases, impressed me with admiration of their uniformity, and I saw, with wonder, the resources of nature when left to herself, or skilfully assisted in her efforts. My faith in pharmaceutic preparations was gradually lessened, and my scepticism went at length so far, as to induce me never to have recourse to them, until moral remedies had completely failed. The success of this practice gives new support, were it necessary, to the following maxim of Dr. Grant: − "We cannot cure diseases by the resources of art, if not previously

acquainted with their terminations, when left to the unassisted efforts of nature."[80]

I regularly took notes of whatever appeared deserving of my attention; and compared with what I thus collected, with facts analogous to them that I met with in books, or amongst my own memoranda of former dates. Such are the materials upon which my principles of moral treatment are founded.[81]

Pinel alluded to a great number of the texts published by British experts on the treatment of the insane, which he obviously read and critiqued according to his experience. Many he found wanting, based as they were on the efficacy of remedies and physics and extravagant claims about the success of their treatments. Despite the censure he recognised the use and potential of moral management developed in the private madhouses of England:

The credit of this system of practice has been hitherto almost exclusively awarded to England. Though it be a department of experimental medicine that is least understood, I trust, that what has been advanced in this section will rescue France from the imputation of neglecting it.[82]

Pinel's moral treatment was based, in the main, upon two factors:
a) A degree of liberty, sufficient to maintain order, dictated not by weak but enlightened humanity, and calculated to spread a few charms ever the unhappy existence of maniacs, (this) contributes, in most instances, to diminish the violence of the symptoms, and in some, to remove the complaint altogether.[83]

b) The use of occupation. He considered that what he termed "mechanical or laborious employment", "active occupation" or the "natural law of bodily labour" was essential to the successful management of "lunatic hospitals". He explained that as:

… the result of the most constant and unanimous experience, that in all public asylums as well as in prisons and hospitals, the surest, and, perhaps, the only method of securing health, good order, and good manners, is to carry into decided and habitual execution the natural law of bodily labour, so contributive and essential to human happiness. This truth is especially applicable to lunatic asylums: and I am convinced that no useful and durable establishments of that kind can be founded excepting on the basis of interesting and laborious employment. I am very sure that few lunatics, even in their most furious state, ought to be without some active occupation.[84]

Pinel goes on to discuss some of the therapeutic effects of occupation including its use in prognosticating patients' re-establishment in community life, and the beneficial institutional consequences of occupational treatment regimes. He goes so far as to indicate the extreme importance, in his view, of physicians studying the occupational nature of their patients; of acting as occupational "therapists":

The scene which is presented in our national establishments by the insane of all descriptions and character, expending their effervescent excitement in antics and motions of various kinds, with out utility or object, or plunged in profound melancholy, inertia and stupor, is equally affecting, picturesque and pitiable. Such unrestrained indulgence of the natural propensities to indolence, to unproductive activity, or to depressing meditations, must in a high degree contribute to aggravate the existing evil. Laborious employment, on the other hand, is not a little calculated to divert the thoughts of lunatics from their usual morbid channel, to fix their attention upon more pleasing objects, and by exercise to strengthen the functions of the understanding. Where this method is adopted, little difficulty is experienced in the maintenance of order, and in the conduct and distribution of lunatics, even independent of many minute and often ineffectual regulations, which at other places are deemed indispensably necessary. The return of convalescents to their primitive tastes, pursuits, and habits, has always been by me considered as a happy omen of their final complete re-establishment. To discover those promising inclinations, a physician can never be too vigilant; nor to encourage them, too studious of the means of indulgence.[85]

Pinel, not only recommends that physicians should be occupationally aware, but also provides an indication of the Governor's duties as an occupational "therapist":

At the commencement of convalescence, and upon the dawn of returning reason, it frequently happens, that the taste of the individual, for his former pursuit of science, literature or other subjects unfolds itself. The first ray of returning talent ought to be seized with great avidity by the governor, and tenderly fostered, with a view of favouring and accelerating the development of the mental faculties. Numerous facts might be mentioned to confirm the importance of this maxim.[86]

Pinel had a great regard for the Governor of Bicêtre whom he judged as a moral and caring person with great skill in the exercise of his calling. An important aspect of the Governor's approach to the humane management of the patients was to involve them in domestic and attendant duties with other patients. Apparently such occupations was also used in the treatment of the mentally ill in other parts of Europe such as Holland and Spain. Whereas today such practice might be regarded by some as exploitation, at that time it was innovative indeed and appears, at least in the instances cited, to have been done with the patients' improvement in mind. In this way the practice of engaging patients in occupation meets the criteria of being regarded as a therapeutic process, as well as being cost effective. Pinel, whose moral treatment approach using occupation was greatly influenced by the governor, reports on its effectiveness as a therapeutic tool:

The method which he (the Governor) adopted for this purpose was simple, and I can vouch my own experience for its success. His servants were generally chosen from among the convalescents, who were allured to this kind of employment by the prospect of a little gain. Averse from ʌctive cruelty from the recollection of what they had themselves experienced; – disposed to those of humanity and kindness from the value, which for the same reason, they could not fail to attach to them; habituated to obedience, and easy to be drilled into any tactics which the nature of the service might require, such men were peculiarly qualified for the situation. As that kind of life contributed to rescue them from the influence of sedentary habits, to dispel the gloom of solitary sadness, and to exercise their own faculties, its advantages to themselves are equally apparent and important.[87]

Pinel considered that, not only should the treatment using occupation differ from patient to patient, it should differ according to diagnosis in much the same way of twentieth century occupational therapists who take a remedial approach. In prescribing the type of occupation he considered most efficacious, Pinel divided the patients in his care into three main categories, melancholics, that is, people experiencing depressive illness; mania, people suffering from a bipolar disorder; and dementia and ideotism, that is those with degenerating or congenital disorders. Excerpts describing his occupational approaches to patients suffering melancholia or mania are as follow:

Melancholics

About their environment he recommended that 'melancholics, ought to be allotted a part of the establishment commanding open and cheerful scenery, and adjoining to the grounds or gardens, where it is intended to engage them in the pleasing exercises of horticulture'.[88] The basis of his treatment of the melancholic was 'the urgent necessity of forcibly agitating the system; of interrupting the chain of their gloomy ideas, and engaging their interest by powerful and continuous impressions on their external senses.[89]

> *The fanciful ideas of melancholics are much more easily and effectually diverted by moral remedies, and especially by active employment, than by the best prepared and applied medicaments. But relapses are exceedingly difficult to prevent upon the best founded system of treatment.*[90]

Pinel demonstrated his innovative approach by telling a case history:

A working man, during an effervescent period of the revolution, suffered some unguarded expressions to escape him, respecting the trial and condemnation of Louis XVI. His patriotism began to be suspected in the neighbourhood. Upon hearing some vague and exaggerated reports of intentions on the part of government agents to prosecute him for disloyalty, he one day betook himself in great tremour and consternation to his own house. His appetite and sleep forsook him. He surrendered himself to the influence of terror, left off working, was wholly absorbed by the subject of his fear; and at length he became fully impressed with the conviction that death was his unavoidable fate. Having undergone the usual treatment at the Hôtel Dieu, he was transferred to Bicêtre. The idea of his death haunted him night and day, and he unceasingly repeated, that he was ready to submit to his impending fate. Constant employment at his trade, which was that of a tailor, appeared to me the most probable means of diverting the current of his morbid thoughts. I applied to the board for a small salary for him, in consideration of his repairing the clothes of the other patients of the asylum. This measure appeared to engage his interest in a very high degree. He undertook the employment with great eagerness, and worked without interruption for two months. A favourable change appeared to be taking place. He made no complaints nor any allusions to his supposed condemnation. He even spoke with the tenderest interest of a child of about six years of age, whom it seemed he had forgotten, and expressed a very great desire of having it brought to him. This awakened sensibility struck me as a favourable omen. The child was sent for, and all his other desires were gratified. He continued to work at his trade with renewed alacrity, frequently observing, that his child, who was now with him altogether, constituted the happiness of his life. Six months passed in this way without any disturbance or accident. But in the very hot weather of Messidor, (June and July) year 5, some precursory symptoms of returning melancholy began to shew themselves. A sense of heaviness in the head, pains of the legs and arms, a silent and pensive air, indisposition to work, indifference for his child, whom he pushed from him with marked coolness and even aversion, distinguished the progress of his relapse. He now retired into his cell, where he remained, stretched on the floor, obstinately persisting in his conviction, that there was nothing left for him but submission to his fate. About that time, I resigned my situation at Bicêtre, without, however, renouncing the hope of being useful to this unfortunate man. In the course of that year, I had recourse to the following expedient with him. The governor, being previously informed of my project, was prepared to receive a visit from a party of my friends, who were to assume the character of delegates from the legislative body, dispatched to Bicêtre, to obtain information in regard to Citizen –, or upon his innocence, to pronounce upon him a sentence of acquittal. I then concerted with three other physicians whom I engaged to personate this deputation. The principal part was assigned to the eldest and gravest of them, whose, appearance and manners were calculated to command attention and respect. These commissaries, who were dressed in black robes suitable to their pretended office, ranged themselves round a table and caused the melancholic to be brought before them. One of them interrogated him as to his profession, former conduct, the journals which he had been in the habits of reading, and other particulars respecting his patriotism. The defendant related all that he had said and done; and insisted on a definitive judgement, as he did not conceive that he was guilty of any crime. In order to make a deep impression on his imagination, the president of the delegates pronounced in a loud voice the following sentence. 'In virtue of the power which has been delegated to us by the national assembly, we have entered proceedings in due form of law, against Citizen –: and having, duly examined him, touching the matter whereof he stands accused, we make our declaration accordingly. It is, therefore, by us declared, that we have found the said Citizen, a truly loyal patriot; and, pronouncing his acquittal, we forbid all further proceedings against him. We furthermore order his entire enlargement and restoration to his friends. But inasmuch as he has obstinately refused to work for the last twelve months, we order his detention at Bicêtre to be prolonged six months from this present time, which said six months he is to employ, with proper sentiments of gratitude, in the capacity of tailor to the house. This our sentence is entrusted to Citizen Poussin, which he is to see executed at the peril of his life. Our commissaries then retired in silence. On the day following the patient again began to work, and, with every expression of sensibility and affection, solicited the return of his child. Having received the impulse of the above stratagem, he worked for some time unremittingly at his trade. But he had completely lost the use of his limbs from having remained so long extended upon the cold flags. His activity, however, was not of long continuance; and its remission concurring with an imprudent disclosure of the above well intended plot, his delirium returned. I now consider his case as absolutely incurable.[91]

Mania

For patients experiencing acute manic episodes he advocated a place for sensory deprivation as opposed to the sensory stimulating environment described for melancholics. Pinel recommended that:

The most furious and extravagant maniacs, it will be proper to confine in the most retired part of the building, where their cries and howlings will not reach beyond the gloom and secrecy of the place, and where no external object can be presented to excite or aggravate their fury. Those subject to periodical mania, may, during their lucid intervals, be liberated from their gloomy residences, and be permitted to associate with the convalescents. In order to avoid relapses, and to effect a permanent and perfect cure, the insulation of periodical maniacs is an important object in every well regulated hospital.[92]

The basis of his occupational treatment for patients with mania, following the acute phase of their illness was 'laborious or amusing occupations (which) arrest their delirious wanderings, prevent the determination of blood to the head by rendering the circulation more uniform, and induce tranquil and refreshing sleep.' With this prescription he found 'Convalescent maniacs, when, amidst the languors of an inactive life, a stimulus is offered to their natural propensity to motion and exercise, are active, diligent and methodical'.[93]

Pinel was very keen to establish outdoor occupations at Bicêtre, and suggested that agricultural work has an instinctive, natural attraction for many people. So strong was his belief in this therapy that, although it was not possible to set up an outdoor area for the purpose at that time at Bicêtre, he recommended that every lunatic asylum should have a large area of land given over to a "sort of farm" worked by the patients, and with the profits going to their support.[94]

I was one day deafened by the tumultuous cries and riotous behaviour of a maniac. Employment of a rural nature, such as I knew would meet his taste, was procured for him. From that time I never observed any confusion nor extravagance in his ideas. It was pleasing to observe the silence and tranquillity which prevailed in the Asylum de Bicêtre, when nearly all the patients were supplied by the tradesmen of Paris with employments which fixed their attention, and allured them to exertion by the prospect of a trifling gain. To perpetuate those advantages, and to ameliorate the condition of the patients, I made, at that time, every exertion in my power to obtain from the government an adjacent piece of ground, the cultivation of which, might employ the convalescent maniacs, and conduce to the re-establishment of their health. The disturbances which agitated the country in the second and third years of the republic, prevented the accomplishment of my wishes, and I was obliged to content myself with the subsidiary means which had been previously adopted by the governor; that of choosing the servants from among the convalescents.[95]

Four examples are provided which demonstrate some of the successes and failures Pinel met with using occupation as a principal treatment regime, and some of his reflections on the extreme complexity of its effective use:

An old literary gentleman, whose incoherent and incoercible loquacity I could sometimes with difficulty follow, was at intervals subject to a rude and gloomy taciturnity. If ever a piece of poetry which at any time had given him great satisfaction, recurred to his memory, he would become immediately susceptible of close attention, and his judgement appeared to recover its usual vigour. At those times, he would compose verses not only accurate in point of order and method, but enriched with appropriate images, and happy sallies of humour and fancy. As I could only bestow a few occasional hours upon experiments of this kind, it is not very easy to determine the quantum of benefit that might have resulted from the continued or frequently repeated application of the same means.

A musician, who had become insane in consequence of the revolution, was deprived of the power of connecting his ideas, and he mingled with his unmeaning monosyllables the most absurd and fantastic gestures. Upon the commencement of his convalescence, he once expressed himself as if he had a confused recollection of his favourite instrument. I took an early opportunity to send to his friends for his violin. It seemed to have a very soothing effect upon him, and he continued to amuse himself with music for several hours every day for eight months, when his recovery was rapidly advancing. But about that time, was admitted into the asylum, another maniac, who was exceedingly furious and extravagant. Frequent encounters with this new comer, who was permitted to ramble about the garden without restraint, again unhinged the musician's mind, and overwhelmed its returning powers. The violin was forthwith destroyed; his favourite amusement was forsaken; and his insanity is now considered as confirmed and incurable. An instance equally distressing and remarkable of the contagious influence of acts of maniacal extravagance upon the state of convalescents; and a strong proof of the necessity of insulation![96]

A celebrated watchmaker was … infatuated with the chimera of perpetual motion, and to effect this discovery, he set to work with indefatigable ardour. From unremitting attention to the object of his enthusiasm coinciding with the influence of revolutionary disturbances, his imagination was greatly heated, his sleep was interrupted, and, at length, a complete derangement of the understanding took place

Following the watchmaker's admission to Bicêtre:

Nothing could equal the extravagant overflowings of his heated brain. He sung, cried, or danced incessantly; and, as there appeared no propensity in him to commit acts of violence or disturbance, he was allowed to go about the hospital without control, in order to expend, by evaporation, the effervescent excess of his spirits …

… To this state of delirious gaiety, however, succeeded that of furious madness. He broke to pieces or otherwise destroyed whatever was within the reach or power of his mischievous propensity. Close confinement became indispensable. Towards the approach of winter his violence abated; and, although he continued to be extravagant in his ideas, he was never afterwards dangerous. He was, therefore, permitted, when ever he felt disposed, to go to the inner court. The idea of the perpetual motion frequently recurred to him in the midst of his wanderings; and he chalked on all the walls and doors as he passed, the various designs by which his wondrous piece of mechanism was to be constructed. The method best calculated to cure so whimsical an illusion, appeared to be that of encouraging his prosecution of it to satiety. His friends were, accordingly, requested to send him his tools, with materials to work upon, and other requisites, such as plates of copper and steel, watch-weels, &c. The governor, permitted him to fix up a work bench in his apartment. His zeal was now redoubled. His whole attention was riveted upon his favourite pursuit. He forgot his meals. After about a month's labour, which he sustained with a constancy that deserved better success, our artist began to think that he had followed a false route. He broke into a thousand fragments the piece of machinery which he had fabricated at so much expense of time, and thought, and labour; entered on the construction of another, upon a new plan, and laboured with equal pertinacity for another fortnight. The various parts being completed, he brought them together, and fancied that he saw a perfect harmony amongst them. The whole was now finally adjusted: – his anxiety was indescribable: – motion succeeded: – it continued for some time: – and he supposed it capable of continuing for ever. He was elevated to the highest pitch of enjoyment and triumph, and ran as quick as lightening into the interior of the hospital, crying out like another Archimedes, 'At length I have solved this famous problem, which has puzzled so many men celebrated for their wisdom and talents.' But, grievous to say, he was disconcerted in the midst of his triumph. The wheels stopped! The perpetual motion ceased! His intoxication of joy was succeeded by disappointment and confusion. But, to avoid a humiliating and mortifying confession, he declared that he could easily remove the impediment, but tired of that kind of employment, that he was determined for the future to devote his whole time and attention to his business …

> *... Close attention to his trade for some months, completed the restoration of his intellect. He was sent to his family in perfect health; and has, now for more than five years, pursued his business without a return of his complaint.*[97]

The breaks in this excerpt are short sections of the story which do not relate to occupation.

Finally, Pinel provided a cautionary tale of 'convalescent inactivity aggravated by neglect of encouraging the patient's taste for the fine arts':

> *The gloomy and irritable character of maniacs, even when convalescent, is well known. Endowed, in most instances, with exquisite sensibility, they resent with great indignation the slightest appearances of neglect, contempt or indifference, and they forsake for ever what they had before adopted with the greatest ardour and zeal. A sculptor, a pupil of the celebrated Lemoin, was defeated in his endeavours to be admitted as a member of the academy. From that moment he sunk into a profound melancholy, of which the only intermissions consisted in invectives against his brother, whose parcimony he supposed had arrested his career. His extravagance and violence rendered it necessary to confine him for lunacy. When conveyed to his apartment, he gave himself up to all the extravagances of maniacal fury. He continued in that state for several months. At length a calm succeeded, and he was permitted to go to the interior of the hospital. His understanding was yet feeble, and a life of inactivity was not a little irksome to him. The art of painting, which he had likewise cultivated, presented its renascent attractions to him, and he expressed a desire of attempting portrait painting. His inclination was encouraged and gratified, and he made a sketch of the governor and his wife. The likeness was striking; but incapable of much application, he fancied that he perceived a cloud before his eyes. He allowed himself to be discouraged by a conviction of his insufficiency to emulate the models of fine taste, of which the traces were not yet effaced from his memory. The talent which he had discovered, his disposition to exercise it, and the probability of rescuing for his country the abilities of so promising a youth, induced the board of Bicêtre to request of him a pledge of his genius; leaving to him the choice of his subject, that his imagination might not be cramped. The convalescent, as yet but imperfectly restored, shrunk from the task which was thus imposed upon him; requested that the subject might be fixed upon, and that a correct and proper sketch might be given him for a model. His application was evaded, and the only opportunity of restoring him to himself and to his country was thus allowed to escape. He felt exceedingly indignant; considered this omission, as an unequivocal mark of contempt; destroyed all the implements of his art; and with angry haughtiness declared, that he renounced for ever the cultivation of the fine arts. This impression upon his feelings so unintentionally communicated, was so profound, that it was succeeded by a paroxysm of fury of several months' continuance. To this violence again succeeded a second calm. But now the brilliant intellect was for ever obscured, and he sunk irrecoverably into a sort of imbecility and reverieism, bordering upon dementia. I ordered him to be*

transferred to the hospital infirmary, with a view of trying the effects of a few simple remedies, combined with the tonic system of regimen. Familiar and consolatory attentions to him, and such other assistance as his case appeared to suggest, were recurred to, more as they were dictates of humanity than as probable means of recovery. His taste for the fine arts, with his propensity to exertion of any kind, had for ever disappeared. Ennui, disgust with life, his gloomy melancholy and apathy made rapid progress. His appetite and sleep forsook him, and a colliquative diarrhoea put an end to his degraded existence.[98]

Pinel's research provided evidence of other places that used occupation in the treatment of the mentally ill during the eighteenth century. One was a madhouse in Amsterdam where patients were engaged in domestic work in much the same way as at both the Retreat and Bicêtre. Pinel noted Thouin's observation:

It is remarkable that in a house containing so many residents there should be so few hired servants. I never saw more than four or five permanent domestics there. All the others are taken from among the convalescents, who, impressed by respect for the governor, are eager in the offer of their services to those who stand in need of them. Having themselves experienced similar attentions from their predecessors, they are the more zealous in the fulfilment of this duty. Servants of this description are never wanting as there are almost as many able convalescents as there are patients who require their assistance. This economical practice is adopted in all the hospitals of Holland. Hence it happens, that maniacs are there better treated and at much less expence of officers and servants than in the hospitals of this country.[99]

Another institution using occupation was a public asylum in Saragossa, in Spain. There "the charms of agriculture" were used as an "antidote to the wanderings of the diseased imagination". Pinel described the daily activity of the Spanish inmates. 'In the morning may be seen the numerous tenants of that great institution, distributed into different classes and awarded their respective employments' by "intelligent overlookers". The overlookers, who were, it would seem, the equivalent of today's occupational therapists, directed the patient's occupations, guided and watched over their conduct. The whole day was filled with 'salutary and refreshing exercises' broken by short periods for 'rest and relaxation'.[100] Some of the patients were 'kept in the house as domestics of various orders and provinces: others, work at different trades in shops provided for the purpose. However, the "greatest number":

… spread themselves over the extensive inclosure belonging to the hospital, and engage, with a degree of emulation, in the soothing and delightful pursuits of agriculture and horticulture. Having spent the day in preparing the ground for seed, propping or otherwise nursing the rising crop, or gathering the fruits of the olive, the harvest or the vintage according to the season, they return in the evening calm and contented, and pass the night in solitary tranquillity and sleep.[101]

Hence it happens, that those whose condition does not place them above the necessity of submission to toil and labour, are almost always cured; whilst the grandee, who would think himself degraded by any exercises of this description, is generally incurable.[102]

The Spanish nobless ... whose pride of birth and family presents unsurmountable obstacles to a degradation so blessed and salutary, seldom recover the full and healthy possession of a deranged or lost intellect.[103]

In Italy employment of patients was valued as therapy. Vincenzio Chiarurgi (1739-1820) instigated that and disposed of the use of mechanical restraint at St Boniface mental hospital in Florence. In Germany, too, Johann Reil prescribed occupations for mentally ill patients. He believed that they should be graded and varied according to changes in the patients' condition.[104]

Pinel was not alone in recognising psychological factors as a basis for insanity. Indeed, the 6th rule of the ancient Regimen was concerned with commonsense interventions to reduce passions or affections of the mind or soul. He was, however, probably the first to advocate that psychological treatment was the most effective kind for disorders which are psychologically caused. To him insanity was a moral (mental or psychological) condition, so it appeared logical to use psychological methods. Such was Pinel's success with moral therapy that he used medical treatments only as a last resort. Bynum, in *Rationales for Therapy in British Psychiatry,* suggests that the relationship between causation and treatment is a two-way affair, the exclusive use of moral management giving weight to the supposition, that, for most mental illness there is no organic cause.[105] It is noteworthy that, building on some of John Locke's earlier work, psychology had advanced during the period, not only through its championing by some physicians, but also with the work of philosophers like the Scottish, David Hume (1711-1776), Frenchman, Etienne Condillac (1715-1780), and German, Immanuel Kant (1724-1804).[106]

It was appropriate that Pinel's revolutionary text was published at the end of the Age of Enlightenment. In a sense it epitomised the culmination of ideas about the importance of observing and treating individuals in terms of their mental health. It provided a starting point for medical specialists by challenging them to study mental illness in a more rigorous and accountable way. In addition it clearly identified that behavioural problems were often psychological in nature and therefore responsive to treatment of a psychological-occupational kind. It is therefore germane that in the final section of this chapter the emergence of a medical speciality in the field of mental health be considered. This is especially so as from the end of the eighteenth century onwards what they decreed in terms of treatment regimes became very important in the development, or not, of occupational programmes.

Insanity as a medical speciality: Impact on the use of occupation

Within the chapter it has become clear that with the birth of a consumer society at the time of the Enlightenment, entrepreneurs flourished in many spheres. In Britain a buoyant and laissez-faire economy led to the emergence of a thriving service industry providing whatever seemed likely to succeed. The treatment of the mentally ill was a part of that scene, and provided a potentially lucrative domain. Lunacy, which had always been a problem, had become more so in times that had different ideas, values and expectations from previous ones and it only required astute salesmanship and business acumen to create a demand for "madness services". Unlike the financial struggles which often faced general practitioners, a madness expert associated with private custodial care was sure of an ongoing income, for even the poorest patient was paid for by their parish. Financial rewards could be great when catering for the rich as accommodation and extras as well as medical services could be charged.[107]

By the latter part of the century, as the process progressed, specialists of insanity came into being. They were frequently the proprietors of madhouses. Although it was not until 1828 that there was an official requirement for madhouses to have medical personnel in attendance, many reputable physicians, anxious to carve themselves a place in the new medical speciality, became madhouse proprietors. Ticehurst House in Sussex, for example, was founded by Samuel Newington, a surgeon-apothecary, and carried on by his physician son, Charles. One in Leicester was set up by Edinburgh graduate, Dr Thomas Arnold, and prominent physicians, such as Anthony Addington, William Battie, Nathaniel Cotton, Edward Long Fox, and the Monros all kept private madhouses. Their fellows with no medical background proclaimed it better to separate accommodation and milieu from medicine. However, their cries became fewer, as more and more doctors began to take an ever-increasing role in the diagnosis, therapy and legal concerns of the mentally ill.[108]

Perhaps because financial success attracted the ambitious, as the century progressed, it became increasingly possible to be proud of a medical career based on mad-doctoring. Many rose to eminence within the Royal College of Physicians, although they did not, at this time form into a cohesive professional group. Indeed, it was not until the middle of the next century that professional associations and periodicals specific to the speciality occurred. There were however a goodly number of texts written on the subject by physicians. These included publications such as Thomas Arnold's two-volume text *Observations on the Nature, Kinds, Causes and Prevention of Insanity;*[109] Andrew Harper's *Treatise on the Real Cause and Cure of Insanity;*[110] John Ferriar's *Medical Histories and Reflections;*[111] William Pargeter's *Observations on Maniacal Disorder;*[112] Alexander Crichton's *Inquiry into the Nature and Origin of Mental Derangement;*[113] William Perfect's *Select Cases in the Different Species of Insanity, Lunacy, or Madness, with*

Modes of Practice as Adopted in the Treatment of Each;[114] John Haslam's *Observations on Insanity;*[115] William Battie's *A Treatise on Madness,*[116] and John Monro's reply to Dr Battie's Treatise.[117]

There was a downside to Pinel's and Tuke's moral treatment, as far as physicians were concerned. Successful therapy, inclusive of occupation, was not dependent on them. It required 'common sense and unprejudiced observation', and 'most of all a willing and sensitive staff'. For example, 'Pinel's case histories were filled with patient-keeper interactions; much less frequently did he record direct interaction with himself'. That factor challenged the growing medical interest in and control over the insane and raised several questions about the potential role of the physician.[118]

Despite that, medical interest and jurisdiction over the insane was clearly increasing, and led to 'physicians almost universally assert(ing) that mental disease had an entirely somatic basis, and thus was accessible to physical remedies'. Adding to that direction, in the Enlightened Cartesian world, when the concept of mind fused with that of soul, there was the need to overcome the assumption held in the very recent past that madness was due to Satanic possession which made clerics rather than physicians the prime candidates for therapists.

In summary, in this chapter the use of occupation has been traced alongside alterations in management as ideas changed about the causes of disorders in mental health. During the period of Enlightenment, in the United Kingdom, the common approaches to care within families and local communities gradually altered towards custodial care in specially designated madhouses. As part of that process the rise of claimed expertise in the cure of madness was the cry of both lay and medical practitioners in the field and many of these advocated the use of interesting and entertaining occupations as part of those cures.

Occupation as treatment was clearly a part of intervention towards mental health in several different situations, in the home, in the community and in state or private madhouses during the Enlightenment. Its usefulness was increasingly recognised and it emerged as a central issue at the end of the eighteenth century through the work of renowned and still highly respected pioneers, Phillipe Pinel, a physician, and William Tuke, a lay specialist. These men in a way, pre-empt ideologically the dual tension within occupational therapy between the medical and the everyday world. It was a very exciting time in the provision of occupation-based services for the mentally ill which led naturally to a period which, so far, has no equal in the extent to which it was used. The story continues in chapter 11.

[1]Clendenning L, compiler. XXXIV Humanitarian Medicine. In: Source Book of Medical History. Dover: 1960, (an unabridged and unaltered republication of the work originally published - London: Constable and Company, Ltd., 1942).

[2]Digby A. Madness, Morality and Medicine: A Study of the York Retreat, 1796-1914. Cambridge: Cambridge University Press, 1985.

[3]Digby. Madness, Morality and Medicine.

[4]Digby. Madness, Morality and Medicine.

[5]Cheyne G. The English Malady: Or a Treatise of Nervous Diseases of all Kinds. London: Strahan and Leake, 1733; The Natural Method of Cureing Diseases of the Body, and Disorders of the Mind Depending on the Body. London: Strahan and Knapton, 1742; An Essay of Health and Longlife. London: Strahan, 1724.

[6]Faulkner B. Cited in: Porter R. Mind-Forg'd Manacles. London: The Athlone Press, 1987; 160.

[7]Rowley W. Cited in: Porter. Mind-Forg'd Manacles…; 160-161.

[8]Scull AT. Museums of Madness: The Social Organisation of Insanity in Nineteenth Century England. London: Allen Lane, 1979.

[9]Porter. Mind-Forg'd Manacles.

[10]Harvey P, ed. The Oxford Companion to English Literature. 4th ed. Oxford: The Clarendon Press, 1967; 200.

[11]Cowper W. Letter to Lady Hesketh. 1786.

[12]Boswell J. Boswell's London Journal 1762-1763. (from the original manuscript prepared for the press, with introduction and notes by Frederick A. Pottle). Melbourne, London, Toronto: William Heinnemann Ltd. 1950. Australian edition: 1951; 77-78.

[13]Boswell. Boswell's London Journal…; 319.

[14]Scull A, ed. Madhouses, Mad-doctors, and Madmen: The Social History of Psychiatry in the Victorian Era. Philadelphia, PA: University of Pennsylvania Press, 1981; 7.

[15]Cheyne. The English Malady.

[16]Blackmore Sir R. A Treatise of the Spleen and Vapours: or, Hypochondriacal and Hysterical Affections. London: J. Pemberton, 1725.

[17]Mandeville B. A Treatise of Hypochondriak and Hysterick Passions. London: Dryden Leech, W Taylor, 1711 and 1730.

[18]Cheyne. The English Malady…; 177.

[19]Cheyne. The English Malady…; 180-181.

[20]Digby. Madness, Morality and Medicine.

[21]Porter. Mind-Forg'd Manacles…; 211.

[22]Pinel P. A Treatise on Insanity. Trans from French by D. D. Davis. Sheffield: Strand, London. Printed by W. Todd, for Messrs. Cadell and Davies, 1806; para 24, 63-65.

[23]Henderson DK. The Evolution of Psychiatry in Scotland. Edinburgh and London: E & S Livingstone Ltd., 1964; 43.

[24]Bynum Jr WF. Rationales for therapy in British psychiatry, 1780-1835. Chapter 2. In: Scull. Madhouses, Mad-doctors, and Madmen…; 41.

[25]Porter. Mind-Forg'd Manacles…; 211

[26]Scull. Madhouses, Mad-doctors, and Madmen.

[27]Bynum. Rationales for therapy…; 40-44.

[28]Porter. Mind-Forg'd Manacles…; 117.

[29]Ward N. Cited In: Porter. Mind-Forg'd manacles…; 123.

[30]Unknown author. De Londres et de ses environs. 1788. Cited in: Porter. Mind-Forg'd Manacles…; 122-126.

[31]Porter. Mind-Forg'd Manacles…; 126-127.

[32]Alldridge P. The Bethlem Royal Hospital: An Illustrated History. London: The Bethlem

and Maudesley NHS Trust, 1995; 24-28.

[33]Bethlem Royal Hospital Archives and Museum. Court of Govenors Minutes. London: 20th June, 1765.

[34]Bethlem Royal Hospital Archives and Museum.

[35]Andrews J. Bedlam Revisited. Unpublished Thesis. Bethlem Royal Hospital Archives and Museum.

[36]Bethlem Royal Hospital Archives and Museum. Bethlem Steward's Account, 24 April-1 May, 1773; Bethlem Steward's Committee Minutes, 17 July, 1779.

[37]von la Roche S. Sophie in London. 1786. In: Williams C. Trans of 'England' section: Tagebuch einer Reise durch Holland und England. London: Jonathan Cape, 1933; 307.

[38]Porter. Mind-Forg'd Manacles…; 121.

[39]Porter R. Disease, Medicine and Society in England 1550-1860. Basingstoke and London: MacMillan Education, 1987; 32–47.

[40]Porter. Mind-Forg'd Manacles…; 131.

[41]Howard J. An Account of the Principal Lazarettos in Europe; with Varios Papers Relative to the Plague: together with further Observations on some Foreign Prisons and Hospitals; and additional remarks on the Present State of those in Great Britain and Ireland. Warrington: Printed by William Eyres, MDCC LXXXIX, 1789; 140.

[42]Henderson. The Evolution of Psychiatry…; 43.

[43]Porter. Mind-Forg'd Manacles.

[44]Porter. Mind-Forg'd Manacles…; 138.

[45]Porter. Mind-Forg'd Manacles…; 1

[46]Porter. Mind-Forg'd Manacles…; 143.

[47]Cited in: Porter. Mind-Forg'd Manacles…; 212.

[48]Pinel P. A Treatise on Insanity…; 63. (Special Edition Pinel on Insanity printed for The Classics of Medicine Library division of Gryphon Editions Ltd., Birmingham, Alabama, 1983.)

[49]Porter. Mind-Forg'd Manacles…; 139.

[50]Porter. Mind-Forg'd Manacles….; 139.

[51]Digby. Madness, Morality and Medicine…; 7.

[52]Porter. Mind-Forg'd Manacles…; 139.

[53]Porter. Mind-Forg'd Manacles.

[54]Harvey. The Oxford Companion to English Literature…; 762.

[55]Porter. Mind-Forg'd Manacles…; 146.

[56]Porter. Mind-Forg'd Manacles…; 144.

[57]Willis F. A Treatise on Mental Derangement, Containing the Substance of the Gulstoian Lectures for May 1822. London: Longman et al., 1823.

[58]Porter. Mind-Forg'd Manacles…; 144-146.

[59]Bockoven JS. Moral Treatment in Community Health. New York: Springer Publishing Co., Inc., 1972; Peloquin SM. Moral treatment: Contexts considered. American Journal of Occupational Therapy 1989; 43(8): 537-544. Paterson C. An historical perspective of work practice services. In Pratt J, Jacobs K, eds. Work Practices: International Perspectives. Oxford: Butterworth-Heinemann, 1997; Wilcock AA. An Occupational Perspective of Health. Thorofare, NJ: Slack Inc., 1998.

[60]Hunter R, Macalpine I. Introduction. In: Tuke S. Description of the Retreat: An Institution near York for Insane Persons of the Society of Friends Containing an Account of its Origin and Progress, the Modes of Treatment, and a Statement of Cases. Originally published in York, 1813. London: Dawsons of Pall Mall, 1964; 19.

[61]Tuke S. Description of the Retreat: An Institution near York for Insane Persons of the Society of Friends Containing an Account of its Origin and Progress, the Modes of

Treatment, and a Statement of Cases. York: Printed by W Alexander, and sold by him; also sold by M.M. and E Webb, Bristol: and by Harvey, and Co; William Phillips; and W. Darton, London, 1813; 22-24.

[62]Hunter & Macalpine. Introduction. In: Tuke. Description of the Retreat...; 25.

[63]Tuke. Description of the Retreat...; 25.

[64]Tuke. Description of the Retreat...; 27.

[65]Foucault M. Madness and Civilization: A History of Insanity in the Age of Reason. New York: Random House, 1973 (original in French, 1961); 247-248.

[66]State of an Institution near York called the Retreat for Persons Afflicted with Disorders of the Mind. 1796; 4. Retreat Archives. Borthwick Institute, York.

[67]Tuke. Description of the Retreat...; 44-46.

[68]Tuke. Description of the Retreat...; 47.

[69]Tuke. Description of the Retreat...; 178.

[70]A Forgotten Worthy. In: The Yorkshire Herald. Friday, July 22, 1892. Retreat Archives. Borthwick Institute, York.

[71]Tuke. Description of the Retreat...; 94-95.

[72]Tuke. Description of the Retreat...; 96.

[73]Tuke. Description of the Retreat...; 51.

[74]Tuke. Description of the Retreat...; 223.

[75]The Retreat Case Notes...; 1, 13. Retreat Archives. Borthwick Institute, York.

[76]Tuke. Description of the Retreat...; 53.

[77]State of an Institution near York...; 9.

[78]Tuke. Description of the Retreat...; footnote, 202.

[79]Pinel. A Treatise on Insanity...; Footnote, 90.

[80]Pinel. A Treatise on Insanity...; Footnote; 108-9.

[81]Pinel. A Treatise on Insanity...; Footnote; 54.

[82]Pinel. A Treatise on Insanity...; Footnote; 107.

[83]Pinel. A Treatise on Insanity...; 90.

[84]Pinel. A Treatise on Insanity...; 216.

[85]Pinel. A Treatise on Insanity...; 216-18.

[86]Pinel. A Treatise on Insanity...; 195-196.

[87]Pinel. A Treatise on Insanity...; 91.

[88]Pinel. A Treatise on Insanity...; 176.

[89]Pinel. A Treatise on Insanity...; 180.

[90]Pinel. A Treatise on Insanity...; 224.

[91]Pinel. A Treatise on Insanity...; Footnote, 224-228.

[92]Pinel. A Treatise on Insanity...; 176.

[93]Pinel. A Treatise on Insanity...; Footnote p.193.

[94]Pinel. A Treatise on Insanity...; Footnote, 194-195.

[95]Pinel. A Treatise on Insanity...; 193-194.

[96]Pinel. A Treatise on Insanity...; Footnote, 176.

[97]Pinel. A Treatise on Insanity...; 68-72.

[98]Pinel. A Treatise on Insanity...; Footnote, 197-200.

[99]Pinel. A Treatise on Insanity...; Footnote, 194.

[100]Pinel. A Treatise on Insanity...; 195.

[101]Pinel. A Treatise on Insanity...; 217-218.

[102]Pinel. A Treatise on Insanity...; 195.

[103]Pinel. A Treatise on Insanity...; 218.

[104]Macdonald. World-Wide Conquests of Disabilities...; 78.

[105]Bynum. Rationales for Therapy..; 41-42.

[106]Macdonald. World-Wide Conquests of Disabilities…; 82.

[107]Porter. Mind-Forg'd Manacles.

[108]Porter. Mind-Forg'd Manacles.

[109]Arnold T. Observations on the Nature, Kinds, Causes and Prevention of Insanity or Madness. Leicester: Printed by G. Ireland for G. Robinson & T. Cadell, 1782-1786.

[110]Harper A. Treatise on the Real Cause and Cure of Insanity; In which the Nature and Distinctions of this Disease are Fully Explained and the Treatment Established on New Principles. London: C. Stalker, 1789.

[111]Ferriar J. Medical Histories and Reflections. Warrington, London; Printed by W. Eyres etc. for T. Cadell, 1792-8.

[112]Pargeter W. Observations on Maniacal Disorders. Reading: 1792.

[113]Crichton A. An Inquiry into the Nature and Origin of Mental Derangement. Comprehending a Concise System of the Physiology and Pathology of the Human Mind. And a History of the Passions and their Effects. London: T. Cadell junior & W. Davies, 1798.

[114]Perfect W. Select Cases in the Different Species of Insanity, Lunacy, or Madness, with Modes of Practice as Adopted in the Treatment of Each. Rochester: W. Gillman, 1787.

[115]Haslam J. Observations on Insanity: With Practical Remarks on the Disease, and an Account of the Morbid Appearances on Dissection. London: Printed for F. & C. Rivington, and sold by J. Hatchard, 1798.

[116]Battie W. A Treatise on Madness. London: J. Whiston & B. White, 1758.

[117]Monro J. Remarks on Dr Batties Treatise on Madness. London: J. Clarke, 1758.

[118]Bynum. Rationales for therapy…; 41-42.

Part 4

Industrial Times

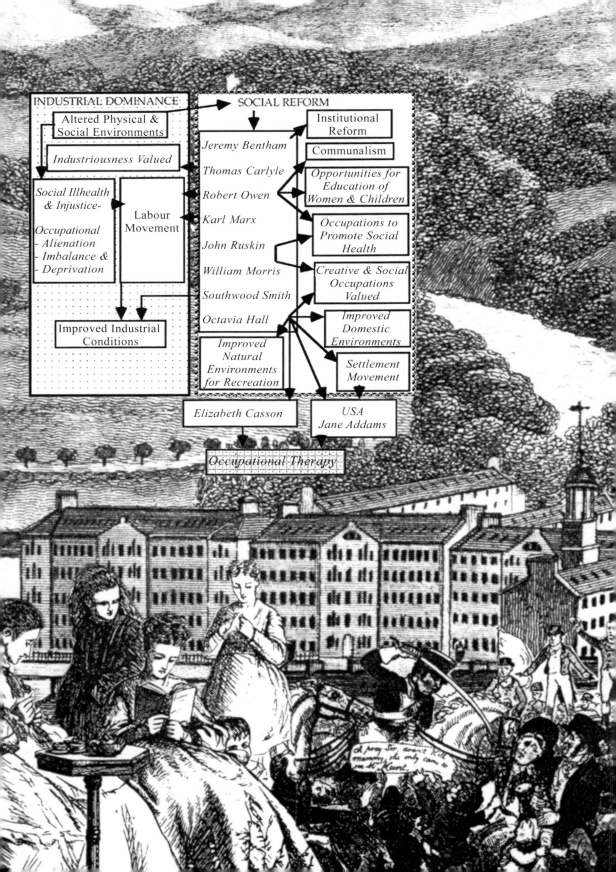

INDUSTRIAL DOMINANCE

Altered Physical &
Social Environments

Industriousness Valued

*Social Illhealth
& Injustice-*

Occupational
- *Alienation*
- *Imbalance &*
- *Deprivation*

Labour
Movement

Improved Industrial
Conditions

SOCIAL REFORM

Jeremy Bentham

Thomas Carlyle

Robert Owen

Karl Marx

John Ruskin

William Morris

Southwood Smith

Octavia Hall

*Improved
Natural
Environments
for Recreation*

Institutional
Reform

Communalism

*Opportunities for
Education of
Women & Children*

Occupations to
Promote Social
Health

*Creative & Social
Occupations
Valued*

*Improved
Domestic
Environments*

Settlement
Movement

Elizabeth Casson

USA
Jane Addams

Occupational Therapy

Chapter 9

Occupation: Ideology and Social Health

Contents

In this chapter an exploration of the industrial era will commence by considering occupation and social health. The ideas and practices that emerged in the nineteenth century remain influential in the present time, and in many cases are still enacted in the daily life of countless numbers of people. As these were largely the result of occupational technology and structural adjustments to the industrial processes, the context of that period is extremely important in tracing the history of occupational regimens for health. The social health of people of the time will be addressed, along with the probable experience of occupational well-being as suggested by the ideologies that emerged during that period. These provide the foundation for occupational therapy's emergence as a separate profession in the twentieth century and are therefore of immense importance. They expressed overwhelmingly, perhaps for the first time, that occupation is more than an economic necessity, and is vital to health. Of course that was touched on in some earlier periods as this history relates, but no generalised understanding or philosophical stance emerged at those times which truly recognised the necessity of meaning and purpose in what people do. It was only when these were almost annihilated by industrial processes that their importance was recognised.

The context

The industrial era began a little earlier than the dawn of the nineteenth century and can be divided into two phases. Both encompassed intense political, intellectual and socio-cultural activity. The first phase, between 1780-1840, saw the French and American revolutions, the Napoleonic wars, the Latin American wars of liberation, a shift in economics from agriculture to manufacturing, and the first phase of the industrial revolution based on steam, coal and iron technologies.[1] The second phase of the industrial revolution in the latter half of the nineteenth century, which Jones describes as the electric revolution, took place against a background of the American Civil and Franco-Prussian wars, imperialism, colonialism, evolutionary theory, and the beginnings of modern information technology, scientific medicine, male suffrage and universal primary education.[2]

By the early 1800s England had emerged as the world's major industrial nation. Powered transport, screw cutting machines and lathes, the discovery of electromagnetism, and the development of modern chemistry amongst other technological achievements changed the lifestyles of the majority of its citizens.[3] Important during the century, in occupational terms was the growth of a new wealthy class of industrialists and traders, and the establishment of trade unions. The unions provided the labouring poor with a 'major institution of everyday self defence' using the weapons of "collective struggle", "solidarity" and "strike".[4] Not surprising in such turbulent times, there were clashes between the classes. In periods of wretched desperation between 1811 and 1816 groups of skilled workers, who described themselves as Luddites, began a wave of machine breaking in the Midland's hosiery and lace industry. Machine breaking, which later spread to the Yorkshire woollen mills, and then the cotton-weavers and cloth finishers in Lancashire and Cheshire was made a capital offence in 1812, and many Luddites were hanged, transported or jailed.[5] On other occasions armed force was used against demonstrations such as those at Spa Fields in London in 1816 and Peterloo in Manchester in 1819, which is depicted in part of the frontispiece to the chapter. Such clashes led to calls for parliamentary reforms concerned with occupational conditions.[6]

After Grey's Reform Bill of 1832, disappointment and discontent aggravated by a bad harvest and economic depression led to the establishment in Britain of a body of political reformers who were mainly working men. They became known as the Chartists, after a people's charter was drawn up which aimed at ameliorating the sufferings of artisans and labourers through parliamentary reform such as universal suffrage for men. In the 1840s extremist Chartists gradually took control and, particularly in the North, skirmishes and rioting took place. That gradually subsided as conditions improved generally and concessions were made in reform bills.[7] Ernest Jones, one of the leaders who advocated force was imprisoned between 1845-1850 for making seditious speeches. Interestingly, whilst in the infirmary of Tuthill Fields prison he used his allowance of paper and ink for letter writing to execute pen and ink drawings, which presumably provided him with some outlet for feelings he could not express in other ways. His drawings contrast a cramped, gloomy Victorian town with factories, church and prison oppressing the populace with the order, space and idyllic environment of a Grecian scene.[8]

During the early period, Napoleon Buonaparte rose to power in France. At home he improved education, revised the law based on the principle of equal citizenship, and aroused a feeling of National unity as he conquered much of Europe. With his defeat at Waterloo and the restoration of many "ancien regimes", constitutional and nationalistic movements were triggered throughout the domains he had conquered as well as many other parts of the world. For all of Europe this was a time of unprecedented challenge and adaptation, as the new industrial structures added another dimension to political change and social unrest.

As a result of the political and industrial revolutions occupational changes of great magnitude occurred. The historian, Hobsbawn, draws attention to the positive aspect of those changes which opened up careers to talent, energy, shrewdness and hard work. Instead of the traditional culture of pre-capitalist society in which people were expected to carry on family occupations despite individual talents or preferences, opportunities to engage in education, business, government service, politics, the professions, the arts and war arose for a greater number and range of people, particularly men in the middle classes. On the negative side, for a variety of reasons, the labouring poor were largely unable to avail themselves of such opportunities. For them, the changes resulted in a reduction in the use of their talents, and long hours and hard work engaged in the meaningless and repetitive tasks of many industrial processes, along with a diminution of their traditional social and ritual occupations, which no longer seemed relevant.[9] Dickens, a novelist who effected change through his powerful storytelling, describes the repetitiveness in his novel *Hard Times*. He wrote:

Time went on in Coketown like its own machinery: so much material wrought up, so much fuel consumed, so many powers worn out, so much money made ... the piston of the steam-engine worked monotonously up and down like the head of an elephant in a state of melancholy madness ... all the melancholy-made elephants, polished and oiled up for the day's monotony, were at their heavy exercise again ... no temperature made the melancholy-mad elephants more mad or more sane. Their wearisome heads went up and down at the same rate, in hot weather and cold, wet weather and dry, fair weather and foul. The measured motion of their shadows on the walls, was the substitute Coketown had to show for the shadows of rustling woods; while, for the summer hum of insects, it could offer, all the year round, from the dawn of Monday to the night of Saturday, the whirr of shafts and wheels. The complement to the machines are the workers - whole humans reduced to Hands.

A race who would have found more favour with some people, if Providence had seen fit to make them only hands, or, like the lower creatures of the seashore, only hands and stomachs. ... A special contract, as every man was in the forest of looms ... to the crashing, smashing, tearing piece of mechanism at which he laboured ... So many hundred Hands to this Mill; so many hundred horse Steam Power.[10]

The revolution also signalled a mass exodus from rural living and diverse rural occupations, to urban crowding in the vicinity of manufacturing works and the necessity to seek employment however uninteresting and poorly paid. The British Poor Law Act, passed in 1834 'for the Amendment and Better Administration of the Laws relating to the poor in England and Wales' was based on Jeremy Bentham's Utilitarian *Fragments on Government*.[11] It was designed to compel people to find employment and reduce the numbers seeking "charity" in "workhouses". Within the Act, relief would only be offered in the workhouse, and able-bodied people seeking relief would be required to earn it in conditions 'less tolerable than that of the lowest labourer outside'.

Workhouses: To deter not succour
Convents: The Work Ethic

The workhouses were made 'as like prisons as possible' with 'a discipline so severe and repulsive as to make them a terror to the poor and prevent them from entering'.[12] With that intent, work assumed a punitive rather than a restorative nature. This could be one of the reasons why occupational therapists have difficulty in associating the history of their profession with the concept of workhouses, despite the charitable nature of their origin and initial intent to better social ill health through occupation. That suggests, once more, how important the social context is in terms of the health giving effects of an occupational approach.

The occupational deprivation and alienation to which workhouse inmates were subjected was further augmented by an austere order of silence and religious discipline designed to stamp out individualism and the possibility of rebellion. Clear, for example, in *Nuns in Nineteenth Century Ireland,* reports that workhouses there did not attempt to solve the many problems women experienced as a result of poverty but to contain and to control by separating them into like groups, often based on moral judgements. It is heartening to read that there was 'considerable traffic out of the workhouse in articles knitted clandestinely by the women to be sold in the markets of the city'[13] as the women perhaps tried to rectify their own insolvency and occupational alienation. Not only women but families too were segregated and their possessions taken away. Despite such measures, and indicative of employment opportunities of the time, the workhouses held 197,179 inmates by the year 1843.[14]

It was a fundamental rule of the system that individuals capable of exertion must never be idle in a workhouse. So men and women were set to manual work about the house and grounds including such tasks as breaking stones and grinding corn. As well, the women were put to house duties, mending and washing clothes, attending the sick and the children, who were also required to occupy themselves. Such engagement in work was the antithesis of occupation as applied in occupational therapy in that it was specifically chosen to be without incentive or motivation, the rules spelling out that 'no pauper shall work on his own account; and no pauper shall receive any compensation for his labour'.[15]

The situation in Ireland was particularly problematic, and because it was not until the nineteenth century that workhouses were established, discussion here will centre on the Irish experience. However much of the ethos and practices there were also true of workhouses in other parts of Britain.

The ploy that applicants for relief could only earn it by labour within a workhouse was hard to apply to Ireland where work was virtually unavailable but, in spite of opposition, the British Government decided to extend it to the recently developed workhouses there. They had been established because in the early 1800s over one-third of Ireland's people were near starvation level, without any state provision for the poor, sick, or old except begging and charity. So great was the problem the British Government set up 114 Royal Commissions and Select Committees of Inquiry between 1800 and 1840 to address it. The Act *For the More Effectual Relief of the Poor of Ireland* eventually passed into law in 1838, resulting in the building of 130 workhouses throughout the country, with accommodation for about 95,000 inmates.[16]

As part of his duties, a Workhouse Master in Ireland had to 'enforce industry, order, punctuality, and cleanliness … read prayers' and:

… provide for and enforce the employment of the able bodied adult Paupers,

during the whole of the hours of labour; to assist in training the youth in such employment as will best fit them for gaining their own living; to keep the partially disabled Paupers occupied to the extent of their ability; and to allow none who are capable of employment to be idle at any time.[17]

An illustration of the unhealthy mindlessness of the occupations used there was a contraption for grinding corn, designed by a Richard Perrott of Cork. Accepted by workhouse Commissioners to keep large numbers occupied at once and to enforce discipline, the machine required over a hundred inmates to walk in a circle manually rotating a large wheel for hours on end. See figure 1.9.1. Thankfully the inhumanity of the instrument and task was recognised and it ceased to be used after about five years.[18]

Still in Ireland, from the 1840s on institutional care for orphans, the aged, the homeless, and the morally deviant was on the increase, largely provided by religious houses. Most of those engaged in a variety of provisions. For example, the Sisters of Charity, amongst other offerings, ran asylums for prostitutes and drunken women, a training school and employment service for domestic servants, primary education for children and night school for adults. Increasing also were the numbers of reformatories and industrial schools. Financed by the government, the industrial school movement first came into operation in 1869. Thirty years later there were 8,422 children in seventy-one industrial schools. Children who were admitted were taught a trade and the products they made were sold.[19]

Magray argues that one compelling reason why women joined religious orders was the nature of the spiritual and material life they offered, which many found very satisfying.[20] As elsewhere, in Ireland during the nineteenth century women were generally seen, as Pope Leo XIII argued, as 'not fitted for certain occupations; a woman is by nature fitted for home work, and it is that which is best adapted to preserve her modesty and to promote the good bringing-up of children and the well-being of the family'.[21] Whilst a growing body of opinion was forming that women could and should have the opportunity to work outside the home there were in fact few openings for them, and the convents provided an important option. 'A great deal of spiritual and mental energy seems to have been demanded by convent life in general, and it is hardly likely that many nuns experienced the lethargy and ennui so vividly and unhappily described by several contemporary women as the lot of the middle-class female confined to home.'[22] Isa Jane Blagden[23] and Florence Nightingale[24] were cases in point.

Convents, in fact, provided women with the chance to effect social as well as religious change. The reorganised church that emerged during the nineteenth century in Ireland and most of Europe was intimately involved with ordinary people rather than the elite or ruling classes. With a caring face 'the Church developed large scale institutions for the care of the sick, the poor, and the destitute, as well as an extensive system of popular education'.[25] Most of these services reinforced a work ethic that gave intrinsic and moral value to occupation.

Indeed, nuns encouraged a new work ethic among the poor. The Monaghan reformatory, run by the Sisters of St Louis, was famous for its attitude towards work. According to a report by one inspector of reformatory and industrial schools, 'the great principle inculcated in this school is that labour is a duty and that it is an obligation to be constantly occupied'.[26] Not only did they preach the beneficial effects of regular work but they also put their beliefs into practical form through the development of small-scale employment schemes. The many convent-run enterprises that sprang up around the country, such as bakeries, laundries, linen schools, woollen factories, and needlework industries, were all aimed at enabling the people to labour for their support rather than having to resort to the common custom of begging.[27] When the Sisters of Charity convent in Benada began to manufacture linen during the 1860s, they believed that the factory would enable:

> … poor women, who would otherwise spend too much time in idleness, with all its vicious consequences, to earn wherewith to supply some of the pressing wants of their families. And such as have not families, to escape by this little addition to their means the poorhouse or beggary.[28]

Employment and unemployment

Women, more than men in agricultural Ireland, experienced underemployment, destitution and disease, and they were more likely to be incarcerated in workhouses. The census of 1851, soon after the famine, found that able-bodied females over fifteen accounted for almost a quarter of all inmates. This number was probably made up of those unwilling to form part of the 3.3% of the adult female work force who sustained themselves as beggars, brothel-keepers or prostitutes. In contrast only 11% of able-bodied males were workhouse inmates.[29] From the beginning of the century, the lack of employment and earning power of women was evident, but it increased as traditional textile production decreased. Dressing flax, spinning, carding, bleaching and similar occupations, or alternatively non-stop knitting of articles for sale had provided employment for many women in the first two decades of the century. In County Down in 1817 a spinner could earn 5 pennies a day, but even if she was particularly industrious, by 1836 that had dropped to 1 penny.[30]

In industrial England, it was often men who experienced that work was hard to find. Industrialists preferred to employ women and children because their labour was less costly, even after 1810 when male wages decreased dramatically.[31] 'In 1838, only 23 per cent of textile workers in Britain were adult males.'[32]

> In the English spinning mills only 158,818 men are employed, compared with 196,818 women. For every hundred men workers in the Lancashire cotton mills there are 103 women workers; in Scotland the figure is as high as 209. In the English flax mills in Leeds there are 147 women for every 100 men workers; in Dundee and on the east coast of Scotland this figure is as high as 280. In the English silk-factories there are many women workers; in the wool factories, where greater strength is needed, there are more men. As for the North American cotton mills, in 1833 there were no fewer than 38,927 women alongside 18,593 men. So as a result of changes in the organisation of labour, a wider area of employment opportunities has been opened up to members of the female sex … more economic independence for women … both sexes brought closer together in their social relations.[33]

From 1780 until it was abolished in Britain in 1933,[34] child labour was a legal reality, although it decreased substantially throughout that time. 'Employed in the English spinning mills operated by steam and water in the year 1835 were: 20,558 children between 8 and 12 years of age; 35,867 between 12 and 13; and finally, 108,208 between 13 and 18.'[35] The children worked for long hours in factories and mines in dull, repetitive tasks that lacked variety. They seldom saw the sunlight and were subject to severe discipline and appalling safety regulations. It was not until 1842 that children under 10 (and women) were prohibited from working in the mines, and 1847 that children's work in textile factories was limited to ten hours per day. The occupational health and safety issues those conditions suggest will be revisited in the next chapter.

Industrial war and occupational utopias

As industry evolved it took its toll on the health and well-being of vast numbers of people throughout Europe. Social activists such as German physician Neumann believed it was a state's duty to look after the health of its workers. He argued, in 1847, that the poor's only property was their labour which was dependent on their health, and that as the state was pledged to protect people's property so it should protect worker's from illness.[36] Another, Eugene Buret, had already complained in 1840 how industry:

> … squandered the lives of the men who composed its army with as much indifference as the great conquerors. Its goal was the possession of riches, and not human happiness. … The industrial war, if it is to be waged successfully, needs large armies which it can concentrate at one point and decimate at will. And neither devotion nor duty moves the soldiers of this army to bear the burdens placed upon them; what moves them is the need to escape the harshness of starvation. They feel neither affection nor gratitude for their bosses, who are not bound to their subordinates by any feeling of goodwill and who regard them not

as human beings but as instruments of production which bring in as much and cost as little as possible. These groups of workers, who are more and more crowded together, cannot even be sure that they will always be employed; the industry which has summoned them together allows them to live only because it needs them; as soon as it can get rid of them it abandons them without the slightest hesitation; and the workers are forced to offer their persons and their labour for whatever is the going price. The longer, more distressing and loathsome the work which is given them, the less they are paid; one can see workers who toil their way non-stop through a sixteen hour day and who scarcely manage to buy the right not to die.[37]

Buret commented that:

We are convinced ... as are the commissioners appointed to look into the conditions of the handloom weavers, that the large industrial towns would quickly lose their population of workers if they did not all the time receive a continual stream of healthy people and fresh blood from the surrounding country areas.[38]

Eugene's harsh criticism was not true of all factory owners as a brief look at the story of the archetypal Victorian industrialist Titus Salt reveals.

Titus Salt: Occupation and social health

In *History Today*, Campbell Bradley tells how Salt, one of the richest and most powerful of the barons of the Yorkshire textile industry, rose from comparatively humble beginnings. He carried with him 'the stern but enlightened values of the Nonconformist Conscience' coupled with 'a belief in every individuals capacity for self improvement'. As Mayor of Bradford, where his first factory had been established, Salt's interest in health and health maintaining occupations was demonstrated by his concern about both cholera and unemployment which were rife. This led him to inaugurate proper systems of drainage and sanitation, soup kitchens, and schemes for emigration to the New World, as well as taking on an extra 100 wool-combers despite substantial losses following a down turn in trade. Bradford, at that time, was the fastest growing town in the western world. Its population of 42,527 in 1831 grew to 103,778 in just twenty years. It also became the dirtiest and most insanitary with an average life expectancy, at birth, of just 18 years, and the greatest proportion of undernourished and crippled children in the country. Whilst in Mayoral office Salt fitted special smoke burners to his factory's chimney stacks to reduce pollution, and tried to induce fellow industrialists to follow his lead. An acceptance of occupation as a necessity for social health was also apparent in his encouraging the establishment of places of recreation as alternatives to public houses, which were morally abhorrent to him. He gave the town a 61-acre park, and was actively involved in the design and building of 'music halls and mechanics' institutes where people could enjoy and improve themselves'.[39]

Salt followed in the Utopian traditions of Owen (who will be discussed later), John Grubb Richardson, a Quaker flax spinner, and another Yorkshire manufacturer, Edward Ackroyd. In his later years, and in preference to living the life of a "gentleman", he set out to build a model industrial community. The motive for Saltaire was both philanthropic and sound business sense. Salt's mill, which came to be known as The Palace of Industry, was enormous, light and airy, with large flues, plate glass windows, and noise minimised by shafting under the floor. At its opening, (figure 1.9.1.) making reference to the dwellings he proposed for Saltaire, he told the 3,500 guests:

> *I will do all I can to avoid evils so great resulting from polluted air and water and hope to draw around me a well fed, contented and happy band of operatives. I have given my instructions to my architects that nothing is to be spared to render the dwellings a pattern to the country.*[40]

Figure 1.9.1:   The opening of Saltaire Mill September 25th, 1853.[49]

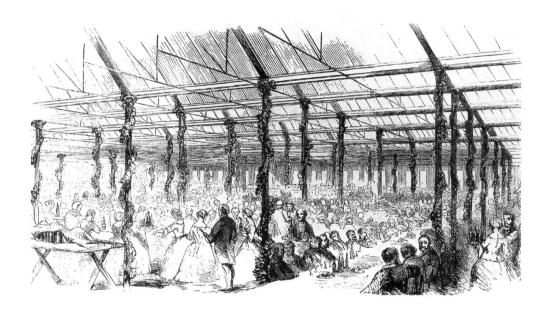

Managers were provided with semi-detached houses, and ordinary workers with three bedroomed cottages, all with water, gas, privy, coal store and ashpit. There was no pub, no pawn shop, and no police station in Saltaire. Instead, and over time, there were churches, public baths and washhouses, almshouses, pensions for the old retired of good moral character, schools, and a hospital. In addition, there were many provisions 'for innocent and intelligent recreation' like works outings, a large park with facilities for cricket and boating, numerous societies, a library, a club and an institute. The latter was 'to supply the advantages of a public house without its evils: it will be a place to which you can resort for conversation, business, recreation and refreshment, as well as for education–elementary, technical and scientific'.[41] Despite a paternalistic, and sometimes harsh attitude to his workforce and the continued employment of children which are at odds with present day values, in general Salt's vision for a healthily occupied town seems to have led to a particularly happy and energetic community. Charles Dickens, visiting in 1857, noted that 'all looked prosperous and happy' and, similarly, another journalist, in 1871 reported 'a better looking body of factory "hands" I have not seen'.[42]

European occupational utopians

The opposite was more often the norm, and as an antidote to the lack of health and well-being, across Europe and the United Kingdom Romanticism flourished in the arts, literature and philosophy. It became an age of romantic protest that rejected the ideas and fruits of the Age the Enlightenment and Reason, and condemned the dehumanisation of industry and capitalism. However a legacy of earlier ideas was retained as Romanticists continued Jean Jacques Rousseau's call for naturalness and authenticity. Nature was depicted as an 'ideal of purity and serenity' or a 'place of wildness and elemental power' where it was possible to find oneself,[43]. In a way, this anticipates an ecological view of health in which natural ways of life and remedies are recommended as prerequisites of health and well-being.

Romanticism, which is essentially conservative, glorified the traditions of earlier times. Not surprisingly, many sought answers by looking to past lifestyles and medieval craft traditions. The Luddites were a case in point, emphasising the importance of maintaining high-quality products, and being opposed to the de-skilling of workers as machinery was progressively introduced. A return to the Guild system was suggested by people with a variety of interests, as the only possible answer to resolve the occupational problems caused by the changed political economy. John Ruskin and William Morris are examples of highly respected and influential authorities that held those views. Their stories appear later in the chapter.

In Germany, during 1848, guild masters and journeymen held artisan congresses to propose alternatives to counter the misery resulting from liberal capitalism, which they saw as destroying the skill, industry, and the human relationships of the workers and society itself. Karl Marlo, a little known authority nowadays but then an ideologist and propagandist force to be reckoned with, expressed the feeling of these assemblies:

> The stability of all social relationships is destroyed; the organic union of the industrial classes is decomposed; and society is divided into two masses of enemies that find their centre of gravity in the bourgeoisie and proletariat. An endless battle for external goods has endangered the inner values of the combatants; avarice on the one side and bitterness on the other have hardened souls against the commands of moral law and even threatened the maintenance

of legal order. All these evils are increasing, for the only remaining law of this endless movement declares: The rich shall become richer and poor poorer.[44]

The liberals in England, he pronounced:

> *... wanted to make work free, and have bowed it under the yoke of capital; they wanted to unchain all powers, and have beaten men down with the chains of misery; they wanted to free the serf from bondage, and have robbed him of the very ground on which he stood; they wanted the well-being of all, and have created only the extremes of poverty and luxury ... they wanted education to be the property of all, and have made it the privilege of wealth; they wanted the highest moral improvement of society, and have plunged it in moral rottenness; in short, they wanted limitless freedom, and have created the most abusive thraldom.*[45]

Marlo, seeking occupational justice, asserted that his colleagues and supporters did 'not aim at founding paradise, but a society in which only the natural world order will set the boundaries to the most free unfolding of all personalities'. He was convinced that it was possible for everyone to 'have a task measured to his abilities and a profit equal to his performance' which would lead to 'a general well-being' and 'productive work' replacing 'unproductive idleness'.[46] Those suggestions were rejected by the Frankfurt Parliament in *Fundamental Rights of German People*,[47] which, like political establishments elsewhere in Europe, including Britain, favoured laissez-faire.

In France also, Utopian visions based on trade guilds were popular. Charles Fourier (1772-1837) envisaged a system of communities (Phalansteries) of some 1,800 people living together as a family and holding property in common[48][49] The Phalansteries Fourier proposed were 'an idealised and restructured vision of agrarian communalism ... which had strong appeal to that first generation of workers ... removed from their traditional rural order' to work in the 'harsh grey life of early factory towns'.[50] Along somewhat similar lines founding anarchist, Pierre Proudhon (1809-1865), argued that workers should emancipate themselves through economic means as part of a radically decentralised social order which would end their capitalistic exploitation[51] A self-educated artisan of peasant origins, his vision encompassed a system of equitable exchange called mutualism[52] which saw 'a return to self regulating communities of skilled craftsmen'[53] financed by free credit. Such schemes of communalism are early examples of community development interests and initiatives, which many health professionals, including occupational therapists, espouse and take part in today.

In Britain, too, the notion of communal living and working was emerging as a basis for social change. The move was led by Welsh born Robert Owen (1771-1858), whose vision of a reformed society can be traced forward to Elizabeth Casson, and to the early days of occupational therapy in the twentieth century through the work of Octavia Hill. The latter's history will be told later in the chapter, but because of this link it is important to also look at Owen's fascinating journey and, as the story unfolds, to reflect on how many of his ideas underlie theories of occupational therapy.[54]

Figure 1.9.2:   Robert Owen against the background of his New Lanark mills
(New Lanark Conservation)

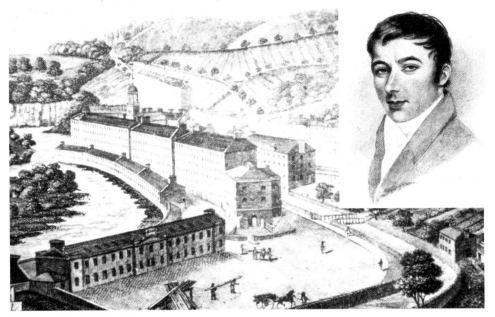

Robert Owen, occupation and social health

Robert Owen was born in a small town in Montgomeryshire where his father was the saddler, ironmonger and postmaster. Owen attended the village school and was such a fast learner that by the age of seven he became something of a pupil-teacher for the younger children because the schoolmaster considered he could teach him no more. Owen balanced his school work with a range of other occupations that he enjoyed such as playing the clarinet and engaging in country dancing, as well as excelling in sports. From those early pleasures he must have established some of his later held beliefs in the importance of early learning and of the need for everyone to have a range and balance of occupations.

On his tenth birthday, equipped with a stagecoach ticket to London and two pounds in his pocket, Owen left home to find employment. For some years he worked, very successfully as a shop-boy in the linen-draper trade, and by the age of eighteen felt ready to take on the challenge of going into the cotton spinning business. Despite difficulties that might have daunted many people he began to achieve success, not only as a cotton spinner, but also as a business manager with radical and humane ideas about workplace organisation. Four years later, such was his reputation that he was invited to join the Manchester Literary and Philosophic Society, by its founder Dr. Thomas Percival. That discussion Society had amongst its members some of the best-known scientists, technologists, and social theorists of the time, and it was possibly there that Owen tried out some of his radical theories about factory management and community life for the first time. He believed that the aim of social institutions should be to make people happy to the extent that they would willingly collaborate with others in the community so that the happiness was sustainable. He argued that society could be reformed without violence to make it more humane and reasonable. To achieve this end, two major changes were essential: the education of everybody from early childhood because each person's character was dependent on their early learning, and the re-development of a sense of communal harmony lost in the upheaval of early industrial capitalism.

On a visit to Glasgow Owen met Caroline Dale, whom he married in 1799. She was the daughter of a rich and philanthropic mill owner, whose factory at New Lanark on the Upper Clyde was generally held to be a model of its kind, but which did not meet all of Owen's exacting standards. Nevertheless he took over the mills and immediately set about changing conditions according to his beliefs, which centred on the need to improve the social well-being of the workers. The process was helped when, in 1813, he entered into partnership with a group of wealthy philanthropists, including Jeremy Bentham the Utilitarian philosopher and a Quaker, William Allen. Their interest and excitement in Owen's work had been generated by two *Essays on the Formation of Character,* published a few years earlier, in which he had explained something of his philosophy and methods.[55]

As part of his practical reforms, Owen addressed many occupational health issues of the time, particularly occupational alienation and imbalance, which was a fact of life for the vast majority. He shortened working hours, and abolished all punishment except fines and dismissal in extreme cases. Within his village he improved the worker's environment by cleaning and paving the streets, adding extra rooms to their one-roomed hovels, improving the goods available in the shops, and discouraging profiteering through the establishment of cooperative buying. He even payed full wages when an embargo on cotton imports forced the mills to close down for months. In part because Owen believed that the nature of communities was created by the nature of their institutions and practices, he refused to employ children under ten years old in the mill and stopped importing pauper child workers from distant parishes which was common practice.

Figure 1.9.3:   The musicians gallery at the New Lanark School
(New Lanark Conservation)

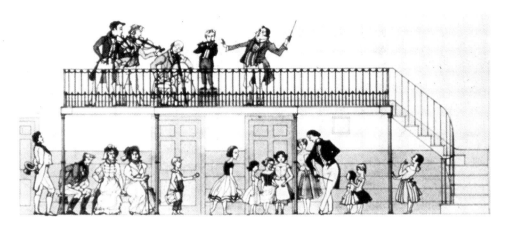

By building sufficient schools for all the children of the community to attend from the day they could walk by themselves until they started work, Owen, whilst still favouring communalism over individualism, in this way encouraged the development of individual talents and potential. By insisting that the schools were also used for evening classes and other community purposes, by both employees and housewives, Owen began to address the products of their previous occupational deprivation. He took these initiatives even further when, in 1816, he opened the Institute for the Formation of Character, which was, in modern parlance, a community centre for discussion, entertainment, enjoyment and leisure. At the opening he reflected on his idea of an enlightened society 'as a society in which individuals shall acquire increased health, strength and intelligence–in which their labour shall be always advantageously directed - and in which they will possess every rational enjoyment'.[56]

Embodying the principles of humanity and good sense emanating from his published essays, which had been widely read, Owen's New Lanark model factory, model village, model schools, and model community were visited by thousands for a decade or more. Princes, politicians, philosophers, philanthropists, and businessmen from home and abroad admired the community. Although his approach was basically apolitical,[57] that interest encouraged Owen to expand the sphere of his ideas into the broader community which was suffering similar social ills to those he had addressed in New Lanark.

He engaged in the reform of working conditions for the masses by, for example, drafting a Bill to forbid the employment of children under 10, and to prohibit night work and reduce hours for those younger than 18. Other cotton manufacturers fought this strongly and successfully and the Bill was watered down, so much so that Owen found difficulty in understanding the morals of his fellow factory owners. Owen also turned his attention to the Poor Law, which many believed would be unable to cope with the influx of unemployed soldiers following the end of the Napoleonic wars.[58] He proposed the setting up of Villages of Cooperation to be situated all over the country that were similar, in many ways, to his New Lanark Community.[59] His plans incorporated the notion of public responsibility for providing both work and a living for all concerned, including that the government should establish public works to employ people in useful occupation. In a widespread publicity campaign Owen published his plan in all the leading newspapers and distributed copies of all of them, by stagecoach, to significant figures in every town in the country. This cost him some four thousand pounds, an enormous sum in the early nineteenth century.

Some of his outspoken comments in the debates that ensued, such as those that showed up atheist ideas also cost him dear. His Quaker partner Allen, for example, was worried about his atheism, and about the casual freedom of the New Lanark schools curricula. Owen was given an ultimatum to bring in more orthodox teachers and to dismiss some of the others. Scripture became compulsory; dancing was banned, and although music was permitted it was to be only in the form of psalms; and all six year old boys and upwards had to wear trousers or drawers under their kilts.

Leaving his son in charge Owen escaped such disappointments, going to America to establish a "community of equality" called New Harmony. Incidentally this became just one of at least sixteen Owenite communities established in America from the 1820s.[60] In his enthusiasm he rushed the development and, when the community failed to live up to his communal ideals he left after only three years, despite having spent, and lost, much of the fortune he had worked so long and hard to build up.

The failure did not, however, change Owen's beliefs that it was possible to put into practice a 'coherent theory of social change'.[61] This was just as well, because when he returned home he found he was regarded as the inspiration of the emerging young Labour Movement, Trade Unions and Co-operative Societies, in all of which his influence remained for a long time.

It can also be argued that he espoused an early, but unknown, creed for occupational therapists or occupational scientists. Many of his ideas were founded on notions about the occupational nature of people that he saw as related to health and well-being, not only in social health terms but with regard to physical and mental health as well:

> … *members of the medical profession know that the health of society is not to be obtained or maintained by medicines;–that it is far better, far more easy, and far wiser, to adopt substantive measures to prevent disease of the body or mind, than to allow substantive measures to remain continually to generate causes to*

produce physical and mental disorders.

When society shall be based on true principles, it will not permit any of its members to be thus made small and imperfect parts of what man might be more easily made to become. It will perceive the great importance of training infants from birth, to become full-formed men or women, having every portion of their nature duly cultivated and regularly exercised.

It will discover that man has not been created to attain the full excellence and happiness of his nature, until all his faculties, senses and propensities, shall be well cultivated, and society shall be so constructed that all of them, in each individual, shall be temperately exercised, and their powers continued and increased by such exercise, until arrested by natural old age.[62]

Owen recognised that the interaction between occupation and health relates to not only exercise but also to the development and expression of each individual's capacities and potential. He went on to argue that individual strengths could be thus utilised to benefit community health and well-being:

It is in the highest interest of all the human race, to which there cannot be a single exception;

1st. That the entire faculties, senses and propensities, should be well cultivated, and at all times duly or temperately exercised, according to the physical and mental strength and capacity of the individual; in order that whatever may be done by each, should be performed in the best manner for the general advantage of all.[63]

For the healthy occupation of body and mind to occur, he argued vehemently for the gaining of extensive understanding of ourselves, society and nature before attempting 'to take one step now in a right course to improve the general condition of society'.[64] In 1841, Owen posed 20 questions to the human race in a paper *Dedicated to the Governments of Great Britain, Austria, Russia, France, Prussia and the United States of America.* Amongst them were:

Is it not in your interest, that each of these individuals should be placed, through life, within those external arrangements that will insure the most happiness, physically, mentally, and morally, to the individual; and the greatest practical benefit to the whole of society?

and

Is it not in the interest of the human race that everyone should be so taught, and placed, that he would find his highest enjoyment to arise from the continued practice of doing all in his power to promote the well-being, and happiness, of every man, woman, and child, without regard to their class, sect, party, country or colour?[65]

To do that, and with a very holistic understanding of the connectedness of body, brain and society, he recommended:

… the discovery of the means, and the adoption of the practice, to prevent disease of body and mind are necessary; … the prevention of disease will be obtained only when arrangements shall be formed, to well educate, physiologically, every man, woman, and child, so as to enable them to understand

their own physical and mental nature; in order that they may learn to exercise, at the proper period of life, all their natural faculties, propensities and powers, up to the point of temperance; neither falling short, nor exceeding in any of them, or discontent and disease must necessarily follow.[66]

His preventive doctrine was based on a belief that 'disease is not the natural state of man' and that in a perfect world, amongst many other changes for the better, 'the physical sciences will have rendered unnecessary all severe, unhealthy or even unpleasant labour' and 'idleness and uselessness will be unknown'.[67]

Robert Owen is considered, by many, to be the father of British Socialism. His immediate legacy, though, was communalism, and just as Owenite Communities had sprouted in the United States, so to did they in Britain. The link with occupational therapy comes about because Octavia Hill's parents were associated with the establishment of an Owenite community near Wisbech in Cambridgeshire, where her father publicly espoused his Owenist views in the newspaper that he owned. There can be no doubt that Owen's beliefs and practical schemes to enable the social well-being of all were a strong influence on Hill's philosophies and life works, which in turn influenced twentieth century occupational therapy and will be considered later. As a preliminary to that story it is important to also consider the views taken by philosophers, social and public health activists throughout the century which have also been influential factors in the development of the profession.

Thomas Southwood Smith, occupation and social health

One of those social and public health activists was another friend of Owen's, the reformist physician, Thomas Southwood Smith, who played a significant role in the history of occupational health. Born in Somerset in 1788 and educated at the Bristol Baptist College, he was to become disillusioned with its harsh Calvinist creed. In particular, he revolted against a religious and social order which debarred 'the poor, the wretched and the sinner from all the amenities of life on earth', before condemning them to eternal punishment. By the age of twenty he had adopted Enlightenment beliefs that he examined in *The Illustrations of the Divine Government,* published in 1816. In that, he argued for the alleviation of suffering and an increase of human happiness no matter what social change was required 'until man in society reflects the benevolent purpose of the Almighty'. That credo sustained him throughout his life and work as a Unitarian minister and a physician who tackled social reform, head on.[68] His mission was faced with tremendous problems.

As a result of the mass movement of people from rural communities into towns and cities, an unbearable strain had been placed on public facilities and infrastructures. Streets, which were largely unpaved and undrained, became quagmires polluted with piled up refuse, whilst available clean water ran dry. There was not enough accommodation to meet demand, so rents rose beyond the means of most labourers who, with their families, were often forced to settle for housing in cellars and subdivided rooms commonly in an appalling state of disrepair with leaking roofs, rotting floors, and sewage disposal problems. Speculators and industrialists who provided new, but usually poorly built housing close to the polluted atmosphere of factories and mills, often perpetuated the situation as that accommodation also quickly became the scene of squalor, misery and disease.[69]

Figure 1.9.4: **Thomas Southwood Smith: Wood engraving by W.J. Linton after Margaret Gillies**
(*The Wellcome Library*)

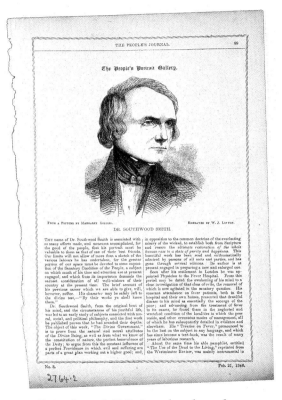

Southwood Smith's early years in Bristol, and Edinburgh where he was a medical student, coupled with many working in Bethnal Green and Whitechapel had given him first hand experience of the state of the housing available to the poor. Addressing a Select Commission of the House of Commons in 1840, he was forthright:

> *At present, no more regard is paid in the construction of houses to the health of the inhabitants than is paid to the health of pigs in making sties for them. In point of fact, there is not so much attention paid to it … (Such) wretchedness (is) greater than humanity can bear, … annihilat(ing) the mental feelings, the faculty distinctive of the human being.*[70]

He argued that priority had to be given to the provision of adequate housing because only following physical improvement could intellectual and moral needs be addressed.

He had two close Quaker friends, William and Mary Howitt, who published *Howitt's Journal*. Within those, in a series of articles written by Mary Gillies in 1847, Southwood Smith's experiences, hopes and aspirations were embodied. *A Labourer's Home* told the story of a labourer and his family coming to Whitechapel from the country, and how he and the doctor (Southwood Smith) watched them sicken and die one by one as they succumbed to the environment. In a follow-up story, *Associated Homes,* Whitechapel "ten years hence" was transformed with well-lit, wide, clean streets, a market, good drains, constant water, and fresh air because the factories had gone. There was also a workers' apartment block, with common rooms and a library, where rooms were let at reasonable rents, and education was provided for men in the evenings. It was gas lit, centrally heated, with hot and cold water on every floor, and centralised refuse disposal. In that Utopian story, the permitted working age of boys was twelve and of girls, sixteen. Southwood Smith laboured hard to turn a vision such as that into reality with the support of many friends and in association with the *Metropolitan Association for Improving the Dwellings of the Industrious Classes*.[71]

Apart from working towards improved housing, Southwood Smith also was a powerful voice in overturning occupational health and safety hazards in industry and the mines. His story about that role will continue to unfold in the next chapter.

Philosophers and social activists: Theorists of occupation for social health

In their Romantic revolt against the emerging industrial world which reduced humans to the status of objects,[72] philosophers of the period began to espouse ideas about the nature of people that were different from those of earlier times. A strong emphasis on individuality emerged along with encouragement of self-expression,[73] and happiness,[74] all of which provides philosophical underpinnings for today's occupational regimens towards social health. These form the basis of many models and frames of reference within occupational therapy.

Jeremy Bentham (1748-1832) was, undoubtedly, one of the most influential men of his time. A prophet of Utilitarianism, a doctrine of the greatest happiness for the greatest number of people, Bentham was directly or indirectly responsible for a great number of reforms. These included changes in representation in government, the abolition of transportation, reform of the Poor Laws, the development of friendly societies, and public health legislation. Typically, when he died, he left his body to a medical school, in such a way as to affect change in legislative policy, so that the Anatomy Bill was soon passed into law.[75]

Figure 1.9.5: **Jeremy Bentham. Line engraving by W J des Hauvents.**
(The Wellcome Library)

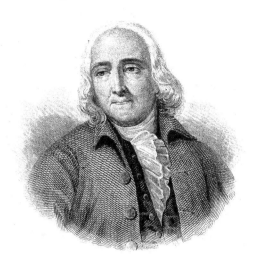

Southwood Smith, who delivered a lecture over his remains, described him as a warrior over 'ignorance, error, prejudice, imposture, selfishness, vice, misery'. Bentham's philosophy, he said, held that there was a close relationship between moral and medical science; and that the object of medicine was 'the mitigation of human suffering and the increase of human happiness'. He based that on the notion that Nature rules humankind with two masters, pain and pleasure, which govern all we do, all we say and all we think. The object of a science of morals was, therefore, to show:

> ... *what is really conducive to happiness; the happiness of every individual man; the happiness of all men taken together, considered as forming one great aggregate; the happiness of all beings whatever, that are capable of the impression: for the science, in its enlarged sense, embraces not only the human race, but the whole of sentient creation.*[76]

In relating Bentham's philosophies to occupational therapy, it is probably right to say that whilst occupational therapists tend not to talk of happiness but of well-being, the aim of much of their treatment is assisting people to enjoy as much as possible their everyday life. Recently that notion has been expanding to embrace communities as well as individuals.

Many nineteenth century philosophers' ideas related to economic conditions, but some of the most influential theories recognised the essential nature of meeting the occupational needs of individuals, and related them to well-being. Several of these theories will be discussed in some depth as they demonstrate the emergence of occupational ideology central to current day occupational therapy, and link its philosophical base with some of the most important and influential of philosophers.

For all philosophers who espoused humanist ideas, the capitalist methods of production that resulted from the triumph of the industrial revolution were repugnant. Many shared similar concerns to those of the social activists already discussed, calling attention to the fragmentation of people through mechanisation, the division of labour, and exploitation which had become the fundamental European experience. People no longer found themselves in community with others, but in a world of harsh individualist competition[77] which prevented their unique capacities, talents and potential from flourishing. Schiller (1759-1805) described it thus:

> Enjoyment was divorced from labour, the means from the end, the effort from the reward. Everlastingly chained to a single little fragment of the Whole, man himself develops into nothing but a fragment; everlastingly in his ear the monotonous sound of the wheel that he turns, he never develops the harmony of his being, and instead of putting the stamp of humanity upon his own nature, he becomes nothing more than the imprint of his occupation or of his specialised knowledge[78]

Philosophers of the time articulated many different and often conflicting points of view about how to overcome the problems, although themes about rediscovering wholeness, and unity with self, others, and nature to overcome the alienating effects of the monumental occupational changes were common. One such was the very influential Thomas Carlyle (1795-1881), who in *Signs of the Times* in 1829 deplored the fact that 'on every hand, the living artisan is driven from his workshop, to make room for a speedier, inanimate one. The shuttle drops from the fingers of the weaver, and falls into the iron fingers that ply it faster.'[79]

Thomas Carlyle's occupational theories

Thomas Carlyle (1795-1881) was born of peasant stock in Dumfriesshire where he attended the Ecclefechan Parish School. Such was his aptitude that he progressed to Annan Academy and then to Edinburgh University at 15 years of age. Before taking to literary work, he returned to Annan as a teacher.[80] In *Chartism* and *Past and Present* Carlyle addressed the vexed issues of work, labour and industry, deploring the democracy and political economy of the day, and advocating a return to medieval conditions under the rule of "strong just men". He reflected:

> There is a perennial nobleness, and even sacredness, in Work. Were he never so benighted, forgetful of his high calling, there is always hope in a man that actually and earnestly works; in idleness alone is there perpetual despair. Work, never so Mammonish, mean, is in communication with Nature; the real desire to get Work done will itself lead one more and more to truth, to Nature's appointments and regulations which are truth.
>
> The latest Gospel in this world is, know thy work and do it. "Know thyself;" long enough has that poor "self" of thine tormented thee; thou wilt never get to "know" it, I believe! Think it not thy business, this of knowing thyself; thou art

an unknowable individual: know what thou canst work at; and work at it like a Hercules! That will be thy better plan.

It has been written "an endless significance lies in work"; as man perfects him self by writing. Foul jungles are cleared away, fair seed-fields rise instead, and stately cities; and withal the man himself first ceases to be a jungle and foul unwholesome desert thereby. Consider how, even in the meanest sorts of Labour, the whole soul of a man is composed into a kind of real harmony, the instant he sets himself to work! Doubt, Desire, Sorrow, Remorse, Indignation, Despair itself, all these like hell-dogs lie beleaguering the soul of the poor day-worker, as of every man; but as he bends himself with free valour against his task, all these are stilled, all these shrink murmuring far off into their caves. The man is now a man. The blessed glow of Labour in him, is it not a purifying fire, wherein all poison is burnt up, and of sour smoke itself there is made bright blessed flame.

… Blessed is he who has found his work; let him ask no other blessedness. He has a work, a life-purpose; he has found it, and will follow it! … Labour is life.[81]
And, he adds 'Every noble work is at first "impossible"'.[82]

Classical economists and German idealists

Antithetical to Carlyle, exponents of the classical economic theory developed by Adam Smith in the previous century provided a different view, which was also aligned with the change to industry. In the nineteenth century this was refined and modified by people such as Jean-Baptiste Says, in France,[83] and David Ricardo (1772-1823) in England.[84] Classical economists called for economic freedom, competition and a laissez-faire government which would promote free trade, labour productivity, and manufacturing, rather than agriculture, as the chief determinant of a nation's economic health and, following this, of people's health.

A classical economist worthy of special note in the context of occupational therapists' views about the relationship of individual choice and meaning to health and well-being is John Stuart Mill (1806-1873). This Utilitarian and Liberal philosopher was a "many sided thinker and writer".[85] He championed happiness,[86] women's suffrage,[87] and individual liberty[88] justice, and freedom to cultivate a self chosen lifestyle as not only necessary for economic and governmental efficiency, but also as a hallmark of a mature society, and of value in itself.[89] Mill held that self-determination and the exercise of choice that does not constrain or disturb the freedom of others, is part of a higher concept of happiness.[90] The links between happiness, health and well-being are central to twentieth century psychology literature[91] and an underlying assumption in occupational therapy practice, which is now receiving some attention as theoretical issues are being addressed in greater depth.[92]

In contrast to classical economics, German idealism was another major philosophical school to emerge in the early nineteenth century from the work of Immanuel Kant (1724-1804), and his follower, Johann Gottlieb Fichte (1762-

1814). This School added significantly to the theory of the centrality of praxis; of "the practical"; of activity, which is the core of occupational therapy philosophy. In the tradition of earlier philosophers, Kant addressed the issue of praxis within his perspective of reasoning. In his *Critique of Pure Reason* he distinguished between "theoretical (or speculative) cognition" and "practical cognition" but concluded that, despite his distinction, reason is "in the last analysis only one and the same", concluding that "everything comes to the *practical*". Fichte, too, stressed the primacy of a practical philosophy, and Friedrich Schelling (1775-1854), another notable idealist, lay even greater emphasis on the practical as well as leaning, in his later work, towards a philosophy of identity.[93,94]

Arguably the most influential philosopher of this time and School was Georg Wilhelm Friedrich Hegel (1770-1831) who reasoned that progress in spiritual and philosophical concepts and insight corresponds to and advances with the direction of social and political history. Like Schelling, Hegel placed the practical above the theoretical. Theory and praxis he asserted are two aspects of humans as individuals, but the truth of theory and praxis is freedom, which can only be achieved at the level of social life and social institutions, through art, religion and philosophy.[95]

Hegel's work inspired many of his followers toward a praxiological philosophy. For example Cieskowski argued that truth had to be realised through praxis or "action"[96] and Moses Hess insisted that "the task of the philosophy of spirit now consists in becoming a philosophy of action".[97] From the point of view of this history it is particularly notable that Hegelian philosophy touched, both negatively and positively, the work of William James, the American Pragmatist whose ideas had a direct bearing on the formative stage of occupational therapy at Hull House in Chicago through the work of John Dewey, Jane Addams, Adolf Meyer and Eleanor Clarke Slagle. Hegel also greatly influenced the young Karl Marx who has played such a large part in world theories and practices of the twentieth century that a section of this chapter is given to discussion of his philosophies. It is appropriate to do that in this history because his philosophy was based on a belief about humans as active and creative beings, which is surprisingly close to what researchers concerned with the nature of people as "occupational beings" are rediscovering at the present time.

Karl Marx's occupational theories

Karl Marx (1818-1883) was born and educated in Germany, but because of his often radical ideas found it expedient to move first to Paris, then Brussels, and finally London in 1849, where he lived until his death. There he engaged in a lifelong collaboration with Frederick Engels, and attended the British Museum Library, daily, for thirty years to carry on his writing. Although he acknowledged Owen's work and communalism as a major contribution,[98] Marx himself is undoubtedly the most influential and best known of socialist thinkers, though he was largely unheeded during his lifetime.[99] Better known for his contribution to communist ideology, its very acceptance by the Eastern Block has led to a lack of appreciation of some of the original ideas on which Marx based his thinking. This was accentuated by the fact that his early writings were not published in English until well into the twentieth century.

The young Marx progressed through interest in Romanticism, Utopian Socialism and Hegelianism. From the latter he maintained a firm belief that humanity makes progress in the course of history. He used this belief as the foundation for his philosophies, whilst differing from Hegel by insisting that freedom and truth are only possible when individuals can act according to their "natural" selves, and are not constrained by the state or capital.

It was in his fundamental theories about human nature and the centrality of praxis that the development of ideas central to many present-day notions about occupational therapy emerged. As early as his doctoral dissertation *The Difference Between the Democritean and Epicurean Philosophy of Nature* (1841) his interest in creative labour (occupation) as the species nature of people started to become evident, as he too maintained the necessity for philosophy to become practical.[100] Marx saw human species nature as a combination of naturalism and humanism. That is, he viewed people in evolutionary terms, as part of nature, and in humanist terms, as beings that create themselves as they act in autonomous, self reflective and adaptive ways, which is how he defined praxis.[101] He argued that as people acquire and develop control over nature they create a humanised environment that produces a wealth of capacities and needs, which become a new starting point for further self-development.[102]

As occupational therapists tend to use praxis in a more limited way when dealing with the rehabilitation of the brain injured, it is useful at this point to consider Marx's definition, especially as the whole concept is so central to the theme of occupational therapists' philosophies. In Bottomore's classic *A Dictionary of Marxist Thought*, Petrovic argues that in Marx's sense, praxis refers to the:

> ... *free, universal, creative and self-creative activity through which man creates (makes, produces) and changes (shapes) his historical, human world and himself; an activity specific to man through which he is basically differentiated from all other beings. In this sense man can be regarded as a being of praxis, "praxis" as the central concept of Marxism, and Marxism as the "philosophy (or better: thinking") of "praxis".*[103]

With that definition in mind it is easy to exchange the word praxis with that of occupation and it becomes clear that Marx considered people to be occupational beings, and that this provided the focus for his future ideas. Whether or not we agree with the results brought about in response to his thinking is unimportant. They do not necessarily make his foundation notions invalid, but rather important to reconsider in the light of further developments.

It was in *Economic and Philosophical Manuscripts*, one of Marx's early works published whilst he was in Paris in 1843, that he developed the notion of creative labour as human's species nature, of people as creative, praxic beings, in both a positive and a negative sense. This concept in particular is similar to how occupational scientists now talk about people as occupational beings. In the positive sense he recognised the developmental and transformative effects of people's engagement in occupation, in life's activities, as he contended that:

> *The animal is one with its life activity. It does not distinguish the aim itself. It is its activity. But man makes his life activity itself an object of his will and consciousness. He has a conscious life-activity ... They (animals) produce only in a single direction, while man produces universally. They produce only under the compulsion of direct physical need, while man produces when he is free from physical need and only truly produces in freedom from such need. Animals produce only themselves, while man reproduces the whole of nature. The products of animal production belong directly to their physical bodies, while man is free in face of his product. Animals construct only in accordance with the standards and needs of the species to which they belong, while man knows how to produce in accordance with the standard of every species and knows how to apply the appropriate standard to the object. Thus man constructs also in accordance with the laws of beauty ... The object of labour is, therefore, the objectification of man's species life; for he no longer reproduces himself merely intellectually, as in consciousness, but actively and in a real sense, and he sees his own reflection in a world which he has constructed.*[104]

Marx's belief in the transformative effects of conscious activity is still evident in later works. In the first volume of *Capital* he wrote:

> *Labour is, in the first place, a process in which both man and nature participate, and in which man of his own accord starts, regulates, and controls the material reactions between himself and Nature. He opposes himself to Nature as one of her own forces, setting in motion arms and legs, head and hands, the natural forces of his body, in order to appropriate Nature's productions in a form adapted to his own wants. By thus acting on the external world and changing it, he at the same time changes his own nature. He develops his slumbering powers and compels them to act in obedience to his sway. We are not now dealing with those primitive instinctive forms of labour that remind us of the mere animal. An immeasurable interval of time separates the state of things in which a man brings his labour-power to market for sale as a commodity, from that state in which human labour was still in its first instinctive stage. We pre-suppose labour in a form that stamps it as exclusively human. A spider conducts operations that resemble those of a weaver, and a bee puts to shame many an architect in the construction of her cells. But what distinguishes the worst architect from the best of bees is this, that the architect raises his structure in imagination before he erects it in reality. At the end of every labour process, we get a result that already*

existed in the imagination of the labourer at its commencement[105]
In various of his writings Marx appeared to see labour as the opposite, rather than a part of praxis. An example is when he described labour as being so alienated from practical human activity that it should be abolished. Sometimes, however, he used labour and praxis synonymously. In some of his work he replaced the word praxis, with "self-activity". However despite the inconsistent terminology, Marx's fundamental idea was that social or occupational reform should aim at transforming labour into self-activity or praxis making a clear distinction between the "realm of necessity" and the "realm of freedom".[106]

Marx is, of course, well known for his belief that so great were the miseries experienced by the rank and file under capitalism at that time, that revolution was certain. Contemporary records justify the foundation for that belief, and he was not alone. Marx was one of many social activists who advocated for a different way of living that was more socially just, and which recognised that people need to find satisfaction in their occupation as well as meeting the other requirements of life adequately. He argued, rather in the way of Carlyle and Dickens that:

> *Labour certainly produces marvels for the rich, but it produces privation for the worker. It produces palaces, but hovels for the worker. It produces beauty, but deformity for the worker. It replaces labour by machinery, but it casts some of the workers back into a barbarous kind of work and turns the others into machines. It produces intelligence, but also stupidity and cretinism for the workers.*[107]

And in the way an occupational scientist or therapist might analyse Marx found that factory work was not fulfilling for the workers. Rather, they were unable to develop naturally their mental or physical capacities, and experienced misery, physical exhaustion, and mental debasement rather than well-being in their daily occupations. He went further in his critique, arguing that workers therefore felt no sense of belonging or of being at home with themselves during their work, which was counter to the needs of their occupational natures.[108]

The idea of workers not feeling at home with themselves when engaged in their labour was a major component of Marx's central concept of alienation.[109] He regarded as potentially alienating any productive, economic, social or spiritual occupations, as well as their products, such as commodities, money, philosophies, laws, social institutions or morals, which estranged people from their natural "creativity".[110] Alienating occupations, he argued, were 'forced upon individuals by the society which they themselves create' and so he particularly saw the division of labour and the limitations imposed by industrial processes as being at fault.[111] Like Ruskin and Morris who followed, Marx deliberated upon the contrast between skilled craftsmen and factory worker who were subservient to machines. He wrote that far from freeing humans from toil, 'the lightening of the labour, even, becomes a sort of torture, since the machine does not free the labourer from work, but deprives the work of all interest'.[112] He envisaged that factory workers:

> *... robbed thus of all real life-content, have become abstract individuals, ... the only connection which still links them with the productive forces and with their own existence - labour - has lost all semblance of self-activity and only sustains life by stunting it.*[113]

Marx perceived this stunting outcome as less than health giving. He suggested a direct illness connection associated with the processes of industrialisation because 'factory work exhausts the nervous system to the uttermost, it does away with the many sided play of the muscles, and confiscates every atom of freedom, both in bodily and intellectual activity'.[114]

Engels, Marx's friend and collaborator, although born in Westphalia and initially influenced by Hegel, Bauer, and Schelling, had for a couple of years worked in Manchester in his father's textile firm. Here he came into contact with the ideas of Robert Owen and Chartism. Their notions were inter-woven with his own belief in the inevitability of revolutionary transformation of the working classes in his book *The Condition of the Working Class in England*[115] which he published in 1845.[116] That influential text also made use of Southwood Smith's 1838 *Report on the Physical Causes of Sickness and Mortality to Which the Poor are Particularly Exposed.*

The interconnectedness of both the lives and thinking of the philosophers and social activists of the nineteenth century continues to amaze me. In particular I am struck by how closely they and their ideas touched on the occupational nature of humankind, and on the necessity for ongoing occupational meaning and satisfaction for everyone. They were driven to these thoughts by being part of a world in which occupational change was instrumental in causing situations which were occupationally alienating, unbalanced and depriving, and which led to occupationally unhealthy and unjust physical and social environments.

Social health and its relationship to what people do continued to be the theme of other influential critics in the second half of the 19th century, and those too, were interconnected. Ultimately most of the major radical thinkers of that period can be said to have influenced the founding ideas that prevailed at the genesis of twentieth century occupational therapy. In that regard, two more important critics remain to be discussed, namely, John Ruskin and William Morris. They carried on the tradition of 19th century British intellectual idealists who resisted ready identification with capitalism, economic expansion and urban industrialisation. Instead they led a moral crusade which began to surface from the middle of the century onwards, towards a rural ideal in which 'human relationships had not been complicated by the cash nexus or the demands of profit'.[117] Paul Rich, in *History Today*, groups them with the earlier idealists into an economic "backwardness" school, which revisited 'medieval social order close to nature' in a search for 'a sense of English cultural and national identity'. Some argue that this ideal had roots deeply embedded in mid eighteenth century romanticism.[118,119] The political reality of that medieval dream, though, was insubstantial, differing widely between the many idealists in different walks of life who espoused it. In fact it was so disparate that at one extreme the young England group of Tories used it to demonstrate the virtues of feudalism. At the other extreme, emergent Socialist and Labour groups used it to demonstrate, through the medieval virtues of a free peasantry, that inequality rather than poverty was the cause of social illness, so allying Marxian views with British socialism and medieval idealism.[120] Both Ruskin and Morris would have to be considered prime examples of that strange mix.

John Ruskin's occupational theories and action

John Ruskin (1819-1900) was the son of a wealthy wine merchant. His father, a self-made man with social pretensions, was excessively proud of his son's apparent prodigy. He provided Ruskin with an extensive education at home and many opportunities to travel throughout Britain and Europe, but few to play or socialise with others of his age. As a child, Ruskin demonstrated interest in a wide variety of subjects and his parents encouraged him in a way that may well have contributed to his later interest in encouraging the occupational talents of others. His father, for example, wrote to him in one of many similar letters:

> You are blessed with a fine Capacity and even Genius & you owe it as a Duty to the author of your Being & the giver of your Talents to cultivate your powers & to use them in his Service & for the benefit of your fellow Creatures.[121]

Ruskin went to Christ Church, Oxford, but despite his talents, and perhaps as a consequence of his individualised education that catered to them, he struggled with the particular demands of a first class degree.

> For those who obtain honours are usually such as would have been high in scholarship without such inducement, who are, in fact, above their trial and take their position as a matter of course and a thing of no consequence. To these the honour is a matter of gratification and of less utility. But the flock of lower standard men of my stamp, and men below me, who look to the honour at the end, and strain their faculties to the utmost to obtain it, not only have to sustain hours of ponderous anxiety and burning disappointment, such as I have seen in some, enough to eat their life away, but sustain a bodily and intellectual injury, which nothing can ever do away with or compensate for.[122]

In addition he was uncertain about his future, with little vocation for a life in the Church which was what his family hoped for. 'Tensions, excitement and the enthusiasms of intensive mental work began to produce their inevitable counter swing into depression and actual physical illness.'[123] His father confided to a friend of the postponement of Ruskin's final examinations, that 'he is not going up for a degree until later which is a great relief to us as he was Killing himself with reading'.[124] A short time later Ruskin withdrew from Oxford indefinitely following 'a short ticking cough … a curious sensation in the throat … a curious taste in the mouth … that of blood',[125] and it was not until some two years later that he completed his degree. During the years of his recuperation he wrote about the links between his occupations and his health and well-being. He said, 'hard mental labour of any kind hurts me instantly'[126] and described how:

> ... *a roughness about the chest ... renders it improper for me to read or draw to any extent, or to do anything that requires stooping, and equally so to take violent or prolonged exercise, or to go out at night, or to saunter in cold galleries, or to talk much, or walk much, or do anything "much", so that I am subject to perpetual mortification in taking care of an absolute nothing.*[127]

> *I have begun a work of some labour which would take me several years to complete; but I cannot read for it, and do not know how many years I may have for it. I don't know if I shall even be able to get my degree; and so I remain in a jog-trot, sufficient-for-the-day style of occupation - lounging, planless, undecided, and uncomfortable, except when I can get out to sketch - my chief enjoyment. I am beginning to consider the present as the only available time, and in that humour it is impossible to work at anything dry or laborious or useful. I spend my days in a search after present amusement, because I have not spirit enough to labour in the attainment of what I may not have future strength to attain; and yet am restless under the sensation of days perpetually lost and employment perpetually vain.*[128]

Following an extensive European tour Ruskin eventually recovered his health, after a stay with Dr Jephson of Leamington Spa who prescribed a simple regimen of regular habits, fresh air and easy occupations. During his time there Ruskin walked twice a day, read, painted, wrote a fairy tale, and put the journal of his travels in order.[129] He returned to Dr Jephson some years later when he became ill once more.

Ruskin did not enter the church, but spent much of his early life as an art critic and writer. He turned to political economy and the need for social reform towards the end of the 1850s, publishing essays on his ideas in the *Cornhill Magazine* in 1860 and *Fraser's Magazine* in 1862-63. These were re-published in *Unto this Last* (1862) and *Munera Pulveris* (1872). In these and other works, such as *Sesame and Lilies* (1865) and *The Crown of Wild Olive* (1866) he advocated a system of national education, the re-organisation of labour and many social reforms. He particularly disapproved of economic policies based on profit alone as he held strongly to the view that wealth was not the only thing worth having.[130]

Without doubt, Ruskin was the foremost progenitor of the Arts and Crafts Movement. In his view, Renaissance attempts to recapture classical symmetry and order was precursory to regimentation in industry, the division of labour, and the division between thinkers and doers that he saw as morally and socially wrong. To right those wrongs he sought to spread enthusiasm for manual labour, and implored his fellow citizens to boycott machine-made goods. As well, in *Unto This Last*, Ruskin urged paternalism from industrialists and the State, the latter by providing minimum welfare guarantees.[131] Additionally, Ruskin set about re-creating a microcosm of medieval society by founding the

Guild of St George to maintain and further the best traditions of country handiwork, agriculture and education. Epitomising the 'quixotic quality of Ruskin's reform', it was built on the principles that 'food can only be got out of the ground and happiness out of honesty' and that the 'highest wisdom and the highest treasure need not be costly or exclusive'.

> *The members of the Guild had originally met in the Owenite Hall of Science in Sheffield to explore their vision of communitarianism. Becoming a miniature feudal kingdom on twenty acres of wooded land, the Guild was so named, in part, because they settled at St Georges Farm in Totley, Yorkshire. They gave a tithe of their fortunes to philanthropic purposes and Ruskin, as a companion of the Guild, contributed generously from his own purse'.*[132]

The Guild, like Shaw's Fabian Society, Ashbee's Guild of Handicraft, Ellis's Fellowship of the New Life, the Arts and Crafts Movement, and similar groupings, attracted a range of middle class men and women from many walks of life in revolt against various conditions of the times. Edward Carpenter, one of their number, observed that what they were opposed to in the period was:

> *… not only commercialism in public life, but cant in religion, pure materialism in science, futility in social conventions, the worship of stocks and shares, the starving of the human heart, the denial of the human body and its needs, huddling concealment of the body in clothes, the "impure hush" in matters of sex, class division, contempt of manual labour, and the cruel barring of women from every natural and useful expression of their lives … carried to an extremity of folly.*[133]

Ruskin, the Guild and other such organisations often had in common spiritual as opposed to material ideals; an appreciation of the simple life, manual labour and the craft traditions of the past; personal and social liberation; and the cultivation of "perfect character".

Figure 1.9.6:   John Ruskin in his study[134]

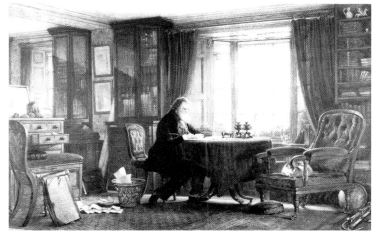

In the Lake District where, from 1872, he made his home at Brantwood overlooking Coniston Water, Ruskin involved himself in local affairs. He expressed strong views about issues of interest to him and instigated practical programmes to promote social well-being by alleviating the social health consequences of a depressed economy and changing occupational circumstances. In accord with his views linking well-being with traditional occupations, he engaged in several industrial experiments. Ruskin acted at times as an intellectual "occupational therapy" entrepreneur addressing issues related to social health and well-being through occupations. This is illustrated by the following story of the revival of the Lakeland spinning and weaving cottage industry with the establishment of the Langdale Linen Company.

Langdale Linen Company: An occupational intervention to improve social health

A condition of tenancy on some farms in Cumbria was to grow flax and to process it into "harden sark". Sark was a shirt style outer garment made from "hards", the coarse fibres of hemp or flax. However by the beginning of the nineteenth century harden cloth, which was so uncomfortable to wear that it was soaked in water and beaten before being worn, had been superseded and by 1812 John Gough reported that few women could spin flax.[135,136]

Ruskin enthused another companion of the Guild, Albert Fleming, with his scheme to revive the occupation, and Fleming's housekeeper, Marion Twelves, after learning to spin became the main instigator of the Industry. A local carpenter made the spinning wheels, and a cottage at Elterwater in the Langdale Valley was acquired by the Guild and named St Martins. At this venue local women learned to spin, and when proficient took a spinning wheel home. They were paid for the thread they produced. Following the acquisition of a second-hand loom, a retired weaver from Kendal went to live and work at St Martins, where the first 20 yards of linen was produced at Easter time 1884. The linen was made up into garments and domestic articles and Marion Twelves taught paying students many forms of embroidery including Greek lace which decorated the objects made, so employing more local women. The fee for the training was defrayed by the Guild. She moved to Keswick to work with Mrs Canon Rawnsley in 1889 at the Keswick Arts Industry. (In John Marsh's book she was Canon Rawnsley's housekeeper and she moved with him.[137]) Later, in 1894, the Guild helped her to purchase Porch Cottage where she established another spinning and weaving industry that she continued until the 1920s.

Mrs Mary Elizabeth Pepper and her mother Mrs Elizabeth Heskett took over at St Martins when Marion Twelves left. In 1901 it moved to High Tilberthwaite farm, then tenanted by Mary's husband Robert.[138] The Misses Dicks founded a branch of the Industry at Troutbeck Bridge where the post office advertised Greek Lace and Art Needlework. This branch and another at the Spinnery,

Bowness continued long after many had given up when foreign products undercut prices after the First World War.[139]

Ruskin's influence was powerful with English friends and associates such as Octavia Hill, who provides an interesting connection from him to the establishment of the first English occupational therapy school, founded at Dorset House in Bristol by Dr Elizabeth Casson. Casson worked as an estate manager for Hill in the rehabilitation of slum tenements in London, which was funded by Ruskin. In that position Casson was engaged in a management role in activity programmes for the "poor" tenants at Red Cross House. It can be surmised that this association had important intellectual consequences for occupational therapists. Casson's experience of the participatory nature of the association between the intellectual social activists and the recipient poor was an important factor in the communal and participatory nature of the training facility that she later established for occupational therapists.

Ruskin's anti-modern critique also shaped the similar vision of William Morris,[140] who in terms of the Arts and Crafts Movement, is the man most associated with Ruskin in the modern day. But that shared interest, along with their notions of creativity as an essential part of social wellness and a subsequent need for reform of society to that end, has linked them together more in the present than in their lifetime. The Arts and Crafts Movement's influence on occupational therapy has long been apparent. This is especially evident in America, where occupational therapy was established earlier in those States where Societies had been established early. Ruskin and Morris's combined influence shaped the direction of the Chicago Settlement programmes, envisioned by Jane Addams and Ellen Gates Starr at Hull House[141] and the establishment, there, of the first formal occupational therapy school in America.

It is therefore timely to trace Morris's story.

William Morris's occupational theories and action

Morris was born in 1834 in Walthamstow to a prosperous family, being the oldest boy of nine surviving children. When he was six they moved to an impressive Georgian house set in 50 acres adjacent to Epping Forest, in which he roamed on his pony, went fishing, and developed an interest in landscape. He had an unusually acute visual memory for form and colour, and detailed images of the English environment were later to be central to 'his creative genius as a poet, painter, fabric designer and inspiration to the Arts and Crafts Movement whose vision transformed the English house and garden' with a revival of rural crafts.[142]

Despite the fairly early death of his father the family remained well-to-do. In later years, Morris, an ardent socialist, was to feel uncomfortable about his father's unabashed capitalism that, however, gave him the freedom to choose his own career. At the time, it also enabled him to attend the newly established Marlborough College where, it is said, he regaled his companions with endless and fanciful medieval tales. He went on to Oxford where he established a life-long friendship with Edward Burne-Jones, who was to become his artistic collaborator. Burne-Jones described how Morris had 'come "tumbling in" on the first evening of a term and "talked incessantly for seven hours or longer"' and how he found him 'different from all the men I had ever met. He talked with vehemence and sometimes with violence. I never knew him languid or tired.'[143]

Figure 1.9.7: William Morris, 1870, by George Frederick Watts

(National Portrait Gallery)

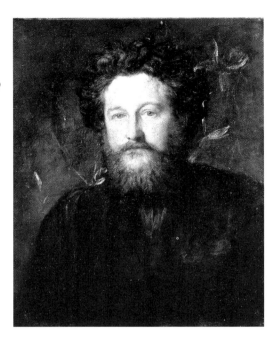

Both Burne-Jones and Morris planned a career as clergymen and discussed establishing a monastic order. Instead they became impassioned by Ruskin's writings, particularly his insight that the art of any period was an 'expression of its social coherence'. They adopted his principle of Truth to Nature and became convinced they must dedicate their lives to art.[144] Morris read Ruskin's *The Stones of Venice* out loud to his friends. To him, the chapter *On the Nature of Gothic Architecture: And Herein of the True Functions of the Workman in Art*, in which Ruskin claimed that workmen experienced a freedom of individual expression within the social milieu of the Middle Ages which was tragically absent in the Victorian age, was a sort of revelation. He converted others with his passion, so that one colleague recalled 'we soon saw the greatness and importance of it'.[145]

Morris attributed Ruskin as being 'the prime mover in the turning of the tide away from a blind faith in materialist progress and towards a perception of the damage to society this implied'. He agreed with his mentor's arguments against the division of labour and the dehumanisation of workers in factories, as well as his attack on the boredom and monotony of the industrial system and the disconnection between labour and leisure which he believed caused "social neurosis". He also shared Ruskin's abhorrence of the distinction between manual labour and intellect: [146]

> *We are always in these days endeavouring to separate the two; we want one man to be always thinking, and another to be always working, and we call one a gentleman, and the other an operative; whereas the workman ought often to be thinking, and the thinker often to be working, and both should be gentlemen, in the best sense* [147]

Morris also read the works of other English social critics, and was 'deeply and lastingly' affected by Carlyle's *Past and Present*. [148]

After graduating he began to study architecture, but within a year, he had joined Burne-Jones in London. Here, prompted by Rosetti, a leader of the Pre-Raphaelite artists, they took up painting. It was through their new mentor that they, at last, met Ruskin, whom Morris impressed with his standard in illuminating manuscripts. As well, during that time, Morris experimented with many crafts, such as embroidery, modelling clay and carving in wood and stone.

After Morris's marriage to Jane Burden, their home became 'the cradle of a craft cooperative that, in 1861, became Morris, Marshall, Faulkner and Company'. He and his colleagues described themselves as "fine art workmen" as they became manufacturers of furniture, stained glass, painted tiles, embroidery, fabrics, sculpture, tapestries, metalwork, jewellery, wall-paintings and wallpapers. [149] In contrast to most men of means of that period, Morris, with the belief that labourers should find similar satisfaction in their work to medieval craftsmen, for many years donned a workman's smock and crafted in like manner. In 1875 he took sole control of the Firm which was renamed Morris & Co. Despite that commercial enterprise, and growing from his notions about the need for meaning in life's occupations, just one year later a passionate belief in socialism began to surface. Morris felt, as did Ruskin, that the best way for working men to regain the dignity, pride and satisfaction in work that had been removed by the industrial process was through integrating politics with art and literature, combined with education. [150] Indeed, on that last point he argued in *Art and Socialism* that:

> *The wonderful machines ... have driven men into mere frantic haste and hurry, thereby destroying pleasure ... they have instead of lightening the labour of the workmen, intensified it, and thereby added more weariness yet to the burden which the poor have to carry.* [151]

Not surprisingly at that time, and particularly amongst members of the working class, there was a deep disillusionment with the main political parties that prompted their interest in revolutionary socialism. But the infant movement was disorganised and small, and became a worthy target for Morris's enthusiasm. He plunged into radical politics with all the zeal of a Utopian as he studied Marx's writings, whilst recognising that the doctrine of socialism had its origins in the social experiments at New Lanark. He then sought to wed others' socialist ideas with the core of Ruskin's and his own beliefs on a worker's right to joyful and useful occupation. This effectively separated Morris from the Fabians and other leading British socialists.[152] Morris had first joined the Social-Democratic Federation.[153] Soon, conflicts within that organisation led him to move on and to form the Socialist League, which campaigned for improved conditions for the working classes and equality for women. When anarchists hijacked that organisation, yet another, the Hammersmith Socialist Society was formed. Political gatherings were held at Morris's home, and notables such as George Bernard Shaw, Oscar Wilde, H.G. Wells, W.B. Yeats and Gustav Holst often frequented these.

Morris supported his beliefs with action. He travelled tirelessly throughout the country giving lectures, speaking at open-air meetings, taking part in demonstrations, and not only editing but selling socialist journals on street corners. He came into frequent conflict with the authorities when they broke up socialist meetings, and often stood surety in court for working-class comrades who were judged more harshly than gentlemen like himself.[154] On one occasion he too suffered arrest.

In one of his lectures, *Useful Work versus Useless Toil*, Morris briefly considered occupation in terms of evolution:

Men urged by their necessities and desires have laboured for many thousands of years at the task of subjugating the forces of Nature and of making the natural material useful to them. To our eyes, since we cannot see into the future, that struggle with Nature seems nearly over, and the victory of the human race over her nearly complete. And, looking backwards to the time when history first began, we note that the progress of that victory has been far swifter and more startling within the last two hundred years than ever before. Surely, therefore, we moderns ought to be in all ways vastly better off than any who have gone before us. Surely we ought, one and all of us, to be wealthy, to be well furnished with the good things which our victory over Nature has won for us.[155]

That he believed the latter supposition to be far from the case is supported by a pithy social analysis of three strata of people in relation to work. Those strata he described as 'a class which does not even pretend to work, a class which pretends to work but which produces nothing, and a class which works, but is compelled by the other two classes to do work which is often unproductive'.[156]

Morris also explained some of his views about misconceptions regarding the value of all work. He was in fact articulating an occupational theory of social health that holds value today and is part of an unacknowledged theory base of occupational therapy and occupational science. He put his critique this way:

It is assumed by most people nowadays that all work is useful, and by most well-to-do people that all work is desirable. Most people, well-to-do or not, believe that, even when a man is doing work which appears to be useless, he is earning his livelihood by it - he is "employed", as the phrase goes; and most of those who are well-to-do cheer on the happy worker with congratulations and praises, if he is only "industrious" enough and deprives himself of all pleasure and holidays in the sacred cause of labour. In short, it has become an article of the creed of modern morality that all labour is good in itself - a convenient belief to those who live on the labour of others.

Let us grant, first, that the race of man must either labour or perish. Nature does not give us our livelihood gratis; we must win it by toil of some sort or degree. Let us see, then, if she does not give us some compensation for this compulsion to labour, since certainly in other matters she takes care to make the acts necessary to the continuance of life in the individual and the race not only endurable, but even pleasurable.

You may be sure that she does so, that it is of the nature of man, when he is not diseased, to take pleasure in his work under certain conditions. And, yet, we must say in the teeth of the hypocritical praise of all labour, whatsoever it may be, of which I have made mention, that there is some labour which is so far from being a blessing that it is a curse; that it would be better for the community and for the worker if the latter were to fold his hands and refuse to work, and either die or let us pack him off to the work-house or prison - which you will.[157]

Morris went on to analyse occupations according to his perceptions of their mental and social health or illness effects, explaining that:

Here, you see, are two kinds of work - one good, the other bad; one not far removed from a blessing, a lightening of life; the other a mere curse, a burden to life.

What is the difference between them, then? This: one has hope in it, the other has not ... What is the nature of the hope which, when it is present in work, makes it worth doing?

It is threefold, I think - hope of rest, hope of product, hope of pleasure in the work itself; and hope of these also in some abundance and of good quality; rest enough and good enough to be worth having; product worth having by one who is neither a fool nor an ascetic; pleasure enough for all of us to be conscious of it while we are at work; not a mere habit, the loss of which we shall feel as a fidgety man feels the loss of the bit of string he fidgets with.

I have put the hope of rest first because it is the simplest and most natural part of our hope. Whatever pleasure there is in some work, there is certainly some pain in all work, the beast-like pain of stirring up our slumbering energies to action, the beast-like dread of change when things are pretty well with us; and the compensation for this animal pain in animal rest. We must feel while we are working that the time will come when we shall not have to work. Also the rest, when it comes, must be long enough to allow us to enjoy it; it must be longer than is merely necessary for us to recover the strength we have expended in working, and it must be animal rest also in this, that it must not be disturbed by anxiety, else we shall not be able to enjoy it. If we have this amount and kind of rest we shall, so far, be no worse off than the beasts.

As to the hope of product, I have said that Nature compels us to work for that. It remains for us to look to it that we do really produce something, and not nothing, or at least nothing that we want or are allowed to use. If we look to this and use our wills we shall, so far, be better than machines. The hope of pleasure in the work itself: how strange that hope must seem to some of my readers - to most of them! Yet I think that to all living things there is a pleasure in the exercise of their energies, and that even beasts rejoice in being lithe and swift and strong. But a man at work, making something which he feels will exist because he is working at it and wills it, is exercising the energies of his mind and soul as well as of his body. Memory and imagination help him as he works. Not only his own thoughts, but the thoughts of the men of past ages guide his hands; and, as a part of the human race, he creates. If we work thus we shall be men, and our days will be happy and eventful.

Thus worthy work carries with it the hope of pleasure in rest, the hope of the pleasure in our using what it makes, and the hope of pleasure in our daily creative skill.

All other work than this is worthless; it is slaves work - mere toiling to live, that we may live to toil.[158]

So powerful is that summation of the requirements Morris saw as necessary for occupation to be health giving rather than a precipitant of disorder, that it could be seen as one of the philosophical statements which underpin occupational therapy practice, just as the words of Adolph Meyer, some 60 years later, with many similar themes are so viewed. In the same paper, Morris also provided health promotive or remedial advice from an occupational perspective at both a social and an individual level. He argued for purpose, variety and meaning in obligatory and self-chosen occupations. Morris also argued for those that were obligatory being engaged in for a short time only, and for balance between those that were physically or intellectually demanding. In his words:

... it follows that labour, to be attractive, must be directed towards some obviously useful end, unless in cases where it is undertaken voluntarily by each individual as a pastime.

... Next, the day's work will be short. This need not be insisted on. It is clear that with work unwasted it can be short. It is clear also that much work which is now a torment, would be easily endurable if it were much shortened.

Variety of work is the next point, and a most important one. To compel a man to do day after day the same task without any hope of escape or change, means nothing short of turning his life into a prison-torment. A man might easily learn and practice at least three crafts, varying sedentary occupation with outdoor - occupation calling for the exercise of strong bodily energy for work in which the mind had more to do. There are few men, for instance, who would not wish to spend part of their lives in the most necessary and pleasantest of all work - cultivating the earth.

One thing which will make this variety of employment possible will be the form that education will take in a socially ordered community. At present all education is directed towards the end of fitting people to take their places in the hierarchy of commerce - these as masters, those as workmen.[159]

His final comment about education meeting the economic priorities of an existing social hierarchy rather than enabling people to live enjoyable, productive lives through well thought out programmes based on their occupational needs and capacities remains true today. That points to a need for those with occupation for health ideals to reassert many of Morris's points of view especially his caution that:

Civilisation ... wastes its own resources, and will do so as long as the present system lasts.

Thus then have the fruits of our victory over Nature been stolen from us, thus has compulsion by Nature to labour in hope of rest, gain, and pleasure been turned into compulsion by man to labour in hope - of living to labour![160]

Perhaps today, one way to tackle that far from health giving scenario would be, like Morris, to challenge the materialism of the dominant social milieu. He did so by disseminating his thoughts about wealth from his occupationally based view of well-being. Reminiscent of many aspects of the World Health Organisation's 1986 Ottawa Charter for Health Promotion, but adding even more weight to the need to call upon the occupational capacities of each individual as well as addressing issues of environment and justice, his argument was that:

Wealth is what Nature gives us and what a reasonable man can make out of the gifts of Nature for his reasonable use. The sunlight, the fresh air, the unspoiled face of the earth, food, raiment and housing necessary and decent; the storing up of knowledge of all kinds, and the power of disseminating it; means of free communication between man and man; works of art, the beauty which man creates when he is most a man, most aspiring and thoughtful - all things which serve the pleasure of people, free, manly and uncorrupted. This is wealth[161]

By the late 1880s, Morris's active participation in politics was slowing down while at the same time his fame as a master of the decorative arts had spread abroad. The Arts and Crafts Movement, which had been named by Thomas Cobden-Sanderson, a bookbinder who lived in Hammersmith close to Morris, was gaining strength throughout the country. Architects, artists and craftsmen campaigned against mass production, and realising a need for strong links with the public organised an Arts and Crafts Exhibition Society, which held regular events from 1888 until the First World War. The Arts and Crafts Movement largely ignored Morris's socialism, remaining constant to his earlier work of promoting a handicraft revival. This was so much so that Morris attacked its 'empty grumbling about the continuous march of machinery over dying handicraft' and its 'various elegant little schemes' for encouraging the public's appreciation of handicraft whilst ignoring the central issue of the degradation of work.[163]

By 1894, when he was 62, although he was still writing, Morris's health was visibly deteriorating and his energy dwindling. He was 'exhausted by a life of extraordinary productivity', diagnosed with diabetes and kidney problems, contracted tuberculosis, and showed signs of upper limb degeneration.[164] One of his physicians, at his death, 'diagnosed his disease as "simply being William Morris, and having done more work than most ten men"'.[165]

In a present era of specialisation Morris's versatility and excellence across so many fields is breathtaking. Morris was gifted with creative talent, which was not only original but also conserved the past and influenced others during his lifetime, and well into the future. He acted according to his philosophical beliefs, which combined business acumen and radical social reform and because of that he has been described as 'a very English revolutionary'.[166] Even so, after he died so to, to large extent, did his "indigenous socialism", with its perspective of meeting all people's occupational needs and capacities. Initiatives for socialist reform then lay with the Fabian Society and the Independent Labour Party, both in some way an anathema to Morris who described them as "gas and water" socialism. Charted by Beatrice and Sidney Webb, the Fabians, whose view was eventually largely accepted, worked towards a future technocratic society administered by managers committed to impartial community service. Although they were critical of industrial capitalism, they linked material with moral progress, and anticipated bureaucratic state socialism as inevitable.[167] Interestingly, Beatrice provides another link in the social activist network of the period as, before her marriage, she worked with the Barnetts at the Toynbee Hall Social Settlement, which will be discussed later.

That shift not withstanding, influential people, as well as many in the general public in the twentieth century, have been inspired by Morris's vision. One of them was leading socialist theoretician, G.D.H. Cole, who in 1959, explained:

> I became a Socialist more than fifty years ago when I read "News from Nowhere" as a schoolboy and realised quite suddenly that William Morris had shown one the vision of a society in which it would be a fine and fortunate experience to live.[168]

News from Nowhere was also responsible, in part, for the post-war socialist vision of Clement Attlee, Prime Minister of the 1945 Labour government. He read and quoted avidly from Morris's Useful Work versus Useless Toil, How we Live and How we Might Live, and A Factory as It Might Be.[169] Indeed, it is reported that in 1953, Attlee wrote to Sydney Cockerell of how he 'was telling a group of foreign socialists the other day how much more Morris meant to us than Karl Marx'.[170]

Women: Occupation and social activism

Socialism and social activism were not the sole preserve of men, and many women were central within the revolutionary groups mentioned above, like Isabella Ford, Annie Besant, Olive Schreiner, and Edith Lees.[171] They provided impetus to the growth of feminism and the place of women in the caring professions. Feminism, amongst the more affluent classes, had been slowly gaining ground since Enlightenment ideas had sparked a more humanitarian view of human needs. One of the earliest texts on the subject was Mary Wollstonecraft's *A Vindication of Rights of Women* published in 1792.[172]

But the lot of most women deemed respectable in the nineteenth century was far from revolutionary. *The Young Lady's Book* of 1876, provided a manual of acceptable occupations described in the terms of those days as 'amusements, exercises, studies and pursuits'. The book was aimed at furnishing 'hints and instruction to the young for a wise occupation of their time - a sensible alternation of useful work and healthful play'.[173] The text dealt with 'what to do and how to do it' and was necessary because of the void which occurred for most young women between finishing with school work and marriage and care of their own home. Even the author of the book describes herself as Mrs Henry Mackarness using her married status in preference to her own name.

One acceptable role for respectable women was the care of the sick which followed the self health traditions of the past. Girls should be taught 'doctoring, nursing and the sister art ... of cooking' wrote Mrs Mackarness, who was 'by no means advocating the new idea of lady doctors'. Indeed she recommended that a woman needed to "doctor herself", manage her own health and 'keep a healthy mind in a healthy body'. To do that she provided a clear occupational prescription amongst her recommendations:

> There are two great rules to be remembered and acted on. That with respect to the organs by which all the functions of our body are governed ..."use keeps them in repair," and "repose prevents them from wearing out."
>
> Each set of muscles should be constantly exercised by active exertion; our lungs by reading aloud, singing, &c., and exercise of all kinds must be properly varied by rest.[175]
>
> ... time can be rightly enjoyed so as to benefit both mind and body. Recreation is in itself a duty and not a waste of time ...
>
> Recreation to the mind is what sleep is to the body, and must ..."form an integral part of human life". But in like manner, as too much sleep is injurious to the body, so is too much recreation injurious to the mind; it must, as it were, be the silken thread on which the duties of life are strung.[176]

Despite the commandment that 'the smallest home duties must come before any other occupation', another kind of voluntary work with some similarity to occupational therapy was to 'teach and work for the poor' who 'were so tenderly confided to our care by Divine command'. Women were inveigled especially to assist those 'who were unable from delicate health or any other cause to go to school'. Such work was thought to be particularly attractive because of the praise and gratitude that followed. Mackarness concluded:

> To visit the sick, clothe the naked, feed the hungry, and instruct the ignorant, is the grave side of our lives. On earth we each have our mission; but we must take it as it is given us - some have only to stand and wait, others to be actively employed - but each individual life has some influence on another, and each individual has his own one or ten talents accorded him. Let us beware how we use them: they are not to be buried, but increased and multiplied.[177]

Taking those strictures into another dimension, several women made an enormous impact on the health and well-being of people in unfortunate circumstances—the poor and destitute, the sick, the insane and mentally incapacitated, and those in prison. Four or five, in particular, stand out. Elizabeth Fry, Florence Nightingale and Octavia Hill from the United Kingdom, and Dorothea Dix and Jane Addams from the United States whose stories will be told, briefly or at some length in the history. In this chapter how Fry, Hill and Addams adopted an occupational vision in their social activist practices will be told, and in subsequent chapters the contribution of the other two will be addressed. They can all be regarded as pioneers of the service industries which have been, largely, the vocation or field in which women have been employed in the twentieth century, and of which occupational therapy is part. Some also had a direct influence on the ideology or formation of that modern profession.

Elizabeth Fry: Occupation and social activism for social health

Elizabeth Fry, nee Gurney, (1780-1845) who is well known for effecting prison reform, was born in Norwich, one of eleven children of a wealthy Quaker family. She married Joseph Fry, a banker and tea merchant. The Society of Friends, as Quakers are more correctly called, are well known for pacifism, social reform, and support of philanthropic ventures of many kinds,[178] not least in establishing humane and occupationally based programmes for treatment of the insane. For Fry, it was the preaching of William Savery, an American member of her faith, which reinforced and gave form to her own desire to bring comfort to those less fortunate than herself.

With unflagging devotion, throughout her life she worked to alleviate the appalling conditions of women in prisons. From 1813, Fry regularly visited women and their children in Newgate gaol, aiming to see that they were properly fed and clothed, segregated from men, and supervised by women, teaching them and providing them with purposeful occupations.[179,180] In 1817, in company with others, she formed an association for the improvement of conditions of women prisoners in other gaols as well as Newgate. As a result of her earlier experience, the reforms continued to include the introduction of various forms of occupation and manual labour for inmates, so that "a place of abject misery" soon became "an industrious community" that was recognised in the House of Commons. There a report stated that 'the benevolent exertion of Mrs Fry and her friends ... by the establishment of a school, by providing work, and by encouraging industrious habits produced the most gratifying change'.[181] Fry was also interested in nursing and set up an institution in Bishopsgate for the training of nurses, some of whom went to the Crimea with Florence Nightingale with whom she was friendly. Nightingale attended the nursing school at Kaiserworth set up by Theodor Fliedner and his wife, who had been inspired by Fry's work.[182] As well Fry continued her crusade of comfort for the unfortunate in many venues. She travelled around the United Kingdom and Europe, rather like John Howard had done in an earlier century, visiting prisons, asylums and homes of detention, and making recommendations for improvement. Indeed, for 25 years she visited every prison ship with women convicts bound for Australia arranging instruction and occupation.[183] Her reports, pamphlets, and magnetic personality enlisted public sympathy along with official acceptance of the need for inquiry and reform.[184]

Like Dorothea Dix, somewhat later, Fry was horrified at the numbers of mentally ill who were imprisoned like criminals, which story continues in chapter 11.[185]

Figure 1.9.8: **Octavia Hill, 1899, by John Singer Sargent.**
(National Portrait Gallery)

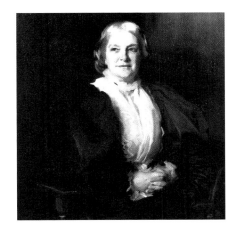

Octavia Hill: Occupation and social activism for social health

Octavia Hill, whose contribution is not widely known today, was in her time as influential and revered as Florence Nightingale. She was an unassuming woman who, like the others, did not seek glory or fortune for herself, and is only now being rediscovered as a gem of the nineteenth century. She is recorded in encyclopedias as a founder of the Open Space Movement and the National Trust. For me, she is the once missing link between nineteenth century social activists and the development of occupational therapy in England.[186]

Born in 1838, Octavia was the third of five daughters born to Carolyn and James Hill, who were themselves quite remarkable. Carolyn was the daughter of Thomas Southwood Smith discussed earlier. She was also a Pestalozzian teacher and brought up her children according to the view that 'a child should be placed in circumstances where it can neither do harm nor suffer harm; then it should be left to its own devices'.[187] She contended that 'Nature has done what is needful for us … with regard to the functions which maintain the being in animal existence'. However, she considered the 'development of the mind' to be 'dependent on the action of the human mind upon it', and identified that there was a similar dependence of spiritual and intellectual functioning on the physical. Carolyn also held the belief that 'no one is totally deficient in any faculty; the difference between individuals is, that the faculties exist in them in different proportions; and probably, under a perfect education, they would be developed according to their original powers.'[188]

Carolyn and her husband were staunch supporters of Owenism. James Hill, who was a business man, became bankrupt following the development of an Owenite Community near Wisbech, and the collapse of his newspaper which he had established to express his views about much needed social reform. Following bankruptcy James had a mental and physical breakdown, and when Hill was five his wife assumed responsibility for the family with some help from her father. A far from wealthy man Southwood Smith inspired by his example, and 'his daughters and grand daughters accepted it almost as a family tradition, that they should be in the vanguard of movements to improve the lot of the poor'. Hill, therefore grew up 'in a household in which the serious topics of social reform were the staple of family conversation'. This was coupled with a religious conversion to Christian Socialism which 'only increased her conviction that she was under an absolute moral duty to engage in whatever course of action might be open to her'.[189] Family values were to be very influential in Hill's future directions.

Following a free and creative country childhood, but one far from affluent, when Hill was thirteen the time came for her to move to London and to start work. First she assisted her mother at a Ladies Cooperative Guild established to provide employment for distressed gentlewomen by the Christian Socialist Movement led by Frederick Maurice. Overwhelmed by the 'full weight of London's misery and desolation' caused in large measure by the industrial revolution, Hill became an ardent admirer of Maurice and embraced his Christian creed which sought to remediate the social ills of the time.

By the age of fourteen she was put in charge of a business which employed Ragged School children making toy furniture. Here Hill began to accumulate knowledge of business methods, which would serve her well in the future. However it is in the way she helped the children to develop and grow through the occupations they pursued that she can be regarded as a pioneer occupational therapist working in community health. The children were from desperately poor and often wretched homes. Some were deformed, some were older than she was, and most were rough and experienced in vice, and accustomed to work according to repressive discipline. Her first act was to remove the rules and regulations pinned to the walls, and when, inevitably, fights or disobedience occurred did not coerce or adopt authoritarian punishment. Instead, she made herself a leader rather than an overseer, sometimes, to illustrate the dignity of labour, doing the children's work in front of their discomforted eyes and concerning herself with every aspect of their well-being.[190]

Horrified by what the children brought to eat for the midday meal she suggested they pool resources and learn how to prepare, serve and eat nourishing food. Any money saved was used for food when the children ran out of funds by the end of a week. At weekends, when the factory closed she took them to the country, as they had no personal or other resources to enable them to use their leisure time wisely or well. Eventually they overcame their fear that wolves and bears might lurk behind the shrubs of Hampstead Heath and responded with enjoyment and laughter to the pleasures and freedoms of open spaces.[191]

The secret of Hill's success was said to be that she treated the children as individuals, knowing what to say to each or how to interest them, and getting to know what they really cared about. She cared so much that it was shattering when, in 1856, the Guild folded and the business was to be closed down. For fifteen months Hill kept the business going, taking the financial responsibility upon her own shoulders, whilst at the same time ensuring that the children became self-supporting. She saw that one or two could train as teachers in infant schools, another in fine needlework, another as a printer and so on. She sought openings for them, and answered all calls from them when they were sick or in trouble, and when she finally gave up the toy making she still concerned herself with her workers' ongoing concerns.[192]

On top of this Hill engaged in other paid employment as, more and more, she took over responsibility for her family. She was employed as secretary and teacher at a working men's college, and worked at illumination and copying in training to become an artist. The latter she did with total absorption for some ten years, as she believed this to be her calling. Her teacher was John Ruskin whom she had admired from afar, then met as part of her work at the Guild, and Hill venerated him. It is obvious that Ruskin respected her and valued their close friendship over many years. Indeed it was with a monetary benefaction from Ruskin, to further the principles of his political economy,[193] that Hill financed the rehabilitation of slum dwellings in London.[194] This is viewed by many as her major contribution to shaping the world of the urban poor.

During the first half of the 1860s all the Hill females were engaged in teaching in a residential girls school they created in their home. Not surprisingly, the school was run on communal lines, with teachers and pupils sharing work and leisure, and growing together. During the second half of that decade Hill established herself as a landlord of numerous pauper tenements within London. She set about shaping and managing them according to her very strong ideals, no doubt her initial inspiration coming from her Grandfather who had also been vitally interested in the improvement of dwellings of the "industrious classes".

Hill's vision started small. In 1864, when she was 26 she wrote:

I have long been wanting to gather near us my friends among the poor, in some houses arranged for their health and convenience. In fact a small private model lodging-house, where I may know everyone, and do something towards making their lives healthier and happier.[195]

She found difficulties in acquiring a property suitable for that purpose, because owners withdrew from the sale when they became aware of her intentions. She ended up purchasing instead, with Ruskin's money, three houses in a court named Paradise Place but which was known locally as Little Hell. In so doing she became the landlady of 'three stinking run-down tenements bursting at the seams with roughs and rowdies'.[196] The tenements were sound but in an appalling state of disrepair, with the only water available collected in open and leaking butts. The tenants, whole families who lived in a single room often with lodgers, were hostile. There was fighting and drunkenness, and children sat listlessly for long hours in the gutters. Rents were in arrears. Most people would despair in such a situation, but Hill exulted in being in a position to create a happier and healthier world for her tenants. She did not believe in charity, as she herself hated to be dependent on anyone, but did believe in fair rents and in meeting the obligations of a landlord in keeping the tenements in good repair. She provided decent water and sanitary arrangements, opened up the washhouses, whitewashed them and all the other shared spaces, repaired windows, and replaced banisters that had been taken for fuel. The only thing she insisted on was regular payment of the rents which she collected herself.

She was never molested as, by herself, she trod the tenements that burly policemen only visited in pairs. Her fairness was respected, as her interest in the tenants became apparent. She secured their cooperation as she shared with them details of her budget, and promised and delivered improvements according to their perceived needs when costs of necessary repairs had been met. She paid the older girls to clean the halls and passages and provided jobs about the tenements for those out of work, and:

… encouraged thrift and industry by starting savings banks. She organised lessons and singing classes for the children, and a working group for married women, who all met in the converted stable behind her house … She organised Christmas parties and summer outings, flower shows, cadet corps and working men's clubs. But she did everything in a way which would encourage self-improvement and discourage dependency[197]

Just as Robert Owen had done in his model village at New Lanark in Scotland,

Hill bought bulk supplies and organised a cooperative store so that her tenants could buy more cheaply. She also provided rooms for community occupations, encouraging social interaction, enjoyment, and the development of skills. 'My strongest endeavours were to be used to rouse habits of industry and effort, without which they must finally sink - and with which they might render themselves independent of me, except as a friend and leader.'[198] Hill made the occupations that took place at the School open to her tenants, and encouraged the students at the School to be responsible for some of the services offered to them. Lord Salisbury said her system was 'to improve the tenants with the tenements'.[199] The way she put it was 'steady and gradual improvement of the people and of the houses'.[200] She explained:

> I should give them any help I could, such as I might offer without insult to my other friends - sympathy in their distresses, advice, help and counsel in their difficulties, introductions that might be of use to them; means of education; visits to the country; a loan of books; a bunch of flowers brought on purpose, an invitation to any entertainment, in a room built at the back of my own house[201]

Overcoming intense opposition and sabotage by other locals, she had a playground made for the children of one of her tenements, and herself spent at least four hours a day for many weeks inspiring and teaching them to play. It was so difficult to overcome their occupational deprivation that she said each day felt 'like so many years', but eventually the children did learn to play, and then became the teachers of the other locals who were invited to join them.[202]

As time went on, by inspiring and training many women in her methods, Hill established far-reaching programmes and influenced social reforms. She published reports on her work and wrote regularly to her fellow workers as part of that process. In a report published in 1869 Hill wrote:

> It is essential to remember that each man has his own view of his life, and must be free to fulfil it; that in many ways he is a far better judge of it than we, as he has lived through and felt what we have only seen. Our work is rather to bring him to the point of considering, and the spirit of judging rightly, than to consider or judge for him[203]

Throughout her life Hill worked so hard that several times she suffered major breakdowns of health, but after time out came back with renewed vigour and more schemes. Her methods were copied in many European countries and in America. At the time of her death she was managing nearly 2,000 houses and flats, and in London today there are still 1,300 houses being managed by the Octavia Hill Housing Trust.

Her idyllic rural childhood, the visits to the countryside with the children of the toy factory, and the establishment of the playground were the foundations for Hill's later battles to save open spaces within cities and country alike so that people had room to breathe, play, recreate and rejoice in the open air. In establishing the National Trust she worked with Robert Hunter of the Commons Preservation Society and with Canon Rawnsley from the English Lake District. Rawnsley had been one of her housing managers in Drury Lane when he was a curate, and it was his housekeeper was so central in the Langdale Linen Company.

Hill's work and ideology were the result of a culmination of influences, all of which embodied ideals about meeting social health needs closely aligned with the occupational natures of people. She is attributed with being a founder of several modern professions including housing management and social work as well as the National Trust, but her links to occupational therapy are only now being recognised and acknowledged within the Octavia Hill Society, and the College of Occupational Therapists. Hill certainly influenced Elizabeth Casson who worked with her as a housing manager early in the twentieth century and who went on to found the first Occupational Therapy School in the United Kingdom. Casson, undoubtedly, carried the values of the nineteenth century social activists discussed in this chapter into her life's work, which will be discussed in the second volume. Occupational therapists can also claim a link with Hill through her influence on the Settlement movement which inspired Jane Addams, an American she met, to set up a Settlement House in Chicago. This house provided the ideology and the venue for the first formal occupational therapy education in the USA.

Before progressing to the story of Jane Addams, a slight detour to Toynbee Hall is warranted, as that Social Settlement appears to have played a part on both sides of the Atlantic in the history being told.

Toynbee Hall

Henrietta Octavia Rowland (1851-1936), an early fellow worker and friend of Octavia Hill, met her husband, the Rev. Samuel A. Barnett (1844-1913), when she had work in connection with St Mary's, Bryanston Square where he was curate. Knowing of Hill's religious persuasion it is perhaps not surprising that Rowland, too, was ardent in the cause of Christian Socialism. Following their marriage in 1873, Rowland matched the young clergyman with experience, zeal, and enthusiasm for the task that lay ahead of them. Together they were to co-author several important texts such as *Practical Socialism* and *Towards Social Reform*, and start the Children's Country Holiday Movement.[204]

Barnett was inspired at Oxford to make his home in the East End of London amongst the poor, whilst maintaining the way of life he and countless others had followed at University. A major influence at Oxford had been Ruskin, who held the post of Slade Professor of the Fine Arts for a time. During that tenure, Ruskin constantly discussed economic and ethical questions in his lectures, and was renowned for his unconventional approach. Once, for example, he set a party of students to mending a road that had fallen into bad repair to illustrate the dignity of labour.

The lasting ties of University friendship were to continue throughout Barnett's life.[205] In 1873, at his wish, he became Vicar of St Jude's, Whitechapel, which the Bishop of London described as 'the worst in his diocese'. Then in 1884 he was appointed as the first warden of Toynbee Hall, a house of residence for men from Oxford and Cambridge who wished to take part in the life of East London and its improvement. Known as a Social Settlement, it was the first of about 50 similar residential settlements throughout Britain.[206]

Barnett held the conviction:
> ... that the things which make men alike are finer and better than the things that keep them apart, and that these basic likenesses, if they are properly accentuated, easily transcend the less essential differences of race, language, creed and tradition.[207]

He expected that the kinds of work that had been carried out by University men in London, would be the sort of activity expected of members of the Settlement. Those that seem most appropriate to this history are listed below:

- *Visiting the inmates of workhouses, whether those who are past work and cannot hope to leave the House again, or those who may yet become self-supporting.*
- *Visiting the casual wards and attempting to rescue the better of their inmates from the company of the depraved.*
- *Attendance in working-men's and boys' clubs; joining in conversation and discussion, helping in entertainments and excursions, conducting men and boys over museums and picture galleries, etc., on Saturday afternoons.*
- *Promoting good musical entertainments or art exhibitions; promoting the opening or beautifying of squares and other spaces.*
- *Advising and assisting boys who have just left reformatory schools; making the necessary arrangements for families about to emigrate, or for persons going to hospitals or convalescent homes; visiting the aged poor and administering pensions to them when pensions have been procured by societies or individuals; arranging and conducting children's excursions, or helping in the scheme recently set on foot for giving children a longer stay in the country; and in other ways carrying out in detail such plans for the welfare of the poor as experienced persons think desirable.*
- *Various kinds of social intercourse, participation in amusements or entertainments, &c.*[208]

Barnett was later to reflect on the twenty-six years since he and his wife established their home in Whitechapel, saying that they had been attracted by 'its poverty and ambitious to fight it in its strongest fortress'. They had found the poor 'in want of more adequate relief', and 'in want of more self-reliance'. Many appeared dependent with 'no heart to make any efforts, regarding gifts with more favour than wages, and with hopes set on begging rather than on earning'. He described many of his neighbours as pauperised - restricting the use of the term to people who were 'incapable of effort and timid of change'.[209]

The residence he founded and led as warden for 12 years was to inspire Jane Addams, and contribute to the establishment of Social Settlements in the United States. Indeed he and his wife were among the earliest visitors to Hull House.[210]

Jane Addams: Occupation and social activism for social health

Jane Addams was born in 1860 into a well-to-do family in Illinios. She is reported to have had a 'normal, active, rural childhood', eventually graduating from Rockford with one of the first bachelors degrees awarded by the College. After rejecting the thought of marriage and a family, which she believed was not possible to combine with a career, and finding that medicine was not for her, she took a few years to discover the important calling she had determined upon at a young age. It was during her second visit to Europe with Ellen Gates Starr, a co-founder, that she decided to establish a Settlement House.[211]

Addams found herself fascinated by the mission work going on in London, and especially by Toynbee Hall. She told her sister Alice:

> It is a community for University men who live there, have their recreation and clubs and society all among the poor people, yet in the same style they would live in their own circle … It is so free of "professional doing good," so unaffectedly sincere and so productive of good results in its classes and libraries so that it seems perfectly ideal.[212]

The visit to the Settlement acted as a catalyst and Addams vowed to establish something similar in a poor section of Chicago on her return to America. Her vision was to work with the poor, sharing and improving the neighbourhood[213] and working 'to provide a centre for a higher civic and social life; to institute and maintain educational and philanthropic enterprises, and to investigate and improve the conditions in the industrial districts of Chicago'.[214] Although Hull House borrowed something from Toynbee Hall, it was part of a national movement in which more than four hundred social settlements were established in American cities by 1911. Its founders were unaware of others when they made their decision, but on learning about the New York settlement they saw their venture as part of the wider crusade.[215]

The works of Ruskin and Morris, whose photographs were later to have pride of place at Hull House, also influenced Addams. She knew of various of Ruskin's projects aimed at helping the working class and had read his *Unto This Last*, which in *100 Years at Hull House*, was described as 'the little book in which he indignantly attacked the evils of the industrial city and sketched out a reform program'.[216] Addams was also familiar with works of other social reformers in Britain. These ranged from Carlyle to the Christian Socialists, who she saw as confronting the problems created by the urban, industrial age, and in their own ways attempting to spiritually awaken the intellectual as well as the working class. In that regard, it is interesting to note that Addams recognised how, despite a young life apparently filled with diverse and interesting occupations, she, herself, had experienced some occupational dissatisfaction. When mentioning that in a paper given to the Ethical Culture Societies in Plymouth, Massachusetts in 1892 she explained that her involvement in the Settlement Movement was to redress such problems at both ends of the social divide. Applying her own experience to that of other educated young people, Addams was aware that lack of occupational opportunity was not restricted to the poor. She reported that her own life, 'so sincere in its emotion and good phrases and yet so undirected, seems to me as pitiful as the other great mass of destitute lives'. She felt that because of the social and occupational expectations of their class, gender, or both, the well-to-do had 'been shut off from the common labor by which they live which is a great source of moral and physical health. They feel a fatal want of harmony in their lives, a lack of coordination between thought and action'. The latter, she argued, could be provided if they were given 'a proper outlet for active faculties'.[217][218]

Such beliefs led to Addams and Starr being involved with others in the establishment of the Chicago Arts and Crafts Society.[219] In doing this they followed the lead of Charles Norton, the first professor of fine arts at Harvard, who is credited with transporting his close friend Ruskin's, and Morris's ideologies to America. There, because the Puritan work ethic was so central to American culture, their conceptualisation of a "pre-industrial craftsperson" found 'particularly fertile ground'. However the Trans-Atlantic interpretation of their work made little distinction between modern and pre-industrial work habits, and the Arts and Crafts ideology became largely interpreted from an individualistic rather than a social focus. Lears suggests that 'American craft leaders were neither as articulate nor as clear headed as Ruskin and Morris', and that they:

> ... were hampered from the outset by their class interests and anxieties, their individualist and idealist assumptions about the nature of social reform, and above all by their own underlying ambivalence toward modern culture and its progressive creed. Like many of their British counterparts, they allowed their quest for wholeness to centre on the self alone. The ideal of joyful labor, when it was not submerged by aestheticism, became a means of personal revitalisation rather than a path to renewed community. In part a reaction against therapeutic self-absorption, the revival of handicraft ultimately became another form of therapy for an overcivilised bourgeoisie.[220]

At Hull House, Addams accepted the inevitability of the industrial system, and sought to revitalise working class lives by education towards personal fulfilment outside of work,[221] and Starr sought to enable immigrants to find solace in art.[222] They followed the creed adopted by other Arts and Crafts' leaders and progressive contemporaries and echoed the catch cry of much of the 19th century,[223] that 'labor! all labor is noble and holy'.[224] Their stance was largely inevitable as, in the new roles being undertaken by women, it made sense for them to establish positions in which they could exercise and demonstrate previously untapped capacities and potential in a way that was adaptive, socially accepted, and politically expedient. Even if they recognised that massive social change was called for, establishing themselves as professionals, and bringing a feminine, caring, moral viewpoint to the workforce was, in itself, sufficiently challenging.[225]

The Ruskin and Morris influence, though, did inspire the establishment of a "Labor Museum" at Hull House. Here the leaders planned to preserve the great array of artistic talent and craft skill that immigrants had brought with them to America, which was rapidly becoming extinct. The younger generations had little appreciation of their seniors' skills and artistic heritage, especially as they were often employed in meaningless uncreative jobs. So, to restore confidence and pride in their cultural background some of the older skilled artisans were employed as teachers.[226]

That initiative probably fostered the idea of a programme directly related to this history. Hull House was, in the next century, to provide classes for attendants and nurses of the insane to learn about "invalid occupations". In 1908, the first Special Course in Curative Occupations and Recreation was offered at the hands of Julia Lathrop, Rabbi Hirsch and Dr Graham Taylor.[227] This course was a forerunner to the Henry B. Favill School of Occupations, which started in 1915 and continued until 1920, and is said to be the first formal school of occupational therapy.[228] It incorporated a programme of study in curative occupations and recreation, having developed from a Community Workshop for cases of 'doubtful insanity' whom the courts considered might return to usefulness if given a 'proper environment and trade'.[229,230]

In summary, the ideologies that emerged during the industrial revolution provide the foundation for the idea that occupation could be used to maintain and restore health, which is the essence of twentieth century occupational therapy. In Britain they were both philosophies relating to the very nature of societies themselves, and the need for individuals to grow and develop their individual potentialities. In the United States of America, on the other hand, the individual message was stronger, and it was that view which eventually pervaded much of occupational therapy. The issues, which will be considered a little more in chapter twelve, colour the history of occupation in physical health and in mental health which are the subject of the next chapters.

[1]Jones B. Sleepers, Wake! Technology and the Future of Work. Melbourne: Oxford University Press, 1995; 11-13.
[2]Jones. Sleepers, Wake!…; 11-13.
[3]Random House. Timetables of History. 2nd revised edition. New York: Random House, 1996.
[4]Hobsbawn EJ. The Age of Revolution 1789-1848. New York: World Publishing Co., A Mentor Book, 1962; 250.
[5]Jones. Sleepers, Wake!
[6]Hobsbawn. The Age of Revolution.

[7]Girling DA, ed. New Age Encyclopedia. Sydney and London: Bay Books, 1983; vol 6: 203.

[8]Jones E. A Prisoners Drawings, Tuthill Fields, 1849. London: British Library: Add MS 61971A, ff 28 & 29 EJ.

[9]Hobsbawn. The Age of Revolution…; 226.

[10]Dickens C. Hard Times. Australia: Penguin, 1981; Introduction: 24-5.

[11]Bentham J. Fragments on Government. 1776. In: Burns JH, Hart HLA, eds. A Comment on the Commentaries; and, Fragment of Government. London: Athlone Press, 1977.

[12]Thompson EP. The Making of the English Working Class. London: Penguin, 1963; 295-6. (quote of Assistant Commissioner of the Poor Law).

[13]Clear C. Nuns in Nineteenth Century Ireland. Dublin: Gill & Macmillan, 1987; 8.

[14]Jones. Sleepers, Wake!…; 20.

[15]O'Connor J. The Workhouses of Ireland: The Fate of Ireland's Poor. Dublin: Anvil Books, 1995; 103.

[16]O'Connor. The Workhouses of Ireland.

[17]O'Connor. The Workhouses of Ireland…; 225.

[18]O'Connor. The Workhouses of Ireland…; 103.

[19]Magray MP. The Transforming Power of the Nuns: Women, Religion, and Cultural Change in Ireland, 1750-1900. New York/Oxford: Oxford University Press, 1998; 78-79.

[20]Magray. The Transforming Power of the Nuns.

[21]Cited in: Daly MF. The Church and the Second Sex. London: Geoffrey Chapman, 1968; 66.

[22]Clear. Nuns in Nineteenth Century Ireland…; 138.

[23]Blagden IJ. Freeman's Journal. 11th June, 1853.

[24]Anderson EG. Fortnightly Review. NS, xv: London: 1874; 590.

[25]Magray. The Transforming Power of the Nuns…; 128.

[26]Abstract of reports of inspectors of reformatory and industrial schools - Ireland 1871-83, File Monaghan, St.L/M. In: Magray. The Transforming Power of the Nuns…; 101.

[27]Official annals, vol 3, Benada Convent, 1863, SOC/M. In: Magray. The Transforming Power of the Nuns…; 101.

[28]Official annals, vol 3, Benada Convent, 1863…; 101.

[29]Clear. Nuns in Nineteenth Century Ireland…; 29.

[30]Clear. Nuns in Nineteenth Century Ireland…; 14.

[31]Buret E. De la misere des classes laborieuses en Angleterre et en France, 2 vols. Paris: 1840; vol 1: 36-7. In: Livingstone R, Benton G, trans. Karl Marx Early Writings. London: Penguin Classics; 293.

[32]Jones. Sleepers, Wake!…; 20.

[33]Schulz W. Die Bewegung der Produktion, eine geshichtlich-statische Abhandlung. Zurich and Winterthur: 1843; 65. In: Livingstone & Benton. Karl Marx Early Writings…; 291.

[34]Children and Young Persons' Act, 1933.

[35]Schulz. Die Bewegung der Produktion…; 65. In: Livingstone & Benton. Karl Marx Early Writings…; 291.

[36]Marti-Ibañez F, ed. Henry E. Sigerist on the History of Medicine. New York: MD Publications, Inc., 1960.

[37]Buret. De la misere des classes laborieuses…; vol 1: 362. In: Livingstone & Benton. Karl Marx Early Writings…; 292, 294-5.

[38]Buret. De la misere des classes laborieuses…; vol 1: 20. In: Livingstone & Benton. Karl Marx Early Writings…; 292.

[39]Campbell Bradley I. Victorian values: Titus Salt: Enlightened entrepreneur. History Today. May 1987; 30-36.

[40]Salt T. Address at the Opening of Saltaire's Mill. Cited in: Campbell Bradley. Victorian values: Titus Salt...; 33.

[41]Salt T. Circular on Saltaire's institute. Cited in: Campbell Bradley. Victorian values: Titus Salt...; 33.

[42]Campbell Bradley. Victorian values: Titus Salt...; 30-36.

[43]Staines J. Romanticism: An idea and its legacy. The Hutchinson Dictionary of Ideas. Oxford: Helicon, 1995; 453.

[44]Marlo K. Cited in Weiss J. Conservatism in Europe 1770-1945: Traditionalism, Reaction and Counter-Revolution. London: Thames and Hudson, 1977; 61.

[45]Marlo. Cited in Weiss. Conservatism in Europe 1770-1945...; 63.

[46]Marlo. Cited in Weiss. Conservatism in Europe 1770-1945...; 63.

[47]Weiss. Conservatism in Europe 1770-1945...; 64.

[48]Harvey, Sir P, ed. The Oxford Companion to English Literature, 4th edition. London: Oxford University Press, 1967; 310.

[49]Fourier C. Theory of the Four Movements, 1808 [1968], Oeuvres de Charles Fourier, vol 1 Paris: Editions Anthropos; Le Nouveau Monde Industriel et Societaire. 1829.

[50]Weiss. Conservatism in Europe 1770-1945...; 60.

[51]Proudhon PJ. The Philosophy of Misery. 1846.

[52]Ostergaard G, Proudhon P-J. In: Bottomore T, ed. A Dictionary of Marxist Thought. 2nd ed. Oxford, UK: Blackwell Publishers, 1983; 451-452.

[53]Weiss. Conservatism in Europe 1770-1945...; 60.

[54]The details of this story are based on Cole's description for The Robert Owen Bicentenial Association: Cole M. Robert Owen until after New Lanark. In: Robert Owen: Industrialist Reformer, Visionary, 1771-1858. London: Robert Owen Bicentenary Association, 1971.

[55]Owen R, the Socialist. Essay on the Principle of the Formation of Character etc. London: Cadell & Davies, 1813.

[56]Owen R. The address to the inhabitants of New Lanark. The Institute for the Formation of Character. January 1st 1816. In: Owen R. Works of Robert Owen: Volume 1 (Pickering Masters Series). London: Pickering & Chatto (Publishers Ltd.), 1993; 120-142.

[57]Harrison J. Robert Owen and the communities. In: Robert Owen: Industrialist...; 27.

[58]Owen R. Report to the Committee of the Association for the Relief of the Manufacturing and Labouring Poor. 1817.

[59]Owen R. Report to the County of Lanark. 1820.

[60]Harrison. Robert Owen and the communities...; 27.

[61]Harrison. Robert Owen and the communities...; 27.

[62]Owen R. Works of Robert Owen: Volume 3: Book of the New Moral World. (Pickering Masters Series). London: Pickering & Chatto (Publishers Ltd.), 1993; 156.

[63]Owen. Works of Robert Owen: Volume 3...; 156.

[64]Owen. Works of Robert Owen: Volume 3...; 157.

[65]Owen R. Paper: Dedicated to the Governments of Great Britain, Austria, Russia, France, Prussia and the United States of America. London, 1841. (New Lanark Conservation).

[66]Owen. Paper: Dedicated to the Governments.

[67]Owen. Paper: Dedicated to the Governments.

[68]Guy Rev Dr JR. Compassion and the Art of the Possible: Dr. Southwood Smith as Social Reformer and Public Health Pioneer. Octavia Hill Memorial Lecture. December 1993. Cambridgeshire: Octavia Hill Society & The Birthplace Museum Trust, 1996; 2-4.

[69]Guy. Compassion and the Art of the Possible...; 13.

[70]Southwood Smith. Address to Select Commission of the House of Commons. London:

1840. Cited in: Guy. Compassion and the Art of the Possible…; 14.

[71]Guy. Compassion and the Art of the Possible…; 15.

[72]Fischer E. Marx in his Own Words. London: The Penguin Press, 1970.

[73]Staines J. Romanticism: An idea and its legacy. The Hutchinson Dictionary of Ideas…; 453.

[74]Bentham J. An introduction to the principle of morals and legislation. 1789. In: Burns JH, Hart HLA, eds. The Collected Works of Jeremy Bentham. Oxford: Clarendon, 1996.

[75]Southwood Smith T. A Lecture Delivered Over the Remains of Jeremy Bentham, Esq., In the Webb-Street School of Anatomy and Medicine on the 9th June, 1832. London: Effingham Wilson, 1832: 72, footnote.

[76]Southwood Smith. A Lecture Delivered Over the Remains of Jeremy Bentham…; 30.

[77]Fischer. Marx in his Own Words.

[78]Schiller F. On the Aesthetic Education of Man, in a Series of Letters. Wilkinson EM, Willoughby LA, Trans. Clarendon Press, Oxford, 1967; Sixth letter; 35.

[79]Carlyle T. Signs of the times. 1829. Cited in: Craig D, ed. Introduction to Dickens C. Hard Times. London: Penguin, 1981; 25.

[80]Harvey. The Oxford Companion to English Literature…; 145.

[81]Carlyle T. Past & present: Work. 1843. In: Knight C. Half Hours with the Best Authors. London: Frederick Warne & Co., circa 1900; p. 220.

[82]Carlyle. In: Knight. Half Hours with the Best Authors…; 221.

[83]Says JB. Traite d'economie politique. 1903.

[84]Ricardo D. Principles of Political Economy and Taxation. 1817.

[85]Cohen B. John Stuart Mill (1806-73). In: Kuper A, Kuper J, eds. The Social Science Encyclopedia. London and New York: Routledge, 1989; 527.

[86]Mill JS. Utilitarianism. 1863.

[87]Mill JS. On Liberty. 1859.

[88]Mill JS. On the Subjection of Women. 1869.

[89]Norton AL, ed. John Stuart Mill. The Hutchinson Dictionary of Ideas. Oxford: Helicon, 1995; 350.

[90]Cohen. In: Kuper & Kuper. The Social Science Encyclopedia…; 527.

[91]See for example: Argyle M. The Psychology of Happiness. New York: Methuen & Co., 1987; Strack F, Argyle M, Schartz N, eds. Subjective Well-Being: An Interdisciplinary Perspective. Oxford: Pergamon Press, 1991.

[92]Wilcock AA. An Occupational Perspective of Health. Thorofare, NJ: Slack Inc, 1998.

[93]Bottomore. A Dictionary of Marxist Thought.

[94]Norton. The Hutchinson Dictionary of Ideas…; 197.

[95]Bottomore. A Dictionary of Marxist Thought.

[96]Cieskowski A. Prolegamena zur Historiosophie. Berlin: Viet, 1838.

[97]Hess M. The European Triarchy (1842) and in Philosophy of Action.

[98]Marx K. Thesis on Feuerbach. First published by Engels as appendix to Ludwig Feuerbach and the End of Classical German philosophy, 1888 1845.

[99]McLellan D. Karl Heinrich Marx. In: Bottomore. A Dictionary of Marxist Thought…; 340-343.

[100]Marx K. The Difference Between the Democritean and Epicurean Philosophy of Nature. Doctoral dissertation; pt. 1, ch. IV.

[101]Markovic M. Human nature. In: Bottomore. A Dictionary of Marxist Thought…; 243-246.

[102]Markovic. Human nature. In: Bottomore. A Dictionary of Marxist Thought…; 245.

[103]Petrovic G. Praxis. In: Bottomore. Fischer. Marx in his Own Words…; 435.

[104]Bottomore TB, trans and ed. Karl Marx: Early Writings. London: C.A. Watts, 1963; 127-128.

[105]Marx K. Capital 1. 1867. Moscow: Foreign Languages Publishing House, 1959. Great Britain: Lawrence & Wishart; 799-800.

[106]Economic and Philosophical Manuscripts and German Ideology Grundrisse and Capital.

[107]Fischer. Marx in his Own Words…; 20.

[108]Fischer. Marx in his Own Words…; 37-51.

[109]Petrovic G. Alienation. In: Bottomore. Marx in his Own Words…; 11-16.

[110]Marx. Economic and Philosophical Manuscripts, 1844. In: Bottomore. Karl Marx: Early Writings.

[111]Mohun S. Division of labour. In: A Dictionary of Marxist Thought…; 155.

[112]Marx. Capital…; 422-424.

[113]Fischer. Marx in his Own Words…; 43-44.

[114] Fischer. Marx in his Own Words…; 43-44.

[115]Engels F. The Condition of the Working Class in England. Leipzig: Otto Wigand, 1845.

[116]Jones GS. Friedrich Engels. In: A Dictionary of Marxist Thought…; 176-177.

[117] Rich P. Victorian values: The quest for Englishness. History Today. June 1987; 25.

[118]Yates N. Victorian values: Pugin and the medieval dream. History Today. September 1987; 33-40.

[119]Rich P. Victorian values: The quest for Englishness. History Today. June 1987; 25.

[120]Yates. Victorian values: Pugin and the medieval dream.

[121]Burd VA, ed. The Ruskin Family Letters. 2 volumes. Cornell University Press, 1973; 209.

[122]Cook ET, Wedderburn A, eds. The Library Edition of the Works of John Ruskin. 39 volumes. London, 1903-12; vol 1: 383-384.

[123]Hunt JD. The Wider Sea: A Life of John Ruskin. London: Phoenix /Orion Books 1998; 74. (First published in GB by JM Dent & Sons Ltd in 1982).

[124]Cook & Wedderburn. The Library Edition of the Works of John Ruskin…; 454.

[125]Cook & Wedderburn. The Library Edition of the Works of John Ruskin…; 259.

[126]Cook & Wedderburn. The Library Edition of the Works of John Ruskin…; 389.

[127]Cook & Wedderburn. The Library Edition of the Works of John Ruskin…; 376-7.

[128]Cook & Wedderburn. The Library Edition of the Works of John Ruskin…; 68-9.

[129]Hunt JD. The Wider Sea…; 119-122.

[130]Harvey. The Oxford Companion to English Literature…; 716.

[131]Jackson Lears TJ. No Place of Grace: Antimodernism and the Transformation of American Culture 1880-1920. New York: Pantheon Books; 1981.

[132]Harvey. The Oxford Companion to English Literature…; 716.

[133]Rowbotham S. Victorian values: Commanding the heart, Edward Carpenter and friends. History Today, September, 1987; 41-46.

[134]Hamilton J (Duchess of), Hart P, Simmons J. The Gardens of William Morris. NSW, Australia: Hodder Headline Australia Pty. Ltd., 1998; 32.

[135]Rollinson W. The Lake District: Life and Traditions. London: Weidenfeld & Nicolson, 1996; 21.

[136]Gough J. The Manners and Customs of Westmorland and Adjoining Parts of Cumberland, Lancashire and Yorkshire. Kendal: 1912.

[137]Marsh J. The Westmorland Lakes: In Old Photographs. Stroud, Gloustershire: Alan Sutton Publishing Ltd, 1992. (Rawnsley was a co-founder of the National Trust with Octavia Hill).

[138]Denyer S, Martin J. A Century in the Lake District. London: The National Trust, 1995; 37.

[139]Marsh. The Westmorland Lakes: In Old Photographs.…; 2, 79.

[140]Jackson Lears. No Place of Grace.

[141]McCree-Bryan ML, Davis AF, eds. One Hundred Years at Hull House. Bloomington &

Indianapolis: Indiana University Press, 1990.

[142]Hamilton, Hart & Simmons. The Gardens of William Morris…; 27.

[143]Hamilton, Hart & Simmons. The Gardens of William Morris…; 28.

[144]Hamilton, Hart & Simmons. The Gardens of William Morris…; 32.

[145]MacCarthy F. William Morris: A Life for Our Time. New York: Faber & Faber, 1994; 69.

[146]MacCarthy. William Morris: A Life for Our Time…; 70.

[147]Ruskin J. The Stones of Venice. Vol. 2. 1853. Cited in: MacCarthy. William Morris: A Life for Our Time…; 71.

[148]MacCarthy. William Morris: A Life for Our Time…; 71.

[149]Hamilton, Hart & Simmons. The Gardens of William Morris…; 42.

[150]Hamilton, Hart & Simmons. The Gardens of William Morris…; 47-48, 67.

[151]Morris W. Art and socialism. In: Morton AL, ed. Political Writings of William Morris. London: Lawrence and Wishart; 110-111.

[152]Jackson Lears. No Place of Grace.

[153]Hamilton, Hart & Simmons. The Gardens of William Morris…; 80.

[154]Hamilton, Hart & Simmons. The Gardens of William Morris…; 81.

[155]Morris W. Useful work versus useless toil. In: Cole GDH, ed. Centenary Edition. William Morris. Stories in Prose. Stories in Verse. Shorter Poems. Lectures and Essays. New York: Edited for Nonesuch Press, Bloomsbury. Random House, 1934; 609.

[156]Morris. Useful work versus useless toil. In: Cole…; 609.

[157]Morris. Useful work versus useless toil. In: Cole…; 603-604.

[158]Morris. Useful work versus useless toil. In: Cole…; 604-605.

[159]Morris. Useful work versus useless toil. In: Cole…; 616.

[160]Morris. Useful work versus useless toil. In: Cole…; 610.

[161]Morris. Useful work versus useless toil. In: Cole…; 608.

[162]MacCarthy. William Morris: A Life for our Time…; 484.

[163]Jackson Lears. No Place of Grace.

[164]Hamilton, Hart & Simmons. The Gardens of William Morris…; 84.

[165]MacCarthy. William Morris: A Life for our Time…; Introduction, vii.

[166]Hamilton, Hart & Simmons. The Gardens of William Morris…; 84.

[167]Wrigley C. Historians and their times: The Webbs: Working on trade union history. History Today. May, 1987; 51-55.

[168]MacCarthy. William Morris: A Life for our Time…; Introduction, xvi.

[169]MacCarthy. William Morris: A Life for our Time…; Introduction, xvii.

[170]MacCarthy. William Morris: A Life for our Time…; Introduction, xviii.

[171]Rowbotham S. Victorian values: Commanding the heart…; 41-46.

[172]Wollstonecraft M. A Vindication of Rights of Women. London: J. Johnson, 1792. Reprint with introduction by Kramnick MB, ed. Harmondsworth, England: Penguin Books, 1975.

[173]Mackarness Mrs H. The Young Lady's Book: A Manual of Amusements, Exercises, Studies and Pursuits. London: George Routledge and Sons, 1876; 465.

[174]Mackarness. The Young Lady's Book…; 1, 5, 10.

[175]Mackarness. The Young Lady's Book…; 8.

[176]Mackarness. The Young Lady's Book…; 264.

[177]Mackarness. The Young Lady's Book…; 465.

[178]Hoggart R, ed. Oxford Illustrated Encyclopedia of People and Cultures. Oxford: Oxford University Press, 1992; 256.

[179]Girling. New Age Encyclopedia…; vol 12: 58.

[180]Isaacs A, ed. Macmillan Encyclopedia. London: Macmillan, 1990; 476.

[181]Henderson DK. The Evolution of Psychiatry in Scotland. Edinburgh and London: E &

S Livingstone Ltd, 1964; 82.

[182]Macdonald EM. World-Wide Conquests of Disabilities: The History, Development and Present Functions of the Remedial Services. London: Bailliere Tindall, 1981; 89.

[183]Girling. New Age Encyclopedia…; vol 12: 58.

[184]Girling. New Age Encyclopedia…; vol 12: 58.

[185]Henderson. The Evolution of Psychiatry in Scotland…; 82.

[186]This story was told as part of the 1999 Sylvia Docker Lecture. The Australian Association of Occupational Therapists Conference. Published: Wilcock AA. Creating self and shaping the world. Australian Occupational Therapy Journal, 1999, 46(3): 77-88.

[187]Moberly Bell E. Octavia Hill; A Biography. From a typescript version made with permission of Constable and Co, available at the Octavia Hill Birthplace Trust, Wisbech, 1986; 7.

[188]Hill CS. Memoranda of Observations and Experiments in Education. London: Vizetelly & Co, 1865: 15-27.

[189]Whelan R, ed. Octavia Hill and the Social Housing Debate. London: IEA Health and Welfare Unit, 1998; 3-4.

[190]Moberly Bell. Octavia Hill…; 19.

[191]Moberly Bell. Octavia Hill.

[192]Moberly Bell. Octavia Hill.

[193]Hunt. The Wider Sea.

[194]Isaacs. Macmillan Encyclopedia…; 574.

[195]Letter to Mrs William Shaen. In: Darley G. Octavia Hill: A Biography. London: Constable, 1942; 75.

[196]Whelan. Octavia Hill and the Social Housing Debate…; 5.

[197]Whelan. Octavia Hill and the Social Housing Debate…; 6.

[198]Hill O. Cited in: Whelan. Octavia Hill and the Social Housing Debate…; 6.

[199]Salisbury Lord. Article in the National Review 1883. Cited in Darley G. Octavia Hill: A Biography…; 225.

[200]Hill O. Management of houses for the poor. Charity Organisation Review, January 1899; 25, (new series); 21.

[201]Hill. Cited in: Whelan. Octavia Hill and the Social Housing Debate…; 7.

[202]Moberly Bell. Octavia Hill.

[203]Hill O. Four years management of a London Court. In: Whelan. Octavia Hill and the Social Housing Debate…; 64. (First published in MacMillans Magazine, July 1869).

[204]Girling. New Age Encyclopedia…; vol 3: 154.

[205]Aitken WF. Canon Barnett, Warden of Toynbee Hall: His Mission and its Relation to Social Movements. London: S.W. Partridge & Co., 1902; 28.

[206]Girling. New Age Encyclopedia…; vol 26: 138.

[207]Samuel A. Barnett (1844-1913), English clergyman who founded the first social settlement, Toynbee Hall, Whitechapel, London, and the one after which Hull House was patterned.

[208]Aitken. Canon Barnett, Warden of Toynbee Hall…; 130-131.

[209]Aitken. Canon Barnett, Warden of Toynbee Hall…; 131.

[210]Bryan & Davis. 100 Years at Hull House…; 61.

[211]Bryan & Davis. 100 Years at Hull House…; 1-4.

[212]Bryan & Davis. 100 Years at Hull House…; 4.

[213]Bryan & Davis. 100 Years at Hull House…; 4, 6.

[214]Bryan & Davis. 100 Years at Hull House…; 15.

[215]Bryan & Davis. 100 Years at Hull House…; 5.

[216] Bryan & Davis. 100 Years at Hull House…; 4.

[217]Addams J. The Subjective Necessity for Social Settlements. Plymouth, Massachusetts: Paper to the Ethical Culture Societies, 1892.

[218]Wilcock. An Occupational Perspective of Health…; 174-175.

[219]Jackson Lears. No place of Grace…; 67.

[220]MacCarthy. William Morris: A Life for Our Time…; 604.

[221]Jackson Lears. No place of Grace…; 79-80.

[222]Starr EG. Art and labor. In: Addams J. Hull House Maps and Papers. NewYork: Thomas Y. Crowell, 1895.

[223]See, for example: Link AS, McCormick RL. Progressivism. Arlington Heights, Illinois: Harlan Davidson, Inc., 1983; Resek C, ed. The Progressives. Indianopolis and New York: The Bobbs-Merrill Company, Inc., 1967.

[224]Pressey EP. New Clairvaux Plantation, Training School, Industries and Settlement. Country Time and Tide 3; February 1903: 121-22; This community was named after St Bernard of Clairvaux, a 12th century hero of simplicity.

[225]Wilcock. An Occupational Perspective of Health.

[226]Washburne MF. A labor museum. In: Bryan & Davis. 100 Years at Hull House…; 74.

[227]Breines E. Origins and Adaptations: A Philosophy of Practice. Lebanon, NJ: Geri-Rehab, Inc, 1986.

[228]Henry B Favill was a Chicago physician with an interest in social issues.

[229]Favill J. Henry Baird Favill: 1860-1916. Chicago: Rand McNally, 1917; 87.

[230]Wilcock. An Occupational Perspective of Health.

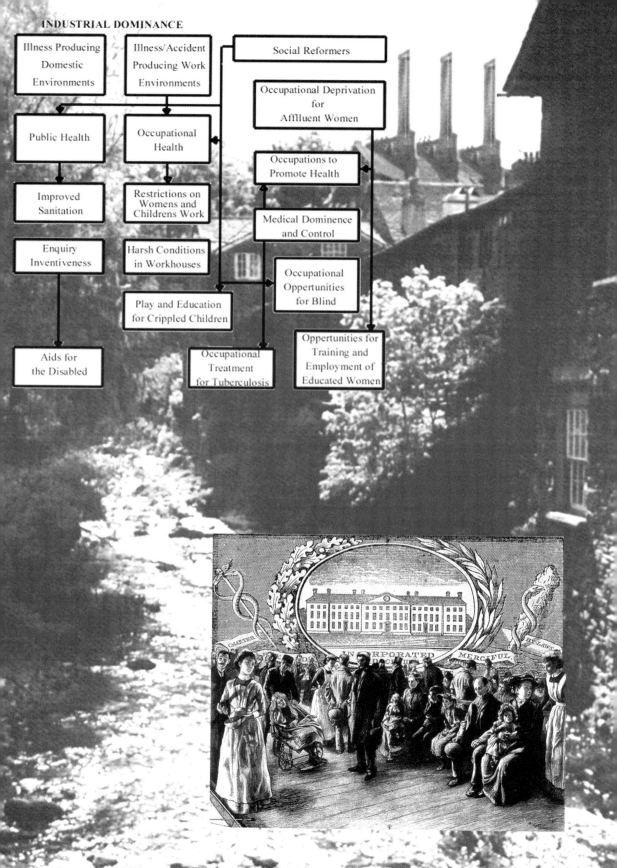

INDUSTRIAL DOMINANCE

- Illness Producing Domestic Environments
- Illness/Accident Producing Work Environments
- Social Reformers
- Occupational Deprivation for Affluent Women

- Public Health
- Occupational Health
- Occupations to Promote Health

- Improved Sanitation
- Restrictions on Womens and Childrens Work
- Medical Dominence and Control

- Enquiry Inventiveness
- Harsh Conditions in Workhouses
- Occupational Oppertunities for Blind

- Play and Education for Crippled Children

- Aids for the Disabled
- Occupational Treatment for Tuberculosis
- Oppertunities for Training and Employment of Educated Women

Chapter 10

Occupation for Physical Health In Industrial Times

Contents

The image many people hold of physical health and well-being during the industrial times of the nineteenth century is of unwashed, puny, debilitated, enfeebled individuals who were susceptible to infections and subject to mechanical injury as a result of unsafe environments. Quite rightly, that picture points to the importance of public health initiatives to correct inequities in work practices and to change domestic and industrial environments so that they were cleaner and safer. As some occupational therapists are employed in that area, it is appropriate to look at the history of that development.

There is also a more reassuring picture of the health care of the period. The literature of the time portrays family doctors charitably ministering to the needs of the poor, knowing everyone, and caring enough to ride out in the dead of night to work through the "crisis" of a child dying of pneumonia. It is a time, somewhat sentimentally viewed, when a more holistic notion of health was part and parcel of medical care, with doctors being seen as wise counsellors, and friendly authorities on all aspects of what would be good for people in their everyday lives. A period just before the miracles of modern medicine but with similar ideology it is likely that some burgeoning of 20th century occupational therapy practices may be visible. Indeed, it was possible that the ideas discussed in the last chapter about the importance of industriousness and the links being made between people's occupations and their well-being influenced physicians working towards physical health. In this chapter, therefore, some discussion will centre on the attitudes and advice of physicians in that vein, as well as initiatives in preventive medicine and occupational health and safety. To that end it is important at the outset to update the history of the medical profession in what was to be a time of immense importance to the founding of occupational therapy.

The state of medicine

The industrial period was a time when the development of large public health care institutions, and the growth of teaching hospitals and schools of medicine in universities, were indicative of the medical profession's changing status in society. The impetus for this process differed somewhat from place to place. In France the "Revolution" is said to have precipitated a sudden transformation and discontinuity between the modest origins, limited activities and aspirations of eighteenth century practitioners and those of the nineteenth century,[1] whilst in the United Kingdom the development was slower and less affected by political events. An example of the change there towards modern practice is provided by the emergence of the general practitioner as family doctor. They developed from the eighteenth century surgeon-apothecaries and man-midwives as a result of the struggle for monopoly in medical care between various groups of medical men, and others whom they categorised as quacks.

Early in the nineteenth century, medicine had not many more answers than it had two centuries before. But probably for both personal and altruistic reasons, there was a determination amongst the medical profession to improve their status and opportunities by curbing the careers of lay practitioners who were still patronised by the masses. However action was slow because, as in earlier times, there was conflict between the different branches of medicine: physic, surgery and pharmacy. Such division was often the topic of debate in the new and radical medical journal, the *Lancet*, founded in 1823 by the surgeon son of a Devonshire farmer, Thomas Wakely. Not one to pull his punches, in his editorials Wakely accused the medical corporations 'of neglecting their duties' and abusing their powers. He also claimed that London hospitals were 'nests of nepotism' where patients 'suffered neglect, mistreatment and hamfisted surgery'. He argued that, notwithstanding honest general practitioners who could barely make a respectable living, medicine would never advance to a prestigious position in society whilst fragmented into 'antagonistic and obsolescent branches'.[2]

The established Colleges' of Physicians and Surgeons remained dominant forces for the first half of the century despite new standards of medical education and waves of reformist agitation. During that time the British Medical Association was founded for general practitioners, who increasingly had well regarded medical degrees and held public positions in the Poor Law, public hospitals and lunatic asylums, for example, and numerically dominated high flown metropolitan practitioners. The Medical Act of 1858, plus subsequent legislation, maintained the Colleges and the tripartite division of English medicine, but established a single public register of all legally recognised practitioners, under the guardianship of the General Medical Council. The Act excluded the unqualified, making it a legal offence for those not registered to represent themselves as medical practitioners, which disqualified them from holding public medical office but did not stop them from practising.[3]

Figure 1.10.1: A group of emaciated and starving physicians lamenting their lack of work. Wood engraving after G.Du Maurier, 1875.

(The Wellcome Library)

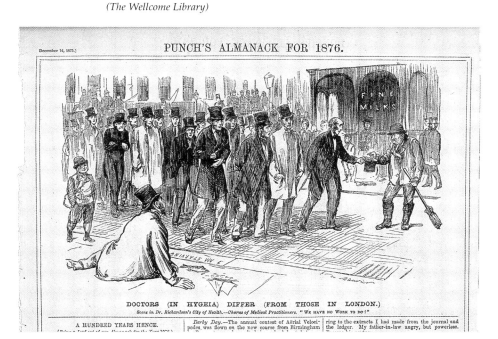

For London's elite physicians and surgeons, established in secure and prestigious consultancy positions within hospital medicine and practice in Harley Street, combined with teaching, there was no diminution of status. For provincial doctors there were few prospects of reaching those heights. Their pedestrian practice depended, to a great extent, upon supply and demand. Because of growing numbers of training opportunities and graduates and a highly competitive market, very few were well off. Most were overworked, carrying bad debts, and making ends meet by becoming Friendly Society or Poor Law doctors. Friendly Societies, largely established because of fear of the workhouse, provided medical care to working men usually in return for a weekly contribution, which was often 1 penny. Because of a lack of effective therapies doctors had to work at patient relationships, developing a comfortable bedside manner and making home visits at any time of the day or night.[4]

For the very poor, medical care was most often associated with workhouses and workhouse hospitals. In Ireland, for example, from the 1840s, hospitals, hospices, and institutions that cared for the handicapped, old and sick were on the increase. Initially, in workhouse hospitals, unqualified and inexperienced people such as the pauper inmates themselves were employed as nurses, with no qualified person to exercise direction. Eventually, despite some reluctance on the part of the Poor Law Commissioners, in 1861 Sisters of Mercy began to be employed as nurses, first at the Limerick workhouse, and then throughout the country.[5,6,7] The employment of any female inmates as nurses was phased out except by special permission of medical officers.[8]

A survey of illness in the 1841 census in Ireland revealed that men were vulnerable to 'fevers, colic, croup and most other infectious diseases', while women were prone to 'consumption and to "wasting, decay and debility"' probably as a result of 'insufficient food and exhaustion'. The high mortality of girls in post-Famine Ireland has been attributed to females not being as well fed as males 'because they were not as economically valuable as their brothers'. Women also made up the larger population in workhouse blind asylums. According to the 1881 census, the numbers of males and females born blind was similar, but girls were more prone to acquired blindness from scarlatina, measles, smallpox, and ophthalmia.[9]

Apart from everyday practice, the nineteenth century was a period of invention and exploration in medicine as it was in other walks of life. Some of the notable discoveries or gains which had consequences for occupational therapy in the next century were physiologist, Claude Bernard's investigations concerning paralyses and vasomotor nerves, as well as the all important notion of homeostasis. Also important were Rudolf Virchow's pathological and microscopic investigations, which enabled a description of thrombosis, and the "Father of English Neurology", John Hughlings Jackson's investigations of the cerebral cortex and movement. Hugh Owen Thomas's inventions of splints and other orthopaedic apparatus and Sir Charles Bell's interest in motor and sensory stimuli, and the treatment of injured hands were also significant.[10,11] In 1817, the first orthopaedic hospital was established, followed by others throughout the country. Whilst insufficient to meet many needs, other aspects of care were provided by organisations like the Shaftesbury Society, the Invalid Children's Aid Association, some local associations for the disabled, and a few institutions providing training and employment.[12]

Medicine, health care and women

On a very different track, another significant development was the redefining of nursing as a career suited to "ladies of birth and breeding"; one that challenged medicine in a way that made it eventually reflect on the nature of its humanity as doctors and nurses, daily, worked alongside each other. Florence Nightingale (1820-1910) comes to mind as the embodiment of that significant change. Nightingale, who is well known for her challenges to the medical profession which, ironically, debarred women from medicine until the 1870s, was the younger of two children brought up in a wealthy, cultured home. She reported suffering extreme boredom, to the point of madness, as a personal and general condition of ladies of her class.[13] At least in part to counter the occupational alienation, deprivation and imbalance she experienced, and against the advice of family and friends, at the age of 25 she decided to undertake a nursing career, which, at that time was extremely difficult for a lady of her circumstances. She took a six-month course at the Institute of Protestant Deaconesses at Kaiserswerth in Germany, and then further training with the Sisters of the St Vincent De Paul Society in Paris. In 1853 Nightingale became superintendent of a Harley Street Home for Gentlewomen during Illness. Her now legendary work at Scutari, during the Crimean War, led to fundamental changes in nursing and medicine and in 1860 the Nightingale School for Nurses at St Thomas's Hospital, London was founded. It is tragic to reflect that she spent the last fifty-three years of her life as a recluse, and that perhaps her early years of an occupationally deprived childhood may have been more influential than one would have supposed.[14]

Women like Nightingale, who challenged the customs of the times to pursue a career in the health field, were instrumental in eventually opening up occupational opportunities for other "respectable" women which were health giving. That in itself may be considered an act of socio-political occupational therapy, one which opened the door for other professions in health to come into being and for women to be able to make good use of their capacities.

A brief look at those expanding opportunities is worthwhile, as they too are an integral aspect of occupational therapy's history. Change would not have occurred without the efforts of pioneering women seeking occupational meaning in a world to which they had been largely denied for so long. *Cassell's Household Guide* of the late nineteenth century provided many articles about the range of employment opportunities opening up for women, including those in health care. One article about nursing explained that without doubt the reason for the 'many complaints against hospital nursing' was:

> *... the fact that for centuries it has been left in the hands of a very low and uneducated class whilst now the advancing spirit of the day is attracting towards it women of a higher social standing and educational culture.*[15]

The greatest obstacle to its adoption was difficulty in getting suitable training and of finding employment afterwards. That was not because of lack of places of employment in need of trained nurses but because 'many changes must take place before women of the middle and upper-middle classes, or, indeed, any women of decency and refinement, could study in them with much advantage or comfort'. The article picked out for criticism places where the nurses were expected 'to cater for themselves and to cook their own food, running the risk of being called away before they even had time to eat their poor morsel of badly-prepared food!' It suggested that 'under such circumstances, neither health nor work could long be retained'.[16] The article continued in a cautionary mode, advising that a primary prerequisite to the career was 'sufficiently good health to stand an amount of hard work to which you have never before been accustomed'. That work was not only bodily exertion but also mental 'which draws upon the physical resources as much if not more'. Another consideration was that the work included many unpleasant and disagreeable tasks for "refined and cultivated women". Qualities deemed necessary were great self-control, patience, good temper, and great intelligence and 'a good knowledge of all domestic duties - such as sweeping, dusting, scouring, bed-making, and the rudiments, at least, of cooking'. In addition, to be suited to nursing, it was advised that women needed 'some knowledge about house-linen' such as 'the various kinds of linen, cotton, blankets, feathers, and hair used'.[17]

That medicine became available as a profession for women during that time has already been mentioned. *Cassell's Household Guide* implied that there may be some question in many minds about the propriety of women entering the sphere, but 'the fact that the University of London contemplates admitting them to degrees' made it necessary to provide a paper on the possibilities. Apparently, even if women had all the educational requirements there had been no board in Britain authorised to grant them degrees, although they could be admitted in Zurich or Paris. Training was offered without examination at the Edinburgh Infirmary. In addition, a Female Medical School opened in Brunswick Square in London in 1874, from which students completed their clinical training at the Hospital for Women opened in Marylebone by Mrs Garrett-Anderson. A short bill was passed in Parliament to permit the granting of medical registration without distinction of sex, but without compulsion to admit women. That bill led to the establishment of a women's medical school at Kings and Queens College of Physicians in Ireland, and the availability of clinical instruction at the Royal Free Hospital, London, as well as the step taken by the University of London senate.[18]

Another health career which began to allow women entry was "dispensing chemistry" because of 'the difficulty of obtaining young men as assistants in the trade'. 'By the Pharmacy Act of 1868 women were admitted to the examination, the passing of which constitutes the legal qualification for the practice of the profession.' Additionally, although decrying the lack of suitable women to fill them, superintendent posts in health care facilities were also available. Towards the end of the century there were, apparently, openings for at least 2,000 such qualified women in hospitals, cottage hospitals, convalescent homes, public and private training schools for nurses, penitentiaries, nurseries and creches.[19]

On a less exalted note, on the home front was the career of nursery maid, said to be suited to girls from 'more highly educated circles of society' than that of domestic servants. The article in *Cassell's Household Guide* that described that job made some interesting observations linking occupation with health. Apart from the ability to rise early, being truthful, having a good temper and strong constitution, it was recommended that a nursery maid be a fair needlewoman because a 'young person who has a taste for sewing is generally more companionable to the little folks in the nursery'. However despite the list of chores which could be expected in the job 'the primary consideration should be to secure plenty of time for out-door exercise and recreation', because 'any kind of game which exercises the limbs of children whilst in the open air, is conducive to health'. The paper added that:

> ... *a skilful nurse will know when to enforce habits of order, and when to give way to a natural inclination on the part of children to create confusion ... The impulse springs from a desire to test bodily strength and to acquire knowledge. It needs guiding not checking.*[20]

So, occupational opportunities began to open for more affluent women, which ultimately must have influenced the state of their health. It was also a time when the conditions of work for those less wealthy, and of their domestic environments, came under the spotlight with regards to their experience of health.

Public health

Throughout the nineteenth century, events and reports revealed the appalling state of public health. There were failures in the provision of necessary amenities such as water, sanitation, and waste disposal, made worse by a huge increase in population, industrial pollution, and slum housing. Together, these factors led to regular outbreaks of cholera in plague proportions. Back in the late eighteenth century, Lettsom, a medical contemporary of reformer, John Howard, had warned how overcrowding in slums, combined with urban filth and ignorance, created ideal conditions for epidemics to prevail. No public action was taken to change the situation at that time, except an Act of Parliament which empowered parishes to levy a rate for payment of 'semi-private, semi-public bodies of "commissioners"', to assume responsibility for civic maintenance such as street cleaning and refuse-disposal. The scale of the health risks of the industrial nineteenth century, however, was beyond their scope.[21]

That factor precipitated the growth of public health, the state having to recognise its crucial importance in the nation's well-being. A leader in that change of direction was Manchester born lawyer, Sir Edwin Chadwick (1800-1890) who devoted most of his life to social reform. Influenced by Jeremy Bentham, with whom he had worked, Chadwick was secretary to the New Poor Law Commission for thirteen years from 1834. The Commission made the workhouse the statutory device for controlling the growing numbers of the poor, as well as establishing Poor Law infirmaries alongside the workhouse. Southwood Smith's influential 1838 *Report on the Physical Causes of Sickness and Mortality to which the Poor are Particularly Exposed,* had provided the foundation for Chadwick's 1842 *Report on the Sanitary Condition of the Labouring Population of Great Britain*. This report did a great deal to warn the public of the unhealthiness of urban areas. In contrast to many physicians who held that disease was contagious, being spread by personal contact through the transfer of disease "seeds", Chadwick, and other like-minded sanitarians, were "anti-contagionists". They believed that sickness sprang from contaminated atmospheres such as polluted water, sewage, animal and industrial waste. To ensure public health, they advocated sanitary engineering rather than medicine was necessary. In particular, plentiful supply of clean water for drinking and a system of underground drainage to flush waste out of urban areas was required. A public health act was passed in 1848, which led to the appointment of local Medical Officers of Health, and a general Board of Health was appointed with Chadwick as a member. Parliament, in a series of statutes, empowered the Board to act on issues such as polluted water supplies. The Nuisance Removal Acts of 1855, 1860, and 1863 empowered Medical Officers of Health to investigate environmental health threats such as rubbish tips, slaughterhouses, poisonous fumes, and suspect food establishments, and to prosecute if necessary. The Nation at last had "health police", and those particular aspects were to become the "known" role of public health for a century or more. The death rate dropped. Indeed social engineering initiatives of the nineteenth century, such as those were responsible for a decrease in morbidity and mortality statistics which make those attributable to modern medicine of recent times pale into insignificance.[22,23]

State attitudes had begun to change. Public health issues, dealt with centrally, in some instances challenged individual expressions of liberty. Examples of cases that caused consternation included compulsory smallpox vaccinations, and efforts to contain venereal disease in the British armed forces. In that matter, the 1867 Contagious Diseases Act gave magistrates the power in particular garrison towns and ports to detain and submit to medical examination and treatment, if found to be diseased, any woman suspected of being a prostitute.

Despite the vaccinations, expansion of Poor Law medical services, and the work of many enlightened medical men, such as James Kay-Shuttleworth who published the classic *The Moral and Physical Condition of the Working Classes* in 1832,[24] the medical profession largely took a backseat in the expanding National public health movement. The pages of the *Lancet* had little to say about the issues, centering instead on medicine's internal political squabbles. Porter, in describing medicine's place, points to the fact that 'neither of the two most vociferous public champions of health, Edwin Chadwick and Florence Nightingale ... was a doctor'.[25]

Even though medicine was not the dominant force in early public health, it is indicative of that professions' growing eminence that public health is regarded as one of its branches, often referred to as "Preventive Medicine", and seen as a jewel in its nineteenth century crown. Sigerist recalled that 'Sir William Osler (1849-1919) called the nineteenth century the century of preventive medicine' and went on to explain that there can be:

> ... no doubt that it was in the field of prevention of disease that modern medicine attained its greatest achievements. Our life is no longer shortened by diseases such as leprosy, plague, smallpox, and rabies. Our life expectation is about twice as long as it was half a century ago.[26]

Sigerist theorised that despite an interest across Europe, the new hygienic (health) movement started in England in a practical way because of the country's internal stability and its humanistic, holistic view of ideal health which was based on the earlier classical paradigm of mental and bodily harmony and balance. He held that view for two reasons. First, with an occupational appreciation of health, Sigerist held that 'sport was an integral component of education in England, and where sport is pursued seriously important conditions for personal hygiene are obtained'. Second, England had 'a government which in itself is strong' which was essential to achieving health in the public domain. However, he recognised that medicine could not successfully fight disease alone largely because 'hygiene and public health, like medicine at large, are but an aspect of the general civilisation of the time, and are largely determined by the cultural conditions of that time'. As the industrial revolution dominated the cultural conditions of the century, occupational health issues became particularly important.[27]

Occupational health

Even Chadwick's interests in the public's health encompassed more than drains and clean water. With Bentham he advised on healthful home planning, and in "occupation for health" terms he recommended the provision of public recreation grounds, and investigated the working conditions of children in factories.[28] In the previous chapter the latter was shown to be a matter of debate in social health. It also became an issue of great importance in occupational health. In fact the whole topic of occupational health was central to reformers" thrusts and parrys as industry became dominant in the economy. Other occupational health reformers included physician, John Aiken, who in his *Description of the Country from 30-40 Miles round Manchester,* drew attention to the deleterious effect of the cotton mills upon the health of child employees.[29] Sir John Simon (1816-1904), another Medical Officer of the General Board of Health, centred his endeavours on the health conditions of industrial workshops and homes within the City of London, and surgeon, Sir James Paget (1814-1899), investigated the loss of working hours according to types of disabilities.[30] Their interest was hardly surprising within the context of that time. As the Reverend John Guy, in the 1993 Octavia Hill Memorial Lecture reminded his audience 'Except for God the most popular word in the Victorian vocabulary must have been work'.[31]

Work had undergone radical transformation over a couple of generations. In the previous century John Wesley had accepted that child labour was an integral and worthwhile aspect of family life and economy, whereby children learnt adult skills from their parents and carried on their various roles and traditions. In the world of industrial manufacturing children went out to work, often having to endure a harsh regime of managers, foremen and supervisors employed by a new elite, the factory owners. Some, like Robert Owen, were "enlightened" humanitarians. Others embraced the doctrines of laissez faire and resisted even the notion of 'statutory limitation upon their employment policies and their treatment of the workforce' which led to a large part of it being exploited and, worse still, unable to protest. Even medical men like physician Edward Holme denied, in 1818, that 23 hours of labour for children might prove harmful, and surgeon Thomas Wilson dismissed the necessity of children being permitted recreation.[32]

Reports from the manufacturing sector highlighted that it was rife with occupational diseases and accidents. Dicken's description of Coketown provides a contemporary view of conditions in industrial Britain, which not only tells of environmental horrors and unsafe machinery, but also of occupational boredom and alienation which are often pre-determining factors in illness and accidents:

> It was a town of red brick, or of brick that would have been red if the smoke and ashes had allowed it; but, as matters stood it was a town of unnatural red and black like the painted face of a savage. It was a town of machinery and tall chimneys, out of which interminable serpents of smoke trailed themselves for ever and ever, and never got uncoiled. It has a black canal in it, and a river that ran purple with ill-smelling dye, and vast piles of building full of windows where there was a rattling and a trembling all day long, and where the piston of the steam-engine worked monotonously up and down, like the head of an elephant in a state of melancholy

madness. It contained several large streets all very like one another, and many small streets still more like one another, inhabited by people equally like one another, who all went in and out at the same hours, with the same sound upon the same pavements, to do the same work, and to whom every day was the same as yesterday and tomorrow, and every year the counterpart of the last and the next.

These attributes of Coketown were in the main inseparable from the work by which it was sustained; against them were to be set off, comforts of life which found their way all over the world, and elegancies of life which made, we will not ask how much of the fine lady, who could scarcely bear to hear the place mentioned. The rest of its features were voluntary, and they were these.

You saw nothing in Coketown but what was severely workful.[33]

Dickens is a reliable source for contemporary information because he based his stories, which were carefully researched, on real issues that complicated the social fabric of the time. He drew on the work of his friends for particular intelligence, which he then transformed into the detail of his magical tales. One of Dickens' friends who was a useful resource, and is relevant in this section of the history, was Southwood Smith. He has already been spoken about in the last chapter as a champion of housing reform and the grandfather of Octavia Hill. It should also be noted in this chapter that he wrote about a physician's traditional interest in the maintenance of health, in his work titled *The Philosophy of Health or the Exposition of the Physical and Mental Constitution of Man, with a View to the Promotion of Human Longevity and Happiness.*[34]

In that, and reflecting some of the occupational ideologies apparent in the last chapter, Southwood Smith approached health from a functional perspective. He argued that 'the object of structure is the production of function' and that 'the sole object of organic life' is 'to maintain it in a condition fit for performing its functions'. He added that 'two functions, sensation and voluntary motion, are combined in animal life. Of these two functions, the latter is subservient to the former: voluntary motion is the servant of sensation, and exists only to obey its commands'.[35] With that as a foundation it makes sense that he considered the development of capacities through use to be a principal source of pleasure and a means of prolonging life. Indeed he combined those notions when he argued that 'there is a close connection between happiness and longevity … to add enjoyment, is to lengthen life',[36] supporting that belief with a physiological premise by maintaining that:

… pleasure resulting from action of the organs is conducive to their complete development, and thereby to the increase of capacity for affording enjoyment; … but also … to the perpetuation of their action, and consequently to the maintenance of life; it follows not only that enjoyment is the end of life, but that it is the means by which life is prolonged.[37]

He went on to explain that:

- *It is, in fact, THE PLEASURABLE CONSCIOUSNESS WHICH CONSTITUTES THE FEELING OF HEALTH.* (his emphasis) *… It is interwoven with the thread of existence; it is secured in and by the actions that build up and that support the very frame-work, the material instrument of our being.*[38]
- *Organs of sense, intellectual faculties, social affections, moral powers, are superadded endowments of a successively higher order: at the same time they are the instruments of enjoyment of a nature progressively more and more exquisite.*[39]
- *The amount of enjoyment which is thus secured to every man, and which every man without exception actually experience in the ordinary course of an ordinary life … would be beyond his power to estimate.*[40]
- *Any attempt to exalt the animal life beyond what is compatible with the healthy state of the organic, instead of accomplishing that end, only produces bodily disease. Any attempt to extend the selfish principle beyond what is compatible with the perfection of the selfish, instead of accomplishing the end in view, only produces mental disease.*[41]

Southwood Smith's holistic vision of medicine coupled with his highly developed social conscience resulted in an interest in and an activist approach to occupational health. The 1832 reformed House of Commons appointed him as one of three parliamentary commissioners along with Edwin Chadwick and the economist Thomas Tooke to look into the issues of concern. Southwood Smith ensured that a questionnaire on the health of employed children was sent to medical practitioners in Lancashire, Derbyshire, and Cheshire, the hub of industrial England. In a supplementary report of the findings of the Commission, the incidence and nature of industrial disease and injury in the early nineteenth century are spelt out. It identified respiratory problems induced by dust and yarn particles in overheated and ill-ventilated mills, the notion of fatigue and monotony as dangers, as well as the risks of accident from operating unprotected machinery.[42]

The work of the commission was incorporated into the Factory Act of 1833 in which children under the age of nine were not permitted to work in textile mills, and under thirteen could not work for more than eight hours a day, and not at night. They were to receive a minimum of two hours schooling each working day and were to be medically inspected. Despite problems in its administration as well as substantial opposition from those with vested interests, the Act was successful in regulating by age, educational attainment, and health, and in promoting ongoing debate about the issues, led in Parliament by the Earl of Shaftesbury, another friend of Southwood Smith. The debate was also carried forward through social narrative by noted authors of popular novels who identified with the problems of the labouring classes and sought to influence legislative reform.

The Blue Books of the Factory Commission reports provided source material for novelists such as radical Frances Trollope and devout Charlotte Tonna.[43] The best known, however, was Charles Dickens who used them as well as personal commentary from Southwood Smith in classics like *Oliver Twist* and *Bleak House*. Almost certainly, in the latter, the young doctor Allan Woodcourt who devoted his life working for the poor of London's slums, is drawn from Southwood Smith:

> *We had a visitor next day. Mr Allan Woodcourt came … I believe - at least I know - that he was not rich. All his widowed mother could spare had been spent in qualifying him for his profession. It was not lucrative to a young practitioner, with very little influence in London; and although he was, night and day, at the service of numbers of poor people, and did wonders of gentleness and skill for them, he gained very little by it in money.*[44]

Conditions in mines were not addressed by the Factory Act, and it was not until 1840 that a Royal Commission of Inquiry was established. Tooke and Southwood Smith were two of the commissioners empowered to report on conditions. The first report addressed the ages of children employed, whether they and women worked underground, and the conditions of employment such as hours, wages, meal-breaks, food, clothing, holidays, accidents, and health. It found that 10 or 12 hours a day was usual, that children as young as six were employed underground in certain pits, the youngest often sitting alone for long periods, in total dark and damp conditions, opening and shutting ventilation doors. Some pushed the coal carriages as they were pulled by youths. Teenage girls worked underground alongside the men, some crawled, hauling coal-sledges, with belts round their waists and chains passing between their legs. At the coalface some worked naked "but for their caps". Many of the women and children suffered rheumatism caused by continuous damp and appeared old and worn beyond their years. Southwood Smith's medical evidence told how the work produced fatigue, extraordinary muscular development, stunted growth, crippled gait, and skin disorders providing an unequivocal link between occupation and ill health.[45]

In order to overcome public and official scepticism about the authenticity of the reports Southwood Smith engaged Margaret Gillies, an illustrator and with whom he "shared a home", to help people who could not visit the mines to see how bad conditions were. Despite gender and class difficulties Gillies recorded scenes of the horrendous, humiliating labour carried out by women and children in the mines with sketches, drawn on the spot. Her illustrations were a unique addition to an official Blue Book. Those, coupled with Southwood Smith's direct and explicit account of conditions in the mines, shocked the nation.[46]

Figure 1.10.2: **Drawing by Margaret Gillies of "three young children hurrying or drawing a loaded wagon of coals. The child in front is 'harnessed by his belt or chain to the wagon: the two boys behind are assisting in pushing it forward."[47]**
(The Wellcome Library)

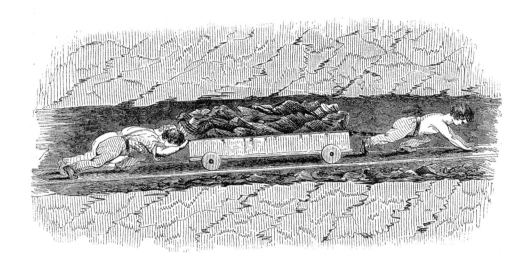

Dickens confessed that he sobbed as he read the Blue Book, which inspired him to visit Cornwall to "see for himself", and to write his most famous story, *A Christmas Carol*. A passage within it, when the Ghost of Christmas Present takes Scrooge to see a family of Cornish tin-miners in their hut on a desolate moor, was a tribute to Southwood Smith.[47] What is fascinating is that the short passage tells of a time of joyous ritual occupation associated with Christmas, certainly in a bleak and desolate place but not of conditions in the mines, perhaps implying that the good doctor's work was beginning to make a difference in the lives of those he sought to help. It also provides a sense of the power of ritual and celebratory occupations even in the life of people who are deprived:

> *And now, without a word of warning from the Ghost, they stood upon a bleak and desert moor, where monstrous masses of rude stone were cast about, as though it were the burial - place of giants; and water spread itself wheresoever it grew but moss and furze, and coarse rank grass. Down in the west the setting sun had left a*

streak of fiery red, which glared upon the desolation for an instant, like a sullen eye, and frowning lower, lower, lower yet, was lost in the thick gloom of darkest night. "What place is this?" asked Scrooge. "A place where Miners live, who labour in the bowels of the earth" returned the Spirit. "But they know me. See!"

A light shone from the window of a hut, and swiftly they advanced towards it. Passing through the wall of mud and stone, they found a cheerful company assembled round a glowing fire. An old, old man and woman, with their children and their children's children, and another generation beyond that, all decked out gaily in their holiday attire. The old man, in a voice that seldom rose above the howling of the wind upon the barren waste, was singing them a Christmas song - it had been a very old song when he was a boy - and from time to time they all joined in the chorus. So surely as they raised their voices, the old man got quite blithe and loud; and so surely as they stopped, his vigour sank again.[48]

Despite clamorous opposition of mine-owners in the House of Lords, such as Lord Londonderry - one of the wealthiest, public outrage forced parliament to move on the issues. In 1842 the Act 'to prohibit the Employment of Women and Girls in Mines and Collieries, and to regulate the Employment of Boys' reached the statute book. Londonderry, in his attack had especially condemned Gillies' woodcuts which 'found their way into the boudoirs of refined and delicate ladies who were weak-minded enough to sympathise with the victims of industry'. Sadly, for Southwood Smith and the other commissioners, the mine-owners' opposition did water down the bill somewhat, but, for the first time, women were included in employment legislation. Their work in mines, along with that of boys under the age of ten, was prohibited, although it was a long step by step process to effective general legislation governing mine safety. Southwood Smith lived long enough to witness the passing of the Act for the Regulation and Inspection of Mines in 1860, which increased to the age of twelve the prohibition of boys working in the mines unless they could already read and write by the age of ten. It also provided rules governing ventilation, safety lamps, and the shoring of galleries.[49]

Another practitioner particularly worthy of note on the occupational health front, was Charles Turner Thackrah (1795-1833), whose approach was less radical and more in keeping with those taken in the present day. Thackrah, at the age of sixteen, had entered an apprenticeship with a surgeon apothecary of Leeds, which was followed by a short training at Guys Hospital where he found he had a forte for scientific investigation. Early in 1817 he began practising on his own account gaining the position of town surgeon (parish doctor) to Poor Law patients, and at the request of the Leeds Workhouse Board successfully investigated and reported on the lodging houses frequented by the poor of the area. The founder of the Leeds Medical School, Thackrah was a scholarly man, who proved to be an able experimental researcher with a keen interest in preventive medicine. No doubt, in the modern day he would have excelled in the field of epidemiology.[50]

Regarded as a father of industrial medicine, Thackrah is best known for his text *The Effects of the Principal Arts, Trades, and Professions, and of Civic States and Habits of Living on Health and Longevity*. Here he demonstrated his keen observation skills on the effects of occupation and social factors across a broad spectrum of ages and the community. To carry out his task he visited places of employment, investigating and analysing occupational processes, hazards, materials, and environments aiming to immediately remove or diminish the "injurious agents" in many occupations.[51]

Despite its scientific nature the text has an occasional descriptive passage which sets the scene. The example below provides an eloquent testimony to the occupational nature of humankind and goes on to establish the basis for his probing:

> *If we turn our view from man to his works, we see the wilderness converted into towns and cities, roads cut through mountains, bridges carried over rivers and even arms of the sea, ships which traverse the globe, lakes converted into corn fields, forests made into pasture, and barren rocks covered with timber; - in a word, we see the face of the world changed by human will and human power.*
>
> *If we look immediately at home, we observe the wonders which science and art have effected. We see large buildings, manufactures of almost every kind, and substances so changed, re-formed, and combined, that nature could scarcely know her own productions. We admire the inventions of science, alike in their minuteness and their size, their accuracy, and their extent of operation.*
>
> *These, and works like these, are assuredly wonderful. But while we admire, let us examine. What are the effects of these surprising works - effects, I mean physical and moral? I say nothing of the wealth they produce or have produced, for wealth is good or evil according to its application: I refer to the health of the millions who spend their lives in manufactories or live by trade, civic arts and professions. I ask if these millions enjoy that vigour of body which is ever a direct good, and without which all other advantages are comparatively worthless? I ask if they attain the age of agricultural workers?*
>
> *To the first inquiry, the mere appearance of a civic population affords a reply. Take indifferently twenty well fed husbandmen, and compare them with twenty townsmen who have equal means of support, and the superiority of the agricultural peasants in health, vigour, and size will be obvious. Medical men, moreover, have daily proof of the ill effects on the human constitution, which employment produce. They find a number, a variety, and a complexity of diseases, which are little known in country practice, and which, though not directly fatal, greatly reduce the powers of life.*[52]

Like Ramazzini, in an earlier century, Thackrah considered intellectual occupations as potentially unhealthy as well as those with more obvious causations, stating that 'great exertions of the brain, combined with sedentary habits and late hours, do certainly tend to produce a delicate state of health'.[53]

Some of the factors causing that were, he said, for the mathematician, 'hours of abstract thought'; for the poet, 'nights of passion, excessive excitement of the imaginative faculties, and irregularity of living'; for the student, 'days of reading'; and in general, ambitiousness, emulation, and envy. The counter measures he recommended were: to reduce the amount of time spent in studious pursuit to no more than 6 hours; to take regular exercise which increased the circulation, such as gymnastics or gardening; and to take care with the timing and mode of eating.[54]

Thackrah was very thorough, addressing over 350 different occupations, from medical men to milliners, wheelwrights to worsted-spinners, fishmongers to founders, and accountants to cattle-dealers, so it is of interest to view, if only in brief, an example of how he recorded his report. Not surprisingly, as a medical man, he considered agents which he found injurious to particular organs. So, for example, those agents he found injurious to the digestive organs he grouped under the following headings: excess of food; defect of proper food; bent sitting posture; long standing; pressure of the chest on the stomach; great muscular efforts; steam; high temperature, common atmospheric impurities, dust and gaseous impurity of the atmosphere; and anxiety and mental application. For each of those he added examples of the occupations at particular risk, like for "anxiety and mental application" he saw merchants, professional men, and students as especially at risk, and for "great muscular effort", porters and millers. As well he gave the particular results of specific injurious agents, for example for those engaged in occupations demanding a bent sitting posture he saw the results as 'defect in the blood's general circulation - Congestion, especially of the system of the vena portae - Functional disorder of the liver – Indigestion - diarrhoea, and other diseases of the mucous membranes of the intestines – piles - fistula in ano'.[55]

As to the question of manufacturing accidents, which is often the focus of present day practice, Thackrah determined that 'these are less frequent than we should expect'. Indeed, he found that the proportion "killed or maimed" decreased every year, because manufacturers were generally attentive to obvious hazards. A major finding on the other hand was that the majority had their constitutions impaired by premature labour, by excess of labour, and by intemperance. Those who lived to old age were so enfeebled that they had to find alternative light employment, or live out their lives in a workhouse.[56]

Whilst the main thrust of public and occupational health was preventive, there was also a recognition, throughout the century, in more affluent society, that the pursuit of positive health was also a wise move. That sentiment continued the ideas of earlier centuries and, as in those times, it embraced occupation for health. Recognition of the need to exercise was part of that, and the following of gymnastics continued to grow.

Gymnastics

At the genesis of occupational therapy in the 20th century and for several decades on, dancing, games and physical exercise were considered important occupations in which students received training. Acceptance of the health value of physical occupations like those in therapy stemmed from the nineteenth century. Then the use of gymnastics to maintain good health began to include women as well as men in much the same way as had been the case in classical times.

It was part of the self health tradition, which drew heavily on that earlier time. By late in the century, in *Cassell's Household Guide*, callisthenics, (the name derived from the Greek kalos (beautiful) and sthenos (strength)), was featured. It appears that it was no longer a fashionable virtue for ladies to be helpless or inactive:

> *Lack of exertion leads to irregular muscular action, which if well directed and regular, invigorates the system. Exercise is now recognised as to be as great a necessity in woman's education as in mans: we are learning that many bodily defects and much of her weak health is attributable to the want of it … exercise is absolutely necessary … curing as it does many deformities of mind and person.*[57]

The importance of physical exercise to maintain health and perfect beauty was recognised, the Guide describing how callisthenics secured "physical beauty", developed limbs and muscles, made joints flexible, gave strength and power, and ensured graceful carriage, erect bearing, and "freedom to the figure". See Figure 1.10.3 for a depiction of nineteenth century ladies callisthenics. In the same vein dancing, too, was recognised as a natural exercise that strengthened the body and was a source of health.[58]

Figure 1.10.3: Nineteenth century callisthenics: A health giving occupation for ladies[59]

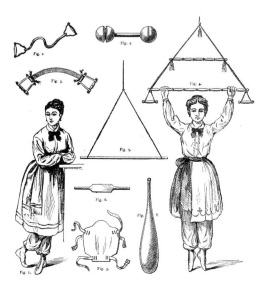

Swedish born Pehr Henrik Ling (1776-1839), mentioned briefly in an earlier chapter, is widely regarded as being responsible for the restoration of interest in physical exercise and gymnastics. His ideas were derived from the holistic notion of the ancients that health was *men's sana in corpora sano* - a sound mind in a healthy frame. In 1813, the Swedish Government set up the Royal Central Institution for Gymnastics in Stockholm and supported it by annual grants of money. Ling was established as Director in that year and held the post until his death 35 years later.[60]

Ling formulated a system of therapeutic exercises and movements in accordance with the "laws of motion" and the belief that there were three fundamental or vital phenomena that needed to be included in a comprehensive system. The first which he called the "Dynamical phenomena", included the mind, moral and intellectual powers; the second, "Chemical phenomena", included secretion, nutrition, and so on; and the third, "Mechanical phenomena", included voluntary and organic motion such as respiration, mastication, and circulation. He argued that those phenomena in combination and harmony influenced "every vital act"[61] and that a state of health was dependent upon them. Any serious derangement in any of them always resulted in disease. To re-establish harmony he prescribed an increase in the activity of those organs with functions related to the decreased or weakened phenomena observing that:

> ... the physician has accordingly to regulate, not only the medicine and food requisite for the sick; but also exercise, position during rest, the manner in which the irritable mind is to be calmed, &c. Due attention to all these matters is necessary to constitute a rational treatment of disease.[62]

Ling proposed some laws, which seem relevant to occupation in general. These were:

- *Every just attempt to develop the powers of the human being - mental and corporeal - is an education.*
- *Correct movements are such as are founded on the natural constitution and temperament of the individual to be developed thereby.*
- *The organism can only be said to be perfectly developed, when its several parts are in mutual harmony; corresponding to different individual predispositions.*
- *The development of the human body must be contained within the limits of the creative faculties, mental or bodily, with which each individual is endowed.*
- *Such a faculty may be blunted by want of exercise, but can never be utterly annihilated.*
- *Perfect health and physical power consequently are correlative; both are dependent upon the harmony of the several parts.*
- *In corporal development, commencing with the simplest, you may gradually advance to the most complicated and powerful movements; and this without danger, in as much, as the pupil has acquired a knowledge of what he is capable, or not capable.*[63]

Until his death in 1839 Ling endeavoured to educate nearly a hundred "gymnasiarchs" in the practice of his system. He recognised two of his students, Branting and Georgii, as being particularly able to carry on his objectives, and along with Ling's son-in-law, a physician they continued his work in Stockholm. Georgii also practised in London,[64'65] where American born Phokion Henrich Clias (1782-1854) had earlier introduced Ling's ideas.[66] Ling's gymnastics were also offered at a gymnasium in London that was opened in 1840 by a Lieutenant Ehrenhoffin, presumably one of his former students. The ideas took root, and the London School Board introduced Ling's system of Swedish gymnastics into London girls' and infants' schools in 1881, whilst centres in Birmingham, Manchester, Liverpool and Bristol began training teachers in the system.[67] Ling had not been alone in his interest. Throughout Europe similar initiatives were afoot, led by Friedrich Jahn, Truls Har Felius, Adolph Spiess, Eduard Henoch, and Archibald Maclaren, a physician who practised and used gymnastics therapeutically.[68]

Physicians with an occupational perspective for healthy living

Some physicians, like Maclaren, espoused what could be called an occupational perspective to medicine and health. Whilst not calling it by that name they were concerned with what people did in their daily lives and advised them about the positive or negative effects of their "doing". According to the socio-cultural expectations of the period, in their writings they frequently took a moral tone and often were remarkably judgemental and patronising. In *Medical and Surgical Directions for Cottagers and for the Domestic Practitioner*, for example, came the recommendations to pray, read the bible and worship; to be temperate in all things including passions and sinful desires; to partake of scotch oatmeal and 'Robinson's Patent Groats ... instead of tea and butter which are very dear'; to keep beds warm in winter with hot bottles or stones; and to remove low spirits 'take every now and then, when low, a dose of opening physic; and talk with cheerful friends, and, if you can, change the scene, go out to see your friends'.[69]

Notwithstanding that all-knowing tendency, much advice and many prescriptions anticipated occupational therapy. The writings of two well-respected and well-known physicians demonstrate an appreciation of a strong relationship between health and how people spend their time. They are Dr Samuel Smiles who was an advocate for political and social reform and best known by the general public for his views on self-help, and Dr James Johnson who was described as *Physician Extraordinaire to the King*, (William IV).

Samuel Smiles (1812-1904) and *Self-Help*

It seems particularly relevant to consider, if only briefly, the work of Samuel Smiles because he was a physician with a dual interest in health and in occupation. From his writing it appears that, to him, the concept of occupation embraced paid employment, personal growth and self improvement through education, exercise, and mental attitude. National health and well-being were as a result of energetic and committed use of capacities and opportunities.

Figure 1.10.4:   Samuel Smiles by Sir George Reid.
(National Portrait Gallery)

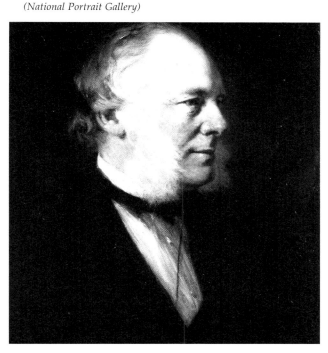

Smiles was born at Haddington in 1812, and received his medical education in Edinburgh. His career was varied, and he devoted his spare time to advocacy of political and social reform along the lines of the Manchester School, which was the name given by Disraeli to the followers of Bright, a Quaker, and Cobden. These men were the members of parliament representing Manchester, and leading representatives of the emerging manufacturing class in English politics after the Reform Act of 1832. Their advocacy led to the repeal of the Corn Laws in 1846.[70] So despite a popular image of conservatism that was somewhat ridiculed or suspect to many Victorian socialist reformers, Smiles did, in fact, emerge from the left wing background of Chartism and the Anti Corn Law League, and held radical views, particularly where concerned with issues of public health.[71]

As a young man Smiles had met and been influenced by Chadwick and Southwood Smith and, not surprisingly, wrote forcefully to facilitate changes to improve the health of populations and individuals. For example, tongue in cheek, he proclaimed:

> When typhus or cholera breaks out, they tell us Nobody is to blame. That terrible Nobody! How much he has to answer for. More mischief is done by Nobody than by all the world besides. Nobody adulterates our food. Nobody poisons us with bad drink ... Nobody leaves towns undrained. Nobody fills jails, penitentiaries, and convict stations ... When people live in foul dwellings, let them alone, let wretchedness do its work; do not interfere with death.[72]

On different health lines, and, perhaps more in keeping with occupational therapy, Smiles' definition of health was decidedly functional and reminiscent of Southwood Smith's. Health, he wrote is 'the natural and easy exercise of all the functions—constituting a state of actual pleasure. The usual, the permanent, the natural condition of each organ, and of the entire system, is pleasurable'.[73] Smiles earliest work was aimed at children's nurture and management, highlighting their need for physical exercise in abundance.[74] He also wrote the stories of industrial leaders and "humble", self-taught students whose work he admired. A prolific writer, much influenced by phrenology, Smiles is, perhaps, best known for Self-Help, which was published in 1859.[75] This text, with the title adopted from that of a lecture given by American reformer R.W. Emerson several years earlier, was extremely popular and was translated into many languages. Writing about the same time that John Stuart Mill and Charles Darwin were putting forth their controversial beliefs, Smiles expounded a doctrine much more acceptable to the masses, indeed, in the spirit of Carlyle, 'something that was old and profoundly true ... the gospel of work'.

In Self-Help, Smiles advocated the combined development of physical, moral and intellectual capacities. With regard to "his day", he regretted that physical exercise had 'somewhat fallen into disrepute ... very much to the detriment of the bodily health'.[76] But it was physical and manual occupation that he recommended to right that wrong. 'Training in the use of tools in a workshop' he suggested for the leisure class:

> ... would teach young men the use of their hands and arms, familiarise them with healthy work, exercise their faculties upon things tangible and actual, give them some practical acquaintance with mechanics, impart to them the ability to be useful, and implant in them the habit of persevering physical effort.

For the youth of the labouring classes he advocated literacy education and for both the combination of "physical work" with "intellectual culture".[77]

He took a phrase, 'not what I have, but what I do is my kingdom' as a motto for another of his books, Thrift[78][79] Smiles' doctrine held notions close to the concepts that are the basis of occupational therapy and anticipated an enabling approach. He advocated that people owe their 'growth chiefly to that active striving of the will, that encounter with difficulty, which he (or she) calls effort'. For Smiles, self-help was the basis of the "genuine" growth of individuals and communities in that 'it constitutes the true source of national vigour and strength'. Help from without is often 'enfeebling in its effects, but help from within invariably invigorates'.

Committed to national education, particularly "continuing" or "adult" education, Smiles was less concerned with social improvement than with mental and physical effort.[80] An example of the views which he advanced and which relate occupations to health reads:

> The brain is cultivated at the expense of the members (limbs), and the physical is usually found in an inverse ratio to the intellectual appetite. Hence, in this age of progress, we find so many stomachs weak as blotting paper, hearts indicating "fatty degeneration", - unused, pithless hands, calveless legs and limp bodies … The mind itself grows sickly and distempered … It is, perhaps, to this neglect of physical exercise that we find amongst students so frequent a tendency towards discontent, unhappiness, inaction, and reverie … The only remedy for this green-sickness of youth is abundant physical exercise, - action, work, and bodily occupation of any sort.[81]

Along the same lines but ahead of his time he recognised that 'the thorough aeration of the blood by free exposure to a large breathing surface in the lungs, is necessary to maintain that full vital power on which vigorous working of the brain in so large a measure depends'. He advocated, therefore, the need to secure a 'solid foundation of physical health' before making a 'sustained application' to mental pursuits.[82]

Smiles also discussed what would now be recognised within the profession as occupational balance, in the sense of a balance between the use of basic faculties rather than the culturally determined "work, rest and leisure". In comparison with the "leisured class" he described one advantage of the "working class" as being:

> … that they are in early life under the necessity of applying themselves laboriously to some mechanical pursuit or other, - thus requiring manual dexterity and the use of physical powers. The chief disadvantage … that they are too exclusively so employed, often to the neglect of their moral and intellectual faculties. While the youths of the leisure classes, having been taught to associate labour with servility, have shunned it, and have been allowed to grow up practically ignorant … It seems possible, however to avoid both these evils by combining physical training or physical work with intellectual culture.[83]

Although there is little information about if or how he recommended occupation in the treatment of his patients, it is probable that he did to some extent, and so it would appear that Smiles was but one step away from articulating "occupational" treatment along the lines of the next century.

James Johnson and *The Economy of Health*

James Johnson followed a different path. He continued the tradition of the *Regimen Sanitatis* by considering the preventive as well as the curative aspects of lifestyle factors, but held a medical view of health as the absence of illness rather than as a positive state of wellness. He was aware of Smiles' work and referred, somewhat dismissively, to his colleague's definition of health. His criticism was that although it 'might be true, if we were in a state of nature' in the conditions of the times there was scarcely 'such a thing as perfect health'. 'Rather than the pleasurable condition described by Dr. Smith' Johnson saw health as, 'often a negative, rather than a positive quality—an immunity from suffering'. His somewhat jaundiced perspective made him proclaim instead that as:

> *... there is no such thing as moral perfection in this world:—neither is there physical perfection. Man brings with him the seeds of sickness as well as of death; and, although, in their early growth, these seeds may be imperceptible, yet so many noxious agents surround us, that we rarely arrive at maturity before the foul weeds become cognizable, and disorder usurps the place of HEALTH!*[84]

Despite Johnson's dismissal of Smiles "natural" health definition he advocated subjection of 'all our actions, passions, pleasures, and labours to laws, in imitation of those which Nature has established'.[85] He also recognised the mind-body link arguing that disorders of the body 'are engendered and propagated, to a most frightful extent, by moral commotions and anxieties of the mind'. In like manner he understood that occupation could prevent disorders of body and mind, stating that 'corporeal exertion especially when aided by any intellectual excitement or pursuit, can obviate the evils that ensue to soul and body from these causes'. He added, pre-empting the notion of the links between occupational deprivation and ill health, that 'as man rises in rank and riches, he becomes deprived - or rather he deprives himself - not of the means, but of the inclination to embrace the protection which this principle holds out'.[86]

In *The Economy of Health* Johnson made some preliminary observations, which are worth noting as they are much more holistic than most medical texts of today. They included: "the chief ingredient in happiness", "power, riches, fame, beauty, &c without health", "religion, philosophy, materialism", "public health of hygiene", and "Spartan gymnastics".[87] Johnson also developed a theory of human development in which the lifespan was divided into "ten septenniads". Within those developmental stages Johnson advocated different occupations as exercise. In the first septenniad from 1-7 years, he considered, as well as the state of the brain and internal organs, the dangers of early mental exertions, physical and moral education, food, clothing, exercise, sleep, habits and manners, order, regularity and punctuality:

> *During the first Septenniad, exercise may be left almost entirely to the impulses of Nature. The great modern error is the prevention of bodily exercise by*

Figure 1.10.5: James Johnson. Lithograph by T Brigford
(The Wellcome Library)

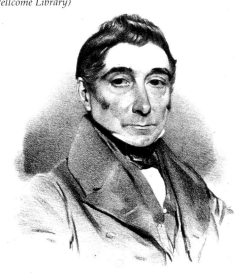

too early and prolonged culture of the mind. In the first years of life, exercise should be play, and play should be exercised. Towards the end of the first Septenniad, some degree of order or method may be introduced into playful exercise, because it will be essential to health in the second and third epochs. Even in this first epoch, exercise in the open air should be enjoined, as much as the season and other circumstances will permit.[88]

In the second Septenniad from 7-14 years, Johnson discussed how school traditions influence health. He included interesting ideas about the "education of females", the "mania for music" and various aspects of the value and use of "time". He argued for occupational balance between mind and body particularly during school days because:

... one radical evil is sure to pervade the system of education pursued therein—namely, the disproportion between exercise of the mind and exercise of the body—not merely as respects the sum total of each species of exercise, but the mode of its distribution.

He added a caustic remark on the changing social demands that appear somewhat similar to our own, saying 'the grasp at learning is preternatural, over-reaching, and exhausting. It is engendered and sustained by the diffusion of knowledge, the density of population, and the difficulty of providing for families.' In schools he believed the lessons and periods of study were too long, the consequence being 'languor and fatigue of the intellect'. Again reminiscent of the *Regimen Sanitatis* he recommended 'small portions of learning at a time' punctuated with periods of play, adding, 'what is lost in letters will be gained in health'. No school, he wrote, 'should be without a playground; and no playground without a gymnasium of some kind, for the lighter modes of athletic exercise'. He blamed the German gymnast Volker for the introduction of over enthusiastic gymnastics whilst suggesting that 'every salutary measure that was ever proposed, has been *abused*; but this forms no just grounds against its *use'.*[89]

During discussion of the third Septenniad from 14-21 years, he noted the change required in the passage from school to work force, including ideas about the "evils of arts and manufactures", and "insalubrious avocations and professions". It was in that stage of development, also, that Johnson believed 'the seeds of female diseases are chiefly sewn'. These were effected by a 'deficiency of healthy exercise of the body, in the open air; and of intellectual exercise in judicious studies'. He blamed socio-cultural factors for this deficiency like the fact that the higher and middle classes prized too highly 'effeminacy of shape and feature', which resulted in 'the pallid complexions, the languid movements, the torpid secretions, the flaccid muscles, and disordered functions, (including glandular swellings,) and consumption itself'. He recommended that 'the hoop and the skip-rope might usefully supersede the harp and guitar, for one hour in the day'. [90]

The adult years between 21 and 56 Johnson divided into five Septenniads. In these he touched on phrenology, imagination, judgement and ambition, activity of the body as an antidote to depression of the mind as "the great principle in hygiene", "temperance and exercise the grand preventives and correctives", "the baleful effects of sedentary habits", and "inactivity the parent of irritability". In the first phase of the adult septenniads Johnson claimed that 'a stock of temperance and exercise laid in at this period will return fifty per cent more of profit in the course of life, than if attempted at any other epoch subsequently'. He equated a youth of *labour* (industry) with an age of *ease* (independence) claiming that 'exercise, in the early years of life, is more certainly followed by freedom from pain in the advanced epochs of existence, than economy is followed by competence'. He told a short cautionary tale:

> *There was a time when a gentleman walked - because he could not afford to ride - and then he was seldom ailing. A period came when he kept his carriage - because he could not afford to walk - and then he was seldom well. He hit on a remedy, that combined the economy of TIME; with the preservation of health. Instead of jumping into the carriage, on leaving a house, he started off at a quick pace, that kept the horses on a trot after him. When well warmed with walking, a little fatigued, or straitened for time, he sprang into the carriage, closed three of the windows, and read, till he arrived at the next rendezvous, after which, the same process of alternate pedestrian and passive exercise was reiterated. Now this is a combination of the two kinds of exercise which I had proved by experiment, many years previously, to be extremely salutary. It is one which the rich can command without sacrifice - even of dignity; - and which many others might employ with very little sacrifice of that valuable commodity - TIME, - and with great advantage in respect to health'.*[91]

Readers are reminded that riding in a carriage was frequently prescribed as a health-giving occupation. During the middle years of life, Johnson explained, 'exercise produces neither pain nor pleasure, it is, nevertheless, necessary to health - but it is at this period that it is too much neglected'.[92]

In the ninth and tenth septenniads from 56 to 70 years he discussed both the desire for retirement and the fatal effects of too early a retirement as well as "dilapidation of the whole frame" and "consolations of old age". In those later years 'the muscles lose their aptitude for motion - the sinews their elasticity - and then rest is little short of sensible pleasure'.

Johnson's concern for occupational balance appears pertinent today, particularly when he argued that exercise and avocational occupations were more conducive to both success and health than a life composed solely of work and rest. Interestingly, he noted that 'this is particularly the case with females; and affords an additional reason for our sympathy and kindness to the more amiable, as well as the most industrious (I had almost said *oppressed)* half of the human race!'

'Any exercise', he said 'as in the various kinds of manufactures or handicrafts, is better than no exercise at all of the body'. He added, however that the benefits were poorly understood:

> We are told, indeed, that exercise strengthens the muscles, and the whole body; - and, on the other hand, that indolence debilitates. This is a very imperfect view of the subject. If strength was the only salutary result of exercise - and if debility was the only consequence of its desuetude, little would be gained by the one, or lost by the other, comparatively speaking. But there are other consequences of a far more important nature. The brain and the nervous system furnish a certain quantum of excitability to the muscles, and to all the various organs and structures of the body; and this excitability ought to be expended in the exercise and operations of these various parts—if health is to be insured. But if, on the one hand, this sensorial power or excitability be expended on mental exertions, the other, or corporeal organs, must necessarily be deprived of their stimulus, and their functions languish, as a matter of course. Hence the innumerable disorders of those who work the brain more than the body! The remedy cannot be found, in this class by forcing the body to exercise, after the brain and nervous system are exhausted. Bodily exercise, under such circumstances, will only do injury. They must curtail the exertions of the mind and increase the exercise of the body.[93]

Johnson certainly appeared concerned about moral or bodily ill health caused by lack of occupation and exercise of mind or body experienced by members of the upper class and others who had no "avocation or pursuit", and for whom "indolence and ennui" were common. He believed, on the one hand, that confinement and inactivity of both limbs and mental faculties without the power or space for stretching them was a problem for immense numbers of people in the civilised world, resulting in irritability or 'excitability of the brain and nervous system'. On the other hand, if lack of physical exercise was combined with mental exertion Johnson maintained that the equilibrium of the circulation became disturbed causing blood to accumulate in some organs.[94] If accumulating in the brain it was the cause of 'headaches, confusion, loss of memory, giddiness, and other affections, so common among sedentary people', and if in the liver it "deranged" 'the whole of the digestive organs, and through them almost every function of mind and body'.

Johnson's prescription to overcome congestion and irritability was carefully graded occupation to equalise the circulation and the excitability:

> *If the individual's circumstances will permit him to engage in any pursuit that may occupy his attention and exercise his body, it will prove one of the most powerful means of counteracting the original cause of many of his sufferings. Unfortunately there are but very few, whose circumstances will permit them to embark in any new pursuit. Yet it is in the power of a great many to engage in a systematic exercise of the body, in some mode or other, if they will only summon resolution to make the experiment. The languor and listlessness attendant on the disorder are great obstacles to this plan; but they should be urged to it by all the eloquence of their medical attendants. Some caution, however, is necessary here. The debility and exhaustion which supervene on the most trifling exertion deter most people from persevering, and therefore, the corporeal exercise must be commenced on the lowest possible scale, and very gradually increased. Thus, a person whose sedentary occupations confine him to the house, might begin by going once to the top of the stairs the first day, twice the second day, and so on, till he could go up and down the same path many times each day[95]*

Among his holistic views of health, Johnson held strong opinions about the value of spas and the health giving environments and occupations, which were part of the total experience of "taking the waters". That topic, with some of his views, will be considered next.

Occupational dimensions of spa treatments

As in earlier times, spas continued to be used for the treatment of various ailments. As well as those at Bath and Buxton, others were established during the nineteenth century, such as at Harrogate, Droitwich, and Leamington Spa, which was patronised by Queen Victoria.[96] Some people, however, continued to travel to European spa resorts. Johnson, in *Pilgrimages to the Spas in Search of Health and Recreation*, gave lengthy descriptions of the daily life and occupations followed in the resorts.[97] He described not only 'the general outlines of a life that may be led at a much frequented watering-place, (but also) … the great diversity of enjoyments that may be procured at these places'.[98]

Johnson explained how 'the patients meet early in the morning on the public walks and at the wells. There they interchange their wishes and hopes for recovery.'[99] At Kissengen, "early" was six o'clock in the morning when a band marched and played through the middle of the town to the "Jardin de Cure", summoning 'eight hundred or a thousand invalids' to their 'morning potations'.[100] At the morning venue:

> ... plans for the amusements of the day are discussed, appointments for shorter or longer excursions made, according to the strength and inclination of each individual; and these excursions, this enjoyment of the open air, contribute a great deal to heighten the salubrious efficacy of the wells. A cheerful mind exercises the most happy influence on the body.[101]

After the bath, patients dispersed to their breakfasts then usually indulged in a few hours rest, or took some walking exercise.[102] After a one o'clock dinner, 'and perhaps a cup of coffee,' 'the plans formed in the morning are executed, each patient trying the strength he has regained' with "promenades in the garden", or "excursions into the country". The evenings were spent in the garden, the conversation halls, theatre, and gaming tables, at one of the parties that were formed in every bathing establishment, or "dancing".[103]

Johnson attributed successful treatment to more than the waters, in many ways anticipating the benefits attributed to therapeutic occupations in the next century. He recognised that it was 'the whole moral and physical conditions' surrounding the patients which effected mental and corporal improvement. Indeed these, he said, 'makes easy work for the mineral waters'. Additionally he recognised as therapeutic:

- *Hope itself, though often resting on fallacious and exaggerated histories of cures, contributes much to the accomplishments of even marvellous recoveries.*[104]
- *The change of scene and air - of food and drink - of rising and retiring - of exercise and conversation.*[105]
- *The enlivening influence which a temporary residence at some watering-place exercises on the mind of the visitor, ... which the best endeavours of the regular physician can seldom effect at home.*[106]
- Disengagement *'as much as possible from the trammels of their professional and domestic occupations and relations, (which allows "persons not labouring under serious disorders") to enter this new world with renovated spirits.*[107]
- *A common purpose, the same society, the participation of the same amusements and pleasures, facilitate the formation of many interesting connections. The opportunity for mutual intercourse are numerous: the social meetings are not hampered by the trammels of ceremony, and we readily acknowledge and enjoy mental and social talents wherever we meet with them.*[108]

Despite the advantages, Johnson warned that:

> ... many diseases - especially organic ones - are aggravated by the journey to a distant spa - by the imprudent use of the water - by the warm or hot bathing - by the enthusiasm or rather hydromania, of the spa-doctor.[109]

William Morris experienced a European spa resort from a patient's point of view. Because of a particular health problem being experienced by his wife, Morris visited the twenty-one mineral springs of Ems. Here he found 'a whole industry of medicine and tourism' growing up around the spas, but which had been known for their curative properties at least since the time of the Romans. The waters, which were carbonated and alkaline, were used in the treatment of "les maladies de femme" as well as chronic catarrh, bronchitis, and laryngitis.

Three of the Ems springs were for drinking. The waters, which were dispensed each morning in cut-glass Bohemian tumblers, were described by visitors 'as warm and mawkish with a distinctive taste of weak beef tea'. Other spring water was used for bathing. That was collected, cooled and distributed into 'more than a hundred individual bathing cabinets'. William Morris is caricatured taking the waters in figure 1.10.6. There was, in addition:

> ... a vapour bath, a powerful uterus-douche, applied for disorders of the uterine system, and the pride of Bad Ems, the natural ascending douche, the Bubenquelle, a fountain half an inch in diameter rising from the bottom of a basin, when a stop-cock was turned, to a height of between two and three feet. This fountain, applied strictly under medical supervision, entered the body via the vagina and was claimed to be effective in the treatment of sterility and discharge from the womb.

As well as the baths, and water consumption, recreational occupations were provided, such as a piano and gaming tables where 'the patients and their companions whiled away the time with rouge et noir and roulette'.[110]

Figure 1.10.6: Cartoon of William Morris taking the waters.[72]

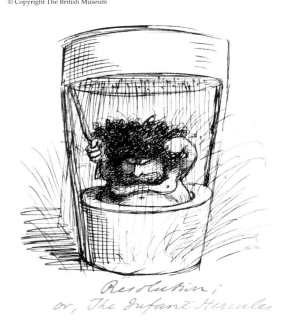

Seawater bathing also became popular in the nineteenth century for health reasons, and not only to effect the improvement of arthritic conditions and bone disease, which rheumatology historians have noted.[111] Its popularity was such that it was included as a topic in *Cassell's Household Guide*. The editors of the *Guide* note that:

> *This custom, however, which is on the whole a most salutary and beneficial one, has not been introduced by the dictates of the physician; as the public themselves have, in the majority of instances, selected the sea-coast as their healthful retreat quite apart from any advice of the medical faculty.*

Particular diseases or conditions which sea-bathing was supposed to improve included constipation, dislocations and sprains, respiratory diseases, scrofula, headaches caused by nervous depression, neuralgia, anaemia or young women's hysteria, digestive problems and, sometimes, paralysis. The editors, despite describing the health benefits of salt water bathing, also recognised it as bracing and strengthening to the system generally, but warned that there were dangers attached to it which were being ignored. That was especially the case when wrongly applied for those with disorder of the cardiac system, hepatic congestion, or enfeebled constitutions.[112]

Occupation as therapy for the physically handicapped

Macdonald, who clearly held a view of occupational therapy as an adjunct to medicine, suggested that because 'medical experts had seemed too busy to be able to apply enough personal interest and attention to it' that 'occupational treatment had not been very fully extended' during the last decades of the nineteenth century.[113] Despite that being largely the case there were, however, a few pointers of things to come, particularly in the treatment of tuberculosis and the blind. Indeed prescription of occupation for specific effect in physical medicine was becoming a reality.

As part of that there was a growing interest in the importance of occupation as a psychological as well as an exercise phenomena in humane interventions concerned with health enhancing, remedial and curative therapies for the physically handicapped or diseased. In 1880 for example, Lady Brabazon, the Countess of Meath, offered a grant of money for materials to any infirmary or workhouse that would engage their patients or inmates in occupation, mainly as "diversional therapy" it appears. The scheme consisted of teaching the infirm and crippled to 'employ their idle hands usefully, and in this way "beguile many a weary hour, and add zest to their lives"'.[114] In view of the general attitude of the times about "industriousness" and its moral value, as well as the credit given to a relationship between happiness and health, the notion of diversion should not be immediately assumed as derogatory, as is sometimes the case today. Rather, it suggests that its proponents viewed the inclusion of diversionary occupation as health giving and remedial. That notion is supported by nineteenth century practices in mental health to be considered in the next chapter.

The last decades of the century saw the beginnings of a movement towards the rehabilitation of crippled children, which was precursory to rehabilitation as a whole. It started, as many health-enhancing movements had before with the notion of education. Much of this particular initiative has been laid at the door of Mary Augustus Ward (1851-1920), a well known novelist born in Hobart, Tasmania who is credited with the earliest establishment of a play centre and educational opportunities for disabled children.

A relative of Matthew Arnold, Ward went to school in England, settled in Oxford, and in 1872 married Thomas Humphry Ward, an academic and journalist. She was a member of the highest literary circles of the day in which she was best known for her very successful novel *Robert Elsmere,* written in 1888. She was also an indefatigable social worker and philanthropist who established a Social Settlement at Bloomsbury, whilst, surprisingly, opposing an 'extension of the franchise to women'.[115] Frederick Watson in *Civilisation and the Cripple* noted:

> *Of all the educational pioneers, the name of Mrs Humphry Ward is pre-eminent in connection with the earliest schools for physically defective children. Her daughter, Mrs Trevelyan, has truly written, "the author of "Robert Elsmere" was indeed no armchair philanthropist, but with an inborn energy and creative force succeeded against a constant handicap of ill-health in turning her dreams into practical realities. The "New Brotherhood" of her novel became embodied during the "nineties first in University Hall, Gordon Square, and then in the actual Bricks and mortar of the Passmore Edwards Settlement … of which she was the guiding spirit and which now bears her name."*
>
> *The first "play centre" was opened there in 1897, and in 1899 Mrs Ward organised the first public day school for crippled children. When the Education Act of 1918 was passing through Parliament Major John Hills was asked by Mrs Ward to try and make education for physically defective children compulsory. She was too well aware that the crippled child from infancy onwards was relegated to the easy chair and regarded as being physically incapable of attending the village school, and grew up unable to read and write. The difficulties of teaching invalid children were obvious, though their capacities are frequently highly developed.[116]*

One aspect of intervention with the physically handicapped in which occupation was used in some ways similar to the twentieth century was with those who were blind. Similar was the recognition of their need to experience satisfaction and meaning in their lives through purposeful use of time, and the careful choice of occupations and adaptations, which made their "doing" possible. Dissimilar was the economic focus, which has been largely ignored and, in some cases, deplored by some therapists during the twentieth century.

Occupation and the blind

It was in France that the blind's need for special educational facilities were first recognised in the 18th century, as discussed in an earlier chapter. In 1801, the pupils of Hauy's School (des Jeunes Aveugles) were moved to the Paris Blind Asylum, the hospital des Quinze-Vingts. Here, it is reported, their education languished.[117]

In 1815 L'Institution des Jeunes Aveugles was again separated from L'Hospital des Quinze-Vingts and, run by an energetic and devoted Dr. Guillie, was immediately successful. Guillie obtained new instructional apparatus, and new type to print embossed books and music. He also taught a wide range of handcrafts such as spinning, weaving, knitting, chair caning, rope, shoe, and harness making.[118] Guillie, in the way of many modern day occupational therapists, looked for strengths to develop within the people he sought to help rather than handicap to overcome. In *An Essay on the Instruction and Amusements of the Blind*, he wrote of the "faculties" which were often to be found in those so handicapped, noting that some were very clever in business, and others 'excellent poets, or learned musical composers'. He provided examples of the success stories of two of his pupils. One of them became 'Grand Master of the University, Professor of Mathematics in the Lyceum of Angers, where he teaches with the greatest success', and the other became notable in 'the philosophy of the French language'. Careful observation provided the insight that the blind often attained that 'facility of analysis and decomposition' when allowed to self develop, in preference to being taught the 'processes and formulas of reasoning' used by sighted people.[119] Perhaps of particular interest, Guillie also described adaptations for particular occupations, some of which are quoted and illustrated below.

Figure 1.10.7   Spinning: (Plate VII: in Guillie, 1819)
(British Library)

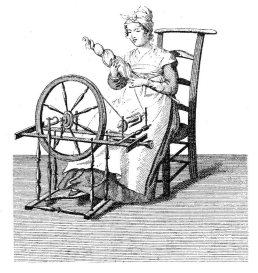

SPINNING does not offer the same difficulties as knitting; nevertheless, the blind must have great practice to be able to spin evenly. As they are always inclined to bend forward, it is proper to keep their distaff high, and as near the head as possible; the left hand being placed above the yarn, as with those who can see. This hand holds the distaff, not only to support it, but to distribute and cull the yarn, which passes through the left hand to be rounded off; the two hands, being thus brought near together, can, much more easily than if they were insulated, stop any knots that are formed, without the Spinner being obliged to suspend the motion of the foot. He must make the wheel turn gently, in order that the thread may not be too much twisted, which would necessarily happen if the yarn was not given out in proportion with the motion of the wheel. It is, consequently, better that the wheels of their machines should be a little smaller than they commonly are, that the rotation of the bobbin may not be more accelerated than is necessary.[120]

**Figure 1.10.8:   Catgut whips:
(Plate XV: in Guillie,
1819)**

(British Library)

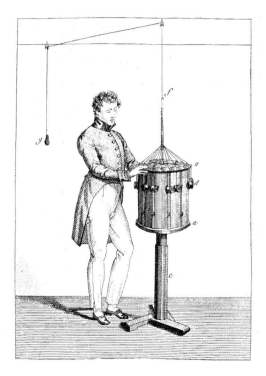

The manufacture of whips in the loom is no longer lucrative, since machinery has been invented by which a single man can make a great many at once. Nevertheless, as the blind can never make whips with the machinery, without assistance, as they did formerly with the frame, we think proper to describe it, that those who wish to make use of may be able to copy it.[122]

Figure 1.10.9: **Weaving:**
(Plate XVI: in
Guillie, 1819)

(British Library)

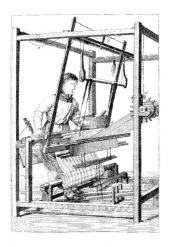

If there is any profession that is eminently suitable to the blind, it is that of weaving, which they have only been put to, however, since the translation of the establishment, though there had been for a long time, in the spinning house of the hospitals, among the other workmen, a blind man who supported his family by the produce of his labour.

Except setting the warp, for which sight is indispensable, there is no part of weaving which the blind cannot execute: they fix themselves the pieces on the looms: they prepare and dry the warp without burning the threads. They manufacture sail-cloth, of which sacks and sails are made, and worked napkins. We have even contrived to teach them to make cotton handkerchiefs of different colours.[123]

Figure 1.10.10: **Straw Chair-bottoms:**
(Plate XVII: in Guillie,
1819)

(British Library)

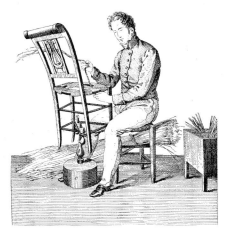

The making straw bottoms for chairs is a mode of industry which the blind perform with ease. … The blind man being seated with his hands on a level with the upper part of the chair-bottom, he fastens the first straws on the side of the back of the chair, and continues turning it round every time he adds a straw.

The blind can work plain or coloured straw equally well; but the work which suits them best is that of the coarse chairs that are used in the churches or public walks.[124]

Guillie is said not to have been very successful in helping his pupils become self-supporting when they left the institution. In that respect, when Dr Howe, a pioneer of work among the blind in America, made a tour of the European Schools in 1833 he was disappointed despite finding the children both happy and well-cared for. He came to the conclusion that though the School looked good the system was a failure because only about 5% were able to support themselves on leaving. Not much later the School replaced handcrafts with training in piano tuning which was more successful in terms of future employment.[125]

The story of the adoption of piano tuning is interesting. Two students at the institution 'got into trouble for tampering with the action of the school piano'. Despite that they 'obtained permission to buy the wreck of an instrument and keep it in the institution'. Eventually they restored it to a playable condition, one of the students, Montal, afterwards becoming one of the best known piano tuners in Paris.[126]

In Britain the four educational establishments for the blind which were founded in the 18th century were added to substantially throughout the nineteenth. Most were charitable concerns but were also in large part self-supporting.[127] Table 1.10.1 lists the British Institutions for the Blind, which spread the length and breadth of the country.

Aberdeen (1812)	Armagh (1854)	Bath (1850)
Belfast (1831)	Bolton (1867)	Birmingham(1845)
Bradford (1861)	Brighton (1842)	Bristol (1793)
Cardiff (1865)	Carlisle (1872)	Cheltenham (1858)
Cork (1843)	Devonport (1860)	Dublin(1810-1858)**
Dundee (1869)	Edinburgh (1793)	Exeter (1838)
Glasgow (1827)	Hull (1868)	Inverness (1866)
Leeds (1866)	Leicester (1858)	Limerick (1834)
Liverpool (1791)	London (1799 - 1881)*	Manchester (1827)
Newcastle (1838)	Norwich (1805)	Nottingham (1843)
Plymouth (1860)	Preston (1867)	Sheffield (1879)
Southsea (1864)	Stockport (1867)	Sunderland (1877)
Swansea (1865)	Wolverhampton (1882) Worcester (1866)	
York (1833)	(NOTE: * London had six institutions. **Dublin had four)	

Table 1.10.1: Institutions for the Blind in the United Kingdom and founding date

There were four classes of such institutions. About 36% were schools for resident pupils and about 26% were workshops, mostly for non-residents. About 24% were a combination of the two, where a workshop was attached to a school and in which some of the pupils continued to work after leaving school and, as well, other blind workers were taken. The final about 12% were asylums in which residents may remain for life. In 1886, there were about 891 male and 676 female school students taught by 74 seeing and 53 blind teachers; 886 males, 204 females and 27 boy workshop attendees instructed by 57 teachers; and 188 male and 309 female asylum dwellers. The age of admission varied, with asylums taking residents from the age of five upwards, resident schools from six to sixteen years, resident school/workshops from eight to twenty-one years, and workshops from fourteen to forty years. Apart from those establishments there was the Mission to the Outdoor Blind which was a Scottish organisation situated close to Glasgow which visited over 1000 people in their own homes. The society also looked after 20 children in the Board School, and helped some to start in trades. Upwards of 50 were engaged in trading concerns, and 52 found employment in dockyards, foundries and such like.[128]

Obtaining remunerative employment was one of 'the most important and, at the same time, one of the most difficult to be solved' despite the fact that there was 'scarcely any trade or profession, except, perhaps, that of painting, in which the blind have not distinguished themselves'.[129]

Figure 1.10.11: Blind school, Southwark. Lettering on the cornice includes: 'Articles manufactured by the indigent blind. Hearth Rugs' and on the left side 'For sale articles manufactured here". Coloured engraving by R. Acon, 1829, after T.H.Shepherd.
(The Wellcome Library)

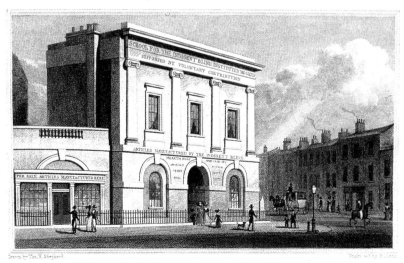

In most schools music was taught, and almost all the larger ones expected their musical pupils to obtain situations as organists, teachers, or tuners. Armitage, the Secretary to the *British and Foreign Blind Association for Promoting the Education and Employment of the Blind*, who considered that independence rather than special workshops was the ideal, suggested that 'the piano and the organ are the principal instruments by which a blind man may expect to earn a living'. He considered that piano tuning was especially valuable because even someone without early musical training could take it up. What was required, apart from three or four years of experience, was 'average intelligence, fair mechanical dexterity, a good ear, … perseverance, and determination to succeed'. A good tuner would probably be able to earn from 50 to 100 pounds a year, which was far more than any other trade.[130]

Another possible source of independence was through the making of baskets, which some did independently of any workshops or charitable assistance. In the workshops, it was the most frequently chosen trade, being selected by 41 institutions despite being difficult and requiring several years' apprenticeship. One of the greatest difficulties to overcome was in maintaining a basket's shape, which if not mastered made the work unsaleable. However, it had the potential to generate a good income of up to 50 pounds a year, especially if the maker was employed in a workshop. Bath was one of the few institutions that taught it to girls, and the women living in that asylum, were known for making 'very beautiful and fine fancy baskets'.[131]

Chair caning was also popular being used in 26 institutions, mat making in 23, wool-work in 20 and brush making in 18. Brush making and chair caning did not pay nearly so well as basket making, but were easier to learn. Whilst very few were able to brush-make at home because of the cost and wastage of the materials, chair caning, suiting both men and women, was a trade that could be practised away from a workshop. In the case of making mats, there was so much competition from prisons that it was scarcely worth while except working for orders. Bedding-making, which term included all upholstery work such as palliasses, hair mattresses, flock and feather beds, was remunerative and an excellent trade for the blind as it was easily learnt by adults of either gender, women earning better wages at sewing the ticking than by knitting. Like brush making it was quite unsuited for work at home because it required so much space. It was practised more in the Scottish than in the English institutions, like rope making. Other occupations taught were knitting, sewing, making "feather and hair cleaners", and weaving carpets. As a rule, the work done was sold from the workshops and, in addition to that, many sold other articles that the purchaser would expect to find in a similar shop.

On a more prosaic note, wood chopping was a popular occupation in London. A considerable number of blind men engaged in it at home, and if they had family members to tie the bundles for them they could earn fair wages.[132]

However, those who became blind after learning their trade, were recommended to continue with it if possible. For the many for whom it would not be possible, it was recommended that they be encouraged to learn 'the kind of employment for which they show most aptitude'. Probably unacceptable to our ears, was the understanding that for some the choice might be begging.

> *The only excuse that can be offered is that it is really difficult, if not impossible, under present conditions, for all those to find employment who are capable of work and anxious to do it; and the free life of the streets offers more attractions to many of these poor people than the workhouse; yet it cannot be too often repeated that begging is in the highest degree demoralising, both to the beggar and to the children or others who assist them.*

Beggars used 'various ways of attracting the notice and compassion of the passers-by' such as 'pretending to sell laces or matches', playing 'a barrel-organ, or some other musical or non-musical instrument', and loud bible reading in a public thoroughfare when footsteps approached. However, apparently, 'the beggar's trade (was) not so profitable as it used to be … since people have found out that they generally do far more harm than good by giving to such persons'.[133]

Some additional light is thrown on the system of training in vogue at that time from the 1874 report of the School for the Indigent Blind in Southwark. That year, workshops were set up in part of the basement for past students to continue their training. Until then, a six-year period had been fixed as the duration of a pupil's stay. It stated in the report that:

> *… mental and industrial training commence together [at the age of 10]. After the first year more time is given to the latter than to the former, and the fourth year, if fair progress has been made in the schoolroom, almost the whole time is devoted to industrial pursuits.*[134]

At the turn of the century "Massage", which had been traditionally practiced by the blind in Japan, was added to the occupations most often followed in Britain as a means for them to make a living. Fox, an ophthalmologist, in an paper which discussed the issue, provided an insight into his profession's interest in meeting, at least, the economic occupational interests and needs of their patients. He wrote:

> *The very important question of providing employment for intelligent blind persons is now occupying, more than ever, the attention of all who are interested in their welfare, and certainly none is more solicitous for their welfare than the ophthalmologist. He is, however, too often at a loss when a hopeless case of blindness comes under his notice, as to what occupation he should recommend the poor sufferer to pursue. Organ playing, music teaching and piano tuning are fairly remunerative to the blind; but all do not possess the necessary qualifications, and it is not always easy to find such occupation for those who have the requisite ability. It is well, therefore, that we can confidently recommend the systematic, careful training of capable, healthy blind persons in the art of massage as a remunerative employment for them.*[135]

When the 'Institute for Massage by the Blind' was founded in London eminent members of the medical profession enthusiastically received it. By 1906, when Fox's paper appeared, there were 21 masseuses and 15 masseurs listed as graduates of the institute whom, he said, were providing great satisfaction to those who employed them.[136]

Occupation and tuberculosis

The prescribed use of occupation as therapy for tuberculosis, as distinct from any economic considerations, was introduced in Scotland in the last decade of the Century by Dr Robert Philip to his patients at the Royal Victoria Dispensary and the Royal Victoria Hospital, Edinburgh.[137] Philip observed, clinically, that, although many patients may seem to improve, 'prolonged continuance of resting is fraught with unsatisfactory results'. He noted that many patients:

> ... put on weight in large amount. Often they become heavy and corpulent. But it is commonly mere fat. The skin textures remain pallid and toneless. The muscular tissues remain soft and flabby and the individual himself is far from physiologically fit.[138]

He instigated a programme of graduated work that he described in a paper, *Rest and Movement in Tuberculosis*, published in the British Medical Journal some twenty years after the programme began. 'We instituted classes for physical movement and respiratory exercises in connection with the Royal Victoria Dispensary for Consumption ... In addition to this measured walks of varying amount and gradient were prescribed, exactly as we prescribe medicines.'[139] The length and gradients of walks taking different routes from the Dispensary were measured and calculated so that they could be prescribed appropriately to an individual case, rather as is the situation with some cardio-vascular rehabilitation programmes in the present day. As 'no accident was traced to the adoption of active movement instead of rest' they continued and extended it. Walking alone was no longer considered sufficient, so a programme of regulated work and recreation was devised:

> When the patient is able to walk five miles a day, including the ascent of gradients, he may be promoted to graduated physical labour, or permitted to engage in such outdoor recreations as riding, mild golf, croquet, fishing and shooting.[140]

The amount of activity was determined precisely for each individual and carried out without undue haste and under careful, ongoing observation to ensure that no clinical signs of overactivity occurred. If they did not the activity levels were gradually increased, the patient advancing through the programme of therapeutic exercise and occupation in a series of classified stages. Patients received a badge of a different colour to denote the stage reached, presumably to ensure staff's easy identification of under or over activity and maybe as a simple device to raise patient's awareness of their progress. Philip as described the stages:

I. Resting stage. (White Badge).
On admission to the hospital all patients are prescribed complete rest, lasting from a few days to several weeks according to the individual case.

II . Stage of regulated exercises. (Yellow Badge).
This includes:
1. Walking varying distances from ? to 5 miles - (a) on the level; (b) on sloping
    ground.
2. Various respiratory exercises once or twice a day.
3. Other forms of movements to improve carriage of shoulders, head, chest, &c.

III. Stage of regulated work.
The work was chosen with a view to utility and with due regard to the patient's individual case and to his past trade. This stage is sub-divided into four grades (A,B,C,D).
IIIA. (Pale Blue Badge).
• Picking up papers, leaves and other light rubbish in the grounds.
• Knitting, sewing, drawing.
IIIB. (Green Badge).
• Emptying garden waste-boxes, and assisting to carry away rubbish.
• Carrying light baskets for various gardening purposes.
• Light painting work (gates, fences, furniture, &c.).
• Wiping shelters, setting tables and laying cloth in patients' dining-room.
• Cleaning silver, cleaning brasses, towel rails and taps.
IIIC. (Deep Blue Badge).
• Raking. Hoeing. Mowing. Sweeping leaves. Drawing two-wheeled barrow with
    assistance. Other gardening jobs requiring a similar amount of exertion.
• Heavier painting work.
• Sweeping shelters. Scrubbing floors. Cleaning boots. Cleaning knives.
• Assisting in laundry (folding clothes, &c.). Washing and drying dishes.
111D. (Red Badge).
• Digging. Sawing. Carrying heavy baskets for various garden purposes.
• Wheeling and drawing full wheelbarrow, and other heavy gardening work.
• Drawing bathchair. Bathing other patients.
• Mangling. Window-cleaning. Polishing floors. Sweeping and cleaning
    courtyard.
• Carpentering. Joinering. Attending boiler. Engineering.
N.B.- In III. B, C, and D patients make their own beds and go errands if necessary.[141]

Philip described how the:

> ... *system produces a fine procession of persons, some just emerging from the serious sickness, and others at varying stages of advance towards perfect recovery - the patients severally and literally "working out their own salvation".*

He concluded that:

> ... *the scheme has worked admirably. The progressive improvement in the majority of the patients has been striking. Physically, the results are registrable from day to day in satisfactory fashion.*
>
> *These include a progressive sense of well-being, keenness to live and work, healthy appetite and digestion, return of fresh colour to face and skin, and gain in weight*[142]

Philip recognised that the programme was not effective for all patients, particularly those with advanced disease. However, he believed that for most, given sufficient time, it was successful. At the end of treatment, those who participated acquired a superior level of health to that they experienced even prior to their illness.

The physical environment, and aids to daily living

W.A.F. Browne, a nineteenth century physician, exhibited an exceptional understanding of people as occupational beings. He applied that understanding to the treatment of the insane, which is described, in detail, in the next chapter on mental health. He also made suggestions that preceded the notion of accessibility of environs for the physically disabled. He wrote, for example, in his text *What Asylums Ought to Be* that:

> ... *it is absolutely necessary that a large portion of it should be built of one storey only ... The paralytic will not then be endangered in ascending or descending the stairs ... while free egress to the open air, to the grounds or gardens is enjoyed by the patient.*[143]

Although that appears to be a rare example of appreciating the difficulties faced by those with physical disability, the spirit of exploration and invention which permeated the times did extend to adapting daily objects for use by the handicapped. It was often people of a creative nature, in comparison to being of a scientific or "medical" bent, who demonstrated an interest in solving apparently mundane problems for people with disability. Artists sometimes portrayed those examples. Theodore Gericault, for example, pictured an early kind of wheelchair, in *A Paralytic Woman*. In it a well-to-do lady sits facing backwards whilst a porter pulls the heavy chair with large wooden wheels through the streets.

Figure 1.10.12: An invalid strapped into a special chair. Coloured lithograph.
(The Wellcome Library)

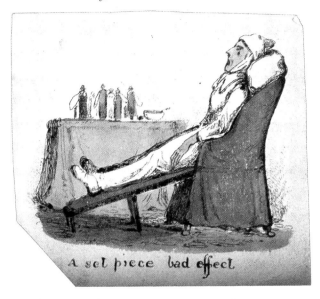

A set piece bad effect

Francisco Goya, the Spanish artist, provided another example. In the early nineteenth century he sketched people who lived on the streets in both Spain and France including some who were physically disabled and used crutches. In one drawing titled *Beggars Get About on Their Own in Bordeaux* he depicted a man suffering from "elephantiasis" getting about on a low profile cart which consisted simply of a board and four wheels. He also sketched a beggar using a cart pulled by a dog, and another, using a more sophisticated model, obviously a self-propelled vehicle with 2 large wheels at the front and a small one at the rear for steering.[144]

The century was certainly a period when people gloried in their creative and entrepreneurial talents, willing to show off their ideas and inventions, however simple they might appear now. Showy pieces of furniture adapted for particular function were just one aspect of the inventive flair. These centred on mobility aids, such as wheeled chairs, similar to those described below which appear to have borrowed heavily from the designs of Merlin whose life and work were discussed in an earlier chapter.

The Invalid or "Gouty"' Chair was made by an unknown hand. The late Georgian style dates it as an early nineteenth century example made to Merlin's design which derived from that of Grollier de Serviere's. The mechanism was simply attached to a conventional armchair, which was a very popular idea throughout the period. Sometimes very grand, the Gouty Chair was made of:
Show-wood grain of mahogany and beech veneered with mahogany, the seat,

back and elbow-cushions stuffed and covered with black hair-cloth edged with gimp. The chair is raised on three mahogany wheels with brass tyres, the two forward ones worked by winches on the arms, the rear one castoring freely …

The front wheels have brass bushes running freely on a fixed iron axle. A brass contrate gear of 48 teeth is screwed to the outer face of each and is engaged by a brass gear of 24 teeth fixed near the lower end of an upright iron spindle. The upper ends of the two upright spindles are housed in the scroll ends of the arms and are reduced to squares to accept a pair of iron winches with brass pipes and mahogany knobs. Sitting in the chair, the user may move at will by turning winches at once or separately. The winches may be taken off when not in use. The wheels may be arrested by pushing down the mahogany knob seen at the front of the seat to the user's right. This causes a pair of iron detents to drop into spaces between the teeth on the large wheels.[145]

Some chairs, both by Merlin and by other makers, had reclining backs, leg extension boards, adjustable tables or reading desks. The "Invalids Wheelchair", described as a Merlin Chair, which was a recliner with leg board, was manufactured by Thomas Chapman of Soho and signed on the hub cap. The first entry for Chapmans' as manufacturers of Invalid Beds, Chairs, &c., in the Post Office Directory was in 1838. It appears that by 1847, when the notice was extended to read 'manufacturer of fracture & invalid beds, chairs, spinal carriages, desks, dressing cases', the firm occupied at least two premises and, possibly remained in business until around 1862.[146]

This type of chair was generally known as a Merlin chair from about 1814 as it is thought to have been devised by him. A similar, but more expensive chair also attributed to Merlin was known as the "Morpheus Chair", but as is the case with the Gouty Chair, no examples signed by Merlin are known. He did invite "all Artists of Genius" to take drawings of his "Morpheus" and "Gouty" chairs, amongst other items, and the leading makers of mechanical furniture of this type, such as Morgan and Sanders, and William Pocock, are known to have taken up his offer. One particular version was described as a:

Reclining armchair with show-wood mahogany frame, the seat, back and elbow cushions stuffed and covered with golden-brown cut moquette edged with green gimp. The seat may be drawn forward, allowing the back to recline. There is provision for a leg board to be drawn out from under the seat, to make a full length couch. The Chair may stand on four casters of conventional size fitted to its legs, but is also fitted with two large detachable mahogany wheels with brass tyres and mahogany hoops for the hands and a large detachable brass castor at the rear.

The hoops on the large wheels for the occupant to hold avoided the need to grasp a dirty tyre and anticipate modern designs. With castor or castors at the rear it was an ancestor of the 20th century hospital wheelchair.[147]

In 1814 William Pocock was a leading manufacturer of furniture and inventions for invalids. He achieved popularity early in the nineteenth century and received Royal Patronage. He was one of many makers specialising in multi-purpose portable campaign furniture produced for the Peninsular War. His range included are various reclining beds, a chair for elevating one or two legs, and a type of Merlin Chair manufactured with "an elegant and modern appearance" … and with an additional reading-stand.[149]

Apart from wheelchairs and specially designed furniture, other attempts were made to make life easier for people with disability, sometimes produced by themselves. In an interesting text titled *Enchiridion, Or A Hand For The One-Handed*, George Derenzy published an account of his inventions and adaptations to assist those with only one hand to manage their activities of daily life. This was prompted by his own handicap and the needs of other soldiers similarly disabled as a result of their profession. He began with a letter addressing his Royal Highness, Frederick Augustus, Duke of York, Commander in Chief:

> *Sir, the attention which your Royal Highness has invariably shewn to the necessities and comforts of the British Army, encourages me to offer to your Royal Highness's notice the following page, illustrative of a set of instruments, to the invention and improvement of which I was originally induced to turn my attention, by the inconveniences I found myself continually exposed to, in my own person, in consequence of the loss of my right arm, at the battle of Vittoria; and on the perfecting of which I have since bestowed considerable time, in the hope of enabling some of the numerous individuals who, from the chance of war, or accident, may be in similar circumstances with myself, to derive the same benefit from the use of them that I have done.*
>
> *In bringing before your Royal Highness anything connected with the cause of humanity, I feel convinced that but little apology is necessary; it is this conviction which has emboldened me to introduce myself on your Royal Highness's notice, and I gladly avail myself of the opportunity it affords me, to declare that I have the honour to be, with the most heartfelt zeal, and attachment,*
>
> *Most respectfully*
> *Your Royal Highness's*
> *devoted and obedient*
> *humble servant*
> *George Webb DERENZY*
> *1 Robert Street, Adelphi*
> *LONDON, July 1st, 1821*[150]

In his text Derenzy observed 'that the real worth of anything is seldom known to the party who may be in actual possession of it', and that:

> *… a sound mind in a sound body, is the greatest good that can fall to the lot of any human being; yet it is granted to millions who are not conscious of any positive happiness from it: let, however, calamity or disease impair either the operations of the mind, or the functions of the body, and their inestimable importance is immediately made manifest.*[151]

He observed that people with the use of both hands 'never pause amidst the various avocations of the day' to give thanks for their ongoing function until, after suffering disease or accident which renders one hand useless, the loss is ever apparent in 'a thousand painful instances of daily and inevitable occurrence'. His own experience led him to devote considerable time and effort to "contriving and perfecting" a set of instruments which would enable independence, negating the assistance of a servant or friend.[152]

He explained that the adaptation with most utility was often the most simple, as has been found true during the twentieth century. Indeed, some of the aids he devised are similar to those made by occupational therapists in more recent times, whilst some, like the "quill holder" are products of his time.

> *The Quill holder is a very simple instrument, by applying which to the stem of the universal joint, and ivory vice, and fastening the whole to the table, a pen may be made or mended, and a pencil pointed, by only one hand, with as much ease and expedition, as if two were employed in doing it. The instrument must be placed on the defective side; so as to make the table support the arm - to nib the pen with one hand.*[153]

The lead cushion 'will be found, simple as it may appear, useful in many instances to a one-handed person; such as in confining papers, or letters in the same manner as a vice', but may, indeed, have been preferable because it was easier to re-arrange. The lead forming the base was about four inches long and half an inch thick. It was covered with lint, which could be renewed if soiled when, for example, it was used on a dressing table for removing soap off a razor or drying it.[154]

Very reminiscent of the "Nelson Knife" was Derenzy's knife and fork instrument. He explained that 'the knife is curved in the form of a cheese cutter, and terminates in four prongs that act as a fork: it cuts by pressure, and as quickly as any other knife can accomplish'. There were three blades in the set, which were made to fit the same handle, which contained a spring to hold them tightly.[155]

Derenzy had his aids manufactured by a London surgical instrument maker, J. Milliken of the Strand, and his price list tabulates the range of his "one-handed apparatus":

	Pounds/	Shillings/	Pence
1. Wash-hand Tray, complete		18	0
2. Ivory vice, Ball & Socket, etc	1	6	0
3. Lather Box	3	6	
4. Lead Cushion	1	6	
5. Syringe, etc.	8	6	
6. Nail File	1	6	
7. File holder	7	0	
8. Boot hooks	10	6	
9. Plated egg-cup	7	6	

10. Steel Egg holder		4	6
11. Pen-knife, etc., etc.,		10	6
12. Pen-holder, & ivory to nib the pen upon		6	0
13. Pen nibber		6	6
14. Heavy ruler		4	6
15. Small steel vice		7	0
16. Hat-stick, complete		10	6
17. Knife and Fork, etc.	1	1	0
18.Nut Cracker, etc.		4	6
19. Card holder	5	0	
20. Neat Mahogany Case for the above	1	0	0
Total Amount	10	4	0

Extra Articles if required.

A pair of steel clamps for wash-hand tray		4	6
' ' plated ' ' ' '		7	0
A pair of nail brushes ' ' '		3	6
A sponge ' ' ' '		10	6
A tin japanned case ' ' '		3	6
A silver egg cup	1	14	6
A steel blade and fork		3	6
A plated ' ' ' '		6	0
A Morocco leather case for a set of knives etc.		4	0
A plated nut-cracker, etc.		9	6
A plated nut card holder		18	6[156]

In summary, a goodly proportion of the work now carried out by occupational therapists to enable people with disability to live fulfilled and independent lives appears to have begun to gain momentum during the industrial period, but was largely carried out outside the medical profession. However there was also a growing interest within their ranks in the illness consequences of paid work, especially among those with serious social or moral concerns about the economic and materially driven values of the time. That led to the development of scientific management specialists and industrial psychologists as well as medical and lay specialities concerned with occupational health and safety. However, as care of physical illness came increasingly to be seen as the exclusive domain of the medical profession, the number of lay or alternative practitioners declined. It was not until the next century that they were replaced with new and different health care specialists who grew under the sponsorship of medicine by accepting its authority. Except for that multiplication of specialties and sub-specialties over the ensuing 140 years, by the 1850s the essential structure of the present medical profession had been created, cemented by the Medical Acts of 1858 and 1886.[157] Occupational therapy could be claimed to be one such sub-specialty.

The evolving dominance of the medical profession, and its distancing from "trade", was dependent on the strength brought about by its unification. Jewson argues that that brought with it a change from the client centred practice of earlier centuries to doctor dominated practice.[158] That was to have implications for occupational therapy in the early days, and resulted in prescribed, "expert" type of practice preceding the current adoption of an enabling approach. Indeed, the prescribed use of occupation as treatment was already a fact, at least in terms of tuberculosis, and the use of occupation as an instrument of health became much more reliant on association with medicine.

[1]Gelfand T. The decline of the ordinary practitioner and the rise of the modern medical profession. In: Statum S, Larson DE, eds. Doctors, Patients and Society: Power and Authority in Medical Care. Ontario: 1981; Waddington I. The Medical Profession in the Industrial Revolution. Dublin: Gill & Macmillan, 1984.

[2]Porter R. Disease, Medicine and Society in England 1550-1860. Basingstoke and London: MacMillan Education, 1987; 48-60.

[3]Porter. Disease, Medicine and Society in England 1550-1860...; 48-60.

[4]Porter. Disease, Medicine and Society in England 1550-1860...; 48-60.

[5]Magray MP. The Transforming Power of the Nuns: Women, Religion, and Cultural Change in Ireland, 1750-1900. New York/Oxford: Oxford University Press, 1998; 78.

[6]Burke H. The People and the Poor Law in Nineteenth Century Ireland. Dublin: WEB, 1987; 162-163.

[7]Report of the Irish Poor Law Commissioners for 1861; 394-417.

[8]O'Connor J. The Workhouses of Ireland; The Fate of Ireland's Poor. Dublin: Anvil Books, 1995; 180.

[9]Clear C. Nuns in Nineteenth Century Ireland. Dublin: Gill & Macmillan, 1987; 11, 28.

[10]Macdonald EM. World-Wide Conquests of Disabilities: The History, Development and Present Functions of the Remedial Services. London: Bailliere Tindall, 1981; 85-86.

[11]Bell Sir C. The Hand; Its Mechanism and Vital Endowments as Evincing Design. London: Bell and Dalby, 1865.

[12]Central Council for the Disabled. A Record of 50 Years Service to the Disabled from 1919-1965. London, 1969; 3.

[13]Woodham-Smith C. Florence Nightingale. London: The Reprint Society, 1952; 71.

[14]Henderson DK. The Evolution of Psychiatry in Scotland. Edinburgh and London: E & S Livingstone Ltd, 1964; 82-84.

[15]Cassell's Household Guide to Every Department of Practical Life: Being a Complete Encyclopaedia of Domestic and Social Economy. New and revised ed. London, Paris & New York: Cassell, Petter & Galpin, c1890; vol. I: 380.

[16]Cassell's Household Guide...; vol. I: 380.

[17]Cassell's Household Guide...; vol. I: 380.

[18]Cassell's Household Guide...; vol. I: 350.

[19]Cassell's Household Guide...; vol. I: 174, 379.

[20]Cassell's Household Guide;...; vol. I: 182-183.

[21]Porter. Disease, Medicine and Society in England 1550-1860.

[22]Girling DA, ed. New Age Encyclopedia. Sydney and London: Bay Books, 1983; vol. 6: 150.

[23]Porter. Disease, Medicine and Society in England 1550-1860.

[24]Kay-Shuttleworth J. The Moral and Physical Condition of the Working Classes. Manchester: 1832.

[25]Porter. Disease, Medicine and Society in England 1550-1860.

[26]Marti-Ibañez F, ed. Henry E. Sigerist on the History of Medicine. New York: MD

Publications, Inc. 1960; 16.

[27]Marti-Ibañez. Henry E. Sigerist on the History of Medicine…; 22-24.

[28]Macdonald. World-Wide Conquests of Disabilities…; 88-9.

[29]Aiken J. Description of the Country from 30-40 Miles Round Manchester. 1795. In: Guy Rev Dr. JR. Compassion and the Art of the Possible: Dr. Southwood Smith as Social Reformer and Public Health Pioneer. Octavia Hill Memorial Lecture. December 1993. Cambridgeshire: Octavia Hill Society & The Birthplace Museum Trust, 1996; 5.

[30]Macdonald. World-Wide Conquests of Disabilities…; 88-9.

[31]Houghton W. Cited in: Guy. Compassion and the Art of the Possible…; 5.

[32]Guy Rev Dr. JR. Compassion and the Art of the Possible…; 5.

[33]Dickens C. Hard Times. Australia: Penguin; 1981; 65.

[34]Southwood Smith T. The Philosophy of Health or the Exposition of the Physical and Mental Constitution of Man, with a View to the Promotion of Human Longevity and Happiness. Volume 1. London: Charles Knight, MDCCCXXXVI 1836-7.

[35]Southwood Smith. The Philosophy of Health…; 73.

[36]Southwood Smith. The Philosophy of Health…; 101.

[37]Southwood Smith. The Philosophy of Health…; 75.

[38]Southwood Smith. The Philosophy of Health…; 81-82.

[39]Southwood Smith. The Philosophy of Health…; 85.

[40]Southwood Smith. The Philosophy of Health…; 88.

[41]Southwood Smith. The Philosophy of Health…; 92.

[42]Guy. Compassion and the Art of the Possible…; 2-4, 6.

[43]Guy. Compassion and the Art of the Possible…; 7.

[44]Dickens C. Bleak House. London: Pan Books Ltd., 1976; 259-260.

[45]Guy. Compassion and the Art of the Possible…; 8-9.

[46]Guy. Compassion and the Art of the Possible…; 10.

[47]Guy. Compassion and the Art of the Possible…; 11.

[48]Dickens C. A Christmas Carol. London: Peerage Books. 1991; 607.

[49]Guy. Compassion and the Art of the Possible…; 12.

[50]Meiklejohn A. The Life, Work and Times of Charles Turner Thackrah, Surgeon and Apothecary of Leeds (1795-1833). Edinburgh and London: E & S Livingstone Ltd, 1957.

[51]Meiklejohn. The Life, Work and Times of Charles Turner Thackrah.

[52]Thackrah CT. Effects of the Principal Arts, Trades, and Professions, and of Civic States and Habits of Living on Health and Longevity: with particular reference to the Trades and Manufactures of Leeds: and suggestions for the removal of many of the agents, which produce disease, and shorten the duration of life. (Originally published: London: Longman, Rees, Orme, Brown & Green, 1831). In: The Life, Work and Times of Charles Turner Thackrah…; 2-3.

[53]Thackrah. Effects of the Principal Arts…; 187.

[54]Thackrah. Effects of the Principal Arts…; 187-189.

[55]Thackrah. Effects of the Principal Arts…; 194-196.

[56]Thackrah. Effects of the Principal Arts…; 205-207.

[57]Cassell's Household Guide…; 25-26.

[58]Cassell's Household Guide…; 25.

[59]Cassell's Household Guide…; 25.

[60]Georgii A, ed. Ling's Educational and Curative Exercises. London: Renshaw, 1875; 17.

[61]Georgii. Ling's Educational and Curative Exercises…; 22.

[62]Georgii. Ling's Educational and Curative Exercises…; 23.

[63]Georgii. Ling's Educational and Curative Exercises…; 21-22.

[64]Georgii. Ling's Educational and Curative Exercises…; 23.

[65]Georgii. Ling's Educational and Curative Exercises…; 19-20.

[66]Goodbody J. The Illustrated History of Gymnastics. London: Stanley Paul, 1982; 16.

[67]Goodbody. The Illustrated History of Gymnastics.

[68]Macdonald EM. World-Wide Conquests of Disabilities: The History, Development and Present Functions of the Remedial Services. London: Bailliere Tindall, 1981.

[69]Medical and Surgical Directions for Cottagers and for the Domestic Practitioner. London: William Freeman, 1864; 38.

[70]Harvey P, ed. The Oxford Companion to English Literature. Fourth edition. Oxford: Clarendon Press; 762.

[71]Briggs A. Victorian values: Samuel Smiles: The gospel of self-help. History Today, May 1987; 37-43.

[72]Briggs. Victorian values: Samuel Smiles…; 37-43.

[73]Southwood Smith. The Philosophy of Health.

[74]Smiles S. Physical Education: or the Nurture and Management of Children. Edinburgh: Oliver & Boyd, 1838.

[75]Harvey. The Oxford Companion to English Literature…; 113, 178, 739, 762.

[76] Smiles S: Self-Help; With Illustrations of Character and Condut. London: John Murray, 1859; 241.

[77]Smiles: Self-Help; 243-244.

[78]Smiles. Thrift. 1875.

[79]Briggs. Victorian values: Samuel Smiles…; 37-43.

[80]Briggs. Victorian values: Samuel Smiles…; 37-43.

[81]Smiles. Self-Help…; 241.

[82]Smiles. Self-Help…; 245, 247.

[83]Smiles. Self-Help…; 243-244.

[84]Johnson AJ. The Economy of Health. 2nd edition. London: S. Highley, 1837; 14.

[85]Johnson. The Economy of Health…; 20.

[86]Johnson. The Economy of Health…; 107.

[87]Johnson. The Economy of Health.

[88]Johnson. The Economy of Health…; 17.

[89]Johnson. The Economy of Health…; 24-25.

[90]Johnson. The Economy of Health…; 50.

[91]Johnson. The Economy of Health…; 64-65.

[92]Johnson. The Economy of Health…; 144.

[93]Johnson. The Economy of Health…; 145.

[94]Johnson. The Economy of Health…; 146.

[95]Johnson. The Economy of Health…; 147.

[96]Kearsley GD, Glyn J. A Concise International History of Rheumatology and Rehabilitation: Friend and Foe. Royal Society of Medical Services, 1991; 4.

[97]Johnson J. Pilgrimages to the Spas in Pursuit of Health and Recreation with an Inquiry into the Comparative Merits of Different Mineral Waters:- the Maladies to Which they are Applicable and Those in Which they are Injurious. London: S. Highley, 1841.

[98]Johnson. Pilgrimages to the Spas in Pursuit of Health…; 62.

[99]Johnson. Pilgrimages to the Spas in Pursuit of Health…; 61-62.

[100]Johnson. Pilgrimages to the Spas in Pursuit of Health…; 177.

[101]Johnson. Pilgrimages to the Spas in Pursuit of Health…; 61-62.

[102]Johnson. Pilgrimages to the Spas in Pursuit of Health…; 62.

[103]Johnson. Pilgrimages to the Spas in Pursuit of Health…; 62, 177.

[104]Johnson. Pilgrimages to the Spas in Pursuit of Health…; 2.

[105]Johnson. Pilgrimages to the Spas in Pursuit of Health…; 2.

[106]Johnson. Pilgrimages to the Spas in Pursuit of Health...; 61.

[107]Johnson. Pilgrimages to the Spas in Pursuit of Health...; 61.

[108]Johnson. Pilgrimages to the Spas in Pursuit of Health...; 61.

[109]Johnson. Pilgrimages to the Spas in Pursuit of Health...; 2.

[110]MacCarthy F. William Morris: A Life for Our Time. New York: Faber & Faber, 1994; 233.

[111]Kersley & Glyn. A Concise International History of Rheumatology and Rehabilitation.

[112]Cassell's Household Guide...; 211-214.

[113]Macdonald. World-Wide Conquests of Disabilities...; 111.

[114]Marr HC. Journal of Mental Science, July, 1899.

[115]Harvey. The Oxford Companion to English Literature...; 871.

[116]Watson F. Civilization and the Cripple. London: John Bale, Sons & Danielsson, Ltd., 1930; 32.

[117]Ritchie JM. Concerning the Blind. London: Oliver & Boyd, 1930; 10.

[118]Ritchie. Concerning the Blind.

[119]Guillie Dr. An Essay on the Instruction and Amusements of the Blind. London: Sampson Low, Marston and Co. Ltd. Reprint 1894 ; 29-30. (originally published 1819).

[120]Guillie. An Essay on the Instruction and Amusements...; 130.

[121]Guillie. An Essay on the Instruction and Amusements...; 135.

[122]Guillie. An Essay on the Instruction and Amusements...; 140.

[123]Guillie. An Essay on the Instruction and Amusements...; 142.

[124]Guillie. An Essay on the Instruction and Amusements...; 144.

[125]Ritchie. Concerning the Blind...; 11.

[126]Ritchie. Concerning the Blind...; 11.

[127]Armitage TR. The Education and Employment of the Blind: What it Has Been, Is, and Ought To Be. 2nd edition. Pall Mall: Harrison & Sons, 1886; 93-109.

[128]Armitage. The Education and Employment of the Blind.

[129]Armitage. The Education and Employment of the Blind.

[130]Armitage. The Education and Employment of the Blind.

[131]Armitage. The Education and Employment of the Blind; 60.

[132]Armitage. The Education and Employment of the Blind.

[133]Armitage. The Education and Employment of the Blind...; 59.

[134]Report of the School for the Indigent Blind in Southwark. 1874 . Cited in: Richie. Concerning the Blind...; 15.

[135]Fox LW. Massage, An Occupation For the Blind. Reprinted from 'Opthalmology' October 1906. London: Welcome Library, 1906.

[136]Fox. Massage, An Occupation For the Blind.

[137]Groundes-Peace ZC. An outline of the development of occupational therapy in Scotland. The Scottish Journal of Occupational Therapy 1957; 30: 16-39.

[138]Philip R. Collected Papers on Tuberculosis. London: Humphrey Milford: Oxford University Press, 1937, 133-134. (Originally published as: Rest and Movement in Tuberculosis. British Medical Journal, 24th December, 1910).

[139]Philip. Collected Papers on Tuberculosis...; 133-134.

[140]Groundes-Peace. An outline of the development of occupational therapy in Scotland.

[141]Philip. Collected Papers on Tuberculosis...; 142-143.

[142]Philip. Collected Papers on Tuberculosis...; 143.

[143]Browne WAF. What Asylums Were, Are, and Ought To Be. Being the Substance of Five Lectures Delivered before the Managers of the Montrose Lunatic Asylum. Edinburgh: Adam and Charles Black, 1837; 183-184.

[144]Covey HC. Social Perceptions of People with Disabilities in History. Springfield, Illinois: Charles C. Thomas. 1998; 47, 50-51.

[145]French A. John Joseph Merlin. An Ingenious Mechanick. London: Iveagh Bequest, Kenwood, Greater London Council, 1985; 73-74.

[146]French. John Joseph Merlin…; 75.

[147]French. John Joseph Merlin; 75.

[148]Pocock W. Furniture and Inventions for Invalids. Double-paged advertisement, 1814.

[149]Pocock. Furniture and Inventions for Invalids.

[150]Derenzy GW. Enchiridion or a Hand for the One Handed. London: T.G. Underwood, 1822; lll-V.

[151]Derenzy. Enchiridion or a Hand for the One Handed…; 9-10.

[152]Derenzy. Enchiridion or a Hand for the One Handed…; 10-11.

[153]Derenzy. Enchiridion or a Hand for the One Handed…; 36.

[154]Derenzy. Enchiridion or a Hand for the One Handed…; 23.

[155]Derenzy. Enchiridion or a Hand for the One Handed…; 42-43.

[156]Derenzy. Enchiridion or a Hand for the One Handed…; 59-60.

[157]Loudon I. Medical Care and the General Practitioner 1750-1850. Oxford: Oxford University Press, 1986; 1-5.

[158]Jewson N. Medical knowledge and the patronage system in 18th century England. Sociology 1974; 8: 369-385.

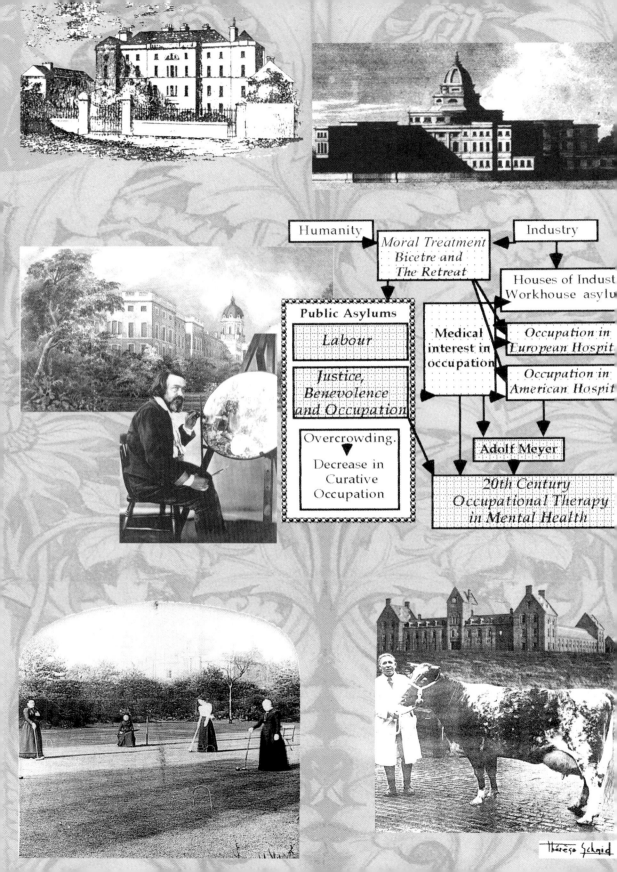

Humanity → Moral Treatment Bicetre and The Retreat ← Industry

Moral Treatment Bicetre and The Retreat → Public Asylums

Industry → Houses of Indust. Workhouse asylu

Public Asylums
Labour
Justice, Benevolence and Occupation
Overcrowding. Decrease in Curative Occupation

Medical interest in occupation

Occupation in European Hospit

Occupation in American Hospit

Adolf Meyer

20th Century Occupational Therapy in Mental Health

Thérèse Schmid

Chapter 11

Justice, Benevolence and Occupation in Mental Health

Contents

In this chapter the story of occupation for mental health is continued. The nineteenth century was, without doubt, the time in history when the use of occupation to treat the mentally ill was at its zenith. There is so much written about the many occupational programmes that were established in Asylums, that only a few have been chosen to consider in depth. These appear outstanding in both the extent of practice and the philosophical ideas behind the treatment.

At the start of the nineteenth century, with industry entrenched as the dominant economic milieu, there was a dovetailing of what had been, and what would be again, substantially divergent views of approaches to care. The largely unsuccessful remedial "physic" regimes of medicine gave way to moral management, the use of purpose built environments and therapeutic occupation. Over this time medicine exerted an ever increasing influence within the domain of mental illness. However in order to do so doctors had to accept a consultant role in the use of occupation as therapy that was, in the main, carried out by people without a physician's training. Perhaps because of that, the majority of physicians did not give up their search for a treatment more fitted to their practice base, and so the dominance of moral, occupational regimes was relatively short lived, in a way similar to rehabilitation medicine in the 20th century.

It is important at this point to clarify just what moral treatment was thought to be in the nineteenth century. W.A.F. Browne, in 1837, described it this way:

> *All recent writers on insanity have spoken loudly in praise of moral treatment ... Each of them attaches a different meaning to the word. Employment is the panacea of one, amusement is the specific of another, classification is advocated by the third. Now were every lunatic busily engaged in a suitable occupation: were recreations adapted to the disposition or previous predilections of all provided; was classification even on a broad basis which I would assign, universally adopted, moral treatment if confined to one or all of these ... would be imperfect and comparatively inefficacious ... they are merely parts of the system for the whole.*
>
> *Every arrangement, beyond these for the regulation of animal functions, from the situation, the architecture and furniture of the buildings intended for the insane to the direct appeals made to the affections by means of kindness, discipline, and social intercourse, ought to be embraced by an effective system of moral treatment.*[1]

Whilst that holistic vision is accepted as the boundaries of moral management, this chapter will, of course, largely concentrate on unveiling the occupational elements.

Because the trajectory of moral treatment was upwards at the start of the nineteenth century it is essential to pick up its story at the beginning of this chapter. Moral treatment influenced the next important phase of treatment of the mentally ill, which was the establishment of lunatic asylums as an essential component of therapy. It was within asylums during this time that occupation played an important role as part of moral treatment in the Western World. Several examples of its use will be provided from North America and Europe as well as the United Kingdom.

Having earlier considered Pinel's use of occupation at Bicêtre in Paris, it is timely to build upon Tuke's 1815 account of the use of occupation at the Retreat in York. In the interest of continuity that story will be told in its entirety before returning to discuss the development of asylums in general, and the use of occupation in some of the others.

Occupational treatment at the Retreat

Figure 1.11.1: Samuel Tuke (1784-1857) Etching by C. Callet
(The Wellcome Library)

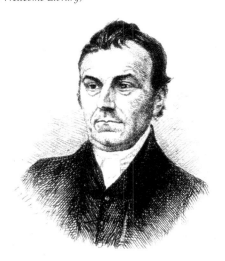

Samuel Tuke's text about the treatment provided at the Retreat provides examples about the use and importance of occupation within moral therapy in early nineteenth century England.[2] In part, as a basis of that use, was a recognition that people may be able to effect their own cure by particular occupations; that engagement in occupation was a natural way of overcoming illness. Tuke, who is pictured in figure 1.11.1, illustrated his belief in the possible effects of occupation by describing the case of "a person of great respectability" who told him of his own unfounded depression and inability to attend to any aspect of his life to the point of physical and mental "emaciation". The man eventually overcame his problems by applying himself to mathematics even though it caused him to experience "indescribable labour and pain". Tuke observed:

> *Perhaps few persons, in the situation which I have described, would have had the courage to form such resolution; and still fewer, the fortitude to perform them. The case, however, certainly points out what may possibly be done; and how important it is, in a curative point of view, to encourage the patient in steady mental pursuit.*[3]

Presumably the perceived difficulty of self motivation to overcome disorder led Tuke to recognise the need for an outside agency to enable renewed engagement in therapeutic occupation. He not only specified the need to use occupation as part of the moral treatment regime, but that any one of a range of people working at the Retreat might be instrumental in facilitating particular patients' engagement in whatever had meaning for them.

Whilst both moral and medical treatment were considered part of the therapeutic process, the first was proving more successful at that time. Tuke considered occupation the most effective form of treatment in terms of the patients learning to exert control for themselves over their mental disorder. 'Of all the modes by which the patients may be induced to restrain themselves, regular employment is perhaps the most generally efficacious.'[4] To have that therapeutic potential he advocated three special properties of the occupations:

That they made physical demands upon the patient

That they were pleasurable for the patient, and

That they counteracted the particular disease manifestations by engaging opposite kinds of capabilities.

In his words:

> ... those kinds of employment are doubtless to be preferred, both on a moral and physical account, which are accompanied by considerable bodily action; that are most agreeable to the patient, and which are most opposite to the illusions of his disease.[5]

Restraint was common in custodial care during the period, and deemed absolutely essential by many experts, so it is not surprising that Tuke explained how this was managed at the Retreat. He described how occupation was used as a form of "self restraint", which he saw as preferable to restraint from outside force or commonly used forms of coercion such as fear, which may have enabled patients to restrain themselves from "mad" behaviour. In the case of fear, he questioned possible detrimental effects because it conflicted with people's apparent need for self-respect. Self respect he saw as a strong motivating factor closely associated with successful occupation, so it was with that in mind that he suggested that occupation aimed at maintaining self respect could be used as a form of restraint. That meant that it was not only beneficial in terms of patient comfort but could be used as a treatment strategy aimed at cure:

> That fear is not the only motive, which operates in producing self-restraint in the minds of maniacs, is evident from its being often exercised in the presence of strangers, who are merely passing through the house; and which, I presume, can only be accounted for, from that desire of esteem, which has been stated to be a powerful motive to conduct.
>
> It is probably from encouraging the action of this principle, that so much advantage has been found in this Institution, from treating the patient as much in the manner of a rational being, as the state of his mind will possibly allow. The superintendent is particularly attentive to this point, in his conversation with the patients. He introduces such topics as he knows will most interest them; and which, at the same time, allows them to display their knowledge to the greatest advantage. If the patient is an agriculturist, he asks him questions relative to his art; and frequently consults him upon any occasion in which his knowledge may be useful. I have heard one of the worst patients in the house, who, previously to his indisposition, had been a considerable grazier, give very sensible directions for the treatment of a diseased cow.
>
> These considerations are undoubtedly very material, as they regard the

comfort of insane persons; but they are of far greater importance, as they relate to the cure of the disorder. The patient feeling himself of some consequence, is induced to support it by the exertion of his reason, and by restraining those dispositions, which, if indulged, would lessen the respectful treatment he receives; or lower his character in the eyes of his companions and attendants[6]

Just as Pinel had found sensory stimulation to be an object of occupational regimes with depressed "melancholic" patients, so to did Tuke describe the necessity for and effectiveness of a variety of occupations in their treatment, and the importance of distraction from their symptoms:

In regard to melancholics, conversation on the subject of their despondency, is found to be highly injudicious. The very opposite method is pursued. Every means is taken to seduce the mind from its favourite but unhappy musings, by bodily exercise, walks, conversation, reading, and other innocent recreations. The good effect of exercise, and of variety of object, has been very striking in several instances at this Institution.[7]

At the Retreat, no aspect in the choice of occupation appeared insignificant. We read, for instance in the example below, about "mathematics and natural science" being deemed suitable topics for patient's reading, whilst "works of imagination" were thought ill-advised because of their supposed similarity to hallucinations and delusions. Also, interestingly, Tuke describes the use of animals as therapy:

There certainly requires considerable care in the selection of books for the use of the insane. The works of imagination are generally, for obvious reasons, to be avoided; and such as are in any degree connected with the peculiar notions of the patient, are decidedly objectionable. The various branches of the mathematics and natural science, furnish the most useful class of subjects on which to employ the minds of the insane; and they should, as much as possible, be induced to pursue one subject steadily.[8]

The means of writing, are, … sometimes obliged to be withheld from the patient, as it would only produce continual essays on his peculiar notions; and serve to fix his errors more completely in his mind. Such patients are, however, occasionally indulged, as it is found to give them temporary satisfaction; and to make them more easily led into suitable engagements.[9]

The superintendent has also endeavoured to furnish a source of amusement, to those patients whose walks are necessarily more circumscribed, by supplying each of the courts with a number of animals; such as rabbits, sea-gulls, hawks, and poultry. These creatures are generally familiar with the patients; and it is believed they are not only a means of innocent pleasure; but that the intercourse with them, sometimes tends to awaken the social and benevolent feelings.[10]

There was also some almost contemporary understanding about the use of occupations that have meaning for the patient in the suggested choice of those that had been previously pursued to a significant degree and to which they were attracted. Tuke advised that 'any branch of knowledge with which the patient has been previously acquainted, may be resumed with greater ease; and his disposition to pursue it will be encouraged by the competency which he is able to exhibit'.[11] He also observed that 'the inclination of the patient may generally be indulged, except the employment he desires obviously tends to foster his disease'.[12]

Tuke recounted a case history of a less than affluent patient suffering from melancholia to illustrate the efficacy of occupation and the critical role played by a "therapist" guiding its application. In the story Tuke recognised that when such therapy was less than maximally effective it could be seen, in some part, as due to lack of an effective approach by the therapist and lack of time given to the treatment because of fiscal constraints:

Some years ago, a patient much afflicted with melancholic and hypochondriacal symptoms, was admitted by his own request. He had walked from home, a distance of 200 miles, in company with a friend; and on his arrival, found much less inclination to converse on the absurd and melancholy views of his own state, than he had previously felt.

This patient was by trade a gardener, and the superintendent immediately perceived, from the effect of this journey the propriety of keeping him employed. He led him into the garden and conversed with him on the subject of horticulture; and soon found that the patient possessed very superior knowledge of pruning and of the other departments of his art. He proposed several improvements in the management of the garden which were adopted, and the gardener was desired to furnish him with full employment. He soon, however showed a reluctance to regular exertion and a considerable disposition to wandering, which had been one of the previous features of his complaint. The gardener was repeatedly charged to encourage him in labour, and to prevent his leaving the premises. But, unhappily, the superior abilities of the patient, had excited a jealousy in the gardener's mind, which made him dislike his assistance; and it may therefore be presumed, that he obeyed his instructions very imperfectly.

The poor man rambled several times from the grounds of the Institution; which, in his state of mind, excited considerable anxiety in the family. Of course it became necessary to confine him more within doors. He frequently, however, walked out; and the superintendent took many opportunities to attend him into the fields or garden, and to engage him for a time in steady manual labour. As his disorder had increased, it became difficult to induce him to exert himself; but even in this state, when he had been some time employed, he seemed to forget his distressful sensations and ideas, and would converse on general topics with great good sense.

In this truly pitiable case, the superintendent several times tried the efficacy of long walks, where the greatest variety and attraction of circumstances were presented; but neither these, nor the conversation which he introduced were able to draw the patient so effectually from the "moods of his own mind," as regular persevering labour in the garden. It is not improbable, however, that the superior manner in which the patient was able to execute his work, produced a degree of self-complacency which had a salutary effect; and that, had his education enlarged his curiosity, and encouraged a taste and observation respecting the objects of nature and art, he might have derived much greater advantage, as many patients obviously do, from variety of conversation and scenery.

The circumstances of this patient did not allow him a separate attendant, and the engagements of the superintendent were too numerous and important, to permit him to devote to this case the time and attention which it seemed to require. He has frequently expressed to me, the strong feelings of regret, which were excited in his mind, by the unsuccessful treatment of this patient; the case certainly points out the great importance of exercise and labour, in the moral treatment of insanity; more especially in cases of melancholy.[13]

With regards to the last paragraph consideration needs to be given to the idea that a private attendant would act, in some part, as an enabler of challenging and meaningful occupation according to the particular needs and potential of a single patient. Even in a private institution like the Retreat the financial costs of providing sufficient, or even "personal occupational therapists", in the modern way of "personal trainers", was not deemed feasible without private funds. The benefits of being in a position to do so are, however, recognised and encouraged. This, coupled with the notion of the skill of the person applying the therapy which has already been alluded to, suggests a far greater understanding of the relationship between what people do and their mental health than is currently always the case. Those who carried out occupational treatment included physicians, superintendents, their wives, matrons, nurses, attendants, and family members. Whilst their official designation may have differed, their duties clearly included, as a primary consideration, the enabling of individual and meaningful programmes. The occupations used in such programmes often closely resembled those of normal life: paid employment for the men folk, and of domesticity for the women. Tuke described how, in a way similar to several institutions on the continent 'the female patients in the Retreat, are employed as much as possible, in sewing, knitting, or domestic affairs; and several of the convalescents assist the attendants'.[14]

At the Retreat great store appeared to set by its homely, domestic and family orientation. That this remained the case well into the nineteenth century is evidenced by a reminiscence of Elizabeth Pumphrey, the daughter of Thomas Allis, who succeeded George Jepson as superintendent in 1823. She recalled that 'in those olden times, when the numbers were small, … the arrangements (were) those of a family party'.[15] This changed later in the century with 'the Retreat becoming essentially a Medical Institution', which 'unavoidably lost its old-time air of freedom and domesticity, so delightful to remember'.[16]

That early freedom and domesticity is well demonstrated by the story of Hannah Ponsonby who was at the Retreat for 'upwards of 40 years'. She first arrived as a child of twelve to help care for her mother who was a patient there until her death in 1816. Ponsonby then stayed on as Catherine Jepson's "devoted" assistant, becoming the Matron when Catherine retired with her husband. As Matron she would have taken responsibility for the women patients' occupations for 18 years as she remained in that post until 1841.[17] (See Figure 1.11.2 for a portrait of Hannah Ponsonby.)

Figure 1.11.2: Hannah Ponsonby
  (Borthwick Institute, York)

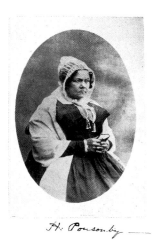

Pumphrey also recalls how, when she herself returned from day-school, she often found her mother '"next-door" among the patients':

> ... *contriving some little pleasure for them - getting worsted and needles for our (MW) to knit (MW preferred having old material to knit, not deeming herself worthy to use new)taking a fresh mince pie to one whose appetite (or will) needed tempting - a tract or book for another - perhaps some pieces of silk or ribbon for one Marg C - who made pincushions or for another, Anne E, who made scissors sheaths, for sale - another knit firm silk sides for round pincushions - another made worsted strings on a "lyre" by which to hang pincushions, key, or scissors - often all three - One decorated her black dress with buttons and coins sewed on.*[18]

Making an appropriate choice of occupation was part of the process of meeting individual needs, as criteria and the therapeutic requirements could differ from patient to patient. Tuke recognised this:

> *The attendant will soon perceive what kind of employment or amusement, is best adapted to the different patients under his care. He will observe that those of the most active and exciting kind, will be best adapted to the melancholy class, where they can be induced to engage in them; and that the more sedentary employments, are generally preferable for the maniacal class. No strict rule, however, can properly be laid down on this subject.*[19]

The Institution's rules about occupation

As the century progressed and knowledge changed or, perhaps, increased with experience the once simple rules and instructions for those working at the Retreat were expanded and altered. Attendants and servants received a copy of the instructions when they entered employment that they returned, with keys and other articles under their care, when they left. There was an expectation that the book of rules would be "frequently perused" and followed.[20] By 1842 in the *Rules for the Government of Attendants and Servants of the Retreat York with Instructions as to the Management of the Patients* particular duties concerning the occupation of patients were listed. Those included:

33. - Exercise and Occupations. It is expected that attendants will, as much as possible, complete the cleaning of rooms, furniture, and utensils under their charge by eleven o'clock; so as to be able to devote from one to two hours before dinner, as well as the whole, or greater part of the afternoon, to joining in the exercise and amusements, and superintending the occupations of the patients.

34. - All patients the state of whose health allows it, must daily, when the weather permits, take a moderate amount of exercise in their respective airing courts or pleasure grounds, both in the morning and afternoon; and those who can be allowed that privilege, are to be taken for walks into the country at such hours as may be appointed by the Resident Surgeon for the men, and by the Matron for the women.

35. - Outdoor Attendant. - The attendant who has the care of the patients who are occupied in the open air, whilst directing and joining in their pursuits, must be very vigilant that they do no injury to themselves or others, or to the buildings or other property. For the full attainment of the object in view, there will be the need for the exercise of patience and equanimity, and for thoroughly kind and considerate conduct and deportment. No patient must be taken out to labour without the approbation of the Resident-Superintendent.

36. - The usual hours for labour shall be from half-past eight or nine o'clock, according to the season, to eleven o'clock, when biscuit or some other suitable refreshment may be provided; and when the less robust shall be allowed to return to their day rooms and airing courts. The others are to resume and continue their employment until half-past twelve o'clock, when they are to return, and under the direction of the out-door attendant, clean themselves and prepare for dinner. In the afternoon, they will resume their occupation from half-past two to five o'clock in summer, and till dusk in winter.

37. - During inclement weather, and in the depth of winter, the outdoor attendant will be expected to superintend the employment of his charge in simple mechanical occupations in the workshop. (Another version of the rules had simple pursuits within doors, either in the workshop or elsewhere).

38. - The out-door attendant will have charge of the library; and in the evening he must be present, as much as possible, with those who are allowed access to the reading room; and must endeavour to gather round him, and amuse, as many of the quiet and orderly patients as practicable.

39. - It is expected that the outdoor attendant, in his intercourse with the patients, will punctually observe the foregoing instructions to the attendants, so far as they apply to him. He is to keep a register of the number employed, which he is, once a week, to bring for examination to the Resident Surgeon.

40. - Occupation of the Women. - It is expected that the nurses, (in another version: under the direction of the Matron) *in their several day rooms, will furnish materials for sewing, knitting, and other suitable occupations to their respective charge; and see that they are, as much as possible, actually employed.*

41. - The Matron (in another version: with the advice of the superintendent) *will direct such of the patients as appear suitable to assist in the kitchen, laundry, or sewing room, or in other domestic services. Whilst thus employed, these patients will be chiefly entrusted to the care of the housekeeper and such of the house-servants as they may be assisting; who must exercise a particular but oversight as to their conduct.*
When patients are thus employed, or when they are assisting in bringing things from the kitchen or laundry, they must not be allowed to loiter about the main gallery, or other apartments; but when they have completed their work, must return to their respective day-rooms.

50. - (The upper attendant's) *time shall be devoted to the superintendence of the exercise and occupations of the patients in his department; and he will be expected to do all in his power to promote their comfort; and to join with them in rational and healthy amusements.*[21]

In the 1847 version of the rules the following was added:
There are few patients who may not be engaged in occupations or amusements of some kind, if their wishes are, in these respects, sufficiently consulted, by the attendants and others around them. It is not, however, the amount of work, so much as the exercise of the bodily and mental powers of the patients themselves, which is the object to be kept in view. An asylum should be conducted neither as a workhouse nor as a factory; and whilst those indisposed but able to work, are to be encouraged, the powers of the willing are not to be overtaxed. Fatigue of body and exhaustion of mind are to be equally avoided.[22]

By 1897 the *Rules and Instructions* no longer contained such detail about the occupations of patients but merely included a brief note about exercise. 'Every patient must be encouraged to take a liberal amount of exercise in the fresh air, and as many as possible should walk beyond the grounds at least once a week.'[23]

That may suggest the demise of the dominance of moral treatment and the ascendancy of more medically based ideologies, however, in the 1890 *Instructions to Members of Nursing Staff* it states that:

> ... *nurses should encourage patients to occupy themselves usefully, and, as far as their duties permit, assist in their amusements and other pursuits. Amusements should not be restricted to the more intelligent, but endeavours made to rouse the interest of all patients.*[24]

This may indicate that the staff responsibility for the occupation of patients changed, as this instruction remained in force into the twentieth century.[25] It also provides weight for the contention that occupational "treatment" extended continuously, at the Retreat from, 1796 to the present day; a 200 year history!

Annual Reports

Another source of information about the use and place of occupation towards the health and well-being of patients comes from the Retreat's annual reports. Excerpts from those of 1850 and 1851 are particularly worthy of inclusion as, in them, John Kitching, the Superintendent at that time, summarised the patients' programme of occupations, and its benefits. He maintained that it was of 'great consequence to the happiness and well-being of all who possess any activity or energy that this should be directed to some satisfactory or productive channel'. He added that 'the importance of affording occupation to all the patients whose state admits of it, both in a curative and moral point of view, cannot perhaps be over-estimated'. Because of occupation's moral and remedial characteristics he explained that 'the means of employing and instructing the patients' had 'engaged the earnest attention of the chief officers, and considerable success had attended their efforts'. Only 24% of patients were unemployed for most of the time, and these were largely cases for whom 'bodily infirmity and advanced age render much employment either impracticable or undesirable'[26]

Kitching described the 'great sources of employment existing for the male patients' as 'the various operations of the farm and garden out-of-doors, and literary pursuits indoors'.[27] He regretted that 'the females have not that pleasant variety of occupation and change of scene which the men enjoy in the diversity of their out of doors employments'. To overcome this perceived disadvantage Kitching proposed, in the near future, 'the erection of a spacious and cheerful room, in which the occupation of the females might be more systematically and agreeably carried on under the superintendence of a work-woman'. The advantages of this plan he explained would be to provide the female patients with a change of environment and company and because of this 'that the work would be more cheerfully done'.[28]

In 1851 Kitching reported on an increase of opportunities for patients to take exercise in the grounds and surrounding countryside, as well as the provision of an extra week-day "meeting" similar to that held on Sundays. With regard to patient's time spent away from the Institution he described how 'during the fine weather, drives into the country have been freely afforded to the female patients, and on some occasions, parties have been formed for longer excursions'.[30] In addition to those:

> In the summer, a small party of patients of each sex, with the concurrence of their friends and of the Commissioners in Lunacy, enjoyed the pleasure of a few weeks change by visiting the sea-side. Lodgings were engaged for them in two separate houses at Scarbro', and under the care of competent attendants, they were allowed to ramble about, and follow their own inclinations as far as practicable ... The change was much enjoyed by all who went, and the result was in every respect highly satisfactory.[31]

In both years, the provision of intellectual occupations was addressed by lecture programmes delivered to patients during the winter. These were 'eagerly attended by many of the patients, and the attendants and other servants of the Establishment'. Kitching explained that 'although it is very difficult to estimate the amount of good conferred by this and similar means, the rational pleasure that many of the patients derived from these lectures, must have been a useful interruption to the course of their mental aberrations'.[32] Over and above the lecture programmes, but in similar intellectual vein, new books were added to the library during the year, along with a new library and book-case being 'procured for the use of the female patients'.[33]

In order to offer, organise and implement therapeutic programmes of occupation Kitching recognised the need for appropriately skilled workers to run them on a day to day basis. He emphasised that 'the practical success (of) our efforts depends upon the aptness and ability of the immediate attendants upon the patients, that the measure of success will vary according to the zeal and capacity which these display'. To that end he strongly and urgently recommended that 'in the selection of these assistants to bestow a very prominent regard upon the possession of vigorous and active powers'.[34] He stressed that in no way did that recommendation undervalue those attributes of attendants at present in the service of the Retreat who, he said 'perhaps could not easily be surpassed for their steadiness and moral character'.[35]

The story of one of the Retreat's attendants during that time, provides a glimpse of how the duties concerned with the patient's occupations were interpreted. The story is important in this history for it is the earliest descriptive record found of someone being employed in a full time capacity as an "occupation for health" worker.

James Mason

ames Mason entered service at the Retreat in March 1839 where he was employed as a farmer and outdoor attendant. At that time he was presumably a young man as he continued to work there for at least 36 years, and for the first ten of those lived in and had his laundry taken care of. From 1849, when it appears he went to live outside the Institution, his salary rose from thirty-five to seventy-five pounds per annum including two meals per day (see Figure 1.11.3). According to the descriptions given in the Rules, above, it would be expected that he would work, in the main, as a provider and supervisor of male patients' occupations.

Figure 1.11.3:   Extract from James Mason's employment record at the Retreat
(Borthwick Institute, York)

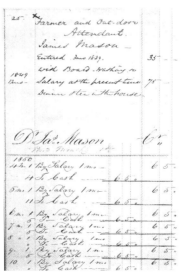

The records of his employment clearly indicate that his principal duty, at least from 1851, and probably earlier, was as an enabler of occupation, to the extent that he could be regarded as a proto-occupational therapist. The main source for this contention is his annual reports to the Superintendent on the occupations of the male patients in his care. In these he described the need to consider the capacities and interests of the patients in the choice of occupations, the beneficial effects of occupation, and the rewards and difficulties of the job. That these reports were considered valuable is testified by the following inclusion in the Superintendent's report dated 1851.

For some information on this head, in regard to male patients, I cannot do better than quote the report of the outdoor attendant, (James Mason,) whose efforts this year to assist me in carrying out this very important branch of treatment, deserve, praiseworthy mention. He says: 'During the past year there have been fewer strong and athletic patients able and willing to work than in some previous years, yet the amount of labour performed by the patients this year may be considered rather more than the average. The number of patients usually employed has been a little increased; endeavours have been made to induce some whose bodily powers preclude the performance of much work, to do a little for the sake of exercise, and some have been employed to considerable advantage, who last year, were reported as unemployed.[36]

Mason's reports were written in a fine copperplate hand and he obviously took great pains over their presentation, as those with too many corrections and the odd ink splotch were replaced with a tidier copy and an occasional change of phrase. In the Retreat Archives kept at the Borthwick Institute of Historical Research copies of the 1870 and 1874 draft reports have been preserved as well as 15 reports on the employment or occupation (Mason used both terms) of the male patients from between 1856 to 1875. Figure 1.11.3 provides an example of Mason's reports.

Figure 1.11.4 **An example of Mason's reports**

(Borthwick Institute, York)

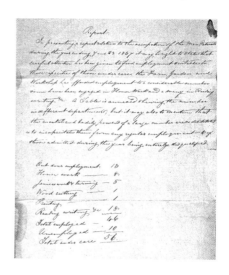

As well, the first of them is presented below in full, except for patient's names, which are omitted. Points from some of the others are then discussed:

Report respecting the employment of the Men Patients at the Retreat for the year ending Sixth Month 1856.

In giving a report respecting the manner of employment of the Men Patients resident in the institution it may be stated that the system of manual labour and mechanical and other employment has been carried out to a greater extent and with more success then during any previous year, many of those who have strength and ability have been engaged in some useful employment, and others less capable have been induced a little exercise, but there is still a considerable number who through advanced age or mental and bodily infirmities cannot be expected to take part in ordinary labour.

In superintending and directing the patients in their employment the past year has been one of more than ordinary anxiety and discouragement, the exercise of great care and attention as well as equanimity of temper has been especially needed to be able to bear the keen sarcasm and the provocation and annoyances which several have caused on many occasions but many have shown willingness and pleasure in taking part in the various occupations on the premises (several) pleasing instances might be named.

In addition to the ordinary work on the Farm, Garden, Pleasure Grounds, and in the house, there has been much extra labour caused by alterations and improvements that have been going forward during the year. One patient assists with the cows. One has been usefully engaged in clipping and dressing the hedges, carting and spreading manure, loading gravel, painting and other labours of the heavier kind. Wood cutting to supply the whole of the establishment with kindling occupies much of one persons time and in Winter especially, the assistance of others is required and the performance of several in the Joiners Shop is very creditable.

The following Analysis shews the manner in which the whole under care have been engaged.

Out door work	*18*
Mechanical work	*8*
Painting	*1*
House Work	*8*
Reading, Writing etc	*11*
Total employed	*44*
Unemployed	*7*
Total under care	*51*

13 of those reported as engaged in bodily labour have also devoted considerable time to reading and some have engaged in various kinds of occupations

Outdoor work of heavier kind	*10*
(list of patient's names)	
ditto of lighter kind	*6*
(list of patient's names)	
Mechanical Work	*8*
list of patient's names	
Painting	*1*
(patient's name)	
Reading Writing etc	*11*
(list of patient's names)	
Reading and other employment	*13*
(list of patient's names)	
Unemployed	*6*
(list of patient's names)	

6mo 12 1856
James Mason[37]

From the tables that Mason included in all of his fifteen reports a composite version has been drawn up (Table 1.11.1).

From this it can be seen that he cared for between 49 to 61 patients presumably on a daily basis, and that the number increased as the years passed. Whether the increase was a result of Mason's effectiveness, for economic reasons, or simply reflects an increasing number of patients within the Retreat is hard to judge. Certainly many patients stayed for years and may have required little input in their daily occupations if they had been chosen wisely in the first place. The one patient involved in "printing", for example, was the same for thirteen years, and was, presumably both interested and capable in what he did. Something occurred to break this continuity for, in 1870, the patient was only engaged occasionally in printing, then in subsequent years in woodsplitting, then housework, then book binding, and then reading. Possibly this implies a loss of interest in printing, less need for printing by the Institution, or simply loss of skill or physical dexterity as a result of the ageing process. The latter thought is supported by the apparent, although slight, decrease over the time span in manual work with a concurrent, slight increase in sedentary occupations such as reading and writing. Indeed, in 1867 Mason notes that 'the mental and bodily powers of a large number are so debilitated as to incapacitate them from

Table 1.11.1: **Type of male patient's occupations, and numbers engaged in them at the Retreat between 1856 and 1875**

(Borthwick Institute, York)[38]

	1856	1857	1858	1859	1860	1861	1862	1864	1867	1869	1870	1871	1873	1874	1875
Outdoor work	18	14	14	17	19	17	13	14	13	14	14	13	12	14	13
Tailors work							1								
Printing	1	1	1	1	1	1	1	1	1	1					
Housework	8	4	5	5	6	5	5	7	8	7	7	6	9	8	6
Read/writing	11	19	17	17	14	16	18	18	18	21	22	26	20	20	24
(Reading plus other occs)	13	15	13	16	16	16	15	16	16	12	13	11	13	16	15
Woodcutting		1	1	1	1	1	1	1	1	1		1		1	
Joinery /mechanical work	8	5	4	3	3	3	3	4	5	2	3	1	3	2	3
Painting							1								
Totals															
Employed	44	44	42	44	44	43	43	45	46	46	46	47	44	45	46
Unemployed	7	9	8	6	5	9	9	7	10	11	11	13	13	13	14
Undercare	51	53	50	50	49	52	52	52	56	57	57	61	57	58	60

any regular employment', and in his 1871 report, he makes specific comment that 'the number capable of manual labour or much physical exertion has been decreasing for a number of years'.

It is probable that Mason's particular bent or skill was geared towards agricultural work as his designation of "farmer" implies. But that his education was not confined to manual tasks is also apparent from his written reports, which were clear, legible and well written. One would imagine that this made him very useful in his particular attendant role as it enabled him to be flexible according to the differing occupational requirements of patients according to illness, age, ability, or interest. Despite the circumscribed nature of the table we learn, for example that in 1862 some were 'engaged in such a variety of occupations as to make it difficult to give a particular account'. In 1873 some of that variety included pumping water, book binding, fancy work, netting, and botany, and a year later that 'the cultivation of Plants and Flowers is a favourite occupation with several of the men patients'.[39]

The table provides an indication that whilst some patients were engaged mainly on sedentary tasks others engaged in both manual occupations and those of a more intellectual nature during their leisure time. Mason recorded, for example, in 1859 that 'sixteen of those who are reported as being employed in outdoor work and other bodily labour also employ themselves more or less in reading and some are diligent in employing their leisure time to advantage'. In 1862 he reported that 'the library has been in constant use and the books, periodicals, and newspapers have been a source of much amusement and instruction'.

As well as tabling the number participating in particular types of occupation, Mason reported on the necessity to match each patient's needs and abilities with what they did. He writes about having found for them 'work as much as possible suitable to their inclinations',[40] and that he had given "constant attention" to 'induce such as are qualified to do something suitable to their capacities'.[41] In several reports he mentions taking into account the patient's 'position in society, the previous habits and dispositions' as well as their 'mental and bodily capabilities'.[42]

Mason obviously recognised, or had been advised of, the intrinsic health benefits of engagement in occupation. Not only did he attempt to provide appropriate occupation but also saw that engagement, of itself, could be therapeutic, socially, physically and mentally. These he alluded to in statements such as 'constant care has been bestowed to induce some whose labour is but of little value to do a little for their own particular benefit',[43] and 'some have been induced to do a little for exercise and their own individual benefit'.[44]

In reporting on the rewards of the job he often noted, as in the 1858 report, 'the voluntary exertion and interest taken' by the patients, and also that 'many have evinced much kind feelings and willingness'. It is however obvious that, just as current therapists could enlarge on the difficulty of working towards engaging people in meaningful occupation when they are ill or handicapped, so, despite the rewards, Mason did not find the job easy. In 1857 he notes that his work took an 'unusual amount of forbearance and equanimity of temper but also a very watchful demeanour both in conduct and conversation'. In the following year he noted how the 'sarcastic, bitter and provocative language received has been such as to put the temper to a most severe test, and wound the feelings'.[45]

Occasionally Mason mentions the discharge or death of the patients in his care, such as in 1873 when one died and four left the institution, and in 1875 when six left during year and three others died. On one occasion in 1871 he referred to one man who was "out on trial" and 'subsequently received his discharge'.

The success of the York Retreat from its inception was widely recognised. It encouraged serious observers, and almost all visitors were impressed by its admirable management, which created an atmosphere of humanity, kindness and reason. An 1815 House of Commons Report was enthusiastic about both its humane "moral therapy" and impressive statistics of cure.

Occupation in other asylums

The Napoleonic and Revolutionary Wars, along with increasing civilisation, were blamed for a major increase in the numbers seeking institutional care for mental illness. Porter reports that 'by the 1810s, official figures indicate that around 2,590 lunatics were confined in licensed houses for the mad, and almost as many again in other places of custody such as houses of correction, workhouses and gaols. The real totals were higher.'[46] One private madhouse in Leicester, established by Thomas Arnold MD (Edinburgh), in 1804 did adopt the parameters of moral treatment and it is worth reflecting on that briefly before consideration of Asylum usage. Watts, in *A Walk through Leicester,* described the establishment as 'a spacious house for the reception of lunatics … with a bowling green and teagarden with many small structures erected for the general purpose of amusement'. It had an underground passage across a street to a walled garden for exercise.[47] Arnold authored *Observations on the Management of the Insane and Particularly on the Agency and Importance of Humane and Kind Treatment in Effecting their Cure,* which was published in 1809, some years before Tuke's much more famous text. Amongst his key principles were the following precepts:

- Patients' minds 'should be soothed and comforted ... by kind and gentle treatment'.
- Their use of proper exercise must be diligently regulated and exacted ...
- They should be allowed under certain circumstances ... various amusements and recreation of mind and body.

In 42 years of practice along those lines he claimed two thirds of his patients were cured.[48,49]

Despite such apparent havens, even in heavily populated areas the number of madhouses was variable, and some profited from the obviously increased need by maintaining patients in squalid and overcrowded conditions. Such factors led to a dramatic change of political and societal response to madness. An Act was passed in 1808 that empowered local authorities to establish rate-supported asylums. This requirement was enforced in 1845 by another Act, as only twelve had been set up to that date.[50] Epitomising the change, during the century madhouses eventually all but disappeared, even though "respectable" families continued to confine their sick members in their comparative seclusion. Asylums metamorphosed into mental hospitals, and became the major officially approved option for the treatment of the mentally ill, it being generally understood that people suffering mental disorder needed a place to which they could withdraw from precipitating factors. "Mad doctors" were also transformed, first into "alienists" and then psychiatrists. As the state took over the handling of mental illness much more order was imposed on what had been a haphazard system, and to do that the expertise of medical authorities was called upon. From then until the present day 'the character and course of mental illness was ... shaped irrevocably by medical intervention'.[51] That point is important as occupation would only be deemed useful in treatment as long as medicine did not develop other therapeutic approaches with which occupation was incompatible, and as long as doctors continued to recognise its benefits. That proved to be the case for a greater part of the century.

In 1841, despite the Retreat leading the field in introducing and using occupation as treatment, Samuel Tuke wrote of a colleague's extensive, systematic, successful and influential endeavours in particular regard to "labour" as distinct from pleasurable activities:

> In turning to the subject of labour in connection with the management of the insane it is due to the memory of the late Sir William Ellis, to bear in mind, that to him we are indebted for the first extensive and successful experiment to introduce labour systematically into our public asylums. He carried it out at Wakefield, with a skill, vigour and kindliness towards the patients, which were alike creditable to his understanding and his heart. He first proved, that there was less danger from putting the spade and the hoe into the hands of a large proportion of insane persons, than from shutting them up together in idleness, though under the guards of straps, straitwaistcoats, or chains.

He subsequently introduced the system of labour into Hanwell; ... The effect of judicious training on those patients who had been allowed to sink into these and other disgusting habits, had long since been experienced at the Retreat without the extensive introduction of the labour system ... In all these asylums the superintendents expressed their decided conviction of the benefit which in a great variety of ways was derived from the employment of the patients, more especially in out-door labour. The tendency of the patients to injure themselves, or others, was said to be lessened; the number requiring any restraint was diminished; the health and comfort of the patients was increased, and some pecuniary profit was derived to the establishment.

I would, however, observe here, that the introduction of the system of labour into asylums, is not primarily to be contemplated as a means of pecuniary profit, but as a means of promoting the cure and the comfort of the patients. Much has been said in favour of amusing occupations for the insane; and they are certainly not to be overlooked, especially those which require active exertion in the open air ... It is true the patient is not capable of all rational perceptions and considerations, or he would not be under care; but there are few, except the demented, who are not, to a considerable extent, under the influences to which nature or habit has subjected them in a healthy state; and the cultivation and extension of the remaining healthy feelings and associations, forms one of the most important parts of moral management.

It is twenty-four years since the first experiments of Dr. Ellis at Wakefield were made; and during the last ten years the labour plan has been adopted extensively in many other of our public asylums in England, Scotland and Ireland. The system has been also introduced at Siegburg (Germany) and at Winnenden. In both these Institutions, the active exercise of the limbs forms a part of the regular medical prescription and though this exercise may be more in the form of recreation, on the part of the higher classes, labour in the garden and grounds is distinctly prescribed for them, with reference to its influence on the mind as well as the body. The question whether labour can and ought to be introduced into our public asylums, may therefore be considered as settled.[52]

Such was Tuke's accolade of the work of William Ellis, with regard to occupational treatment, that the next section of the chapter will discuss his major offering, before looking at a few of the other asylum programmes in England. Tuke also regarded highly the work being done in Scottish asylums on this front, and so discussion of what was happening there, and in Irish and Welsh Asylums will follow. In particular the ideas and direction taken by W.A.F. Browne, whose objectives for treatment in asylums - justice, benevolence and occupation - have been used as the title of the chapter, will be considered.

William Ellis: Wakefield and Hanwell

In *A Treatise on the Nature, Symptoms, Causes and Treatment of Insanity*, Ellis explained that 'recent parliamentary returns show, that there are in England 12,668 Pauper Lunatics and Idiots; and the Insane alone, including the different classes of society, cannot be estimated at fewer than 10,000'. He blamed imbalanced lifestyles for its prevalence, offering the argument that for members of affluent society 'the brain and nervous system are kept in a state of constant over-excitement, whilst the frame is debilitated, from the muscles being rarely called into proper and regular exercise'. Amongst the poor he recognised excess of alcohol, 'exposure to cold, the want of common necessaries of life, and other results of extreme poverty' as major causal factors.[53]

Ellis also acknowledged that there was a sparsity of effective medical remedies, and that those available were principally 'of use in the early stages of the disease'. He recognised also that moral treatment was far from easy, calling for forbearance and 'constant, never-tiring, watchful kindness' on the part of those providing it.[54] That led to his call for "proper persons" to be selected as attendants and that they must be well remunerated:

> *When the harassing and irksome nature of the duties of the attendants of the insane, and the importance of those duties being properly fulfilled, are considered, it is obvious, that such an amount of remuneration should be proposed as should induce persons of character and respectability to offer themselves as keepers and nurses.*[55]

In his account of the management of the asylum at Hanwell, Ellis traced the steps by which employment of patients gradually increased, until, at the time of his writing, 454 out of 610 were 'regularly at work; and many of them at trades, with which they were totally unacquainted until they were taught them in the institution'. The process had not been without opposition:

> *When the system was commenced by myself and my wife, on the opening of the Asylum for the West Riding of Yorkshire, at Wakefield, so great was the prejudice against it, that it was seriously proposed, that no patient should be allowed to work in the grounds outside the walls without being chained to a keeper. Another suggestion was, that a corner of the garden should be allotted for their labour, and that they should dig it over and over again all year round. The kind feeling and good sense of the people in the neighbourhood soon overcame these prejudices; and not only did they witness with pleasure the unfortunate patients engaged in their works in the grounds of the institution, but they were delighted to meet them emerging from its bounds, and, by a walk in the country, and a little intercourse with their fellow men, preparing to enter again into society*[56]

Although some prejudices about employing patients were overcome there remained 'insuperable objection to their making anything for sale out of the institution' on the grounds that it would disadvantage those people employed within the industry and 'shopkeepers in the metropolis'.[57]

Ellis was one who deemed the idea of asylum to be central particularly for those in the early stages of illness. 'When the exciting cause cannot be removed, the patient should be placed in circumstances calculated as much as possible to produce a complete interruption to the train of thought' including withdrawal from routine habits and society of friends. He wrote: 'I know of no means of accomplishing this more effectually than by sending the patient on an excursion into a fine country, mountainous if possible: the air, the scenery, and the exercise, all have a salutary influence.' He thought, however, that a medical attendant and medical remedies should accompany patients.[58] Indeed, Ellis believed that a patient's mind had to be distracted from the "excitation" deemed to be causing the disorder. That belief led to him becoming a driving force in establishing labour as the principal treatment at Wakefield and Hanwell, and advocating its use in Asylums throughout the country.

On the arrival of each patient at Hanwell, as much information as possible was gathered from overseers, relatives and friends. Patients were then assigned a ward, stripped, cleaned and dressed in asylum dress before being seen by the house surgeon who ascertained their general state of health. He then called in the physician who prescribed the moral and medical treatment, and after a few days of observation 'an attempt is made to induce him to employ himself, and to become, as it were, one of the family'.[59]

Most of the staff employed at Hanwell were associated with the programme of occupational treatment. 'The medical and moral treatment of all the patients is under the immediate direction of the resident physician and the matron.' Ellis explained that the 'keeping in order of so complex a machine' required 'the constant and anxious watchful attention of the superintendent and matron: there is not a single movement which does not directly emanate from them'. As well as the attendants and nurses 'the wife of the house surgeon … assists in … the employment and moral treatment of the females'. To the storekeeper was given the responsibility of obtaining supplies such as hemp, twine, coir, leather, pottle, woodstraw, willow, and bristles needed for the work.[60] The female storekeeper also:

> … apportions to the respective female nurse the articles for the employment of their patients, and collects them and takes an account of them in detail when manufactured. Every morning and afternoon she collects the female patients, to be employed in out-door work, and sends them, under the charge of proper female nurses, to the gardener, with a written paper containing their numbers. He employs them, under the care of the nurse, in such portion of out-door work as may be desirable; and the female storekeeper, each morning and afternoon visits the females at work out of doors, and takes care that they are properly attended to by the nurse, under whose immediate charge they are placed.[61]

Ellis described the female "workwoman" as a very important person in the institution.

... after breakfast she is always employed in cutting out, arranging, superintending the making, and selling the various articles, which are to be disposed of in the bazaar. Many of the patients in the Asylum at Hanwell have been reduced to pauperism solely from their insanity; and others of them have been in the habit of employing themselves in fine needlework. A considerable difficulty was felt in finding suitable occupation for such patients; the ordinary sewing and mending, which were wanted for the institution, were disliked, and there appeared no means of procuring for them work suited to their tastes. With a view to obviate the evils of idleness in this class, the matron hit upon the plan of establishing a bazaar. She borrowed from the treasurer twenty-three pounds eighteen shillings; this she laid out in the purchase of a few articles in the first instance as patterns, and in the buying of requisite materials. These are made up and worked by the patients, and sold by the workwoman to visitors at the bazaar, or are sent off to order. The scheme has answered beyond the most sanguine expectations.

Ellis added that:

It is hardly possible to conceive the benefit which the patients have derived from this employment: It is congenial to their previous habits, it excites a great interest; many of them select and contrive with as much anxiety the various patterns, as if they were exclusively to derive all the profit from their sale. One poor women who had been insane a long time previous to her admission in 1831, ... and whom no persuasion could previously induce to work on the establishment of the bazaar, spent her time in minutely working collars and ladies' dresses. This employment was of her own selection, and it so absorbed her attention that the irritability by degrees wore off; and after having for a long time past exhibited no symptom of insanity, she was discharged cured. Others take charge of particular portions of the work, and employ under them patients, with less mental powers than themselves. In fact there have been many contrivances for the happy occupation of patients, but I do not think any have been more beneficial than the bazaar.[62]

With some of the profits they bought a finger organ for musical concerts and use in the divine service. This added to the workers' self respect and 'raises them in the moral scale'.[63]

But before that could occur, Ellis advised that following admission:

The first step on the part of the medical man, is to gain the confidence of the patients by kind treatment, and a solicitude for their welfare ... To engage their attention on some new object, either by affording them useful employment or attractive recreation, is the next step to be pursued.

One of the reasons he held that view was his belief that:

... where the mind has no opportunity of employment on objects of importance, it will either busy itself about trifles, or sink into apathy, or allow itself to wander unchecked in idle reveries. In Hogarth's picture of Bedlam, the straw crown was not the mere symbol of madness; the making it, however

valueless, tended to the happiness of the patient, and was an act of practical wisdom.[64]

However he warned:

... though we know that nothing tends to the restoration of the weakened brain, or of a weakened limb, so much as moderate exercise; yet, if that exercise be commenced too soon, much mischief is often the result ... In many cases, particularly amongst the industrious poor, whose previous habits have rendered such a system of quiet, and an abstinence from physical labour irksome, a desire is frequently expressed to be permitted to work before the exercise would be prudent.[65]

Figure 1.11.5: William Ellis 'Occupational Treatment Plan.'

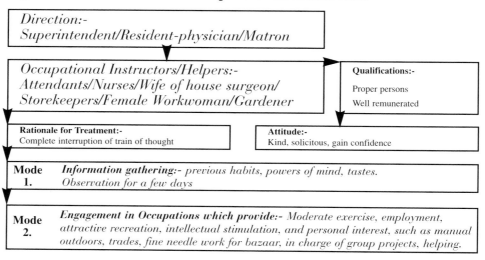

Ellis, who recognised from experience the 'immense difference, both in physical and mental powers and habits' there is between people,[66] described the "first object" in evaluating an individual's mental state was to carefully ascertain what had been his 'previous habits and powers of his mind; what has been the state of his sentiments and passions; and what has been his general conduct'. He went on to explain that:

Considerable tact is required in adapting the particular kind of occupation to the tastes of the patients. They are usually more inclined to work at the trades to which they have been brought up, than to turn their attention to pursuits entirely new. Most men seem to have a natural fondness for farming and gardening, and these occupations have this great advantage, that there are certain portions of the labour in them, in which a violent or suicidal patient may be employed, without being entrusted with any tools by which he might either injure himself or others. But so important do I consider diverting the mind by employment, that where the patient cannot be induced thus to occupy himself, or where occupation is too mechanical to keep the mind interested, I do not hesitate, with proper precautions, to intrust him with tools, even where an inclination to suicide or violence exists. And though I have adopted this plan in numbers of cases, no accident has yet ensued, and it has frequently been the means of the patient's complete recovery.[67]

The considerable tact that he called for, plus "a little management and address", was needed particularly when trying to engage in "bodily labour" those of high social standing used mainly to "mental exertion". But recognising the many values of manual work in the open air, Ellis argued:

This is exceedingly beneficial; for in addition to the moral advantage derived from the mind being diverted, there is an actual physical good, by the exercise turning the blood and vital energy to the supply of muscular power, and preventing excess of circulation in the internal organs. Of course many will be found to whom such an employment would be irksome; but whatever be the rank of life, or the difference in outward circumstance, man is still the same being.[68]

So much did Ellis believe in manual, outdoor work that when patients were first admitted:

In the first instance, out-of-doors employment is generally tried; the patient is put under the especial charge of one of the servants, and set to work on the ground in such a way as to avoid any danger of his injuring himself or others.

As "his character" became more known he may have worked with an attendant who shared his trade or one which he would like to know. The choice was considerable, including blacksmithing, bricklaying, joinering, tinning, shoemakering, tailoring, brushmaking, twine-making, pottlemaking, basket making and coopering. Patients were rewarded with a little tea, tobacco, beer, or some other luxury.[69] If patients chose to be "idle" but were in 'good health, and in a proper state to work, they are allowed no beer, and every little indulgence is withheld'. With that incentive most soon found the benefits of employment.[70]

Usually about 55 male and 33 female patients were engaged in gardening and farming working with two gardeners and a farmer. One dairymaid had a staff of 'four to six female patients' who assisted the farming man with milking about 16 cows. The bread and beer for "the family" of 660 were made by one female with the help of eight patients. The washing for the 612 patients was achieved by a laundry maid helped by 16-20 patients. Of the two nurses employed in the female wards, it was the junior who took the patients to work outdoors, whilst the others sewed, mended, spun twine, or made baskets or pottle. Of the two keepers in each male ward, one was a mechanic who, with the agreement of the superintendent, after early morning ward duties took a selection of patients from his own and other male wards to his workshops or about the hospital. Those not selected worked with the other attendant in tasks such as picking coir or twine spinning.[71]

Despite Ellis's belief in the efficacy of outdoor work he saw the necessity to also encourage "intellectual faculties":

In a well-regulated institution, every means ought to be invented for calling into exercise as many of the mental faculties as remain capable of employment. We must remember that the happiness of man, whatever be his situation in life, consist in the proper and harmonious exercise of all his powers, moral, mental, and physical ...

The library is a source of great amusement; and as the books are distributed on Saturday, the reading of them sometimes to one another, sometimes alone, serves to occupy the mind, and keep the patients quiet on Sunday - by far the most difficult day in the week to manage them. The patients on that day not having their ordinary employment, and not being previously accustomed to amuse themselves with mental occupations, suffer from ennui; and the result of their idleness is a greater quantity of vice and mischief on that day than on any other day of the week.[72]

The effectiveness of "mental employment" received excellent press in the *Chambers' Edinburgh Journal* of June 8th 1844, in which it was reported:

INSANITY CURED BY MENTAL EMPLOYMENT

A carpenter was admitted as a patient into the asylum at Wakefield. He had previously made several attempts at self destruction, and was then in a very desponding state. After the diseased action had subsided, great dejection still remained. He was, however, most fortunately placed under the care of the gardener, who was then constructing a grotto or moss house in the grounds. The contriving of the building offered a scope for his ingenuity and taste. He was consulted on the arrangement of the floor, which was formed of pieces of wood, of different kinds, set in various figures. He was furnished with tools, though he was, of course, most carefully watched. He took so great an interest in the little building, that the current of his thoughts was changed - all his miseries were forgotten; and his recovery took place in the end of a few months. He very justly attributed his restoration to the "moss house".[73]

Figure 1.11.6: William Ellis (1780-1839) Lithograph by WL Aldous
(The Wellcome Library)

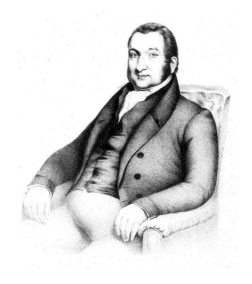

Ellis's place at Hanwell Asylum, by the time of that article, had been taken by Dr John Conolly, who disclosed that it was after a visit to Glasgow Asylum that he first realised the importance of the study and treatment of mental disorders. At that point he 'unconsciously devoted to the cause of the insane', and was soon to become an influential force within psychiatry.[74] An *Illustrated London News* of 1843, reported on the inclusion of "hospital utility" occupations as well as recreations, exercises and hobbies as a major part of the Hanwell treatment under his guidance. Indeed Conolly, who adopted Tuke's theories and published a treatise on *The Treatment of the Insane without Mechanical Restraint* became almost as famous as his predecessor for his interest in occupation and "non-restraint".[75] Edward Charlesworth, and Gardiner Hill, who succeeded him at the Lincoln Asylum, also introduced Tuke's recommendations.[76]

As a result of the influence of the Retreat, Hanwell, and Wakefield, by the middle of the nineteenth century asylums throughout England used occupation as treatment. Horton Road and Coney Hill Hospitals in Gloucester for example, like many others, typically employed male patients in the gardens and grounds, as well as tailoring, shoe-making and printing, and female patients in domestic occupations like sewing, knitting, laundry work, and the production of bedding and clothing for the institution. Some patients were engaged in the preparation of appliances for the sick and wounded of various nineteenth century wars. The Richmond District Asylum's programme, again like many others, embraced education, recreations, drama and gymnastics, which were organised by teacher attendants.[77] W.A.F. Browne wrote of the programme at Richmond:

> The Richmond Asylum had 130 out of 377 constantly contributing to the support of the institution and their own restoration. Twelve of the 130 were learning to read. This noble and most philosophical attempt to build the mind anew on the ruins of outraged feeling, or enfeebled judgement, or whatever the form of the injury sustained, by conveying new ideas to the perceptive powers, and by calling up, by means of education, faculties which were previously unknown or dormant, and which may prove to be healthy or antagonist to those diseased - has been made elsewhere; and on a more extended scale, patients have been instructed in the rudiments of science, in drawing, music, have been taught weaving, shoe mending, and other common arts, and have even been tempted to participate in the representation of comedies.[78]

Bethlem Hospital and occupation

Some mention must also be made about Bethlem Hospital during the nineteenth century as its position as the first asylum for the insane makes it interesting to investigate whether or not the growth of moral treatment and the use of occupation affected that bastion of stricter regimes. Russell in *Scenes from Bedlam* describes how, in fact, treatment did change towards more humane and less punitive approaches, including stress on the value of occupation, and how Mrs Forbes, the Matron from 1815, had liberated patients from restraint. In that same year the Asylum had moved to new purpose-built premises at St Georges Fields, the central portion of which is all that remains in the present day, housing the Imperial War Museum. Males were separated from females in two wings on the four floors, which in the beginning were bleak and sparsely furnished.[79][80] At that time it was reported to the Madhouses Committee that walking in the green yards when the weather allowed, and the use of a pack of cards supplied by the apothecary were the only occupations and amusements available to patients, apart from their occasional assistance in 'cleaning and scouring the galleries'.[81]

By the middle of the century comfortable furniture was introduced along with sensory stimulating pictures, flowers, aviaries and animals.[82] Also around mid-century the Asylum's Annual Report recorded that:

> ... the occupations, which were said to fill a considerable portion of the patients' time, were gardening and the workshops for the men, and laundry and needlework for the women. The men formed into groups for digging, sweeping, rolling and weeding in the gardens, while in the workshops they followed the trades of carpenter, smith, cooper, plumber and mason. Apart from washing and ironing, the women sewed men's shirts, women's cap, gowns, shifts and aprons, and also made up pairs of sheets, bed-ticks and pillowcases. To counterbalance all this industry, the amusements consisted of the library, billiard and bagatelle rooms, along with cards, draughts and dominoes, chess and piano playing.

This was confirmed by an article in *The Illustrated London News*, dated March 24th 1860, which reported that although:

> ... the slightest evincement of a wish for healthful employment is cheerfully met by the authorities, there does not seem to exist that feverish desire to utilise the patients - to make them "worth their salt," as it were, which is painfully palpable in some county institutions. In Bethlem those who are able and willing are supplied with light and pleasant occupation about the house ... but no attempt is made to force the inclinations of the patients, or to set them irksome tasks.[83]

The report continued, describing the "female gallery" pictured in figure 1.11.7, which exhibited:

> ... the benefits derived from the absence of coercion and the substitution of amusements and light employments for a dull and rigorous restraint. The first female ward I visited was occupied principally by patients who were approaching convalescence, and it was easy to discern an approach towards sanity not only in the elegance and cheerfulness of the decorations, but also in the recreations and occupations of the denizens of the place.[84]

George Augustus Sala, the reporter, commented on the ballroom at the end of the gallery where balls were held for both male and female patients in the autumn and winter months. 'Both Dr Hoods and Dr Helps join the patients at these entertainments.' He also viewed the ladies' workroom pictured in figure 1.11.8. in the company of Dr Hood where he was impressed and surprised to note that:

> *When Dr Hood pays one of his cheerful visits to the ladies workroom - fitted up with exquisite taste, and where convalescent and docile patients amuse or employ themselves in embroidery, fancy work, and flower-painting in water colours - it is by no means an uncommon occurrence to be asked by one of the inmates to go out "for a day's pleasure".*[86]

Apparently such permission was readily given if the patient was well enough and there was scarcely "a place of amusement in the metropolis", like the "Soho Bazaar" or the "Pantheon", were they did not visit.

Figure 1.11.7:   The Royal Hospital of Bethlem - The Gallery for Women. [85]
(The Bethlem Royal Hospital Archives and Museum)

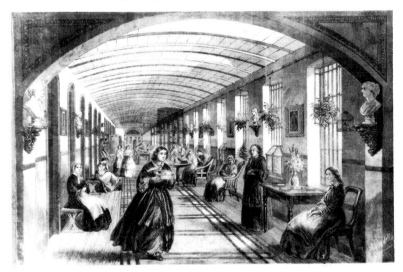

Sala described the male gallery as similar to the women's but without some of "the elegancies" although it too had 'pet birds and animals, cats, canaries, squirrels, greyhounds, &c'. In the spacious saloon at the extremity of that wing was a billiard room which was 'much frequented by the male patients in the evening'. He described how at other times they:

> *... amuse themselves with games at bagatelle, cards, drawing, painting, reading &c. In our Illustration* (shown as figure 1.11.9. here) *is a party playing chess; others are killing time with music, or with that great consolator the tobacco pipe. Still many of the patients take no pleasure in any kind of amusement, but for hours will sit or stand alone wrapt in thought ...*
>
> *The Long Gallery gives access to a very excellent library. ... The library is always well frequented. Many of the patients are highly educated and accomplished men; more than one have been celebrated in intellectual pursuits.*[87]

Some celebrated artists were also patients in the hospital during the nineteenth century and they continued with their artwork whilst confined. Notable examples include Richard Dadd, a patient from 1844 to 1864, and Jonathan Martin who set fire to York Minster in 1829.[88]

Figure 1.11.8: **A workroom in one of the women's wards in the late nineteenth century**
(The Bethlem Royal Hospital Archives and Museum)

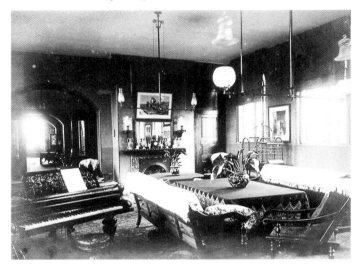

Figure 1.11.9: **The Royal Hospital of Bethlem - The Gallery for Men**[89]
(The Bethlem Royal Hospital Archives and Museum)

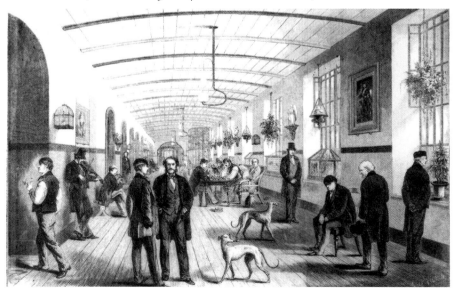

The rules that set out the duties and conduct expected of staff continued throughout the centuries to become more and more explicit, and the nineteenth century was no exception. The Matron in 1815, for example, was detailed to ensure that the able patients assisted the washerwomen in boiling the dirty linen, and by 1837 it was the assistant-keeper's specific duty to 'assist watching the patients employed in the garden'. Just 10 years later duties were spelt out in fifteen-minute intervals, as was the case by that time at the Retreat and Hanwell, but the occupations were less tightly controlled than at the latter. Despite such attempts at improving the services offered, Bethlem suffered a major investigation into its practices in 1851-2. By 1873, although moral treatment was still used, Dr Williams concentrated in his Report on physical treatments such as drugs and shock treatment using "galvinism" or shower baths.[90] However, it seems that occupations were still being used in 1891 as the rules for that year specified that at 9 a.m. 'all the patients selected for employment shall be ready to go with the several Attendants and Servants under whose care they are to be occupied'; that they worked for six days a week, except for Sundays which was for attendance at chapel; and that Tuesdays were for 'taking to the store room articles made by the patients and receiving a fresh supply of work'.[91]

In order to appreciate a more complete picture of what moral treatment achieved within an English county mental hospital, Lancaster Asylum has been chosen as a prime example.

Lancaster Asylum and Samuel Gaskell

The Lancaster Asylum, instituted on the 28th July 1816, was one of the first county asylums to be built under the 1808 legislation. Similar to many other mental institutions, initially its patients were subjected to coercion and restraint, little different from earlier private madhouses. As time went by the principles of moral treatment were adopted, but this was difficult to administer because Lancaster had become one of the largest asylums in England. This was despite the fact that Walton, in his study of asylum admissions in Lancashire in the 1840s, found that large industrial towns and cities had a lower rate of committals because of 'strong family and community solidarity based on shared work experience over generations'.[92] Notwithstanding, Lancaster Asylum in the second half of the nineteenth century, and typical of a pauper asylum of the period, was overcrowded, with more than twice as many patients than was advised for an institution with a curative purpose.

The story of Samuel Gaskell who was appointed as superintendent of Lancaster Asylum in 1840, and a member of the Lunacy Commission in 1849, provides another contribution to the history of occupation for health. He was a committed and energetic exponent of the principles of moral treatment, and the use of occupation flourished under his leadership. However, his particular bent towards good management, discipline, and kindly orderliness, along with his influence on the management of asylums generally as a Lunacy Commissioner, could be said to have resulted in a significant. In the longer term, this was possibly a detrimental influence on the use of occupation as a remedial agent as distinct from an economic one.

Gaskell, the second son of a successful sailcloth manufacturer, was born in Warrington on the northern coast of Lancashire in 1807. There, the well-to-do embraced Unitarianism, a dissenting form of Christianity which views human nature as essentially good. Unitarians are interested in social, personal and moral improvement through self-discipline and self-control. Such convictions are largely compatible with those of moral treatment, so Gaskell's background proved fertile to his adoption of Tuke's doctrine of remediation of insanity, with occupation as part of that process. As many of the influential intelligentsia and industrialists of the times worshipped at the Unitarian Chapel, Gaskell's background beliefs, eventually, proved a support to his career opportunities.[93]

Gaskell had been interested in a medical career since childhood, but a change in family fortunes led to his being, for a brief period, apprenticed to a publisher and bookseller. In 1825, though, he procured a six-year apprenticeship in surgery at Manchester Royal Infirmary, and he qualified with an LRCS and MRCS after a year of residency in Edinburgh. It was when he returned to work at the Infirmary in Manchester in 1834, as resident apothecary, that he came into sustained contact with people suffering mental health problems, as that hospital had admitted lunatics from as early as 1763.[94]

Following his prestigious appointment to Lancaster Asylum as Superintendent, Gaskell set about, with great vigour, to create a more humane and efficient establishment. As a great admirer of Conolly's work he sought to replicate Hanwell's system. Despite the Asylum being overpopulated with pauper inmates, within a year he had abolished all forms of personal restraint such as handcuffs, leg irons or straitjackets. He also made improvements to the patients' living environment, by changes such as enlarging windows and removing bars, adding gas light, demolishing the high walls which fenced in airing courts, as well as improving hygiene procedures, bedding, clothing, and food. He also introduced the other rudiments of moral treatment, not least the inclusion of occupation for as many as possible. Indeed, in a Lunacy Commision Report attached to that of the Medical Officers for 1847 the following statement appears:

Occupation is considered a most important part of the plan of treatment in this Asylum; and we were more than usually gratified by observing the large proportion of patients both male and female, employed in various ways both out of doors and within.[95]

In the Rules, which formed a part of "General Management", directions about the occupation of patients were included just as they were at the Retreat, and other Asylums:

V. Employment of patients.

That during the day, the patients of both sexes be employed, as much as practicable, out of doors, the men in gardening and husbandry, the women in occupations suited to their ability; and that as a principle in treatment, endeavours be continually used to occupy the minds of the patients; to induce them to take exercise in the open air; and to promote cheerfulness and happiness amongst them.

VI. Workshops and tools provided.

That workshops and tools be provided, and artisans and others be encouraged to follow their particular calling and to learn shoemaking, tailoring, and other common and useful trades, and that needlework, straw work and other suitable employments be provided for the women.

VII. Books to be provided.

That an ample supply of books and cheap publications of a cheerful nature (in addition to bibles and prayer books) be provided, and kept up in case of destruction; and that various means of amusement be placed at the disposal of the patients of both sexes, and that they be encouraged to have frequent recourse thereto.

VIII. Airing grounds.

That the airing grounds into which several wards open, be accessible to the patients for at least three hours in the afternoon, of every day when the weather is favourable.[96]

To augment his plans to engage as many as possible in recreation and agricultural employment Gaskell purchased thirty-five acres of moorland, so encouraging a range of outdoor occupations. These included the development of a small farm, building a reservoir, and constructing walking paths for other patients.[97] Apart from such outdoor work, tradesmen were employed to instruct patients as well as to work around the hospital itself. In the 1845 *Report of the Medical Officers* it was claimed that 'amongst the females a striking increase of the amount of work executed is observable. Most of the articles of clothing needed for themselves, and the men, are now made in their department.'[98] It was also noted that 'new workshops and dormitories were ready for use in April, 1845, since which period they have been fully occupied by patients engaged in various trades'.[99] More extensive and organised than any twentieth century occupational therapy department the report describes how:

… in the upper part of this detached building are dormitories for most of the patients engaged in the various trades, and in the lower part are the separate shops of the joiner, blacksmith, plumber, tailor, and shoemaker, as well as a

machine and weaving room: it contains also a commodious dining room for the use of the working party.[100]

Occupations were carried out in wards as well as workshops 'such as the making of mats, floor cloths, rugs, shawls, hats and bonnets, a sufficient quantity of which is made by the patients to supply the wants of the institution'.[101] Whilst many of those initiatives had obvious economic benefits, provision was also made for more restful pastimes such as games, amusements, books, newspapers and, following Tuke's lead, care of domestic animals. At the Retreat Tuke had found that caring for animals provided beneficial effects for patients, appearing to draw them out of their fixations, passions, hallucinations or fears. Gaskell took the ministration aspect of such occupation further by placing young orphans in the care of some of the female patients, to very therapeutic effect.[102] He also persuaded a 'few of the better informed and capable patients' to provide tuition to 'the ignorant' as a means of therapy for both groups.[103]

This led, not surprisingly, to another manifestation of his interest in and commitment to therapeutic occupation. Gaskell established evening classes, at first during the winter months and specifically for those who worked the land and were housed in the separate building previously mentioned. In a short time "schooling" was extended into each ward superintended by the Matron and Chief Attendant. In the classes patients learned to read, write and do arithmetic as many of them were illiterate and innumerate. The custom was for patients to put away their "employment" at four o'clock in the afternoon and attend classes according to their particular level of need. They were instructed by the ward's attendants and nurses, 'aided by a few of the more able patients who act as monitors' and assisted by Mr Danby, the Chaplain. On other days, at the same time, patients were encouraged 'to enter on different recreations and amusements', which in the summer should be 'in the open air as much as possible'.[104]

However, Lancaster Asylum, at this time, housed an increasingly large population of "mentally deficient" patients for whom such classes were unsuitable, so in 1846 Gaskell visited Paris to examine French methods for educating "congenital idiots". On his return he not only broadcast what he had learned to those in the industry but also to a general lay audience. He then set up day-schools in the Asylum to 'quicken the feeble and scanty germs of intellectual power bestowed on these forlorn creatures'.[105] Similar to infant schools, the venture achieved results with which he was well pleased. Indeed, within a year, he proclaimed that 'several idiots, formerly considered incapable of amendment, are not only rescued from a miserable state of existence, but are now orderly, cleanly, and daily engaged in some simple occupation'.[106] Later in his time at Lancaster Gaskell, with like minded others, put his energies into creating the first English Asylum for the "feeble-minded and idiotic" because he considered it inappropriate to mix such patients with 'those attacked with insanity'.[107] He acted on his convictions expediently, because:

A considerable share of the attention of those parties employed in the treatment of mental affections, as well as those engaged in promoting general education, appears at the present time to be attracted to this subject; and there is good reason to hope that, from the united exertions of such individuals, and the establishment of institutions specially adapted to carry out their intentions, a helping hand will be extended to the feeble minded and the idiotic, whom we trust to see ere long raised from their present neglected and degraded state[108]

In many aspects of care Gaskell sought to accentuate the moral treatment side of asylums rather than custodial confinement. For example, he viewed as objectionable the practice of setting 'an attendant to watch over a body of patients, without himself rendering assistance in the work'. To overcome this perceived problem, and remarkably modern in concept, 'an order was issued that everyone taking charge of a number of employed patients, should enter actively on the work, so as both to stimulate their exertions, and render the occupation more productive of benefit as a remedial agent'.[109] Gaskell expected that the behaviour of 'every individual officer or servant' was important to regulate and 'correct disordered mental action' by 'rousing the depressed, soothing the excited, and correcting the irregular', through 'attention to the habits of patients - classification - occupation, amusements, and all the influences arising from the varied duties of social life'. He demanded 'cultivation of kindly sympathies towards patients ... between one patient and another, and thoughout the whole as a body'.[110]

Despite such wisdom, at Lancaster under Gaskell, the emphasis of moral treatment, including the use of occupation as therapy, gradually became more of a method of discipline for difficult patients, and for enforcing the Asylum's routine than to restore sanity. Gaskell's satisfaction in the fact that during his tenure there was no recourse to mechanical restraint despite a large population of criminal patients led him 'to devise and enforce means calculated to prevent ... interruptions to the order, quietude, and well-being of the (patients)' whilst yet 'promoting a more cheerful, contented, and tractable disposition'. His determination and unremitting attention to detail in order to 'secure the most complete order, regularity, and decorum' produced an environment in which both staff and patients knew and complied with what was expected of them.[111] For example, attention to issues such as the use of potentially dangerous implements by patients was carefully monitored according to the amount of use, their diagnosis, and a careful weighing up of safety issues versus possible benefit.[112] Gaskell was rewarded for this approach as it was the "tranquillity and orderly conduct" of the patients, plus their remarkably good physical health, cleanliness, cheerfulness and exemplary behaviour at chapel which was praised by the Lunacy Commission on its inspections. Gaskell's emphasis can be contrasted with that of the Tuke's original view of occupation within moral treatment which, instead of institutional orderliness was aimed at creating a stimulating environment in which routine could be sacrificed to the needs of the individual in order to meet remedial ends.[113]

It was, largely, Tuke's emphasis that became the focus of "occupational therapy" as it was recreated in the twentieth century. On the whole occupation as a restraint was looked upon unfavourably. However as the therapeutic use of occupation diminished it seems that, at least in some instances, it was again replaced by restraint in some asylums. In that regard it is worth noting that in 1911, in the United States, the passage of three bills through the Massachusetts Legislature related to the reintroduction of occupation as restraint in preference to other physical methods. Vernon Briggs explains that the bills proposed the introduction of occupation into mental institutions, along with training in occupation, for attendants.[114]

As with all early moral treatment exponents, Gaskell was extremely sceptical about the place of conventional medical approaches in the treatment of insanity. Scull reports that within the Lancaster Asylum 'on a per capita basis, the nine shillings and one penny that had been spent on medicines in 1833 had fallen to only one shilling and twopence by 1846'.[115] Not surprisingly many doctors found this to be unacceptable. John Charles Bucknill expressed sorrow that medicines were largely excluded from treatment because, he wrote, some are 'scarcely more limited in their curative influence upon recent diseases of the brain, affecting the intellectual functions, than upon any other large class of visceral diseases'.[116] Likewise James Cowles Prichard, a Lunacy Commissioner, objected 'that the attention of medical men has been of late years too exclusively devoted to what is termed Moral Treatment, to the neglect, in some instances, of the resources of medicine'. He added that because 'insanity never exists without a physical cause, namely, some disturbance of the functions of the brain' it follows 'that physical agents ought to be resorted to in the first instance'.[117] As such views became more widespread they arguably led to the neglecting of more obvious aspects of moral treatment, and to not according occupation its due place in the armament of treatment techniques necessary for the health and well-being of those with mental health problems. What could have happened, in contrast, was the melding of medical and occupational approaches which was not to occur across asylums until well into the twentieth century, and then with only limited emphasis on the latter.

As some justification for such an omission, it appears from the limited statistical evidence available that moral treatment, as it was carried out in the large asylums at this time, was less effective than its adherents prophesied. At Lancaster, cures seem to have declined from about 20% before Gaskell's appointment to about 11% five years later. The pattern was similar in other places and is attributed, by those who believed in the effectiveness of moral treatment, on the ever-increasing numbers of pauper patients who were mentally deficient and those with chronic illness of long-standing. To compound the problem Poor Law Authorities, as well as families, sent less and less new cases to asylums.[118] Despite the fact that even Gaskell's kindly disciplinary approach to moral treatment worked well at Lancaster when driven by his commitment and enthusiasm, the results were not sustainable as practice became routine, and resources became strained and then reduced. On his taking up of the Lunacy Commission appointment Lancaster Asylum gradually lost its place in the spotlight as 'an exemplary demonstration of what a reformed asylum could accomplish' by providing a 'more humane and caring environment than most lunatics would have found in either workhouse or the community'.[119]

By 1871 the Rules no longer contained such detail about the occupational aspect of attendants' and nurses' roles. This was despite the fact that it was still recognised that 'in most cases … the patient's mind should be kept employed and active' so that as soon as possible after admission the patient is 'induced to employ herself, or if incapable of any occupation, she must be engaged with some kind of entertainment; and, in doing this, it must be borne in mind that employment is preferable to amusement'.[120] Female attendants were adjured to use 'every exertion to ameliorate and improve the condition of the patients under her charge' not sitting in their own rooms until after the patients had retired to bed. 'At all other times, she must be actively employed in attending on the patients, forwarding their occupations, or cleaning the rooms and galleries'.[121]

Scotland

As in many aspects of medical care Scottish asylums were at the forefront of the use of moral treatment and occupation during the nineteenth century. However, in looking at the overall picture it is important to establish that in Scotland, as in other parts of the British Isles, people with mental illness were often to be found incarcerated in workhouses. MacNiven, in his discussion of reforming mental health commissions in the mid-nineteenth century explains:

> In many counties in Scotland all types of cases of mental illness were received into poorhouses, and in many instances the arrangements for their treatment were quite inadequate. The premises were often small and poorly constructed. The rooms were insufficiently furnished. The wards were often overcrowded. Sometimes two patients occupied the same bed. The bedding of deteriorated patients was often soiled. Restraint was generally used and applied at the discretion of the attendant. Occupation and amusements were seldom provided. Statutory records were not kept in some of the poorhouses. The Commissions (1857) report commented on the high mortality rate in poorhouses as compared with the mortality rate in the chartered hospitals. The Commission strongly disapproved of the tendency to attach wards for mental patients to poorhouses.[122]

The Lunacy Act of Scotland, which required the building and management of district asylums was not enacted until 1857. Nevertheless, seven hospitals were built in Scotland between 1781 and 1839 for the specific purpose of providing accommodation and treatment for large numbers of people suffering mental illness. The asylums were, in chronological order, Montrose Royal Mental Hospital, Aberdeen Royal Mental Hospital, Edinburgh Royal Mental Hospital, Glasgow Royal Mental Hospital (Gartnaval), Dundee Royal Mental Hospital, Perth Royal Mental Hospital (Murray's), and Dumfries Royal Mental Hospital (Crichton). These were originally all non-profit making institutions of high standard. The surplus of the reasonable charges for those who could afford them were reinvested in patient services so that the Boards of Management were able to provide 'for poor patients the most skilful medical attention and advice gratis'.[123] For some of the poorer patients, however the grand and spacious galleries of, for example, Gartnavel Hospital in Glasgow, were overwhelming and oppressive. The Paisley paupers, cases in point, 'wish to get back to Paisley; they feel themselves lost in Gartnavel'.[124] Yet, despite the grandeur and spaciousness, these hospitals too, suffered with overcrowding and economic decline, inevitably followed by lowered standards.

Surprisingly, a social reformer who helped to change the situation was Dorothea Lynde Dix, an American on holiday in Scotland. Born in 1802 and despite an often difficult childhood, by the time she was twenty one Dix had established two schools for infants, the first at the age of fourteen. Her teaching career was interrupted by tuberculosis, which eventually forced her into a different kind of work of a philanthropic nature. Despite ill health, in her late thirties, she agreed to give Sunday school lessons to 20 women confined in the East Cambridge jail in Massachusetts. Appalled by what she found there, not least the housing of the insane with both guilty and innocent inmates, she visited prisons and almshouses throughout many States and addressed their Legislatures on her findings. She advised them of how, with untrained supervision and no treatment facilities, the insane were often caged, penned, chained, naked, and beaten and lashed into obedience. Her interventions led to the founding of new, and the renovation of other, mental hospitals, including two in Canada; one in Nova Scotia and the other in Newfoundland.[125]

In Scotland, on finding the private establishments for the insane guilty of "unconsciously" subjecting hundreds of "miserable" inmates to "bitter bondage", she set about trying to change that situation. After getting no satisfaction from the local officials to whom she spoke she made a hasty visit to London to lay her case before Lord Shaftesbury and the Home Secretary, Sir George Gray. Travelling over-night, and taking no time to dress for the occasion, because the Lord Provost of Scotland was hot on her heels, she accomplished her purpose within a few days. As a result a Commission was set up in April, 1855, to enquire into the condition of the insane in Scotland, which led to the passing of the 1857 Lunacy (Scotland) Act. This revolutionised the treatment of the mentally ill in Scotland.[126]

The Commission found, in a total population of 2,888,742 (according to the 1851 census), approximately 7,403 people who they classified as insane, including 2,603 "congenital idiots". Of these, 657 patients were in 24 licensed private madhouses and a staggering 3,822 were housed in unlicensed establishments, with only 2,132 in the chartered mental hospitals listed above.[127]

In the latter the Commissioners found that 'superintendents had not yet entirely succeeded in their efforts to act upon the modern views of treatment of the insane'. For example, whilst personal restraint had almost disappeared, seclusion was still often used, particularly at Gartnavel. The Commission recommended the building of simpler buildings, and domestic atmosphere and arrangements, because in 'plain domestic buildings a more contented frame of mind is likely to arise, which is highly important and conducive to mental restoration'. Critical also with regard to the provision of therapeutic occupation the Commission found that 'some Medical Superintendents had been content to provide entertainments to the exclusion of more serious occupations'. The entertainments they listed included 'games, frequent excursions, occasional picnics, concerts, lectures, evening parties and dancing; and at the Crichton in Dumfries there were also theatrical performances'. They commented favourably on that Asylum's museum of natural history and its library of 5,000 books.[128] They recommended that:

> ... abundant means of occupation are of the greatest consequence to the well being of the insane ... none are more conducive to recovery than outdoor labour. Hence the importance to every asylum of a sufficient quantity of land to ensure constant employment for the male patients ... there are few better curative agents in the treatment of insanity than agricultural labour.[129]

In 1881, the Commissioners reinforced their early opinion of the usefulness of agriculture stating that;

> For one patient who will be stirred to rational reflection or conversation by such a thing as a picture, twenty of the ordinary inmates of asylums will be so stirred in connection with the prospects of the crops, the points of a horse, the illness of a cow, the lifting of the potatoes, the laying out of a road, the growth of the trees, the state of the fences, or the sale of the pigs.[130]

It could be argued, in the present day and age, that similar benefits might be gained from "souping up" cars, car racing, computer games or the internet, although the advantages of being in the open air, and vigorous physical exercise would be missing from that picture.

Of the licensed madhouses the Commission reported:

> They have few or no means of recreation or occupation, and scarcely any suitable books. The attendants and nurses are not in sufficient number, and their wages are too low to secure the services, or continued stay of efficient persons. Generally, no religious exercises, or other agencies calculated to elevate the moral tone of the inmates are employed, and scarcely anything is done to break the cheerless monotony of their existence.[131]

MacNiven, in his 1960 Presidential Address to the Royal Medico-Psychological Association suggested that:

> The Commissioners of the Scottish Board of Lunacy must have been the greatest upgraders in history. They were never satisfied with the existing conditions in hospitals; they were always suggesting improvements in accommodation, in diet, in the nursing of patients, in their clothing, in the service of their meals, in their amusements and recreations and in their training and management.[132]

The two medical practitioners on the Commission, James Cox and William Alexander Francis (W.A.F.) Browne were zealous, but tolerant, reformers. Both were influenced by philanthropist and phrenologist Dr Andrew Combe. That influence is worth noting in this history as on a visit to Hanwell in 1834 Combe had been particularly impressed by the benefits afforded to patients by useful occupation, and the attention given to their preferences. Taking this impression to heart, as manager of Morningside Asylum, Combe articulated the need to address the individuality of patients. He expressed a concern that even creating order in the daily lives of an institution through common sense and kindness was insufficient in terms of remediation. Such order, he wrote, was 'constantly in danger of falling into lifeless routine … which leaves many a patient to move on in the dull round of disease who, by individual care and attention, might have roused to healthful hope and activity'.[133]

Cox, who was Combe's nephew, had a high regard for moral and industrial training and agreed with the wisdom of the time that asylums were indispensable. However, he questioned their inalienable remedial value, suggesting that even in the best of them 'the patient's life was restricted and there was much in ordinary life, in its change of society, amusements, scenes and circumstances which helped to lift the mind out of its diseased rut and restore it to healthy action'.[134] Browne, the other medical Commissioner, dedicated his book, *What Asylums Were, Are and Ought to Be,* to his friend, Combe.[135] In this he summed up the "whole secret" of moral treatment 'in two words, kindness and occupation'.[136] Indeed, so strong was his belief in, and use of, occupation that he emerges as a significant pioneer in occupational therapy's story.

W.A.F. Browne

Browne was appointed as the first Medical Superintendent at Montrose in 1834. This Hospital already had a history of curative occupation, as the hospital farm was started in 1812 with 2 cows, and was to grow in importance through much of the Hospital's existence providing employment and provisions for its community.[137] Indeed in the 1950s when the Department of Health decreed, in general, the closure of hospital farms, the Montrose farm continued on 'condition that its primary purpose was to be seen as providing therapeutic work for the patients'.[138] The Report of 1826 describes how 'the medical attendants cannot avoid remarking that the want of employment and the tediousness of idleness are constant complaints among the patients'. To overcome this and despite the fact that they did 'not consider cards the most proper amusement … packs of cards were given, with which they (the patients) seemed highly delighted'.[139] In the Hospital's 1828 medical report, the recommendation was made that 'when out of bed, the whole of the insane, ought according to their different states, to be kept in some one employment or another', and also advised the provision of a library. It seems that by 1832 at least, several male patients worked daily in the garden. Music had already been found to be beneficial, so, in that year, a fiddler attended on a weekly basis, and the patients were encouraged to dance, though male with male and female with female.[140] At the time of Browne's appointment there were problems in finding a sufficient supply of work, but despite this a range of occupations were employed in 1834 as shown in Table 1.11.2..

Employment	No
Gardening, &c.	6
Pumping water, &c.	1
Shoemaking	1
Tailoring	1
Weaving	6
Winding yarn	3
Teasing Oakum	18
Spinning	5
Knitting	8
In Laundry	2
In Household matters	2
In opening the outer gate	4
In Fine Work	5
In Transcribing	2
In Reading, Music &c.	8

Table 1.11.2:   Employment of patients at Montrose in 1834

In his first annual report at Montrose in 1835, Browne set down some of his thoughts. They included ideas about "diversion" that are useful to remember, particularly in the context of the day. Diversion was of enormous value at a time when drug therapy was not a real option. He recognised that:

> *Occupation is itself useful in producing sustained and regular habits, but is infinitely more so in arresting the attention and engaging such other powers as are required in the performance of the work, and thus rendering impossible for the*

workman to dwell with the same intensity, at least on those morbid trains of thought which constitute his malady.[141]

He also advocated that it was essential to start a programme of occupation early because 'unless patients are induced to have recourse to some employment very soon after admission, it is found extremely difficult to rouse them from the state of lethargy and abstraction into which they fall'.[142] On a practical level he suggested that 'it was useful to have alternative occupations, one indoor and one outdoor, for each patient', and that it was necessary to have 'separate workshops for the mechanical arts'. He also made use of local community facilities, a harbinger of future trends, reporting that patients attended lectures at the Literary and Scientific Institution. By 1837 he was recommending that patients could engage in community projects on a grand scale, that is, that they 'be employed on public works such as the building of roads near the Asylum'.[143]

In his book he described his ideal asylum. Spacious, and with extensive grounds he pictured galleries, workshops and music rooms all of which were "a hive of industry", the inmates 'actuated by the common impulse of enjoyment, all are busy, and delighted by being so'. He thought useful employment was of more benefit than "frivolous diversions", believing that patients should be paid wages which would accumulate during their hospitalisation and be available to them when they were discharged. Some patients, he saw, would 'act as domestic servants, some as artisans, some rise to the rank of overseers. The bakehouse, the laundry, the kitchens, are all well supplied with indefatigable workers.' There are 'companies of straw-plaiters, basket-makers, knitters, spinners, among the women … weavers, tailors, saddlers, and shoemakers, among the men'. He said 'all are anxious to be engaged, … without any other recompense than being kept from disagreeable thoughts and the pains of illness. They literally work to please themselves.'[144]

> *You may visit rooms where there are ladies reading, or at the harp or piano, or flowering muslin, or engaged in some of those thousand ornamental productions in which female taste and ingenuity are displayed. You will encounter them going to church or to market, or returning from walking, riding or driving in the country. You will see them ministering at the bedside of some sick companion. Another wing contains those gentlemen who can engage in intellectual pursuits … The billiard room will, in all probability, present an animated scene. Adjoining apartments are used as news-rooms, the politicians will be there … One acts as an amanuensis, another is engaged in landscape painting, a third devotes to himself a course of historical reading, and submits to examination on the subject of his studies, a fourth seeks consolation from binding the books he does not read.**

Browne footnoted that '*to exemplify the various modes of engaging the attention of lunatics, it may be mentioned that the manuscripts of these pages were transcribed, and the proofs corrected by individuals in the asylum under my charge'.[145]

Despite his condemnation of the frivolous, it has already been described that Browne advocated drama and music as therapeutic agents. He also had a good word to say on "promiscuous dancing" in that it had 'repeatedly promoted physical as well as physiological changes, and general but wisely regulated intercourse tends to humanise and mollify the asperity of both sexes'.[146]

Longer extracts from Browne's book provide his version of the benefits of employing occupation in the treatment of the insane during the nineteenth century. That he saw it as a remedial tool is made clear by his following assertion: 'I may, with all reverence, compare the employment to that of any other medicine. It must be regulated by the idiosyncrasies of the patients, by the symptoms, the duration and complications of the disease.'[147] Browne suggested that disease of the mind could be thought to reduce the mind to a 'state of childhood' in which 'waywardness', 'impatience of control and compulsory labour', 'capricious desire for gratification', and sometimes 'stubbornness and temper' were displayed. However because 'other characteristics of youth' were present it was possible to employ those to 'communicate strength, or to awaken powers that perhaps require only a proper stimulus to assume their legitimate exercise' towards 'health and serenity of mind'. Sometimes coaxing, bribery or "awe" may be necessary and unavoidable, making 'what is valuable attractive, and what is attractive, valuable' to connect them 'with their comfort and happiness'.[148]

With some remarkably modern concepts he discussed occupation's curative effects as:

- Exercise to the sound part of the mind which simultaneously rests the diseased part
- Producing tranquillity through repetitive action
- A means of imposing of attention and self-control
- Providing a new series of impressions, and
- Using the mind-body interaction in a way similar to conventional medicines.[149]

He also advocated benefits from those treating the patients experiencing the world in which they lived, suggesting a community model, which anticipated those of the twentieth century. He wrote:

> ... it is not only necessary that he who devotes himself to the care of the insane should pass his noviciate in an asylum; or, in the active discharge of his duties, see his patients, as has been recommended, once or twice a-week; he must live among them; he must be their domestic associate; he ought to join in their pursuits and pastimes; he ought to engage them in converse during the day, and listen to their soliloquies in the retirement of their cells.[150]

In attempting to answer the paramount question about whether occupation can cure illness, he put it this way:

> The fact is so evident that the mind must be relieved from sorrow or any other painful impression by distraction that the humanity of resorting to occupation for this purpose is universally admitted. But it may not follow that because the mind is relieved from pain it is consequently placed in the best condition to recover; in other words, (we have to address the question) does employment promote cure?

The presumption that it is capable of doing so is founded upon a very familiar precaution. We do not use a leg or an arm that has been bruised or wounded or is inflamed; we endeavour to save it from exertion, and allow it to rest by employing the other. In prescribing occupation then to the insane, it is proposed to engage the healthy, the unwounded powers and thereby to save those which are pained or diseased, and would be injured by exertion. If a man, who imagines himself an outcast from society, the object of contempt and scorn, be placed at a loom, and induced to produce ten or fifteen yards of cloth per day, it is quite clear, that during the execution of his task, if it be done well, he is forced to exert his whole attention and no little ingenuity and manual dexterity upon the management of the shuttle, beam, etc., that while his mind is so directed, it cannot be under the dominion of its morbid sorrows; that just in proportion to the degree and duration of the occupation will be freedom from disease and the nearer approach to health.

But there are other objects than abstraction gained by this system. It gives regularity to the mental operations, than which nothing can be more conducive to tranquillity: It imposes the necessity of self-command and attention, it communicates new series of impressions, and if judiciously managed, it may be made, by giving tone and vigour to the body, to react on the mind, in the same manner that evacuates, opiates, or tonics do.[151]

He also recognised the negative effects of idleness, monotony, and lethargy at times when patients did not engage in occupation, as on Sundays. Because of that, like others already mentioned, he described religious practice as a therapeutic necessity. It continued 'the regimen by which occupation is provided and by which unhappiness is conciliated, by calling healthy feelings into play' reducing the 'uninterrupted sufferings of self-tormented spirits'.[152]

Because he conceived that when patients are working 'in order to please themselves and having found joy in work, difficulty is found in restraining their eagerness and in moderating their exertions',[153] obviously, he was of a mind that the choice of occupation was important. At the same time, he was not unheedful of the need for a balance between those of a mental and physical nature, nor of the health requirements of exercise. He advised:

In the selection … it is not enough to have the insane playing the part of busy automatons, or to wear out their muscular energies vicariously, in order to relieve the drooping heart of its load. There must be active, and if possible, an intelligent and willing participation on the part of the labourer, and such a portion of interest, amusement, and mental exertion associated with the labour, that neither lassitude nor fatigue may follow …

It ought not to be complicated, for that would discourage: it ought not to be purely mechanical, for that frustrates the end in view: it ought not to be useless and evidently for the purpose of acting as a means of abstraction, for the artifice is often detected, and the patient is disgusted. The utility of every thing ordered should be palpable; and this argument holds out another inducement to engage every individual in the pursuits to which he has been accustomed.[154]

The best rule is to have all descriptions of occupations at command; and where a sedentary one is chosen, or preferable, to suggest walking or swinging as a recreation and interruptions, or to devise means that the necessary amount of exercise be taken.[155]

Browne explained that it is, in part, because of the physical exercise and the holistic concept of flow-on benefits from body to mind, that many asylums used farm work and gardening in the treatment of the insane at that time. This concept has been poorly understood by later occupation for health workers, unionists, and others who have only considered their apparent exploitative nature. Henderson, a founder of twentieth century occupational therapy in Britain, acknowledged that occupation such as 'work in the laundry, in the kitchen, in the sewing room, in the garden or workshops', was used 'as a means of assisting the employees of the hospital organisation'. However he also identified that 'our predecessors had the interest of their patients at heart and knew the value of work in producing happiness and efficiency leading to eventual recovery'.[156] Where later therapists have utilised the same occupations for small, individual projects seldom of an on-going nature, they have failed to recognise the strength and size of the earlier vision, at least how Browne, Tuke, Ellis and others of their persuasion saw it.

With a view to secure the benefit of exercise in the open air, as well as mental concentration, farm labour has been much resorted to, and asylums are surrounded by farms, and parks and garden. The plan is unexceptionable, and wherever it can be carried into effect, will promote the restoration of those engaged.[157]

Far from thinking it right to use them for the economic benefit of the institution alone, Browne recognised when such occupations could and couldn't be used:

But however excellent in certain circumstances, it is quite clear that its application must be partial, that it can only take place during particular seasons of the year, and can include a very small class of lunatics admitted into urban asylums.[158]

Browne's valuing of functional occupation for the 'artisans and tradesmen' who made up the 'greatest proportion of the insane poor' was a sign of the times. Then it was expected that people must earn their own living to survive. The alternative was the dreaded poorhouse and the haphazard charity of the rich. Browne's views reflect this when he argued that:

Whatever the staple trade of the district, its implements, or the means by which it is carried on, should be found in the asylum; and not only this, but every reasonable provision for engaging those workmen, who must be members of every community, and found in every district. Weavers, shoemakers, tailors, gardeners, carpenters, watchmakers, have all been tried for years, and found to work as diligently, and to produce as good articles when confined as when at liberty. I cannot see, nor admit, any limit to the application of the principle.[159]

In the application of labour as a remedy, it is of importance to know what number of patients may be expected to co-operate, and should it be suited to their condition, to work out their own cure. Even in old cases where the mind and muscles have been allowed to slumber, or to struggle in the restlessness of pain for twenty years, wonderful transformations may be accomplished; and so potent and infectious is imitation, so exquisite is the pleasure of being roused to activity, and of being tranquillised by having a specific object to action presented, that two-thirds of those affected may be employed, and the hoary headed lunatic who has dreamed away a quarter of a century may be converted into a busy, bustling, and highly useful personage.[160]

But conceding its practicability, it may be demanded, is it safe? Can the maniac be intrusted with instruments of the most dangerous, and, if he should so incline, deadly kind; which, wielded by the tremendous force that he is well known to occasionally possess, would enable him to sacrifice all around, and then destroy himself? If there be any superiority in the modern mode of studying the dispositions of the insane, it consists in the power of discriminating those who may be allowed to be set free from those who would abuse liberty, and those who may be allowed with impunity to use knives, hatchets, etc., in their ordinary calling, from those who may not.[161]

Mrs Elizabeth Crichton founded and endowed the Crichton Royal Hospital, Dumfries, from funds left by her husband James for charitable purposes. She head hunted Browne when made aware of his "epoch making" although he was only 33 years old.[162] He took up the position as Medical Superintendent when the Hospital was opened in 1839 conducting it according to the great principles of 'justice, benevolence, and occupation'. *The Shipping and Mercantile Gazette* of the day provided a table showing the rates of board and differences between the types of patients, (see table 1.11.3) and explained the advantages of uniting public and private asylums in one facility. Amongst these was the great care taken in the selection of attendants of 'irreproachable character, good education, and of mild but firm disposition'. Their remuneration was, in part, dependent on 'their exertions on behalf of the patients entrusted to their care' whom they were 'not permitted to leave for a single moment, and whom they are enjoined to soothe, encourage, amuse, or employ'. The Resident Medical Officer and the Matron were expected to:

… associate constantly with the Patients, direct their pursuits and employments; suggest and join in their amusements; conciliating their affections and obtaining their confidence, by treating them on rational and enlightened principles; by undeviating kindness, and by a scrupulous attention to the gratification of all their desires, whenever these are compatible with, or conducive to, health and tranquillity.[163]

This is an excitingly early indication of the links between justice, occupation and an enabling approach, which are resurfacing in current literature as important and central to the future of occupational therapy.

PAYMENT PER ANN.	NUMBER OF ROOMS	DIET	LUXURIES	ATTENDENTS	REMARKS
I 10/-	The individuals who are to constitute this class are to be nominated by Mrs Crichton (founder of the hospital)				Accommodation, Diet, &c., is given to this class, which consists of persons of respectability in reduced circumstances, according to what they have been accustomed to.
II 15/-	A public room for 10; a private sleeping room for each; iron bed; no curtains, no carpets, &c.	Animal soap every day; animal food thrice a week; bread, vegetables, &c.	Tea to the females; tobacco and beer to the industrious males	One keeper to 10	Paupers admitted at this rate must be natives of the counties of Dumfries and Wigtown, or Stewartry of Kirkcudbright, are admitted at this rate; 1. is charged in addition for bed and body clothes.
III 18/-	Do.	Do.	Do.	Do.	Paupers who are not natives of the counties of Dumfries and Wigtown, or the Stewartry of Kirkcudbright, are admitted at this rate; 1. is charged in addition for bed and body clothes.
IV 30/- to 100/-	Two public rooms for 10; a private sleeping room for each; with curtained bed,	Animal food every day; tea night and morning; no desert or wine 10 dine together	Wine to the industrious piano, billiards, and society to the well behaved	One keeper 10	In this class a difference will be made in the situation of Rooms, the articles of furniture, &c., according to the Rate of Board; Light in every Room; Baths; hot and cold water in every Gallery of 11 rooms.
V 100/-	A Parlour and Bed-room for each, furnished in American birch	A separate table, with wine, desert, &c., three	Use of a carriage as an indulgence a piano, &c. as a right.	One keeper to 4	Light in every Room, &c. &c.

| VI 200/- | A Parlour and Bed-room of large dimensions, and furnished in mahogany | A separate table, wine, desert, &c., every day | Use of a carriage three time a week, or use of a horse. | One keeper to 2 | Do. |
| VII 350/- | A Parlour and Bed-room, Bathroom, &c., elegantly furnished. | A separate table, wine, desert every day; game in season; plate given. | Use of a carriage or horse every day. | One keeper to each Patient | Do. |

Table 1.11.3:   Established Rates of Board, &c. Crichton Royal Hospital, Dumfries, 1839164

During the 1840s Browne introduced, within the occupation programme, physical exercises in the open air, excursions in an omnibus, attendance at concerts, lectures, readings, theatre and circus, and in-house theatricals in which patients performed.[165] The story of one patient who was encouraged to take part illustrates Browne's skill in enabling meaningful occupation. RC, a serious student of oriental languages, who had been an officer of the East India Company, was admitted in 1843 after withdrawing from life by spending almost five years on the floor rolled up in a carpet. As seven members of his immediate family suffered mental illness, the prognosis was not hopeful. After considerable effort Browne persuaded RC to design a poster for a theatrical production. It was, apparently, remarkably good and led to him attending the play. The next step was successfully encouraging the patient to take part in the next production in which he was, yet again, remarkably good. Browne recorded in the official records that RC was "liberated" in 1846, 'after achieving many triumphs in histrionic and pictorial art'.[166]

Browne kept a substantial library with new works being constantly added; he tempted patients to read by leaving books lying around the galleries;[167] and he boasted that 'the orders for books are as regularly given as prescriptions for medicines'. He also published the first in-house asylum journal called *The New Moon* which was very successful in bringing in funds for further developments such as the purchase of a printing press, and continued to be produced until 1937 when it became the *Crichtonian*.[168] In different directions, and similar to Tuke and Gaskell, he encouraged patients to keep pets such as sheep, rabbits and white mice and some worked in the stables with the horses. The amusements offered in 1840 ranged through backgammon, battledoor and shuttlecock, billiards, cards, concerts and theatre, dances, drafts, drawing, drives, fancy-work, music, picnics, quoits, races, regatta, skittles, singing school, visits to camera and horticultural exhibitions and a menagerie, walks, reading and writing. In addition Christmas and New Years Day were celebrated with special dinners.[169]

There were visiting teachers of music and drawing, and it is interesting to note that in the art therapy programme, of four patients for whom drawing was prescribed it was seen to be the cause of cure for two of them. In the 1847 report Browne proposed to engage another instructress for special embroidery.[170] A further innovation during the next decade was the introduction of a course of lectures on physiology, which provided patients with information about subjects such as the special senses. The goal was to combine amusement with a beginning understanding of some of the sources of delusion and hallucination.[171]

After Browne left Crichton to take up his Lunacy Commissioner position, occupation continued to be used at the Hospital through the century. Some examples of this are that:

- In the late 1850s Dr Gilchrist wrote of the importance of making the patients co-operate actively in the amusements, and a brass band was formed.[172] The 1875 annual report rated the importance of 'curative agencies' - 'the workroom should be first, recreational hall second, the surgery third'.[173]
- Under the same superintendent, Brownhill farm was purchased in 1867, and added to through the years, including a substantial new quadrangle complex of buildings in "old Scotch" style in the last decade of the century. The philosophy behind the agricultural work was simply stated as 'insanity is a disease which demands a stimulus, and there is no stimulant to equal fresh air and exercise … the patients are not in the Asylum for the farm, but the farm has been provided for the patients'. This included the private as well as pauper patients.[174] In 1882, it had been ruled that 'no financial value is to be attached to patients' farm labour, which is prescribed medically and essentially as a therapeutic measure'.[175] The farm operated for that purpose until 1966 when farming outside the hospital no longer offered employment possibilities for discharged patients. This being the case, Dr James Harper, the incumbent Physician Superintendent, issued a memorandum stating that 'hospital farm work has, therefore, practically no value as rehabilitation and the retention of the farm cannot be justified purely on therapeutic grounds'.[176]
- The development of facilities for games. During the nineteenth century these included billiards, lawn bowling, quoits, lawn tennis, badminton, croquet, cricket and football, and in some cases they were to competition standard.[177] The serious intent was manifest by the engagement, for some five years, of a cricket professional as an attendant in 1887.[178]
- By 1880 the most successful of all forms of indoor occupations was wall-paper-hanging, painting, and decorating.[179]
- Dr Rutherford, in 1886, mentioned gardening as being particularly valuable for the treatment of insanity in adolescence.[180]
- An instructress from Finland was employed for a few months in 1895, to teach weaving to patients who were interested.[181]
- During the first hundred years about 40% of those admitted annually recovered. This was largely a result of 'the work-a-day, educational, social,

and recreational activities, which were constantly being expanded and reconsidered with a view to catering for interest and demand'.[182]

At Montrose also, after Browne left to take up his appointment at the Crichton Royal, the occupation programme continued. Lists of work done in 1856 provide an indication of the routine occupation provided apart from amusements and recreation. (Tables 1.11.4. and 1.11.5).

	Made	Mended		Made	Mended		Made	Mended
Bed covers	40	48	Pairs of blankets	148	113	Sheets	72	265
Bed ticks	94	70	Pillows	116	10	Pillow cases	234	149
Quilted sheets	9	0	Quilted coverlets	15	0	Straw mattresses	6	4
Canvas beds	14	9	Canvas dresses	7	13	Feeding aprons	18	5
Smock frocks	6	23	Shirts	182	218	Shifts	146	237
Flannel shirts	102	315	Petticoats	84	216	Drawers	22	102
Stockings	215	2,086	Socks	113	67	Gowns	114	226
Bed-gowns	26	128	Aprons	77	118	Day-caps	156	120
Night-caps	51	73	Stays	14	48	Stocks	48	95
Polkas	7	6	Bonnets trimmed	35	0	Handkerchiefs hemmed	381	160
Towels hemmed	145	75	Window-blinds	46	38	Table-cloths	15	22
Habit shirts	12	30	Binding shoes	34	0	Toilet covers	32	18

Table 1.11.4: List of work done on female side of the House (Montrose)183

	Made	Mended		Made	Mended		Made	Mended
Coats	1	134	Jackets	16	261	Waistcoats	13	329
Trousers, pairs	11	584	Drawers, pairs	30	222	Patent Dresses	4	24
Braces, pairs	18	78	Stocks	6	186	Straw Seat	1	0
Hemp Nets	54	8	Cotton Nets	19	0	Sheep Nets	6	2
Shoes, pairs	1	15	Slippers, pairs	34	73	Oakum picked, 19cwt. 1qr. 24lbs		

Table 1.11.5: List of work done, in tailor's workroom, &c. (Montrose)184

Occupations, apart from work included games like skittles, badminton, archery, golf, football and cricket. Military drill was offered along with classes in reading, writing, singing, and dancing, and a weekly dance. The opening of a new Recreation Hall in 1882 increased the scope of visiting concert parties that already took place, so that even the D'Oyly Carte Opera Company performed there in 1885. Excursions were also a regular feature and surely the most impressive would have to have been the 1887 two day walk which necessitated overnight stays, followed by a train journey to Ballater, before a further ten mile walk to the Highland games at Balmoral before returning the same way. Such social life was reported in the *Sunnyside Chronicle*, the hospital magazine, which started in 1887 and ran, off and on, until the 1970s.[185]

Other Mental Hospitals, apart from Montrose and Dumfries, also ran extensive remedial occupational programmes. Some of these will be described starting with The Glasgow Royal Mental Hospital because it too played a significant part in the story of 20th century occupational therapy. The other programmes will be considered in brief.

Glasgow Royal Mental Hospital (Gartnavel)

When the Glasgow Asylum for Lunatics was opened in 1815, Henderson reports that two rooms were built for the patients' use. In these, they engaged in spinning, knitting and sewing, because according to the Hospital Report of 1817, 'every encouragement (was) given to the exertions of industry, because nothing contributes so much to promote a cure and prevent a relapse'.[186] In addition the report stated that 'two looms have been erected by the superintendent, which made one patient who had been for some years listless, almost to torpor, exclaim that "the house was now altered indeed, it was now worth living in"'.[187] Apparently a year previously, one patient, following much knitting of worsted gloves, was proclaimed cured and happy after being ill for twenty-three years. By 1820, patients, as well as their previous occupations, were engaged in numerous others of a work or recreational nature such as gardening, cobbling, weaving, music, mathematics and games.[188] Indeed they could be punished for non-engagement. Georgina Ferguson and Margaret Gibson, for example, patients during the 1820s, were "rotated" on a special chair for refusing 'to sew or amuse themselves'.[189]

The "rotating chair" was mentioned in an earlier chapter, as a form of treatment adopted in at least one private madhouse during the previous century. It appears to have become established for a short time in various asylums, as mechanisation became revered during the beginning part of the industrial revolution. This was despite no apparent positive results except nausea and vomiting, which did probably quieten patients until they overcame their discomfort. Bearing the above example in mind, at the Glasgow Asylum 'there seems little doubt that the rotating chair was occasionally used as a form of punishment'. This and other forms of restraint and confinement, like the widely used "Glasgow muff" (a leather device which bound the hands and wrists), obviously continued to be used alongside moral treatment for a considerable time.[190]

The regular and habitual use of occupations was part of moral treatment; 'exercise and labour, as appropriate to gender and class, were seen as especially efficacious means of distracting patients from their concerns, as well as sedating them by using up their energies'. The occupations chosen for use tended to differ according to social status in that physical labour was prescribed for pauper patients, while distractions and amusements, such as billiards, were reserved for those who were fee-paying, because 'gentlemen would feel degraded if employed in digging and wheeling'.[191] By the 1830s, the hospital also had the means for weaving, carding, dressmaking, tailoring, shoemaking, carpentry and saddlery.[192] The hospital report published in 1839 explained:

> It was long justly complained of a radical defect in almost all the Institutions for the treatment of the Insane that no proper plan for the employment of lunatics had been adopted. The idea of teaching lunatics to perform any useful handicraft operation would at one time have been treated as altogether chimerical, but by such well-devised occupations as experience has shown to be practicable, this difficulty has been surmounted, and the means have been discovered of affording salutary exercise and amusement to almost every description of the insane, while daily employment is now universally confessed to be one of the most effectual means of promoting their recovery.[193]

The range of occupations grew throughout the century and became available to increasing numbers of patients. Dr Hutcheson, the first resident physician and then physician-superintendent, emphasised the therapeutic value of reading and music.[194] One of the first occupations to be used had been "riding in a carriage" which had long been deemed beneficial for many illnesses as is reflected in interpretations of the *Regimen Sanatatis*. A carriage was purchased early in the Asylum's history, and from the 1820s at least, carriage rides were available for more affluent patients. There was even a carriage simulator consisting of 'a wooden chair the seat of which engages in the teeth of the wheel which in turning impresses upon the patient a movement analogous to the trot of a horse.' Could this be the first example of remedial equipment such as reigned supreme in occupational therapy departments of the 1960s? Carriage exercise was reintroduced, on a more formal basis, by Dr Alexander Macintosh in 1849, and continued until the early twentieth century. This same superintendent solicited some payment be given to patients for their labour, but failed to convince the Directors of the Asylum to take such a step.[195]

In the tradition of earlier times, Hutcheson maintained the distinction between medical and moral treatment. Under "medical", though, he included attention to environment, diet and exercise which are more often associated with the moral treatment approach. With "moral" he prescribed kindness, confidence, healthy occupations and amusements, as well as the absence of all mechanical personal restraint. Indeed, the time between the 1840s and 1870s was one in which the physician-superintendents allied themselves with the non-restraint movement which was becoming powerful within British psychiatric practice, although not always totally successful. From that time "non-restraint" came under increasing attack from some psychiatrists, and restraint came into vogue once more as protection against suicide, violent behaviour, self injury, or even to prevent patients from disturbing others, masturbating or admitting insomnia.[196]

A remarkable book *The Philosophy of Insanity*, first published in Glasgow in 1860 by an unknown author after his second confinement in the Glasgow Royal Asylum, tells a first hand story of labour and amusements as curative agents.[197] Only one copy was known to exist of this "plain, truthful" account written to help fellow sufferers and the general public to better understand the experience of insanity when Dr Frieda Fromm Reichmann found it and had it republished in 1947. In it the author told how:

> For the last two years I have attended the concerts and balls given during the dark months of the year to inmates of Gartnavel Royal Lunatic Asylum; and from what I have seen, and also from what I have heard from the inmates themselves, I know that these meetings have often soothed the excited, cheered the desponding, and turned the mind aside for the time from the corroding task of contemplating its own sorrows, and consequently ministered to the great purpose for which asylums are instituted - the cure of insanity.
>
> That music had almost a magical influence over insanity in days that are long past, history, sacred and profane, testifies; and all that have watched the expression upon the faces of the inmates of this asylum during these vocal and instrumental performances must have seen that time had not robbed the beneficent spirit which presides over sweet sounds of any portion of her entrancing power. Concerts far excel any other description of amusement that can be introduced into an asylum in the universality of their application. They suit both sexes alike, are alike attractive to youth and to age; they soothe the excited - cheer the depressed. And their regular recurrence breaks up that stagnation of the mind consequent upon the monotony which must ever reign within the walls of, and be injuriously felt by all connected with, places of confinement.
>
> ... through the philanthropy of the gentlemen connected with the management of the Glasgow City Hall Saturday Evening Concerts, who attend with the professionals engaged by them gratuitously, these concerts, for arrangement and musical excellence, rank high, and could not easily be surpassed. The calm quiet attention to the music, and the orderly conduct observed by the patients could not be excelled, and is seldom equalled by any assemblage of sane persons; while the feeling of enjoyment which illuminates almost every face is not only a matter of delight but of astonishment.
>
> Here there are people listening to a song and joining in the dance.[198]

He was obviously a man who reflected deeply about what he saw, and probably discussed his opinions and insights with staff he worked with during his own curative occupations. He concluded as other authorities before him had that diversion from a state of madness, even if only for brief periods was beneficial. He held that:

> To attempt to reason anyone out of insane feelings must be nearly always

ineffectual and often mischievous; but to divert the current of thought for however short a time from the fiery channel in which it is flowing must be in every case and under all circumstances beneficial. A very excellent method of obtaining this most desirable end consists in keeping the fingers employed at some light and useful labour, if possible in the field or garden, under the superintendence of a judicious, sympathising person who would regulate the labour to the strength and former habits of the patient.

To female patients this exercise does not apply; but for ladies there is needlework in many a form, and for others there is an abundance of household work in the asylum which is a thousand times better; indeed, get them to assist the nurses and take an interest in the work of the house, and the cure is begun - and it has been well said that anything well begun is half ended.[199]

In recognising the relationship between occupation and sleep as part of a healthy continuum he was both a product of his time and ahead of it. This continuum is still scarcely mentioned in occupational therapy or health promotion literature, and is invisible in that of conventional medicine.

Employment tends to induce sleep, without which every attempt at cure is a mockery. In order that the mind may live in a state of efficiency, we must submit to the semblance of death for at least a fourth part of our existence.[200]

That a wide variety of occupations were available and used at Gartnavel for curative purposes is clear, for this patient's account can surely not be considered as propaganda or self seeking as other reports from asylum staff may be. There is also an indication of the staff being viewed as part of the therapeutic process, of them needing to share experiences with patients for them to be most effective.

Light reading, to those who can enjoy it, must have a very excellent effect; but when reading can be enjoyed, we will find that the mind is progressing toward a cure or has arrived at a silly unsatisfactory stage of convalescence beyond which it is not likely to go. No one whose mind is distracted can settle down to read. If any particular subject is harassing the mind, a reference to it will be found in every sentence, whatever may be the subject upon which the book treats[201]

... in- or outdoor amusements in which a number can join, especially if attendants or other sane people can be associated in the game, cannot fail of being highly beneficial. In all cases of curable sanity the company of the sane is much to be desired.[202]

This patient evidently found horse riding to be the occupation with most meaning for him, and he describes, in great detail, what he most benefited from it:

Although, unfortunately, far from being practical in every or indeed in very many cases, yet there is no exercise or amusement at all to be compared to riding (the more spirited and troublesome the animal is, the better for the purpose) in any case where it is imperative that the mind should be lifted from preying upon its own vitality ...

An afflicted man who can ride well, mounted upon a strong, sound horse which, from its habits, requires constant watching, galloping across country with his eyes fixed upon his horses ears and not quite certain where the next leap may land him - with distended lungs, inhaling as much oxygen in one minute as he would do at his own fireside in five, has very little time to think about, and soon gets as regardless of the troop of blue devils which he is rapidly leaving behind him as the horse which is bearing him so bravely on. There is nothing more exhilarating and, of course, nothing more conducive to bodily and mental health than the motion of a strong active horse to a man who has a sure seat in the saddle and a firm and skilful bridle-hand.

I believe there is even more in this than meets the common eye; and with the certainty of being laughed at by some people and having it set down as an insane notion by others, I will state that a young, spirited horse imparts a portion of that vital energy with which he overflows to a dull, melancholy, wealminded rider. I have felt this, or at least believed that I did so, I may safely say a hundred times. I have often mounted, weak and vacillating, almost afraid to slack the bridle and let the horse go, and after an hour or two of hard riding I have dismounted in mind and body a very different man[203]

Other Scottish asylums

When Samuel Tuke made a visit to Scottish Asylums in 1838 he found that 'at Perth, Dundee and Aberdeen, the men's wards were nearly empty, so large a proportion were in one way or another engaged in labour'. It seems as a consequence of this that in these asylums the 'lowest class of patients' were not the 'dismal-looking objects cringing in the corners of the rooms or squatting on the ground, almost lost to human form' as he had found in many other hospitals. In the Dundee Royal Mental Hospital Tuke records that:

> *... out of fifty-seven men patients of the lower class, twelve were engaged in stone breaking, eight in gardening, thirteen in weaving, one in tailoring, two as shoemakers, whilst a few were engaged in the preparation of tow for spinning, and several in the various services of the house*[204]

Tuke's observations supported those of Browne a few years earlier. He had reported that 'in Dundee Asylum in 1834-35, ninety-two of ninety-six paupers were engaged in various branches of industry, from picking oakum and mending shoes up to flowering muslin and upholstery work'.[205]

Tuke seemed somewhat surprised, when he noted that 'I must not omit to mention that at Aberdeen the manager had succeeded in inducing the higher class of patients to engage in gardening, etc.' From another source, however, it appears that during Dr Macrobin's time as Medical Superintendent of Aberdeen Royal Asylum, between 1830 and 1852, restraint remained in much use. In an inventory, and other records, for the year 1847 it appears that 22 pairs of ankle straps, 10 pairs of bracelets, 10 pairs of iron handcuffs, 24 body belts, 16 straight jackets, 9 sets of bed straps, 2 muzzles, 3 restraint chairs, 1 rotary chair, and 1 hand-barrow for moving patients were in constant use. When Dr Jamieson succeeded Macrobin, a more benign approach was instigated including plenty of fresh air, walking exercise, and occupation to exercise hands and minds.[206]

At the Perth Asylum, it appears that from the start of its history, patients worked in the garden, for in its first report of 1828 it states that for such occupation they were rewarded with tobacco, snuff or tea. However, this might have been overly successful, as seven years later a report states that 'twenty-two to twenty eight patients work on the grounds which requires no small degree of ingenuity to torture - if the term may be used - into forms of usefulness'. The latter was perceived as a necessity to prevent patients feeling 'hurt or affronted at being put to work at anything they could neither see nor value'.[207] The first Report also notes that none were constrained to engage in anything to which they were averse, and nor were any confined to their rooms. About this time, and particularly prior to discharge on apparent recovery, patients were permitted, and indeed encouraged, to regularly attend the market with servants in order to ease the transition between hospital and home.[208]

In the 1850s gardening was extended into floriculture, and also into agriculture with patients being put in charge of cattle. To enable some male convalescent patients to learn job skills considered useful after discharge, a workroom was provided. However, its use did not remain exclusively male, and female patients were also employed in the workroom a year after it became available, as well as doing needlework in the wards. In the treatment of some female patients it was thought that dolls had value and the 1859 Annual Report records how 'a lady with puerperal mania began to recover from the moment she cast eyes upon a doll'.[209]

With regard to recreation and education, during 1836 a curling pond was built and in the 1850s "Lady" patients enjoyed archery for sport, whilst gentlemen went fishing, and also played cricket and football. Educational opportunities for both included a course on economic botany, classes in languages, and lectures about "Galvanism", "Jacobite minstrelsy", "The blood, its composition and uses", "Time, its proper occupation and uses"; "Drugs, their economic botany", and "Coal, its natural history and uses". Pauper patients enjoyed as topics for their classes "music", "psalmody", "religion", "reading", "writing", "arithmetic" and "dancing".[210] Indeed, dancing was considered by the Superintendent to be a 'particularly suitable amusement for Scottish patients'. Towards the end of the century, and with a more participatory approach, patients were given more responsibility in organising their own concerts and amusements, which proved to be of benefit to them.[211]

At the Royal Edinburgh Mental Hospital, as well as the more usual occupations of the times, occupations frequently used in the early to mid 20th century, such as bookbinding, basketry, and communal singing, were being carried on by 1840.[212] The Lunacy Commission Report of 1857 records that the Asylum's furniture was made by the patients,[213] and in the Hospital's own Report, Dr T. S. Clouston wrote that, in 1885, curling had been found to be a valuable occupation for one particular patient. He added, 'I could not help thinking that if I had some medicine in the surgery which would take hold of my patient's brains as curling had done in this case, our recovery rate would be a large one'.[214]

The Elgin Pauper Lunatic Asylum seems to have been responsive to the Commissioner's enthusiastic support of agriculture, as it was used as the chief occupation on the hospital's 70 acres of land, with even the women patients engaging in light work in the fields. The Commissioners' 1863 report was very complimentary:

> Perhaps in no asylum in Scotland has greater progress been made in the treatment of the insane during the past five years than at Elgin … The cultivation of this land, which is all done by the patients, with the occasional assistance of a plough, affords so much out-of-door employment of a kind that pleases and interests them, that a great deal of the beneficial results alluded to must be ascribed to the possession of this land … The superintendent reports that the possession of the land besides being advantageous to the patients, is likewise profitable to the institution.[215]

Bearing in mind what happened to occupational programmes elsewhere in Britain, it can be wondered whether the latter sentiment expressed by Elgin's Superintendent gained prominence in later years, with the therapeutic benefits lapsing into "lip-service" rhetoric.

Further reports of the beneficial effects of occupation include the Brabazon Employment Scheme, which was started at Woodilee Asylum by Miss Aikman in 1898. It was 'managed by twelve ladies each of whom is peculiarly gifted to teach some special subject. It can readily be seen that the work engaged in is both varied and interesting.' Amongst the occupations taught were rug making, lampshade making macrame and drawn-linen work, woodcarving, basket making, and bent ironwork. The medical staff are convinced that 'not only has the work a brightening influence on the patients—it is actually of benefit to their mental condition'.[216]

As well, at the Fife and Kinross District Asylums fifty female patients were occupied in the workroom, "teasing hair" for a firm of upholsterers in Cupar. This is the first report found of labour being done for a firm outside a hospital. The Commissioners' report on Ayr contrasted dramatically. In 1868 they found the patients to be unoccupied and destructive.

In general though, as the century drew to a close, administrative changes resulted in attendants becoming more like companions and less like gaolers. The Commissioners, in 1888, pointed out that this followed on inevitably from the abolition of airing courts and the development of the open-door system, because, in order to know where they were and what they were doing, the onus was on the attendants to keep the patients happily occupied. In the tradition established in Gheel, community care was also utilised as part of the system in Scotland:

> *Ever since the middle of the nineteenth century this system of providing accommodation and treatment for certain groups of mentally ill and subnormal patients has been utilised in Scotland under the more familiar name of "boarding out". The fundamental reason for its introduction was to release more bed space for acutely distressed patients who were urgently in need of hospital treatment; it had the additional advantage of being more economical than hospitalisation.*[217]

Ireland

In Ireland, at the start of the period under question some charity hospitals for the mentally ill existed, but it was not until the 1820s that lunatic asylums were built on a systematic basis, the one in Belfast being established in 1829. Lunatic wards were set up in workhouses some 15-20 years later, and it has been argued that their very existence created the demand that supplied them.[218] They relaced the earlier Houses of Industry, and in many the mentally ill co-existed with "crooks", old people and children. The number of private asylums increased steadily throughout the century, some gender specific, with some managed by Catholic orders and some by Quakers following the Retreat model.[219]

Patients placed in custodial care for mental illness were considered unfit for work outside the asylum. Across the country, although the number of men in this kind of custody exceeded women, the latter were 'in a growing majority among adults confined in the lunatic wards of workhouses', and were more likely to be committed to asylums as dangerous and to die there. As in England the connection between "lunacy" and poverty, hard work, and ill health of women was recognised as a fact. Admission to an asylum was often 'the penultimate step in a process of deterioration'. Particularly at risk were women from places with 'very little industrial employment and where occupations were solitary or semi-solitary' rather than the industrial north east.[220]

At the turn of the eighteenth and nineteenth century one medical authority considered to be an apostle of enlightenment and moral treatment in Ireland was Dr William Saunders Halloran (1765-1825). He was a graduate of Edinburgh who managed the lunatic department in the Cork House of Industry, and had a private asylum called Citadella. Like other advocates, he recognised the value of occupation for maniacal and convalescent patients alike.[221] However, in his *An Enquiry Into the Causes Producing the Extraordinary Addition to the Numbers of the Insane Together with Extended Observations on the Cure of Insanity*, it was apparent that he did not entirely follow the "soft approach" taken by the

Quakers at the Retreat. He did support:
- Friendliness and personal relationships between the patients and the doctor
- The use of circulating swings as a panacea
- Sleep, diet, emetics and laxatives, and
- Entertainment, and physical occupation out of doors.

To advance the latter he designed a special straitjacket for outdoor activity, and leased some acres of farmland where patients are said to have worked happily whilst generating a profit for the institution.[222]

Richmond Asylum in Dublin was the first public establishment for the reception of the mentally ill in Ireland. When it opened in 1815 for 218 patients, a lay person, Richard Grace was appointed "Moral Governor". It was managed according to the principles of Pinel and Tuke. Grace lived in the Asylum with his wife, Anne, who was both Matron and Housekeeper. It was his job to create opportunities for the employment and recreation of the patients, each of whom he was expected to know, and to see each day. The visiting medical officers were Alexander Jackson who, at his appointment, sold Farnham House, his private lunatic asylum, and Hugh Ferguson, who had previously been attached to the House of Industry. They advised the Moral Governor on the subject of occupation and employment, as well as restraint, diet, classification, and discharge. Macdonald explained that the occupations available for the patients included education, recreations, drama, and gymnastics, which were run by "teacher attendants".[223] 'As in the House of Industry Lunatic Asylum with its 370 inmates, cure rates were reported to be high.'[224]

The system of labour became widespread amongst the asylums. By 1843, at Maryborough, where "idiots", "epileptics", "curable" and "incurable maniacs" were housed, more than two thirds of the inmates were engaged in occupation. Fed on a largely carbohydrate diet, of which working men received more than either women or non-workers, most were employed on the farm. Men were also occupied as carpenters, tailors, manufacturers of tin products, and cobblers, and women at spinning, knitting, sewing and domestic chores.[225]

Just as was the case in other British asylums, and exacerbated by the potato famine (1840-1900) and, towards the end of the century, by the struggle for complete independence from England, asylums in Ireland became overcrowded. That made individual relationships between patients and the moral managers or visiting physicians impossible to sustain. This resulted in an imbalance of the amount and type of occupation available to patients, some being totally unoccupied whilst others had to labour excessively. The use of various forms of restraint increased.[226]

By 1855, a laborious task expected of some patients by all asylums except the one at Cork, which had been described as the best managed establishment of its kind,[227] was raising water from wells by pumps. These were worked by 4-6 patients in enclosed sheds which became oppressively hot in summer. The Commission on the Irish District Asylums found 'the description and amount of labour' imposed upon the patients for work of that description 'to be highly objectionable and not calculated to improve either their mental or physical condition'. Also unfavourable was their view of the size and aspects of airing courts. They argued that 'too little reference' had been given 'to obtaining for the patients a cheerful look-out'. Except for felons, they deemed 'cheerfulness, sunniness and space' essential for all inmates. On a positive note, they found that 'music and recreation halls have been provided, and the general evidence of the medical officers is favourable as to their utility in amusing the patients, and relieving the monotony of their seclusion'.[228] By 1862 however, John Blake, the member of parliament for Waterford, following visits to most of the asylums was convinced that there was 'not a single one that can be held up as an example' with regard to "lightening' patients" lives.[229]

In 1869, the first asylum for "idiotic and imbecile children", the Stewart Institution, was built and opened in the grounds of Henry H. Stewart's Asylum for Lunatic Patients of the Middle Classes, in Lucan. It was modelled after Abendberg in Switzerland. Doctor Frederick Pim, the manager, had had some training in English "idiot" asylums before his appointment. He established a programme for his "pupils" in which they engaged in domestic or gardening tasks, needlework or singing. For those for whom it was possible he also offered a programme of basic education in reading, writing, and arithmetic[230]

Wales

At the North Wales Hospital in Denbigh, occupation played an important role in the treatment of patients, and it is of interest that that hospital was to appoint the first trained occupational therapist in Wales in the twentieth century. It was established in the 1840s following the intervention of Doctor Samuel Hinch, who was the Medical Superintendent of Gloucester Lunatic Asylum. In 1842, the same year that the Lunacy Commissioners were set to investigate conditions in asylums, Hitch wrote a letter to the The Times about the particular plight experienced by Welsh pauper insane:

So few of the lower class of the Welsh, except some in towns or the precincts of inns, speak English, and this only for the purpose of commerce, or to qualify themselves for the duties of menial servants, and not to an extent which would enable them to comprehend anything higher, - whilst both the officers and servants of our English Asylums, and the English public too, are equally ignorant of the Welsh language, - that when the poor Welshman is sent to an English Asylum he is submitted to the most refined of modern cruelties, by being doomed to an imprisonment amongst strange people, and an association with his fellowmen whom he is prohibited from holding communication with ... He becomes irritable and irritated; and it is proverbial in our English Asylums that the Welshman is the most turbulent patient wherever he happens to become an inmate.[231]

Hitch became an adviser to the Committee planning the building of the Hospital, which was an obvious necessity as the report of the Commission revealed in 1844. Aimed at relieving 'the most grievous calamity that can befall humanity' and the replacement of 'mechanical restraints and coercion' ... 'by kind management and moral discipline in their own language' the hospital was largely financed by public subscriptions. These included gifts from Queen Victoria, Prince Albert and the Prince of Wales, and 20 acres of land given by Joseph Ablett of Llanbedr Hall. The hospital opened in October 1848.[232]

For many years it was able to follow the foundation philosophy of minimal restraint and kind and humane treatment until, suffering the fate of most similar institutions, the hospital became largely custodial because of 'overcrowding, staff shortages, (and) counties sending patients only when they had severely deteriorated'. Apart from physical care the only treatment available was occupation of an employment, recreational and spiritual nature. As in many other asylums it was the Medical Superintendent who organised the employment and recreation of patients apart from his medical duties and the management and supervision of staff generally.[233]

Figure 1.11.10: The hospital farm at North Wales Hospital in Denbigh[234]

Clwyd. The North Wales Hospital, Denbigh, 1842-1955....;

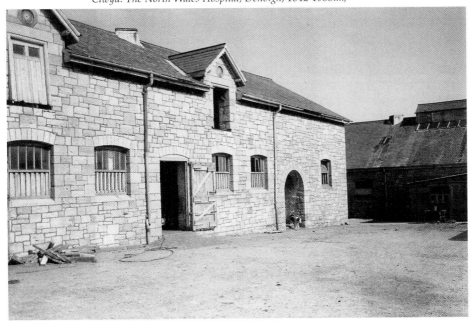

Whilst female patients were occupied in the laundry, sewing room and washhouse, male patients were engaged in the gardens, farm, and tailoring, joinery and shoemaking shops. Over the century the farm, which was extended, became central 'to both the economy of the asylum and the employment of the patients'. (See figure 1.11.10). Patients were involved in preparing grounds for other activities such as bowls and skittles, and as labourers on minor building projects, painting and decorating. Patients unable to participate in such occupations spent endless hours walking aimlessly about the airing courts. Country walks, bowls, skittles and quoits, were popular recreations in the early years, but at first, little was organised in the evenings apart from an Annual Christmas Ball which was originally held in 1852 and continued for about 120 years. By 1864, weekly dances were held and both staff and outside agencies provided entertainment for patients such as concerts and the offerings of a full brass band formed in 1870. Later in that decade, 100 patients were taken to entertainment in the town, 'an experiment which was successful and repeated'. For spiritual activities the original chapel rooms on the top floor of the building were replaced in 1862 by a purpose built chapel with seating for 200 patients. The apparently musical staff employed around 1870 formed a choir, which participated in the chapel services. Indeed, Clwyd reported in his history of the hospital that staff were selected according to their occupational abilities, stating that 'for many years staff were selected according to their size, musical ability, singing or instrumental, sporting prowess, and ability to speak Welsh'.[235]

As a final comment on the use of occupation for mental health during the industrial period a citation from a report of the British Medico-Psychological Association's annual meeting in York, noted in the *Yorkshire Herald* of Friday 22, 1892, is apt. It told of ongoing changes in the system, which was part and parcel of the scene for occupational therapists for much of the twentieth century:

> *It was undoubtedly said and believed by them of old time that all insane persons should be sent to the wards of an asylum, but we, in these latter days, know of a far more excellent way. … We all know that there are many patients who require isolation from home and home surroundings, and special skilled treatment, but whom we dare not take the responsibility of consigning to the wards of an asylum. To meet this defect in the hospital treatment of the insane, many, if not all, of our hospitals have built separate villas in their grounds, each villa carefully designed and planned for the individual treatment of a small group of selected patients.*
>
> *… It seems to me that a marked advance has been attained in our hospital villa treatment of the insane by the increased facilities afforded us of gaining a personal knowledge of and affection for our patients - in learning their individual capabilities, and in directing, guiding, and leading their energies from unhealthy into healthy channels. Our patients are so infinitely happier if they are doing something. Nothing can be worse than listless despondency. It seems to me we ought to study each individual patient's idiosyncrasies and powers; that we ought not merely to believe in theory the truth of the axiom, Find thy work and do it; but we ought to teach our patients some congenial occupation, and see that they have every assistance in gaining the necessary knowledge.[236]*

Occupation as treatment in Europe

W.A.F. Browne wrote that 'on the Continent, a very powerful movement has been made to place the treatment of lunatics upon a true basis'. Knowing of his belief in justice, benevolence and occupation, it would be fair to suggest that he recognised advances towards those ideals. And, indeed, from the latter part of the eighteenth century as well as the early decades of the nineteenth, occupations such as farming, music, weaving, printing and translating, were included as treatment in France, Italy and Spain.

**Figure 1.11.11: Eight women patients in the grounds of Salpetriere.
Lithograph by A Gautier, 1857**
(The Wellcome Library)

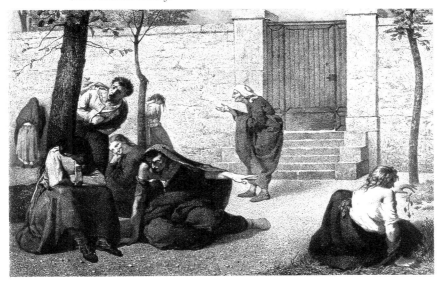

Doctors Fairet and Voisin provided gentleness and affection towards their patients who enjoyed spacious and beautiful grounds outside Paris. Those afforded constant employment in the open air, and there were spacious apartments containing 'all the ordinary means of amusement, music, billiards, &c'. Dr Leuret, another Parisian, working around the 1840s, used several terms to describe the type of occupation treatment he offered to patients with mental disorders, not only "moral treatment" but "manual work", "art and mental work", or "invalid occupations".[237] At Bicêtre, Guillaume Ferrus, as superintendent, carried on working according to Pinel's theories and established a farm attached to the hospital for therapy. He employed 150 patients constantly in levelling, masonry, digging, joinering, blacksmithing, and carpenting.[238] Ferrus, with other doctors like Voisin, Belhomme, Fairet and Seguin established educational facilities for mentally handicapped children at

Bicêtre, Salpetriere and in other European countries. Others of Pinel's students, Jean Esquirol and Jean Georget wrote about their methods and cases.[239]

In the London Medical Gazette of May 23rd, 1835, a reporter provided the public with news of their activities:

> *The French certainly carry their treatment of the insane to a far higher pitch of refinement than we do. The idea of giving a ball in a lunatic asylum, may startle some of our mad doctors; but what think they of the following precedent. On the 7th instant, May 1835, the females of Salpetriere were treated to a grand ball. The insane ladies themselves were entrusted with the getting up of the entertainment. They adorned the ball-room with festoons, garlands and devices; and in the midst they crowned with immortelles, the bust of Pinel, the liberator of the insane from the old system of cruelty and terror. The dancing, it is said, went off with charming effect; the students, intern and extern, did the honours and the festivity was kept up to an hour sufficiently advanced to satisfy all parties, who to do them justice, were indefatigable in their efforts to please and be pleased. It should be added, that the gay scene, (which was appointed and arranged with the most serious object) has been generally attended with good results: it served admirably to fix and amuse the minds of the patients; and several who laboured under melancholia were much diverted for the time from their imaginary woes. M. Esquirol some years ago tried this method with success; but it is to M. Pariset, the physician to Salpetriere, that the credit is due of having so happily ventured on its repetition in the present instance[240]*

Commenting on that event, Browne reflected that dancing 'as both physical exercise, and as recreation' had been introduced into many "well-regulated" British Asylums often on a weekly basis, with excellent results. He added a rider: 'what Esquirol and Pariset have accomplished and experimented with, we (in Britain) have already reduced to a system'.[241]

Browne was obviously well versed in European therapeutic endeavours and also added some other of his observations of practice in Europe:

> *Military exercise has been substituted in some countries (for other outdoor occupations); and however ridiculous it may first appear, that a battalion of lunatics should perform the evolutions of a well-disciplined corps, the moral result has justified the expedient. I confess to have seen the drill-sergeant work miracles.[242]*

> *Where the situation of the asylum affords a commanding view, such as at Charenton, these alleys (ie. covered galleries or verandas) are favourite places of resort, and during summer are frequented not only by the idle saunterer or sentimental gazer, but are crowded with reading-desks and drawing and work tables, and by all those who have wisdom, or are instructed, to associate the pleasures which the beauty of nature affords with the ordinary and obligatory occupations of life.[243]*

Moral treatment in the United States

The Moral Treatment era in America was dominant from approximately 1817 until about 1847, being influenced by the efforts of Samuel Tuke and the programme at the Retreat in York.[244] Evidence of the use of therapeutic occupation in American Mental Hospitals spans the century, though perhaps is more marked during that period. It may well have begun to a limited extent in the previous century under the direction of Philadelphian, Dr Benjamin Rush (1745-1813) who, like Pinel, was inspired by the writings of physician-philosopher, John Locke. Rush is known to have prescribed corn shearing and grinding, and gardening for male patients and churning, sewing, and spinning for female patients.[245]

In view of Tuke's influence, it is not surprising to find that as early as 1813 right up until the 20th century occupation was being used at the Friends Asylum for the Insane, just as it was in the United Kingdom. Dunton, in 1915, reports that Dr Robert H. Chase wrote that:

No feature in the treatment of the insane is more highly valued than occupation, systematically applied and judiciously carried out. Work is a law of our nature which demands expression in the insane no less than in the sane. To understand this one only has to reflect upon the depressing effect of inaction, then turn to the satisfaction and strength that result from the agreeable use of one's mental and physical powers. It may be seen that from the beginning Friends' Asylum made intelligent and continuous effort to give the patients the benefit that comes from employment and rational diversion[246]

In the Chronology which is in the same volume are found many events bearing upon the occupation and diversion of patients, all showing that the hospital authorities were imbued with the idea that occupation was a valuable form of treatment[247]

For example, 'at McLean Hospital: The importance of various forms of diversion, and especially of manual occupation, has been recognised from its (McLean Hospital) very beginning.' (Adolph Meyer found that in 1895 McLean still had some organised recreational activities[248])

In his report for 1822 Dr. Wyman writes, "the amusements provided in the establishment for lunatics, as draughts, chess, backgammon, nine-pins, swinging, sawing wood, gardening, reading, writing, music, etc., divert the attention from unpleasant subjects of thought and afford exercise both of body and mind (and) have a powerful effect in tranquillising the mind, breaking up wrong associations of ideas and inducing correct habits of thinking as well as acting."

Another Superintendent, Dr Bell, in 1839, says that "the experiment of mechanical labour was here first introduced, and the safety, expediency and immense utility of putting tools in the hands of the patients entirely and satisfactorily decided." And again, speaking of occupation as a means of cure, "there is probably no other institution in the world where the value of this has been more fully tested than here". Although later, owing to the class of patients received at McLean, mechanical and agricultural labour was abandoned for "some form of lazy idleness," yet each superintendent has done his share in developing this method of treatment. For the men, since 1834 there has been a carpenter's shop in which woodcarving and cabinet making have been taught; while the women have had lessons in drawing and painting and have done various forms of fancy-work.

In 1836, according to the report for that year, 50 patients worked in the carpenters shop 6 hours a day and made 7,236 candle boxes which were sold ... Later the boxes were not sold, though they continued to be made. In 1836, "100 cords of wood were carted by patients from wharf to house, and 200 cords were sawed, split and piled".[249]

According to medical historian Bockhoven, the Worcester State Hospital in Massachusetts, which opened in 1833, was also important in terms of moral treatment in America, demonstrating 'beyond doubt that recovery was the rule'.[250] An example of the recovery statistics of patients admitted to the Worcester State Hospital between 1833-1852 and used to attract prospective customers is provided as Table 1.11.6.

5 year period	Patients Admitted	Patients Discharged Recovered	Patients Discharged Improved
1833-37	300	211 (70.0%)	39 (8.3%)
1838-42	434	324 (74.6%)	14 (3.2%)
1843-47	742	474 (63.9%)	34 (4.6%)
1848-52	791	485 (61.3%)	37 (4.7%)

Table 1.11.6: **Outcome in patients admitted to Worcester State Hospital who were ill less than one year**
(Data from Annual Reports of the Hospital)[251,252]

Moral treatment was reported as curative by the superintendents of the asylums who ran the programmes, with some hospitals, such as the Hartford Retreat, recording success rates of up to 90%.[253] One of the others was Pennsylvania Hospital for the Insane, a prestigious private institution, which Thomas Story Kirkbride headed for forty years.[254] His annual reports aimed at, amongst others, prospective customers and their families, detailed over fifty occupations available to inmates including light gymnastics, fancy work, magic lantern displays, and lectures. 'Intelligent and educated individuals with courteous manners, and refined feelings' were employed to encourage reading, handiwork and music on the wards to cater to the intellectual and artistic needs of the more cultivated patients.[255]

Moral treatment declined in America, just as it did in Britain despite its reputed success. On both sides of the Atlantic its demise has been linked with overcrowding, as treatment deteriorated into custodial care.[256,257] Peloquin, an American occupational therapist also suggests another factor for the reduction of occupation based programmes, namely that medicine was reconsidering the treatment of insanity in which ideas about occupation did not seem important; the "natural" was overtaken by the "scientific". The success of moral treatment was challenged as exaggeration, and largely disappeared. Peloquin concludes that:

> Moral treatment's decline relates closely to a lack of inspired and committed leadership willing to articulate and redefine the efficacy of occupation in the face of medical and societal challenges. The desire to embrace the most current trend of scientific thought led to the abandonment of moral treatment in spite of its established efficacy. The failure to identify and address the social and institutional changes that had gradually made the practice and success of moral treatment virtually impossible led to the erroneous conclusion that occupation was not an effective intervention.[258]

A closing note about the nineteenth century in the United States must acknowledge that Adolph Meyer gave his first paper there in 1893 to the Chicago Pathological Society. He commented that although one would least expect mention of "occupation" to such an audience, he asked them for suggestions 'as to the tastes and best lines of occupation of American patients', because 'the proper use of time in some helpful and gratifying activity' appeared to him 'a fundamental issue in the treatment of any neuropsychiatric patient'. He found that there was some ward and shop work being carried out at Kankakee and, later, some gardening for women in convalescent cottages, was carried out under the inspiration of Isabel Davenport.

In summary, the age of industry during the nineteenth century saw the dramatic growth of occupational programmes across Britain, Europe and America as one of the central tenets of Moral Treatment. With the establishment of state treatment facilities for the mentally ill, the occupation programmes established were extensive, and apparently more effective than any other regimes before the advent of the medication which is available today. That, in itself, suggests a present day value to augment and extend current programmes which have declined with the closure of institutional care. The century saw the advent of remarkable medical men who pioneered occupational therapy across those formative years and into the twentieth century.

---

[1]Browne WAF. What Asylums Were, Are, and Ought To Be. Being the Substance of Five Lectures Delivered before the Managers of the Montrose Lunatic Asylum. Edinburgh: Adam and Charles Black, 1837; 156.

[2]Tuke S. Description of the Retreat: An Institution near York for Insane Persons of the Society of Friends Containing an Account of its Origin and Progress, the Modes of Treatment, and a Statement of Cases. York: Printed by W Alexander, and sold by him; also sold by M.M. and E Webb, Bristol: and by Harvey, and Co; William Phillips; and W. Darton, London, 1813.

[3]Tuke. Description of the Retreat…; 186.

[4]Tuke. Description of the Retreat…; 156.

[5]Tuke. Description of the Retreat…; 156.

[6]Tuke. Description of the Retreat…; 158-159.

[7]Tuke. Description of the Retreat…; 151.

[8]Tuke. Description of the Retreat…; 183.

[9]Tuke. Description of the Retreat…; 181-182.

[10]Tuke. Description of the Retreat…; 96.

[11]Tuke. Description of the Retreat…; 183-184.

[12]Tuke. Description of the Retreat…; 181.

[13]Tuke. Description of the Retreat…; 152-155.

[14]Tuke. Description of the Retreat.

[15]Pumphrey E. Recollections of the Retreat of 50 years ago. York: Borthwick Institute of Historical Research. Archival material, 1892; 30.

[16]Pumphrey. Recollections of the Retreat…; 22.

[17]Pumphrey. Recollections of the Retreat…; 22.

[18]Pumphrey. Recollections of the Retreat…; 29-30.

[19]Tuke. Description of the Retreat…; 181.

[20]Rules for the Government of Attendants and Servants of the Retreat York with Instructions as to the Management of the Patients etc., 1847. York: John L. Linney, printer, 1847; 24.

[21]Rules for the Government of Attendants…; 17-18.

[22]Rules for the Government of Attendants…; 17-18.

[23]Rules and Instructions. York: Committee of the Retreat, printed by De Little and sons, The City Press, 1897; 10.

[24]Instructions to Members of Nursing Staff. The Retreat, York: 1890; 4.

[25]Instructions to Members of Nursing Staff. The Retreat, York: 1904; 4.

[26]Kitching J. Fifty-Fourth Report of the Friends"Retreat, near York. York: Borthwick Institute of Historical Research, 1850; 17-18.

[27]Kitching. Fifty-Fourth Report…; 17.

[28]Kitching. Fifty-Fourth Report…; 18-19.

[29]Kitching. Fifty-Fifth Report of the Friends'Retreat, near York. York: Borthwick Institute of Historical Research. 1851; 18-19.

[30]Kitching. Fifty-Fifth Report…; 17.

[31]Kitching. Fifty-Fifth Report…; 16.

[32]Kitching. Fifty-Fifth Report…; 16.

[33]Kitching. Fifty-Fifth Report…; 17.

[34]Kitching. Fifty-Fourth Report…; 18.

[35]Kitching. Fifty-Fourth Report…; 18-19.

[36]Kitching. Fifty-Fourth Report…; 17.

[37]Mason J. Report Respecting the Employment of the Men Patients at the Retreat for the Year Ending Sixth Month 1856. York: Borthwick Institute of Historical Research, 1856.

[38]Kitching. Fifty-Fifth Report…; 18-19.

[39]Mason J. Report Respecting the Employment of the Men Patients at the Retreat for the Year Ending Sixth Month 1874. York: Borthwick Institute of Historical Research. 1874.

40Mason J. Report Respecting the Employment of the Men Patients at the Retreat for the Year Ending Sixth Month 1862. York: Borthwick Institute of Historical Research, 1862.

41Mason. Report Respecting the Employment of the Men Patients…; 1874.

42Mason J. Report Respecting the Employment of the Men Patients at the Retreat for the Year Ending Sixth Month 1859. York: Borthwick Institute of Historical Research. 1859.

43Mason. Report Respecting the Employment of the Men Patients…; 1859.

44Mason. Report Respecting the Employment of the Men Patients…; 1862.

45Mason J. Report Respecting the Employment of the Men Patients at the Retreat for the Year Ending Sixth Month. York: Borthwick Institute of Historical Research. 1858.

46Porter R. Mind-Forg'd Manacles. London: The Athlone Press, 1987; 111.

47Watts S. A Walk through Leicester. Leicester: Combe, 1804; 24-25.

48Arnold T. Observations on the Management of the Insane and Particularly on the Agency and Importance of Humane and Kind Treatment in Effecting their Cure. London: Phillips, 1809; 10-13, 55.

49Carpenter PK. Thomas Arnold: A provincial psychiatrist in Georgian England. Medical History 1989, 33: 199-216.

50Porter. Mind-Forg'd Manacles…; 117.

51Scull A, ed. Madhouses, Mad-doctors, and Madmen: The Social History of Psychiatry in the Victorian Era. Philadelphia, PA: University of Pennsylvania Press, 1981; 226-227.

52Tuke S. 1841. In: Russell JI. The Occupational Treatment of Mental Illness. London: Bailliere, Tindall & Cox, 1938; v-vi.

53Ellis Sir WC. A Treatise on the Nature, Symptoms, Causes and Treatment of Insanity, with Practical Observations on Lunatic Asylums and a Description of the Pauper Lunatic Asylum for the County of Middlesex, at Hanwell, with a Detailed Account of its Management. London: Samuel Holdsworth, 1838; Preface, v-vii.

54Ellis. A Treatise on the Nature, Symptoms, Causes and Treatment of Insanity…; 6.

55Ellis. A Treatise on the Nature, Symptoms, Causes and Treatment of Insanity…; 9-10.

56Ellis. A Treatise on the Nature, Symptoms, Causes and Treatment of Insanity…; 8.

57Ellis. A Treatise on the Nature, Symptoms, Causes and Treatment of Insanity…; 311.

58Ellis. A Treatise on the Nature, Symptoms, Causes and Treatment of Insanity…; 190.

59Ellis. A Treatise on the Nature, Symptoms, Causes and Treatment of Insanity…; 307.

60Ellis. A Treatise on the Nature, Symptoms, Causes and Treatment of Insanity…; 191-193.

61Ellis. A Treatise on the Nature, Symptoms, Causes and Treatment of Insanity…; 297.

62Ellis. A Treatise on the Nature, Symptoms, Causes and Treatment of Insanity…; 300-301.

63Ellis. A Treatise on the Nature, Symptoms, Causes and Treatment of Insanity…; 302.

64Ellis. A Treatise on the Nature, Symptoms, Causes and Treatment of Insanity…; 199.

65Ellis. A Treatise on the Nature, Symptoms, Causes and Treatment of Insanity…; 193.

66Ellis. A Treatise on the Nature, Symptoms, Causes and Treatment of Insanity…; 15.

67Ellis. A Treatise on the Nature, Symptoms, Causes and Treatment of Insanity…; 196-197.

68Ellis. A Treatise on the Nature, Symptoms, Causes and Treatment of Insanity…; 198.

69Ellis. A Treatise on the Nature, Symptoms, Causes and Treatment of Insanity…; 308.

70Ellis. A Treatise on the Nature, Symptoms, Causes and Treatment of Insanity…; 311.

71Ellis. A Treatise on the Nature, Symptoms, Causes and Treatment of Insanity…; 305-306.

72Ellis. A Treatise on the Nature, Symptoms, Causes and Treatment of Insanity…; 298.

73'Sir W. C. Ellis on Insanity'. In: Chambers W, Chambers R, eds. Chambers' Edinburgh Journal, Saturday June 8th 1844; no 23: 368.

74Conolly J. Presidential address to the RMPA. Edinburgh. 1858. Cited in: Andrews J, Smith I, eds. Let There be Light Again: A History of the Gartnavel Royal Hospital from its Beginnings to the Present Day. Gartnavel Royal Hospital, 1993; 52.

[75]Conolly J. The Treatment of the Insane without Mechanical Restraint. London: Smith, Elder & Co., 1856.

[76]Macdonald EM. World-Wide Conquests of Disabilities: The History, Development and Present Functions of the Remedial Services. London: Bailliere Tindall, 1981; 87-8.

[77]Macdonald. World-Wide Conquests of Disabilities.

[78]Browne. What Asylums Were, Are, and Ought To Be.

[79]Allderidge P. The Bethlem Royal Hospital: An Illustrated History. The Bethlem and Maudsley NHS Trust, 1995; 10-12.

[80]Russell D. Scenes from Bedlam: A History of Caring for the Mentally Disordered at Bethlem Royal Hospital and The Maudsley. London: Bailliere Tindall & the Royal College of Nursing, 1997; 65.

[81]Madhouses Committee Reports. 1815-16; 36, 92. Bethlem Archives.

[82]Allderidge. The Bethlem Royal Hospital: An Illustrated History...; 10-12.

[83]Sala GA. A visit to the Royal Hospital of Bethlem. In: The Illustrated London News. March 24th 1860; 291.

[84]Sala. A visit to the Royal Hospital of Bethlem....; 291.

[85]Sala. A visit to the Royal Hospital of Bethlem....; 292.

[86]Sala. A visit to the Royal Hospital of Bethlem...; 296.

[87]Sala. A visit to the Royal Hospital of Bethlem...; 296.

[88]Allderidge PH. Pictures at Bethlem. Bethlem Royal Hospital, 1986.

[89]Sala. A visit to the Royal Hospital of Bethlem...; 292.

[90]Russell. Scenes from Bedlam...; 65-66.

[91]Russell. Scenes from Bedlam...; 91-94.

[92]Walton. Cited in: Clear C. Nuns in Nineteenth Century Ireland. Dublin: Gill & Macmillan, 1987; 13.

[93]Scull A, MacKenzie C, Hervey N. The administration of lunacy in Victorian England: Samuel Gaskell (1807-1886). In: Masters of Bedlam: The Transformation of the Mad-Doctoring Trade. Princeton, NJ: Princeton University Press, 1966.

[94]Scull, MacKenzie & Hervey. The administration of lunacy in Victorian England.

[95]Report of the Medical Officers of the Lunatic Asylum for the County of Lancaster. Lancaster: Printed by William Newton, Cheapside, 1847; 9.

[96]Committee of Visitors. Rules for the Government of the Pauper Lunatic Asylum for the County of Lancaster. Lancaster: Printed by W. Newton, 1846; 7-8.

[97]Scull, MacKenzie & Hervey. The administration of lunacy in Victorian England...; 169.

[98]Report of the Medical Officers of the Lunatic Asylum for the County of Lancaster. Lancaster: Printed by William Newton, Cheapside, 1845; 12.

[99]Report of the Medical Officers of the Lunatic Asylum for the County of Lancaster...1845; 6.

[100]Report of the Medical Officers of the Lunatic Asylum for the County of Lancaster...1845; 12.

[101]Report of the Medical Officers of the Lunatic Asylum for the County of Lancaster...1845; 12.

[102]Scull, MacKenzie & Hervey. The administration of Lunacy in Victorian England...; 169.

[103]Report of the Medical Officers of the Lunatic Asylum for the County of Lancaster...; 1848; 6.

[104]Report of the Medical Officers of the Lunatic Asylum for the County of Lancaster...; 1848; 6, 19.

[105]Scull, MacKenzie & Hervey. The administration of Lunacy in Victorian England...; 169.

[106]Report of the Medical Officers of the Lunatic Asylum for the County of Lancaster...; 1847; 5.

[107]Report of the Medical Officers of the Lunatic Asylum for the County of Lancaster…; 1848; 7.

[108]Report of the Medical Officers of the Lunatic Asylum for the County of Lancaster…; 1847; 5.

[109]Report of the Medical Officers of the Lunatic Asylum for the County of Lancaster…; 1845; 11.

[110]Report of the Medical Officers of the Lunatic Asylum for the County of Lancaster…; 1845; 7.

[111]Report of the Medical Officers of the Lunatic Asylum for the County of Lancaster…; 1845; 10.

[112]Report of the Medical Officers of the Lunatic Asylum for the County of Lancaster…; 1845; 13.

[113]Scull, MacKenzie & Hervey. The administration of lunacy in Victorian England…; 173.

[114]Vernon Briggs L. Occupation as a Substitute for Restraint in the Treatment of the Mentally Ill: A History of the Passage of Two Bills Through the Massachusetts Legislature. (1911). New York: Arno Press, 1973.

[115]Scull, MacKenzie & Hervey. The administration of lunacy in Victorian England…; 170.

[116]Bucknill JC. Journal of Mental Science. Cited in: Scull, MacKenzie & Hervey. The administration of lunacy in Victorian England…; 171.

[117]Prichard JC. Cited in: Scull, MacKenzie & Hervey. The administration of lunacy in Victorian England….; 171.

[118]Scull, MacKenzie & Hervey. The administration of lunacy in Victorian England…; 171.

[119]Scull, MacKenzie & Hervey. The administration of lunacy in Victorian England…; 172-173.

[120]Rules and Regulations for the Female Attendants in the County of Lancaster. Manchester: Printed by Johnson and Rawson, 1871; 14-15.

[121]Rules and Regulations for the Female Attendants in the County of Lancaster…; 3.

[122]MacNiven A. The first commissioners: Reform in Scotland in the mid-nineteenth century. Journal of Mental Science 1960, 106(443): 451-471.

[123]Henderson DK. The Evolution of Psychiatry in Scotland. Edinburgh and London: E & S Livingstone Ltd, 1964; 42-43.

[124]MacNiven. The first commissioners…; 451-471.

[125]Henderson. The Evolution of Psychiatry in Scotland…; 89-90.

[126]Henderson. The Evolution of Psychiatry in Scotland…; 92-93.

[127]MacNiven. The first commissioners…; 451-471 (454).

[128]MacNiven. The first commissioners…; 451-471 (458-9).

[129]Scottish Lunacy Commission. Report of The Scottish Lunacy Commission. H.M. Stationary Office, 1857.

[130]Commissioners in Lunacy for Scotland. Annual Report of the General Board of Commissioners in Lunacy for Scotland. H.M. Stationary Office, 1881.

[131]Extract from Report of the Royal Lunacy Commission. 1857. Cited in: Fourteenth Annual Report of the General Board of Control for Scotland for the Year 1927. Edinburgh: His Majesty's Stationery Office, 1928.

[132]MacNiven. The first commissioners…; 451-471. (467).

[133]MacNiven. The first commissioners…; 106, (443): 451-471. (461).

[134]MacNiven. The first commissioners…; 451-471. (463).

[135]Browne WAF. What Asylums Were, Are and Ought to Be. London: Messre A & C Black, 1838.

[136]Browne WAF. What Asylums Ought to Be. Lecture V. In: Scull A, ed. Tavistock Classics in the History of Psychiatry. The Asylum as Utopia. WAF Browne and the Mid-

Nineteenth Century Consolidation of Psychiatry. London and New York: Tavistock/Routledge, 1991; 177.

[137]Presly AS. A Sunnyside Chronicle 1781-1981: A History of Sunnyside Royal Hospital, Produced for its Bi-Centenary. 1981; 43.

[138]Presly. A Sunnyside Chronicle 1781-1981...; 44.

[139]Presly. A Sunnyside Chronicle 1781-1981...; 44.

[140]Groundes-Peace ZC. An outline of the development of occupational therapy in Scotland. The Scottish Journal of Occupational Therapy 1957, 30: 16-39.

[141]Poole R. Memoranda Regarding the Royal Lunatic Asylum of Montrose. Edinburgh: Black, and London: Longmans, 1841.

[142]Poole. Memoranda Regarding the Royal Lunatic Asylum of Montrose.

[143]Groundes-Peace. An outline of the development of occupational therapy in Scotland.

[144]Browne. What Asylums Were, Are, and Ought To Be...; 229-230.

[145]Browne. What Asylums Were, Are, and Ought To Be...; 230-231.

[146]MacNiven. The first commissioners...; 451-471 (465).

[147]Browne. What Asylums Were, Are, and Ought To Be...; 207.

[148]Browne. What Asylums Were, Are, and Ought To Be...; 193-208.

[149]Browne. What Asylums Were, Are, and Ought To Be.

[150]Browne. What Asylums Were, Are, and Ought To Be...; 181.

[151]Browne. What Asylums Were, Are, and Ought To Be...; 93-94.

[152]Browne. What Asylums Were, Are, and Ought To Be...; 209.

[153]MacNiven. The first commissioners...; 451-471 (465).

[154]Browne. What Asylums Were, Are, and Ought To Be...; 94.

[155]Browne. What Asylums Were, Are, and Ought To Be...; 95.

[156]Henderson D. Life and work. Scottish Journal of Occupational Therapy 1957, 30: 7-10.

[157]Browne. What Asylums Were, Are, and Ought To Be...; 95.

[158]Browne. What Asylums Were, Are, and Ought To Be...; 95.

[159]Browne. What Asylums Were, Are, and Ought To Be...; 95-96.

[160]Browne. What Asylums Were, Are, and Ought To Be...; 92.

[161]Browne. What Asylums Were, Are, and Ought To Be...; 96.

[162]Williams M. History of Crichton Royal Hospital 1839-1989. Dumfries and Galloway Health Board, 1989; 19.

[163]The Crichton Institution for Lunatics, Dumfries. In: The Shipping and Mercantile Gazette. June 1839.

[164]The Crichton Institution for Lunatics.

[165]Easterbrook CC. The Chronicle of the Crichton Royal. Dumfries: Courier Press, 1940.

[166]Williams. History of Crichton Royal Hospital 1839-1989...; 25.

[167]Williams. History of Crichton Royal Hospital 1839-1989...; 22.

[168]Williams. History of Crichton Royal Hospital 1839-1989...; 23.

[169]Williams. History of Crichton Royal Hospital 1839-1989...; 22.

[170]Browne WAF. Annual Reports. Crichton Royal Mental Hospital, Dumfries, 1843, 1844 , 1847.

[171]Easterbrook. The Chronical of the Crichton Royal.

[172]Scottish Lunacy Commission. H.M. Stationary Office, 1857.

[173]Williams. History of Crichton Royal Hospital 1839-1989...; 53.

[174]Williams. History of Crichton Royal Hospital 1839-1989...; 37.

[175]Easterbrook. The Chronical of the Crichton Royal.

[176]Williams. History of Crichton Royal Hospital 1839-1989...; 37.

[177]Williams. History of Crichton Royal Hospital 1839-1989...; 56-57.

[178]Annual Report of the Crichton Royal Mental Hospital. Dumfries: 1887.

[179]Groundes-Peace. An outline of the development of occupational therapy in Scotland.

[180]Annual Report of the Crichton Royal Mental Hospital. Dumfries: 1887.

[181]Annual Report of the Crichton Royal Mental Hospital. Dumfries: 1895.

[182]Williams. History of Crichton Royal Hospital 1839-1989...; 53.

[183]Presly. A Sunnyside Chronicle 1781-1981...; 42.

[184]Presly. A Sunnyside Chronicle 1781-1981...; 42.

[185]Presly. A Sunnyside Chronicle 1781-1981...; 45-47.

[186]Henderson DK. Occupational therapy. Journal of Mental Science, 1925.

[187]Henderson DK. Report of the Physician Superintendent for the year 1923. In: The One Hundredth and Ninth Annual Report of the Glasgow Royal Asylum for the Year 1923. Glasgow: James Hedderwick & Sons Ltd., 1924.

[188]Groundes-Peace. An outline of the development of occupational therapy in Scotland.

[189]Andrews J, Smith I, eds. Let there be Light Again. A History of the Gartnavel Royal Hospital from its Beginning to the Present Day. Glasgow: Gartnavel Hospital, 1993; 56.

[190]Andrews & Smith. Let there be Light Again...; 56.

[191]Andrews & Smith. Let there be Light Again...; 56-57.

[192]Groundes-Peace. An outline of the development of occupational therapy in Scotland.

[193]Extract from the annual report of the Glasgow Royal Asylum for the year 1839. Cited in: Henderson. Report of the Physician Superintendent for the year 1923.

[194]Groundes-Peace. An outline of the development of occupational therapy in Scotland.

[195]Andrews & Smith. Let there be Light Again...; 56-59.

[196]Andrews & Smith. Let there be Light Again...; 58.

[197]Unknown Author. The Philosophy of Insanity. With introduction by Frieda Fromm-Reichmann, M.D. London and New York: The Fireside Press, 1947.

[198]Unknown. The Philosophy of Insanity...; 72-73.

[199]Unknown. The Philosophy of Insanity...; 70.

[200]Unknown. The Philosophy of Insanity...; 70.

[201]Unknown. The Philosophy of Insanity...; 70.

[202]Unknown. The Philosophy of Insanity...; 72.

[203]Unknown. The Philosophy of Insanity...; 71-72.

[204]Tuke S. Introduction. In: Maximilian J. Construction and Management of Hospitals for the Insane. (trans. by John Kitching) London: J. Churchill, 1841.

[205]MacNiven. The first commissioners.

[206]Begg RSM. A Short History of Royal Cornhill Hospital. Typed copy of articles originally in: Cornhill Courier. 15th March, 29th March, 12th April, 1966.

[207]Annual Report. Murray's Royal Asylum, Perth. 1835.

[208]Groundes-Peace. An outline of the development of occupational therapy in Scotland.

[209]Annual Report. Murray's Royal Asylum, Perth. 1859.

[210]Marr HC. Journal of Mental Science. July, 1899.

[211]Groundes-Peace. An outline of the development of occupational therapy in Scotland.

[212]Annual Report. Edinburgh Royal Mental Hospital. Edinburgh, 1840.

[213]Commissioners in Lunacy for Scotland. Annual Report of the General Board of Commissioners in Lunacy for Scotland. H.M. Stationary Office, 1857.

[214]Annual Report. Edinburgh Royal Mental Hospital. Edinburgh, 1885.

[215]Commissioners in Lunacy for Scotland. Annual Report of the General Board of Commissioners in Lunacy for Scotland. H.M. Stationary Office, 1863.

[216] Groundes-Peace. An outline of the development of occupational therapy in Scotland...; 22.

[217]Henderson. The Evolution of Psychiatry in Scotland...; 95.

[218]Clear. Nuns in Nineteenth Century Ireland...; 11.

[219]Reuber M. State and Private Lunatic Asylums in Ireland: Medics, Fools and Maniacs (1600-1900). Cologne, Germany: MD Thesis, 1994; 187.

[220]Clear. Nuns in Nineteenth Century Ireland…; 14, 29.

[221]Macdonald. World-Wide Conquests of Disabilities…; 91.

[222]Halloran WS. An Enquiry into the Causes Producing the Extraordinary Addition to the Numbers of the Insane Together with Extended Observations on the Cure of Insanity. Dublin: 1810, 1818; 50, 170-172.

[223]Macdonald. World-Wide Conquests of Disabilities.

[224]Reuber M. State and Private Lunatic Asylums in Ireland…; 69, 73.

[225]22nd Report of Inspector General, 1844, HC 1844 (567) xxx. 69. In: Reuber. State and Private Lunatic Asylums in Ireland…; 91.

[226]Reuber. State and Private Lunatic Asylums in Ireland…; 113.

[227]Reuber. State and Private Lunatic Asylums in Ireland…. 73.

[228]Bucknill JC, ed. Report of the Commission on the Irish District Lunatic Asylums. The Asylum Journal of Mental Science, Vol. II. London: Longman, Brown, Green and Longman, 1855-1856; 393-404.

[229]Reuber. State and Private Lunatic Asylums in Ireland…; 113.

[230]Reuber. State and Private Lunatic Asylums in Ireland…; 179.

[231]Hitch S. Letter to the Times. September 1842. Cited in: Clwyd W. The North Wales Hospital, Denbigh, 1842-1955. Denbigh: Gee & Son, 1995; 13-14.

[232]Clwyd. The North Wales Hospital, Denbigh, 1842-1955…; 14-16.

[233]Clwyd. The North Wales Hospital, Denbigh, 1842-1955…; 16-17.

[234]Clwyd. The North Wales Hospital, Denbigh, 1842-1955…; 77.

[235]Clwyd. The North Wales Hospital, Denbigh, 1842-1955…; 17-21.

[236]Report: British Medico-Psychological Association. Annual meeting in York. The Yorkshire Herald, Friday 22, 1892.

[237]Macdonald. World-Wide Conquests of Disabilities.

[238]Browne. What Asylums Were, Are, and Ought To Be…; 193, 218, 220.

[239]Macdonald. World-Wide Conquests of Disabilities.

[240]London Medical Gazette, May 23, 1835; 288.

[241]Browne. What asylums ought to be. In: Scull Tavistock Classics in the History of Psychiatry…; 219.

[242]Browne. What Asylums Were, Are, and Ought To Be.

[243]Browne. What asylums ought to be. In: Scull. Tavistock Classics in the History of Psychiatry…; 192.

[244]Corsini RJ, ed. Encyclopedia of Psychology, Vol. 2. NewYork: JohnWiley & Sons, 1984; 162.

[245]Macdonald. World-Wide Conquests of Disabilities.

[246]Dunton WR. Occupational Therapy: A Manual for Nurses. Philadelphia and London: W.B. Saunders Company, 1915; 14.

[247]Dunton. Occupational Therapy…; 15.

[248]Meyer A. The philosophy of occupational therapy. Archives of Occupational Therapy 1922; 1: 1-10.

[249]Dunton. Occupational Therapy…; 12-13.

[250]Bockoven JS. Moral Treatment in Community Mental Health. New York: Springer Publishing Company, Inc. 1972; 14.

[251]Bockoven. Moral Treatment in Community Mental Health…; 14.

[252]Wilcock AA. An Occupational Perspective of Health. Thorofare, NJ: Slack Inc., 1998; 170.

[253]Peloquin SM. Moral treatment: Contexts considered. American Journal of Occupational Therapy. 1989, 43(8), 537-544.

[254]Tomes NJ. A generous confidence: Thomas Story Kirkebride's philosophy of asylum

construction and management. In: Scull A, ed. Madhouses, Mad-doctors and Madmen. See: Kirkebride TS. On the Construction, Organisation and General Arrangements of Hospitals for the Insane. Philadelphia: Lindsay and Blakiston, 1854.

[255]Kirkebride TS. Annual report of the Pennsylvania Hospital for the Insane. 1845; 38, 1846; 24-25, 1858; 22-32, and 1869; 26. Cited in Tomes NJ. A generous confidence.

[256]Bockoven. Moral Treatment in Community Mental Health.

[257]Peloquin. Moral treatment: Contexts considered.

[258]Peloquin. Moral treatment: Contexts considered.

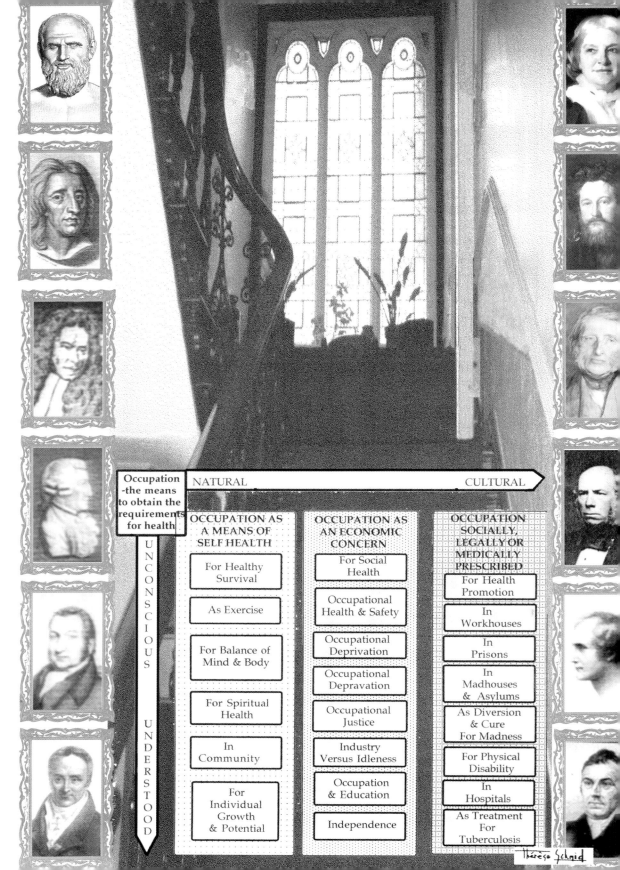

Occupation -the means to obtain the requirements for health

NATURAL — CULTURAL

UNCONSCIOUS — UNDERSTOOD

OCCUPATION AS A MEANS OF SELF HEALTH	OCCUPATION AS AN ECONOMIC CONCERN	OCCUPATION SOCIALLY, LEGALLY OR MEDICALLY PRESCRIBED
For Healthy Survival	For Social Health	For Health Promotion
As Exercise	Occupational Health & Safety	In Workhouses
For Balance of Mind & Body	Occupational Deprivation	In Prisons
For Spiritual Health	Occupational Depravation	In Madhouses & Asylums
In Community	Occupational Justice	As Diversion & Cure For Madness
For Individual Growth & Potential	Industry Versus Idleness	For Physical Disability
	Occupation & Education	In Hospitals
	Independence	As Treatment For Tuberculosis

Thérèse Schmid

Chapter 12

Towards a Profession of Occupational Therapy

Contents

In this chapter the threads of the history of occupational regimes for health up to the twentieth century will be woven together, whilst exploring the particular aspects of occupation's use in the past that the profession of occupational therapy has drawn upon. It is important to consider the total picture such interweaving provides as this will furnish a platform to consider twentieth century directions from a more holistic point of view. This may enable better recognition of the part played by changing socio-cultural contexts, by spiritual beliefs and philosophical mores, by changing technologies, and by advances in medical knowledge, and help clarify what part these and an understanding of the biological effects of occupation play on health. To bring together such a picture of the past, the essence and direction of occupational regimes will be drawn from the text and analysed afresh in comparative terms.

In order to address the issues in a concise yet useful way the chapter will be divided into the three main groupings used in the conceptual map at the start of the chapter. It will then be further subdivided according to major issues, which will include some reference to all the aspects within it. The conceptual map begins the process of grouping the many components of the relationship between occupation and health that emerged during the history. Although not shown in it, because of complexity, some of the concepts cross all groupings in one form or other according to evolving cultural values. As well, and for similar reasons, some modern terms such as "occupational utopias", have not been included in the map whilst others like a "occupational justice" have. Additionally, in that map no particular occupations have been included and some have been so important in the past that they will be referred to again in the chapter. The chapter will briefly consider links to the twentieth century as a way forward to the second volume of the history, as well as some thoughts about the future.

Occupation as a primary mechanism for health

The first concept that needs to be recognised is that occupation is the in-built mechanism that enables humans, and other animals, to obtain the requirements for living, for survival, and for health. That fundamental truth is the essence of occupational therapists' claim that what people do can influence physical, mental, social and spiritual health. It is such a basic mechanism that it has failed to be fully understood for much of human existence and, for much of the time, has been neglected as an important entity by those concerned with human health.

Despite that, in many respects it has been recognised and acted upon, in part almost unconsciously. That accounts for its appearance throughout the centuries in various guises according to the socio-politico-cultural milieu and beliefs, and the extent of medical knowledge. It accounts for the need to supplement the daily occupations of life followed by Greek citizens, when they handed over to their slaves those that were concerned with physiological functioning because they thought them degrading and "less than human". They invented multi-occupational gymnasia to provide physical and mental balance, which they perceived to be essential to health and beauty. Those replaced many of the benefits lost by not engaging in a wide range of everyday occupations.

Occupation as a means to self health

Health has been described as the 'well working of the organism as a whole'. Kass, who defined it that way, added that it is:

> ... a natural standard or norm - not a moral norm, not a value as opposed to a fact, not an obligation, but a state of being that reveals itself in activity as a standard of bodily exercise or fitness, relative to each species and to some extent to individuals, recognizable if not definable and to some extent attainable.[1]

Kass's association of activity with health as a state of being anticipates the idea of people as occupational beings which has provided the impetus for the development of occupational science as a foundation science for the practice of occupational therapy. Occupational science is the rigorous study of people's occupational nature and needs, science being used in the original sense of "knowledge". The science is in line with the profession's initial objectives described by its American founders, which called for 'the study of the effect of occupation upon the human being; and the scientific dispensation of this knowledge' as well as 'the advancement of occupation as a therapeutic measure'.[2]

In terms of self health, whilst many would lay this as the foundation stone of medicine, it can also be recognised as the foundation stone of occupational therapy, and it can be argued that the latter led to the former. Whether one takes an evolutionary or a biblical view of the origins of human life, occupation played an important role in individuals maintaining their own health. It was through their physical toil and rest, mental planning and creativity, social organisation and spiritual fulfilment that early humans maintained or enhanced 'the well working of the organism as a whole'. They naturally engaged in health promoting, illness preventing occupations. Before the advent of physick, blood-lettings, prescriptions, or specific health advisers, people instinctively did whatever made them feel better as well as seeking out substances which appeared to relieve a health problem. The natural engagement through extensive and varied use of their capacities, and the seeking out or the preparation, once found, would have been therapeutic in themselves. These processes and their effects can be conceived as the original forms of self health occupational therapy. It is the taking of the substances sought that are the original forms of self health medicine. With that clearly in mind, it is possible to understand that the notion and practice of self health has been present throughout time. In many cases early humans would have turned to rest and sleep occupations in the initial phases of whatever ailed them, before gradually taking up occupations which were necessary, possible, or made them stronger or feel improved.

Naturally, early humans lived together in small communities which provided protection and succour to them and in which the health of the group was deemed to be at least as important as individual survival. Community health is still fundamental to everyone's health. Yet life became so different between natural and industrial periods that it is often difficult to appreciate how socio-politico-cultural actions can alter community experience so much that individual and community health is at risk because of change within daily occupations. The changes to what and how people engaged in occupations and the environmental developments which support or create those changes have gradually alienated people 'from the most fundamental truth of our nature, our spiritual oneness with the living universe', and our dependence on maintaining its physical health, as well as our own.[3]

Some societies still living a more natural lifestyle, such as some groups of Australian aboriginals, continue to place value on kin and community to the extent that the Australian Aboriginal Health Organisation defined health as 'the social, emotional, spiritual and cultural well-being of the whole community'. They recommend that 'health services should strive to achieve that state where every individual can achieve their full potential as human beings and thus bring about total well-being of their community as a whole'.[4]

For thousands of years, self health mixed with familial and community care was the most used form of therapy. It appeared common sense, became part of folklore, and following the advent of writing, then printing, became the basis of rules of health–the *Regimen Sanitatis*–which were transmitted across the centuries. Within those rules of health occupation, in the form of both activity and rest, was mainly recognised for its potential as exercise, although how it interwove with other aspects of daily life, like food, environment and mood, were also considered.

The exercise benefit of occupation, perhaps the easiest of the health benefits to recognise, became an important basis for Classical medicine. It was initially formulated during Greco-Roman dominance of the Western World before later being incorporated into the *Regimen Sanitatis*. Despite providing the origins of modern Western democracy, philosophy, architecture, science, arts and medicine, people in the Classical world had very different ways of thinking and behaving to today. For example, they were Empire builders who, despite their advanced idea of "the individual", did not hesitate to slaughter all men in a conquered territory. For this sort of ethic to be widely held, and to be successful, it becomes obvious why they gloried in "the physical". It is this latter notion of physical perfection, which ties in with the strongly held views about exercise, that was implemented in the structure of their societies, what they learned, what occupations they valued and encouraged, and how they wrote about and envisaged health. As the great Galen, Burton explained in *Anatomy of Melancholy*, they preferred 'Exercise before all Physicke, Rectification of diet, or any regiment in what kinde soever; 'tis Natures Physician'.[5] Similarly Rhazes (c. 850-925), the renowned Arabian physician, held that 'there can be no better cure than continual business … neither can health be preserved without bodily exercise'.[6]

The Classical view of health which remains the accepted starting place of modern medicine gradually grew out of religious medicine, old peasant taboos, magic and common-sense health care. It provided health rules about such things as urination and cleanliness; rising early; drinking wine mixed with water; extolling industry, justice, and moral behavior, and from the voice of the gods proclaimed work rather than idleness. Hippocrates, known as the father of modern medicine, understood much of the place of "natural" occupation, such as labour, intellectual and recreational pursuits mainly in exercise terms, and like present day occupational therapists recommended particular occupations for particular purposes.

Those ideas survived well past the advent of humanism and the classical revolution of the Renaissance. At that time exponents of "occupation as exercise" again resorted to the idea of gymnasia and physical activities to maintain health, and prevent and remediate illness. In terms of everyday life, Cheyne, the great self health writer of the Enlightenment, was still espousing much the same message as Hippocrates and Galen, with regard to the relationship between people's occupation and their physiological health. He considered, as Dunton did at the beginning of the twentieth century when promoting the profession, that occupation is 'almost as necessary to health and long life, as food itself'.[7] In that spirit of natural health through the exercise of capacities, he equated occupational balance in terms of energy and restfulness rather than work, rest and leisure as is so often espoused in the modern day.

The notion of physical perfection and mind/body balance as it was sought in the gymnasia gave way to notions of spiritual perfection as church and monastic power gained ground during the Middle Ages. Even the rules of health, which remained the basis of medical practice and self health, were subjugated to fit the spiritual values of those days. self health of a spiritual kind embraced notions of labour being necessary for a healthy soul, which was essential for a healthy body and mind. Such a view was particularly useful at a time when medicine had no sophisticated tools to aid recovery from most illnesses. That is particularly so when it is remembered that spirit, mind and body influence each other and so may have appeared effective, in comparison to other interventions, in maintaining physical and mental health. Because disease was often attributed to sin, people needed to engage in "right or wrong" occupations according to the Christian creed.

Labour and commitment, by nature rather than design at that time, called for body and mind being exercised and capacities kept honed and healthy. Labour of a physical nature such as agricultural and household occupations fulfilled spiritual requirements of the church and, by default, physical and mental health requirements also. Prayer, pilgrimages, crusades, and charitable good works contributed further to the well-being of the soul. Despite the overwhelming belief that the divine was above the temporal and that healing was subject to ecclesiastical regulation,[8] some medieval physicians, like Hildegard of Bingen, still prescribed occupation as exercise.

In the nineteenth century there was a resurgence of interest in all things medieval, and particularly in the craft traditions of the time. Ruskin and Morris, leaders of the Arts and Crafts Movement and the Pre-Raphaelites, attributed more to that time and those traditions than design, colour, form, and attractiveness. They recognised the potential of the occupational milieu of the period to meet the needs of people's individual nature through the physical, mental, and spiritual demands of their creative means of employment.

In the tradition of earlier British intellectual idealists, Ruskin and Morris used their own "creative natures" to fight against capitalism, economic expansion and urban industrialisation by revisiting a 'medieval social order close to nature'.[9] In Ruskin's view, the division of labour and that between thinkers and doers, and the regimentation of industry was morally and socially wrong and he sought to spread enthusiasm for manual labour. Morris's vision was shaped by Ruskin, both arguing for social reform against the boredom and monotony of the industrial system, and the dehumanisation of factory workers.

It will be recalled that Morris, in explaining his views regarding the value of all work, articulated an occupational theory of social health that holds value today. It is important enough to the understanding of the place of occupation in self health to reiterate what he said:

> It is assumed by most people nowadays that all work is useful, and by most well-to-do people that all work is desirable … (They) cheer on the happy worker with congratulations and praises, if he is only "industrious" enough and deprives himself of all pleasure and holidays in the sacred cause of labour …
>
> … it is of the nature of man, when he is not diseased, to take pleasure in his work under certain conditions. And, yet, we must say in the teeth of the hypocritical praise of all labour, whatsoever it may be, … that there is some labour which is so far from being a blessing that it is a curse; that it would be better for the community and for the worker if the latter were to fold his hands and refuse to work, and either die or let us pack him off to the work-house or prison—which you will.[10]

The discussion of how Ruskin and Morris's Arts and Crafts Movement influenced the genesis of occupational therapy in America is recalled. However, its place in British occupational therapy has been largely overlooked, perhaps because of the regrets many have held over recent years about the identification of the profession with craft work. But in neglecting that important heritage, the self health needs that can be met through manual and creative work have also been devalued, as well as the social activist connection which suggests a socio-political direction in the future. Those concerns about one important aspect of people's occupational nature lead to the next major theme, in which ideas about occupation lost much of their association with individual or societal health and economic concerns became dominant.

Occupation as an economic concern

As time went on, occupation became viewed as a largely economic phenomenon, which remains the case today. It was no longer based on the natural needs of individuals and communities, but was more and more driven by materialism and sophisticated political agendas, at least from the time of the establishment of city states some ten thousand years ago. As materialism and acquisitiveness began to override simpler satisfactions concerned with meeting personal needs, social status and class distinctions divided occupational opportunities arbitrarily, and so reduced the health giving effects of an occupationally balanced lifestyle. The situation lead, in many instances, to occupationally unjust situations in which people were occupationally deprived, exploited, or alienated by being unable to meet their own occupational potential through developing personal capacities. Occupational injustice was often experienced by the poor who were frequently expected to labour excessively in mundane, boring, and environmentally hazardous environments, or alternatively unable to find employment and meet the other requirements for health. Alternatively many people sought solace in occupations thought to be of a depraved nature according to the values of whatever period it was. The well-to-do could also experience the ill health effects of unbalanced occupation, when they, through societal expectations, were expected to lead pleasure seeking lives which may or may not meet their occupational nature or needs despite appearing to be largely self chosen. All those scenarios had, and have, the potential to be a major predisposing cause of ill health.

The monastic period had provided a health service, which was available to the poor as well as the affluent. Based on spiritual, charitable, industrious and hospitable lines, its demise at the time of dissolution effectively terminated public health services, which were not replaced by alternative provision. In fact, the numbers of the poor, unemployed and occupationally deprived rose sharply as disenfranchised clerics joined their ranks. That situation obviously caused major social ill health, which became apparent quite quickly. Calls from the public demanded action to reduce the numbers of occupationally deprived and depraved. So a hospital aimed solely at occupational illness was established along with four others which assisted unwanted children and the physically and mentally sick. The Renaissance, therefore, saw Royal Charters establishing five hospitals in London. Of that small number, one was to remediate social and occupation illness by occupational means.

Whilst the term hospital was used in a broader sense then that in the present time, the recognition of the need to remediate "occupational sickness" in the time of Edward VI, is a significant milestone. The employment of Art-Masters to develop and to restore skills was a fascinating scenario, even if done, principally for economic purposes. It was probably not until the First World War, in the twentieth century, that anything similar occurred outside the field of mental health. The Reconstructive workshops which then emerged, despite a curative intent following physical or mental trauma, still had an economic purpose - to restore people to a state in which they were able to meet their own economic requirements.

Throughout an extended period, particularly from the time of Renaissance, industriousness appears to have been valued for its own sake, only tailing off in the latter part of the twentieth century. Carlyle's conjecture that 'even in the meanest sorts of Labour, the whole soul of a man is composed into a kind of real harmony, the instant he sets himself to work!' provides some indication of the almost religious fervour that was given to that social more.[11] The Reverend John Guy in 1993 looked back to the nineteenth century and remarked that 'except for God the most popular word in the Victorian vocabulary must have been work'.[12] Despite Morris, amongst others, commenting unfavourably on that view, some aspects of it still carry over in today's clime and certainly remained strong at the period during which occupational therapy was established. There can be little doubt that it was an underlying notion in foundation philosophies of the profession.

Figure 1.12.1: **Occupation driven by materialism and political economy, and the social initiatives that followed the dissolution of the monasteries**

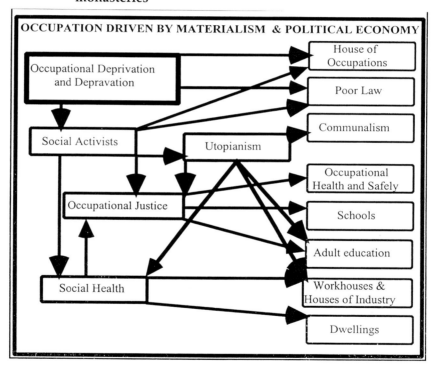

Other initiatives which were set up to remediate social ill health followed over the next centuries inspired, in many cases, by social activists with a vision of how things ought to be. One of the directions they took to demonstrate the possibility of a world in which there was a more egalitarian ethos and in which health, happiness and well-being flourished, was to write about or try to develop their Utopia–their ideal society. Utopianism was evident long before Sir

Thomas More coined Utopia as the name for his ideal state. As Hardy and Davidson recognise in their introduction to papers given at a 1988 international conference on Utopian thought and communal experience held in New Lanark, Scotland, 'the idea of contemplating the perfect society and of seeking to create it in practice has roots that run deep in human history'.[13] It was manifest in stories of the Golden Ages long past in which people were said to be naturally, healthy and happy.[14] At that conference Kumar argued that 'all social theory is utopian', that 'there is nothing wrong or unusual in theories and concepts possessing these ideal qualities', because whilst a theory is a one sided 'exaggeration of certain features of individuals and social life' that is also its value. 'For each new theory is a new way of seeing ourselves.'[15] For occupational therapists, seeing the profession in a new light adds new dimensions to what is or can be offered to individuals or communities who could benefit from an occupational view or intervention towards health. Trying to view the world through utopian spectacles of an occupation for health perspective would provide clues about what an occupationally healthy world would be like.

Utopians in this history have provided examples of how they addressed the occupational nature of people including their social, mental and physical health needs through the realisation of aspirations. Plato and Socrates are examples. They outlined their ideal societies in *Republic* and in *Timaeous* and an example of their occupational bias is their championing of gymnastics from infancy throughout life. That was based on a belief that demanding physical occupation provided for the harmonious and proportional development of the intellect, spirit and body.[16]

More's picture of Utopia, which was discussed in an earlier chapter, clearly illustrated the place of occupation in a healthy and just communal society. Whilst there are some aspects of his vision which tell of problems specific to his times, there are pointers to the sorts of communities that the World Health Organisation of the present time also recommend, if we are to achieve a healthy world and reduce unnecessary illness caused by occupational imbalance due to the excesses of affluent societies on the one hand and deprived societies on the other. More envisioned that a free, simple, and natural way of life in which people engaged in occupations that benefited both themselves and the community. Only necessary work was obligatory, as his Utopia provided no place for the accumulation of wealth and its unnecessary trappings or the 'vain and superfluous' occupations they generated.[17,18]

A whole group of practical utopians and social activists, who played an important part in the life of Britain, and in this story, are central characters in the chapter about occupation and social health in the 19th century. As lines of thought and action can be traced from them to twentieth century occupational therapy, and because some of the connections have recently resurfaced, that story will be briefly revisited.

Robert Owen is the first to be considered. As well as the "father of British Socialism", he is described as a utopian socialist, along with Saint-Simon, and Fourier who are all associated with pre-Marxist socialism and from whom the latter is thought to have had its origins.[19] A network of contacts such as business links to Bentham, friendship links with Southwood Smith, or leadership in the development of Owenite communities, and so through James and Carolyn Hill to their daughter, Octavia, and thence to Elizabeth Casson, permits us to trace Owen's influence to them and thence to occupational therapy's philosophical underpinnings.

As part of his practical reforms, Owen addressed many occupational health issues of the time, particularly occupational alienation and imbalance, which was a fact of life for the vast majority. Some of his views were evident in his address to the inhabitants of New Lanark on the occasion of the official opening of the Institute for the Formation of Character in 1816. We have read how Owen explained his plan for 'a society in which individuals shall acquire increased health, strength and intelligence'–because their labour was always 'advantageously directed' and enjoyable.[20] He advocated that it was, without exception, 'in the highest interest of all the human race' that everyone should be enabled to develop his or her potential according to the physical and mental strength and capacity of the individual.[21]. Not content with proposing the idea, Owen augmented his plan with educational programmes that addressed his workers' previous occupational deprivation and encouraged their talents and potential.

Thomas Southwood Smith, Owen's friend, was Utopian in a different way. Instead of establishing a commercial venture that provided the opportunity to establish a community along his own lines of thought, he sought to change the lot of disadvantaged people generally. To do that he became involved in issues of social and occupational reform that caused him particular concern, and he did so in a creative and effective manner. He not only investigated as part of National programmes aimed at reform, but stirred up sympathy for those vexed issues by making use of the skills and appeal of a popular writer–Charles Dickens, and an artist–Margaret Gillies. Their skills and appeal enabled him to enlist public sympathy towards the causes of public and occupational ill health that he sought to improve.

His daughter, Carolyn, and her husband, James Hill, together established an Owenite community. Carolyn, not surprisingly, maintained her own utopian views with a strong occupational flavour. She, too, recognised the need for individuals to develop their unique capacities whilst also understanding that differences between them were more a matter of degree than deficiency. Being a Pestalozzian teacher, she suggested that improvement could be made through education.[22] That calls to mind the closeness of fit between occupational therapy and education in general, as developing individual's occupational potential is germane to both. It suggests that a closer relationship between the two might be beneficial in more than such things as adaptations for handicapped students, or programmes for children with writing disorders. Making the links clear between occupation and health to students of all age groups through class contact, special texts for use in schools, media or "net" programmes would be ways to increase population awareness.

The Hills' daughter, Octavia, would not have thought to describe herself as a utopian despite seeking to improve aspects of the existing community which did not fit with her view of fairness and the ideal world of her dreams. Her upbringing, following her early formative years mainly spent with her mother and her grandfather, must have been steeped in the philosophies of Owenism and the need to be in the vanguard of social reform to improve the lot of the poor. Indeed, social reform was the staple of family conversation. Her subsequent views were reinforced by her contact with Maurice and conversion to Christian Socialism.[23] That she was influenced by Owen's ideas is evident as, following his initiative, she bought bulk supplies and organised a cooperative store so that her tenants could buy more cheaply. Similar too was the way she provided facilities for community occupations, social interaction, and skill development which was also evident in Elizabeth Casson's psychiatric clinic and occupational therapy school of the next century. Another idea of Hill's appears to anticipate those of twentieth century occupational therapy. This was her determination to rouse habits of industry and effort in her tenants, so that they might become independent of her except as a "friend and leader".[24]

The network of social activists that culminated, in this history, with Casson, also included Hill's close association with Ruskin and the Arts and Crafts Movement ideology. His financial support for her housing schemes and friendship for at least two decades cannot fail to have influenced her ideas. It must be recalled that the Arts and Crafts Movement, as well as trying to improve the visual environment, was aimed at improving the occupational experiences of the masses by overcoming the mental, physical and social ill health caused by the soul destroying employment of the industrial revolution. Hill's other major interest, of preserving the natural environment so that it was available for people to enjoy and refresh themselves, in her own hard times as well as the future, is heartening to those occupational therapists who link practice with ecological models of health. That is surely an important way forward in the twenty-first century when we are called upon to handle the occupational challenges of the information technology revolution.

Since the connections have been made during the process of data gathering for this history, new networks have been established between the British College of Occupational Therapists, Robert Owen's New Lanark and the Octavia Hill Society. In the latter, Elizabeth Casson now features on a mural depicting Octavia Hill's works in her birthplace Musem at Wisbech. The organisation has also provided a seminar on her work for the retired members group, and taken them to view the site of Redcross Hall, Cottages, and "occupational" Garden where Casson worked near the College headquarters in Southwark.

That network of social activists and political reformers link occupational therapy back to a range of associated ideologies which were powerful in their own time, and have had far reaching effects into the present. They include utopian communalism, historical materialism, occupational health and safety reform, education, socialism, Christian socialism, and the Arts and Craft, Settlement, and Open Space Movements, as depicted in figure 1.12.2.

Figure 1.12.2: Occupational therapy and associated ideologies from the 19th century

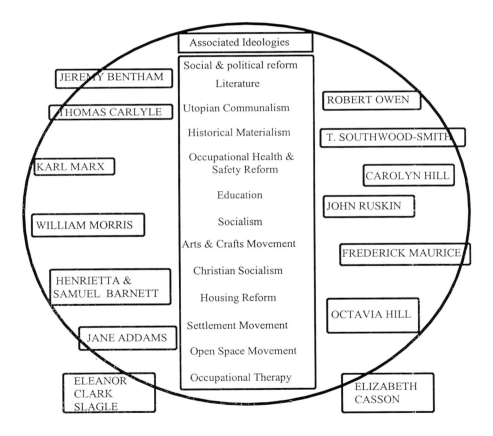

Occupational health

Southwood Smith's major contribution to occupational health issues preceding the twentieth century recalls the long history of interest in the ill health effects of paid work for many people. As paid employment has been the principal means of gaining the other requirements of health, as well as being a major contributor itself, it has always assumed a central place in the occupation and health debate, at least since the time of Hippocrates, and then through Galen, to Ramazzini, Thackrah, and Southwood Smith amongst others. Interest has tended to centre on the detrimental effects of occupation, reflecting medicine's major interest in illness rather than wellness. This, it can be argued, has focussed much of that profession's attention away from the positive attributes of occupation, which has always been the major focus of occupational therapists.

It would be useful for the medical profession to appreciate better the positive aspects of occupation's potential contribution to the prevention and cure of illness, and the promotion of health. On the other side of that same coin, if occupation remains or regains its central place within occupational therapy, a greater understanding by occupational therapists of the potentially negative effects of occupation on health is just as important as understanding the positive effects. In the twentieth century, the impact of paid work was and is the subject of major health intervention as in occupational health and safety legislation, but many other professions take the leading roles, and surprisingly, occupational therapists have less to do with that than other forms of occupation. In a similar surprising scenario, they have little to do with the development of recreational or sporting opportunities for the disabled in the community, although this seems to fit the central premise of the profession, that of using the media of occupation to create, return, or enable people to a state of health or well-being.

The paucity of interest in main stream aspects of occupation for health in recent times perhaps might be blamed, somewhat, for the lack of general understanding of occupation encompassing the range of human doings. The arbitrary division of occupation into separate components such as employment, recreation, home duties, play, education, sport, exercise, rest and relaxation, and even activities of daily living with its many different levels of meaning, has impeded the development of an understanding within health care, medicine, and socio-politically that it is the total combination of physical, mental, social and spiritual doing, the obligatory and the self-chosen, which provides the basis for the health or ill health consequences of occupation in everyday lives. Whilst some parts of those might be more responsible than others for particular effects, it is understanding the holistic picture which provides the foundation for understanding the centrality of occupation as a mechanism for health. For occupational therapists, the division of medical and community services into different aspects of care, according to, say, diagnostic groupings, has further complicated the clarity of the message they need to share with colleagues and community.

Occupational justice

In addressing some of the problems caused by the materialistic, individualistic, and economic focus of the post-medieval world in Britain, social activists inspired some institutional solutions. Perhaps the best known, and deplored, was the establishment of the Poor Law, and later, of workhouses. The intent behind them was commendable and "occupational" in spirit, so it can be questioned what went wrong. One answer might be the same as a previous observation about the lack of holistic understanding of the natural place and purposes of occupation. Other answers might be the emphasis on industriousness rather than meaning, the soul-destroying occupations selected for all and sundry, the obligatory nature of the detention and the work, and lack of attention to encouraging the growth of personal potential.

That scenario leads to the concept of occupational justice, which has emerged from time to time throughout the history. It can be said that whilst some aspects of the Poor Law seemed remarkably generous and far-sighted, other aspects such as the management strategies used in workhouses were far from occupationally just. They used occupation as punishment so that inmates became alienated from their own nature by the system. That deprived them of meaning, purpose, happiness and well-being through their occupations, and prevented them from balancing their mental, social, physical and spiritual needs, and interests. The programmes failed to address the economic issues from a "futures" perspective, in real terms, in that the managers or keepers did not look for, recognise, or attempt to develop individual or communal capacities, and so enable rehabilitation at either level.

That failure occurred despite the enlightened ideas that were being put forward by such people as Locke, Diderot, Hume, Kant, and Voltaire for equality, justice, and liberation from restrictive systems, based on a view of human need for self-expression and the right to happiness and personal fulfilment. Although that was part of an ethos celebrating industriousness, energy, and practical individualism within the thriving agricultural, commercial, and manufacturing sectors, failure was punished by disgrace and destitution.[25]

Occupation, socially, legally or medically prescribed

Although self health remained the basis of health and medical care for many thousands of years, being dominant until the nineteenth century, prescriptive practices at societal, communal and individual levels gradually increased. By the start of the twentieth century prescription was in the ascendant position and occupational therapy as a separate profession arose under that influence as directed by the medical profession. The history though has exposed various types of prescription, which were concerned with occupation and an underlying social, mental, and physical health purpose, which must also be recalled in this summative chapter.

The need for prescription arose as the number and variety of socio-political structures and institutions increased when natural societies developed into agricultural and then industrial ones. Arising with those changes was the need to find different ways of tackling social, mental, and physical issues that caused problems. At first those were more likely to be of a social or communal nature which often had legal ramifications, except for individual providers of medical care whose prescriptions were aimed at individual cure and health maintenance, especially for the more well-to-do. Prescriptive practices then emerged at various levels of society, first as rules to maintain the life and health of citizens by ensuring dominance over warlike neighbours. Later prescriptions focused on behaviours to ensure spiritual salvation. Later again the prescriptions addressed making difficult decisions about how to handle such things as social deviance, aggression, depraved or criminal behaviour, poverty, destitution, dependence, disability and illness. Finally, they were directed towards individual regimes of behaviour to effect change in health status.

Prescriptive practices for health and well-being through occupation are evident, for example, in Sparta's compulsory requirement for its citizens to attend gymnasia for pre-determined periods; in prayer and labour demanded by the medieval church. They are also evident in the requirement for all those who met pre-determined criteria to be subjected to the regime of workhouse life for social, custodial and remedial purposes.

Early prescriptions were often related to apparently obvious notions about occupation being a natural phenomenon. Cooke's 1702 sermon about workhouses being the best charity clearly picked up the idea of the natural health-giving value of occupation as the basis for their establishment and prescription. Readers will recall that he proclaimed that:

> ... *each product of Nature seems industrious by a self conscious Law, and the Labour of each Part is mutual from the expectation of a Reciprical return; so that Nature seems to abhor Idleness, for the same reason that she fears a Dissolution; and the same natural Motive that perswades us to self Preservation, will be sure to instruct our Heads to Project, and our Hands to execute the bussiness of our*

*several Callings, that there may be no Scism in the Body thro' any negligence of
its Members, but each performing its proper Office, the whole may be supported
after the wise design of Nature.*[26]

That idea resonates through prescriptions from many different types of
authorities for many aspects of social, legal, and individual health. John Locke,
for example, recommended that people, as rational creatures, should 'employ
our Faculties about what they are most adapted to, and follow the direction of
Nature, where it seems to point us out the way'. With that idea guiding him, his
prescription was far from what did occur in workhouses or penal institutions,
or, at a later date, in industry. It will be remembered that he recommended that
if people do 'not boldly quarrel with their own Constitution … our proper
Imployment lies in those Enquiries, and in that sort of Knowledge, which is
most suited to our natural Capacities, and carries in it our greatest interest'.[27]

Such understanding of people's occupational nature and needs was
overridden by the power of the economic focus. The material wealth of the few
was to condemn the occupational health of the masses. Although it appears that
there is more understanding of health needs now than in the past, essentially
that remains the case. In the present, the incredibly small percentage of
companies ruling the lifestyles of human populations over the globe means that
there is little change, just a shift from a national to a world population focus. The
material wealth of those few overrides the occupational health needs of many
people by diverting them solely towards economic needs. Wealth, in those cases,
is more important than health; production more important than satisfaction,
happiness, and well-being from using the talents and capacities of each. Such
scenarios imply that occupational therapists will require a very loud voice
indeed to get the message across about the essential links between occupation,
well-being, and health, and totally new strategies to those used in the twentieth
century.

Even well respected activist and vocal entrepreneur William Morris's voice
was listened too for only a short time when he analysed occupations as "good"
or "bad" according to his perceptions of their mental and social health or illness
effects. Readers will recall his explanation that its good effects were threefold, in
that 'worthy work carries with it the hope of pleasure in rest, the hope of the
pleasure in our using what it makes, and the hope of pleasure in our daily
creative skill'. He went on to discuss how hope of pleasure in the work itself
might seem strange to most people even though for:

> *… all living things there is a pleasure in the exercise of their energies, and that
> even beasts rejoice in being lithe and swift and strong. … If we work thus we shall
> be men, and our days will be happy and eventful.*

The lack of appreciation he anticipated was due almost solely to the ill health
giving effects of an economic focus on occupation, as he explained 'all other
work than this is worthless; it is slaves work - mere toiling to live, that we may
live to toil'.[28] On that basis, Morris's prescription argued for occupations that

were purposeful, that is 'directed towards some obviously useful end'; for those which were 'a torment' to be 'much shortened'; for variation and balance between the physical and mental, sedentary and energetic; and for education 'in a socially ordered community' to offer more than 'fitting' people to take their places in 'the hierarchy of commerce'.[29]

Another of the nineteenth century social activists with a prescription for social health was Octavia Hill. Her encouragement of occupation and independence, although prescriptive was tempered with another view recently adopted by occupational therapists, that of enabling clients, and of intervention being client centred. Readers will recall that Hill reminded her helpers of the necessity of remembering that every person has a personal view of his or her own life, 'and must be free to fulfil it'. She argued that as each individual had experienced and felt what others can only see from their own perspective they are the better judges. 'Our work' she said, 'is rather to bring him (or her) to the point of considering, and the spirit of judging rightly, than to consider or judge for him (or her).'[30]

That social prescription which is about enabling rather than imposing is surely true for all people whatever their problems. For some it appears more difficult to act on than others, as is the case for many working with the mentally ill who may take a long time to find their way forward.

Prescription for mental health

Except in European countries, which maintained monasteries that offered sanctuary, communal and legal care for people with mental illness underlay most prescriptions until the advent of mass institutions in the eighteenth and nineteenth centuries. Even after that event, the field of mental health was not a closed shop, and physicians other than those employed in asylums frequently expressed opinions. Especially depression, or melancholia as it was more commonly known, which Cheyne described as 'the English malady', was a subject often addressed by those physicians still interested in health (hygiene) per se. James Johnson was one such and he put forward, as 'the great principle in hygiene', a view that activity of the body was an antidote to depression of the mind.[31] His ideas were in line with the long standing *Regimen Sanitatis*, so it was hardly surprising that he recognised the relationship between occupation and sleep as part of a healthy continuum.

> *Employment tends to induce sleep, without which every attempt at cure is a mockery. In order that the mind may live in a state of efficiency, we must submit to the semblance of death for at least a fourth part of our existence.*[32]

This occupational continuum is an almost forgotten aspect of today's often chaotic temporal lifestyles, and worthy of revisiting in occupational therapy research.

However, as asylums became the focus of care, the primary prescription was detention, if not in those specially designated hospitals, then in workhouse or gaol. Once a resident, and despite the many claims of cure, it does seem that many remained incarcerated for the rest of their lives. That their need for occupation was not immediately apparent seems quite remarkable. The effects of continuous detention in a place in which there was nothing to do must have precipitated many additional illnesses and deaths as well as ensuring little respite from mental disturbances, as remains the case in many places of detention to this day.

It was at that point that some far-sighted physicians, whose profession was assuming dominance in asylums and insanity as an area of medical specialisation, acted as catalysts to bring together the idea of occupation with cure for mental illness. That was to have wide reaching effects, to the extent that occupation became the central focus of curative and maintenance services across most asylums in Britain. Programmes were more extensive than any offered in the twentieth century, and contrary to popular belief they were founded on the notion of therapy rather than economic savings for the institutions. As Kitching, the Superintendent of the Retreat during the 1850s, stated in one of his annual reports 'the introduction of the system of labour into asylums, is not primarily to be contemplated as a means of pecuniary profit, but as a means of promoting the cure and the comfort of the patients'. [33] And, at least, one patient of the period, backed up that professional judgement, when he wrote:

> ... there is an abundance of household work in the asylum which is a thousand times better; indeed, get them to assist the nurses and take an interest in the work of the house, and the cure is begun - and it has been well said that anything well begun is half ended.[34]

Occupational therapists have been heard to reject "maintenance" work within a psychiatric hospital being described as therapy. But, when accounts from that time are considered, the grounds for challenging the practice are less clear cut. Without adequate research to make such a judgement, there may be some truth in the rationale and practice. For example, could self-respect from being part of a workforce of sorts (however poorly remunerated) be more therapeutic to health and well-being, than making or doing something that a therapist recommends, even if that appears to provide meaning? Questions such as that require urgent attention.

Gradually, in line with the industrial materialism evident outside the asylums, the economic focus came to predominate, and the curative effects were largely forgotten in all but a few strongholds. Compounding the process of a decrease in the use of therapeutic occupation was the search, by physicians, for other types of therapy more in line with their training, interests, and control. Coupled with the later preoccupation with discovering curative agents that demonstrate an immediate effect, those factors reduced the extensiveness of occupational treatments until its rediscovery in the next century. Notwithstanding that, its prescription continued in some asylums without break. Montrose hospital, in Scotland, was one such. Its farm, it will be recalled, which started in 1812 with 2 cows, was allowed to remain open on 'condition that its primary purpose was to be seen as providing therapeutic work for the patients' at the time in the 1950s when the Department of Health decreed, in general, the closure of hospital farms.[35,36]

Extensive source material from Pinel and Tuke within this history explained their belief in occupation as a curative agent. Pinel's prescription of occupation increased as his faith in 'pharmaceutic preparations was gradually lessened'. Upholding the "natural health" maxim that 'we cannot cure diseases by the resources of art, if not previously acquainted with their terminations, when left to the unassisted efforts of nature',[37] he attempted to prescribe according to a patient's 'promising inclinations'. His prescriptions had an empirical base drawing as they did upon observation and experience as well as extensive searches of written material. Readers will remember there is nothing cautious about his findings:

> ... in all public asylums as well as in prisons and hospitals, the surest, and, perhaps, the only method of securing health, good order, and good manners, is to carry into decided and habitual execution the natural law of bodily labour, so contributive and essential to human happiness. This truth is especially applicable to lunatic asylums: and I am convinced that no useful and durable establishments of that kind can be founded excepting on the basis of interesting and laborious employment. I am very sure that few lunatics, even in their most furious state, ought to be without some active occupation.[38]

Pinel's research also led him to the observation that the ability and inclination to engage in the everyday occupations of life was a sign of recovery. As he stated in his *Treatise on Insanity*, 'the return of convalescents to their primitive tastes, pursuits, and habits, has always been by me considered as a happy omen of their final complete re-establishment'.[39]

Tuke's prescription, which was equally conclusive, included a combination of physical and mental occupations that had three particular attributes that he believed essential to the therapeutic purpose. You will recall that they were those 'which are accompanied by considerable bodily action; that are most agreeable to the patient, and which are most opposite to the illusions of his disease'.[40] It would, indeed, be fascinating to conduct research into the accuracy of Tuke's beliefs, especially as his last point raises the currently vexed issue of diversional therapy, which is worthy of consideration in the light of its many adherents throughout this history.

Tuke did not prescribe "discussion of their problems" for patients with depressive illness. Indeed, he found that to be 'highly injudicious. The very opposite method is pursued.' He did prescribe every means he could 'to seduce the mind from its favourite but unhappy musings, by bodily exercise, walks, conversation, reading, and other innocent recreations'.[41] He was not alone in believing that cure depended on the patient's mind being diverted from the manifestations of the disease process. The whole notion of Asylums themselves was based on that idea. Admission to them was considered treatment because it provided a place of withdrawal from precipitating factors and the aggravation caused by crazy behaviour.

W.A.F. Browne, it will be recalled, prescribed diversional occupations because of their capacity to arrest attention and engage 'such other powers as are required in the performance of the work' and so make it impossible for the patient to dwell on 'morbid trains of thought which constitute his malady'.[42] Sir William Ellis was another eminent specialist who prescribed that 'when the exciting cause cannot be removed, the patient should be placed in circumstances calculated as much as possible to produce a complete interruption to the train of thought'.[43] Later, in his Treatise, he gave even stronger support when he declared:

> *But so important do I consider diverting the mind by employment, that where the patient cannot be induced thus to occupy himself, or where occupation is too mechanical to keep the mind interested, I do not hesitate, with proper precautions, to intrust him with tools, even where an inclination to suicide or violence exists.*
> *... and it has frequently been the means of the patient's complete recovery*[44]

His belief in the mind being distracted from the "excitation" of the disorder must have been a major influence in his prescribing labour as the principal treatment at Wakefield and Hanwell, and advocating its use in Asylums throughout the country.

At the Retreat the occupational programmes were extended in line with Ellis's ideas. There, readers will remember, Kitching maintained that the patient's programme of occupations was of 'great consequence to the happiness and well-being of all'. He also maintained that "activity or energy" should be 'directed to some satisfactory or productive channel' and that 'the importance of affording occupation to all the patients whose state admits of it, both in a curative and moral point of view, cannot perhaps be over-estimated'.

Those professional views about diversion were backed up by the personal account of a patient written to help fellow sufferers in 1860. He put forward his view that it was 'nearly always ineffectual' to 'attempt to reason anyone out of insane feelings'. Instead he advocated engagement in occupation which kept 'fingers employed at some light and useful labour, if possible in the field or garden' in order to 'divert the current of thought for however short a time from the fiery channel in which it is flowing. (That) must be in every case and under all circumstances beneficial.'[45] That unidentified patient chose the word beneficial to describe the outcome of using occupation in this way. Beneficial – "doing good", stems from the latin – "bene", meaning well. From the same derivation and meaning almost the same thing comes benevolent. That word was also linked with occupation and with justice in Browne's direction for the Crichton Royal Hospital when he became its founding superintendent in 1839.

So occupation was linked with wellness, doing good, and justice within 19th century asylums. It seems appropriate that the final words in this section should be concerned with wellness, with occupation and with justice, as occupational justice to ensure universal health and well-being is an idea which has emerged in occupational therapy during the last decade. Browne's decidedly utopian notions of what asylums ought to be highlighted a vision of 'justice, benevolence, and occupation', which seems a phrase appropriate to adopt across the spectrum of care central to the future of occupational therapy and not just in mental health.

Prescription for physical health

It can be argued that prescriptions for physical health started with the regimens of the classical world based on humoural physiology. The European re-adoption of the classical doctrines of Hippocrates and Galen through Arabic medicine resulted in rules (regimens) of health (Sanitatis) being formulated. Those rules certainly must be the longest surviving prescriptions as, incorporated into the medieval *Regimen Sanitatis Salerno*, the six almost unchanging rules of the "non-naturals" survived into the nineteenth century as the way to maintain health and prevent illness. The standardisation of the rules was so striking that until the Regimen was identified as an entity during the data gathering process of this history, plagiarism seemed alive and well across the centuries.

It will have become clear to readers that the Regimen is central to the history of occupational for health. Rule 2 of the non-naturals encompassed occupation as motion, action, or exercise within primary systems of monastic and secular medical care as a preventive mechanism and as a curative agent. In order to propagate the message the Regimen was provided as individualised prescriptions for the well-to-do; as an integral part of medical textbooks; and as verses for generalised public information.

The rules can be detected in different forms, according to the focus of the expert prescribing them. Pare, for example, a surgeon, described the benefits in fairly mechanical terms as one might expect. He regarded the category of motion as describing occupational exercise such as 'walking, leaping, running, riding, playing at tennis, carrying a burden, and the like'. Its physiological benefits he saw as improved digestion, nourishment, expulsion of wastes, internal cleansing, strengthening of respiration and body-limb function, and increased tolerance.

Cheyne, a physician, provided another version of the same rules for "nervous distemper" in *The English Malady*. He prescribed a regimen of diet and exercise–amusement or entertainment -which 'combine the mind' with 'bodily labour and constant change of air'.[46] Whilst admitting that the kind of exercise was unimportant as long as it included 'continuing actions and motion' which would 'strengthen the solids' he mentioned riding, walking, chaise riding, active games and sports like hunting, shooting, bowls, billiards, and shuttlecock. After sufficient exercise, at the end of the day he further prescribed 'innocent entertaining amusement … to prepare them for their nights rest'.[47]

The ongoing popularity of the Regimen gives rise to the idea that preventive medicine had a higher profile in previous times than was the case in the twentieth century. Lack of effective remedies at that time would have made that good sense. However, it seems that then as now, curative approaches were the more highly valued. Mercurialis during the Renaissance, for example, prescribed "maintenance", "prophylactics" or "Hygiene," as an adjunct to the restoration of health, therapeutics or remedies to cure disease, which in his opinion took pride of place.[48] Like twentieth century occupational therapists, for both preventive and remedial purposes, he prescribed graded activity.[49]

Southwood Smith's holistic vision of medicine, coupled with his highly developed social conscience, resulted in his functional approach to health and activism in matters relating to occupational health. He prescribed with the notion of happiness in mind, along with the development of capacities and longevity. That was based on his belief that 'the object of structure is the production of function' and that 'the sole object of organic life' is 'to maintain it in a condition fit for performing its functions'.[50] In a credo worthy of an occupational therapist, it will be recalled how he described 'pleasure resulting from action of the organs is conducive to their complete development, and thereby to the increase of capacity for affording enjoyment … the perpetuation of their action, and consequently to the maintenance of life'.[51]

By the end of the nineteenth century the prescription of occupation for specific purposes was becoming a reality, within the sphere of physical remedies following illness and in habilitation for the disabled, especially children. The Brabazon scheme, which was started in 1880, for example, consisted of teaching the infirm and crippled to 'employ their idle hands usefully, and in this way "beguile many a weary hour, and add zest to their lives"'.[52] Once again, as in the sphere of mental health, diversion was seen as health giving and remedial.

The prescription of habilitation programmes started, as many health-enhancing movements had before, with initiatives towards providing education for children with disability. The crippled, deaf and blind were particular recipients. Mrs Humphry Ward, the novelist, has been named as a pioneer of the movement, and she became the guiding spirit of the Passmore Edwards

Settlement where the first "play centre" and the first public day school were established for crippled children.[53] The establishment of occupational institutions for the blind was the other major step forward in terms of enabling people with that handicap to engage more fully in everyday life, and to provide for them a wider range of occupational choice than begging, which had been a major employment for many.

Curative prescription of occupation, as distinct from economic considerations, commenced in Edinburgh with Dr Robert Philip when he observed that 'prolonged continuance of resting is fraught with unsatisfactory results' and followed that insight with the establishment of a programme of graduated work 'exactly as we prescribe medicines'. Patients advanced through a programme of therapeutic occupation in a series of classified stages and were rewarded with different coloured badges presumably to ensure the staff's easy identification of under or over activity and perhaps as motivation.[54,55]

John Howard, the philanthropist, has also emerged within the history as a man of great insight, and, perhaps, a founding father of qualitative research. Certainly his observations and meticulous recording of conditions in hospitals and penal institutions noted, possibly for the first time, that acute hospitals had a need for occupational regimes aimed at "daily life" skills, and suitable environments for their implementation. It will be recalled that he observed that 'there are no convalescent wards or sitting rooms, so that patients are often turned out very unfit to work, or the common mode of living.'[56] He also noted access problems at one hospital where 'the staircases are spacious but they are of wood: the rises are too high; and there is no handrail on the wall'.[57]

Perhaps surprising has been the attention given, from time to time in the past, to adaptations to enable mobility and other activities of daily life. What almost appeared to be new inventions in the twentieth century had much earlier prototypes. Examples include using a weighted cushion to stabilise objects, the equivalent of a Nelson knife that George Derenzy devised in the nineteenth century; and the wheeled chairs and specially devised furniture of great beauty and utility fashioned by John Joseph Merlin during the eighteenth century. In similar vein, but both remedial and functional in purpose were the surprisingly modern splints of the surgeon Paré. Such examples seem to give credence to the notion of reinventing the wheel, which may well be true of much of occupational therapy practices for the profession has been fairly negligent in recording or publicising its philosophies, research, and successes.

A last note in this section reflects on the origins of ongoing services for people after acute hospital stays, which can be regarded as the forerunner to rehabilitation. It was as early as the end of the eighteenth century that the need for convalescence became apparent, to allow people to regain their energy and so provide a better chance for them to take up their lifestyles again. Those opportunities are decreasing at present, and research in that sphere may be useful to discover whether or not modern lifestyles have negated the need for such services.

An overview of occupation for health practices throughout history

An overview of the nature of "occupation for health" practices throughout the centuries uncovers the many ways it has been used. Figure 1.12.3 attempts to illustrate different rationales that have been a part of physical, mental, social and spiritual health care over the years. Interestingly there seems to be overlap between most, regardless of the field of care, but particularly between the mental and physical types of occupational intervention, which has been the major focus of occupational therapists in the twentieth century. In contrast, those of a social and spiritual nature that have appeared less prominent since the profession was established appear to run parallel with each other, with little overlap. The lack of programmes in those fields may have less to do with need than the direction in which services have been aimed and positions available, along with cultural mores in line with medicine's focus of approaches.

Figure 1.12.3: Different rationales for occupational intervention within physical, mental, social and spiritual health care over the centuries

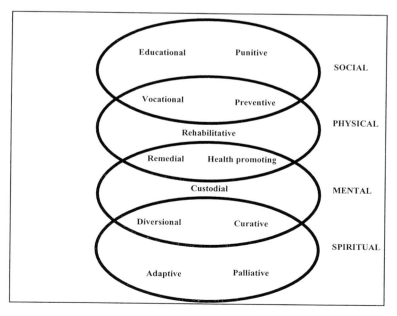

The occupations deemed important throughout time have varied immensely, but those which have seemed to be used more than most for preventive or remedial purposes range from equitation (horse-riding), to walking, gymnastics, picking oakum, farm work, gardening, labouring generally, and listening to or making music. The making of functional objects which are seen as recreational crafts in the present was used in some asylums as therapy but became prominent as part of employment training for people with handicap in the nineteenth century. Craft work, therefore does not appear to have played a long-term significant role in the profession's pre-history, except in so much as making objects such as baskets or pots, and weaving cloth have been, of course, occupations of great significance in the daily lives of people for thousands of years, giving employment and personal development through use of skilled capacities to artisans and many others.

In considering the range of occupations for health used over time, as well as the contexts of their use, a brief return is warranted to the question posed in the introductory chapter about who were the proto-occupational therapists.

Who were the occupational therapists?

Whilst no particular group of people were specifically nominated to theorise, prescribe, provide or enable occupations for health, many different specialists addressed occupation as part of their employment. However, the fact emerged that, just as in other areas of health and social care, the provision of self health was the reality for the masses for most of human existence, as well as being fundamental to later developments. Whilst specialists did emerge from time to time it was not until the narrow focussing of scientific modern health care and social services that it became necessary to create one group of experts who centred on the provision of occupation for health.

The history has identified that individuals themselves, their families, communities and persons of authority within them, such as medicine men, shaman and religious personnel, and many others have advocated and prescribed, or carried out the work at various levels of societies. In some of the Greek States of the Classical period it was the political systems which required a particular regime of occupations to maintain and improve its people's health and strength. From that period the notion of physical exercise and the use of gymnastic occupations emerged as central, and continued to be used. Apart from the state itself, the therapists of classical times were the physicians and the gymnasts, whilst the ideas which gave them credence was put forward by tellers of stories of the gods and adventure sagas, along with notable philosophers and "scientists".

Monks and nuns were the people best qualified to be the occupational therapists of the medieval period because of the spiritual nature of the times which sought the salvation of souls after death in preference to bodily health in the present. They advised, prescribed, sanctioned and enabled all strata of society to engage in charitable and moral occupations along with prayer and pilgrimages for their spiritual well-being and physical labour according to monastic creeds, all of which enhanced, to some extent, their physical and mental health. Nuns continued to provide occupational care, in Ireland throughout the centuries.

Philosophers, physicians, pharmacists, barber-surgeons, lay-practitioners, and literary philanthropists all played a part in new thinking and practices as Renaissance and enlightenment ideas surfaced, and the reformation interfered with or put an end to older models of care. As social health needs became prominent other subsidiary workers became involved in the provision of occupational programmes. Such people had roles as keepers, "basket-men" and attendants in workhouses, gaols and madhouses, others were classified as art-masters when passing on their occupational skills to disadvantaged children in places like Bridewell Hospital–the House of Occupations.

In industrial times social activists, reformers and commentators led the way in focussing attention on the occupational needs of the greater population, whilst some industrialists provided environments which met their ideas of an enlightened and humane view of people's occupational needs. Others put their attention to altering unsatisfactory working conditions.

In asylums, medical personnel, superintendents, attendants, nurses, and others were employed for various duties relating to the occupation of inmates. Pinel and Tuke, who had been the institutors of occupational treatment, only acted as "therapists" spasmodically. Further, although Kitching explained that 'the means of employing and instructing the patients' had 'engaged the ernest attention of the chief officers, and considerable success had attended their efforts', the implementation was mainly left to others who had ongoing and daily contact with patients. Because of that, the importance of engaging people for the job who were kind, had a range of interests and skills, and a good deal of commonsense, was recognised. That some were dedicated to their task is clear from the amazing records kept by James Mason over many years at the Retreat. Those are also testimony to the idea that proto-occupational therapists were part and parcel of the fabric of health care, at least in the nineteenth century.

Attendants such as Mason could not have been successful without the support, or participation of the superintendent or matron, who in that case could be seen to have taken a consultant therapist's role. That notion is supported by a former patient's view, which argued that for occupation to be successfully used in an asylum it had to be 'under the superintendence of a judicious, sympathising person who would regulate the labour to the strength and former habits of the patient'. The same source provided an indication that a participatory approach on the part of the provider was the most effective and therapeutic.[58]

Figure 1.12.4: Proto-occupational therapists throughout time

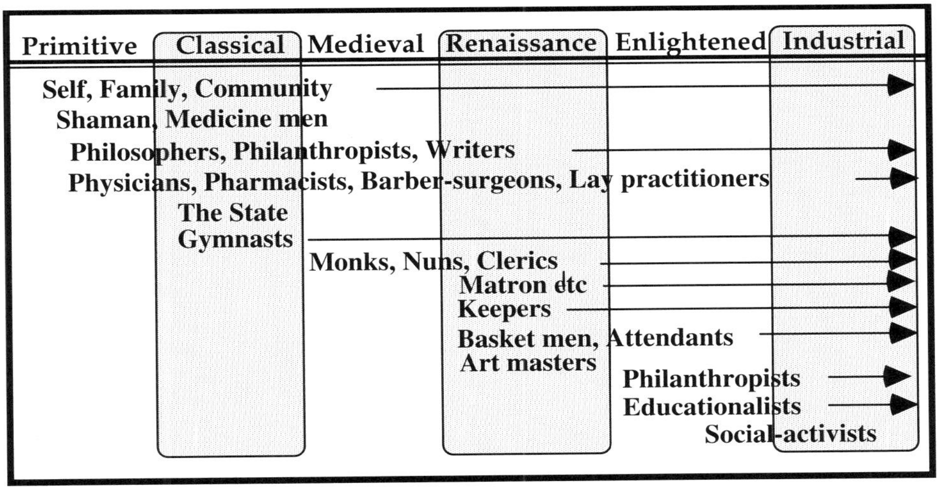

Primitive	Classical	Medieval	Renaissance	Enlightened	Industrial
Self, Family, Community					→
Shaman, Medicine men					
Philosophers, Philanthropists, Writers					→
Physicians, Pharmacists, Barber-surgeons, Lay practitioners					→
The State					→
Gymnasts					→
	Monks, Nuns, Clerics				→
	Matron etc				→
	Keepers				→
	Basket men, Attendants				→
	Art masters				→
			Philanthropists		→
			Educationalists		→
			Social-activists		

Occupation for health ideology

From time to time, some occupation for health ideologies or philosophies were obviously germinating. In classical times, for example, although the socio-cultural context was so different to today, the notion of praxis, mentioned in the introduction, was articulated by prominent philosophers. The idea of humans as praxic beings is remarkably similar to that of humans as occupational beings, and debate still rages about whether praxis is characterised by human activity in all its forms or whether it is one aspect of human nature or action. There is even current disagreement about the extent to which the concept of praxis can be defined or clarified, in similar vein to the attempts being made to define and clarify occupation amongst occupational therapists. Petrovic suggests that, for praxis 'the definitions range from that which treats it simply as the human activity through which man changes the world and himself, to more elaborate ones which introduce the notions of freedom, creativity, universality, history, the future, revolution, etc'.[59] As all of those points can be deemed a potential part of definitions of occupation which could impinge upon the provision and delivery of occupational therapy such ideology from a long past time is still relevant. Occupational scientists studying humans as occupational beings have to take such ideas as those seriously, and if the science becomes a major foundation of the profession they could take occupational therapists well and truly into the political arena. Petrovic argues that if praxis is about 'what human beings really do, then it is evident that there has always been more unfreedom and uncreativity in human history than the converse'. That again raises the notion of occupational justice, and the need to increase awareness generally so that socio-cultural changes aim towards the reduction of occupational deprivation and self-alienation by helping people to reach towards their occupational potential within a humane society which recognises the occupation for health needs of each.

The idea of occupations that were not deemed healthful differed according to context. Of particularly interest are two different versions of occupations that have been viewed as less than human, indeed slaves work! The first was in the classical world when occupations concerned with the physiological requirements of life including much of the creative work of artisans were considered "animal" and so beneath the notice of citizens. It seems a somewhat bizarre notion when war-like occupations were deemed to be worthy of humans. The second was an idea by Morris, referred to earlier, which he developed in response to the soul-destroying effects of industrial work. Morris claimed, in almost direct antithesis to the classical times, that any work that is not creative in nature is slaves work–simply toiling to survive, and surviving only to toil.[60]

The idea of slave's work, in both cases, alludes to the notion that humans have special occupational capacities beyond those of all other animals. However, both pick up different characteristics of occupations as special and distinct from others considered less than human. The two vastly different concepts of what should be the healthful focus of pursuits provide an insight into how even fundamental truths can be seen differently according to the context and specific cultural mores underpinning the perceived needs of human's occupational nature.

Another major occupational idea that has been dominant throughout many centuries, at least in northern climes, is the notion that industriousness is good. That moral judgement is probably founded on the deeper truth about the fundamental relationship between occupation and health. Readers will recall that labour was deemed as important for spiritual health by monastic rule and especially that of St Benedict, which claimed that 'idleness is the enemy of the soul.[61] So for the many hundreds of years of the Middle Ages labour formed a central part of the health providing behaviour of the masses. Whilst some disciplines might take a jaundiced view that it might have been an exploitative ploy on the part of the well-to-do, and there were, obviously, cases in which that was true to the detriment of some people, on the whole it was probably more health-giving than not, for the vast majority.

The idea continued, and it will be remembered that it gained renewed strength in industrial times, when in all probability there was a more than an exploitative element to it in many cases. However physicians were amongst its adherents, and Dr Samuel Smiles is a particular case in point. He raised the notion of industriousness to new heights with his amazingly popular text *Self-Help*.[62] Some of those who were in agreement with his views also linked that occupation for health philosophy with another of considerable importance - namely happiness and well-being.

The notion that happiness was related to health, well-being, and longevity, as well as being the focus and purpose of human life, had been popular from time to time, reaching its zenith in the 18th and 19th centuries. To many battling the physical, mental and social disorders of society the concept might seem a light-hearted and self-centred. Jeremy Benthan's activism, however, which attempted to right a great many of the wrongs according to the creed of Utilitarianism–the greatest happiness for the greatest number of people, suggests that it can be a serious and legitimate creed.[63]

Others who have been central in this history adopted it within the health arena. One such is Thomas Southwood Smith who carried out his occupational health and housing studies as well as his medical practice according to his belief that 'the natural and easy exercise of all the functions' constitutes a 'state of actual pleasure'. 'The usual, the permanent, the natural condition of each organ, and of the entire system, is pleasurable.'[64] In mental health, Sir William Ellis recommended occupational treatment in asylums for the alleviation of suffering to a state of, at least moderate enjoyment, if not happiness.[65]

Such philosophies provide the foundation of modern day occupational therapy. In addition to those ideas, though, are suggestions that a scientific underpinning is also required for people in general to understand it, and for it to be used effectively as therapy.

Locke's argument about what he considered to be the *Division of the Sciences* and the three subsequent research approaches he deemed necessary is particularly exciting. The three sciences he recommended appeared to him to be 'the three great provinces of the intellectual world, wholly separate and distinct one from another'. They included, in closest to modern day terms, biological science, communication science, and occupational science which he called ethics. Readers will recall that he defined science as the means to explore, discover and understand the whys and wherefores of the world as far as it was possible. On this basis, his recommendations were driven by the idea that science should add to knowledge in a way that betters the human experience. In terms of occupational science, which in the modern day explores people as occupational beings, Locke argued for the study of 'all things that can fall within the compass of humane understanding'. In this he included 'that which man himself ought to do, as a rational and voluntary agent, for the attainment of any ends, especially happiness'. That seemed to him to be about 'the things in (peoples) own power, which are (their) own actions, for the attainment of (their) own ends' and 'actions as they depend on us, in order to happiness'.[66]

Pinel, amongst others, in a different vein but in particular reference to therapy, recognised the complexity of using occupation as treatment when he argued for appropriate research and attention. He said, about the provision of occupation that 'a physician can never be too vigilant; nor to encourage them (the patients), too studious of the means of indulgence (the occupations used)'.[67]

The indication that earlier authorities recognised the need for rigorous study of the uses of occupation for health ties in with the directions posed in the twentieth century by the American founders. Their initial objectives called for 'the study of the effect of occupation upon the human being; and the scientific dispensation of this knowledge' as well as 'the advancement of occupation as a therapeutic measure'.[68]

Figure 1.12.5: **Issues that have been addressed in the first volume of the history of occupation for health**

PERIOD	THERAPIST	PURPOSE OF OCCUPATION	FOCUS OF HEALTH & WELL-BEING
Primitive	Self, family, community, shaman, etc	Survival, self-care, individual, communal	Physical, mental, social, spiritual
Classical	The state, writers, philosophers, physicians	Political, health-promotion, philosophical, industrial, communal	Physical, mental
Medieval	Monks, nuns, self, families	Industrial, palliative, self-care, remedial	Spiritual
Renaissance	The Crown, self, families, parishes, physicians, etc	Political, communal employment, self-care palliative, preventive	Social, physical
Enlightenment	Self, physicians etc, madhouse proprietors, keepers	Preventive, industrial, curative, employment, custodial, philosophical, educational	Physical, mental
Industrial	Socio-industrial activists, writers, physicians etc, attendants	Political, economic, punishment, communal, curative, industrial, educational, employment, preventive, adaptive	Mental, social, physical

In this summative chapter the history of occupational regimes for health up to the twentieth century have been woven together. Particular aspects of the past have been revisited to provide an overall picture from which readers may consider twentieth century developments as well as, ultimately, directions for the future. The monumental differences between both philosophies and practices which have occurred with the evolution of civilisation may help the profession and others to recognise the part played by contexts, beliefs, socio-cultural mores, and technologies, as well as advances in knowledge.

Because of the fundamental nature of occupation across the broad spectrum of the everyday lives of all people, whatever their socio-cultural and environmental context, it has been extremely complex to appreciate the scope of the practice of occupation for health prior to the advent of occupational therapy as a profession. To do so has called for an approach unbiased by present day ideas and practices. Getting to that point took time, and it may be that some readers find that a similar open way of considering the material will be necessary. If that can be done, the history may provide a start to recognition of the many ways occupation has been instrumental in effecting change in physical, mental, social, and spiritual health. In turn that may encourage a greater range of questions, research and initiatives to facilitate growth and direction based on in depth and investigative practices.

If that proves to be the case it may encourage others along the path of using history as a method of serious investigation which can inform the present and future as other qualitative research does. Indeed, there are many topics in the history which beg further and closer investigation, and stories to be told which have not been uncovered here. Even though that might be the case, the many extracts, which ensure that the history can be used as a source book may assist future researchers to start their investigations more expediently.

A personal vision for the future of occupational therapy has emerged, in part, as a result of exploring its pre-twentieth century history. That vision is a world in which the different occupational natures of all individuals, whether disabled or not, is recognised in a just and equitable way because occupation is recognised generally as a major, natural mechanism for health, happiness and well-being. When socio-cultural contexts counter the meeting of people's occupational nature, ill health is almost inevitable. Those facts are too poorly appreciated within the socio-economic, political and medical world, as well as populations in general, at the present time. That means that occupational therapists need to return to their illness-preventive and health promoting roots, which were articulated in the long history of the *Regimen Sanitatis*. The profession could even learn from the methods by which that was promulgated as part of health literature, and for both individuals and the population generally through appropriate use of modern media. Changes of understanding are possible. Witness the many variations and uses occupation for health has undergone over the centuries. Most are still valuable, and collectively those ideas would provide powerful support for expanding services appropriately to meet people's health needs.

Self health has proved to be a major part of the profession's history, and that is appropriate as occupational therapists hold dear the notion of helping people to help themselves, of enabling their independence and potential and ultimately of finding their own way forward. Prescriptive practices that circumscribed practice did not appear till late in the piece, and it will be interesting to follow the fortunes of that factor in the next volume.

[1]Kass LR. Regarding the end of medicine and the pursuit of health. In: Caplan AR, Engelhart HT, McCartney JJ, eds. Concepts of Health and Disease: Interdisciplinary Perspectives. Massachusetts: Addison Wesley Publishing Co., 1981.

[2]Certificate of Incorporation of the National Society for the Promotion of Occupational Therapy, Inc. 1917. Then and Now: 1917-1976. Rockville, MD: American Occupational Therapy Association, 1967; 4-5.

[3]The Asian NGO Coalition, IRED Asia. The people centred development forum. Economy, Ecology and Spirituality: Toward a Theory and Practice of Sustainability 1993; Potter VR. Bioethics, the science of survival. Biology and Medicine 1970; 14: 127-153.

[4]Agius T. Aboriginal health in Aboriginal hands. In: Fuller J, Barclay J, Zollo J, editors. Multicultural Health Care in South Australia. Conference proceedings Adelaide: Painters Prints, 1993; 23.

[5]Burton R. The Anatomy of Melancholy. Oxford: Printed for Henry Cripps, 1651; 266-267.

[6]Burton. The Anatomy of Melancholy…; 266.

[7]Cheyne G. Essay of Health and Long Life. London and Bath: Strahan, 1724; 89-91.

[8]Porter R. The Greatest Benefit to Mankind: A Medical History of Humanity from Antiquity to the Present. Harper Collins (first published 1997) Paper back edition, 1999; 110.

[9]Yates N. Victorian values: Pugin and the medieval dream. History Today. September 1987; 33-40.

[10]Morris W. Useful work versus useless toil. In: Cole. GDH, ed. Centenary Edition. William Morris. Stories in Prose. Stories in Verse. Shorter Poems. Lectures and Essays. New York: Edited for Nonesuch Press, Bloomsbury. Random House, 1934; 603-604.

[11]Carlyle T. Past & Present: Work. 1843. In: Knight C. Half Hours with the Best Authors. London: Frederick Warne & Co.; 220.

[12]Houghton W. Cited in: Guy Rev Dr. JR. Compassion and the Art of the Possible: Dr. Southwood Smith as Social Reformer and Public Health Pioneer. Octavia Hill Memorial Lecture. December 1993. Cambridgeshire: Octavia Hill Society & The Birthplace Museum Trust, 1996; 5.

[13]Hardy D, Davidson L, eds. Utopian Thought and Communal Experience. Geography and Management Paper No. 24, Middlesex University, 1989.

[14]Dubos R. Mirage of Health. New York: Harper & Rowe, 1959.

[15]Kumar K. Utopian thought and communal practice: Robert Owen and the Owenite communities. In: Hardy D, Davidson L, eds. Utopian Thought and Communal Experience…; 17-36.

[16]Georgii A. ed. Ling's Educational and Curative Exercises. London: Renshaw, 1875; 9.

[17]More T. Utopia. (first published 1516). Abridged edition. London: Phoenix, 1996; 16-17.

[18]Wilcock AA. Occupational Utopias: Back to the future. Journal of Occupational Science 2001; 1(1): 6-13.

[19]Utopian socialism. In: Bottomore T, ed. A Dictionary of Marxist Thought, 2nd revised ed. Oxford: Blackwell, 1991; 561-2.

[20]Owen R. The address to the inhabitants of New Lanark. The Institute for the Formation of Character. January 1st 1816. In: Owen R. Works of Robert Owen: Volume 1 (Pickering Masters Series). London: Pickering & Chatto Publishers Ltd., 1993; 120-142.

[21]Owen R. Works of Robert Owen: Volume 3: Book of the New Moral World. (Pickering Masters Series). London: Pickering & Chatto (Publishers Ltd.), 1993; 156.

[22]Hill CS. Memoranda of Observations and Experiments in Education. London: Vizetelly & Co., 1865; 15, 27.

[23]Whelan R, ed. Octavia Hill and the Social Housing Debate: Essays and Letters by Octavia Hill. (First published in MacMillans Magazine, July 1869.) London: IEA Health and Welfare Unit, 1998; 3-4.

[24]Hill. Cited in: Whelan. Octavia Hill and the Social Housing Debate...; 6.

[25]Porter D, Porter R. Patient's Progress: Doctors and Doctoring in 18th Century England. Cambridge: Polity Press, 1989; 7-8.

[26]Cooke T. Work-Houses the Best Charity: A Sermon Preacht at the Cathedral Church of Worcester, February 2d 1702. By Thomas Cooke Master of Arts, and Rector of St Nicholas in the City of Worcester. Published at the Request of the Mayor and Aldermen. London (Printed for John Butler, Bookseller in Worcester, and sold by most Booksellers in London and Westminster, 1702; 7.

[27]Locke J. An Essay Concerning Humane Understanding. London: Printed for Tho, Basset, and sold by Edw. Mory at the sign of the Three Bibles in St Paul's Church-Yard. MDCXC; 327.

[28]Morris. Useful work versus useless toil. In: Cole...; 604-605.

[29]Morris. Useful work versus useless toil. In: Cole...; 616.

[30]Hill O. Four years management of a London Court. In: Whelan. Octavia Hill and the Social Housing Debate...; 64.

[31]Johnson J. The Economy of Health or the Stream of Human Life. 2nd ed. London: S. Highley, 1837.

[32]Unknown Author. The Philosophy of Insanity. 1860 (with introduction by Frieda Fromm-Reichmann M.D.) London and New York: The Fireside Press, 1947; 70.

[33]Tuke S. 1841. In: Russell JI. The Occupational Treatment of Mental Illness. London: Bailliere, Tindall & Cox, 1938; v-vi.

[34]Unknown Author. The Philosophy of Insanity...; 70.

[35]Presly AS. A Sunnyside Chronicle 1781-1981: A History of Sunnyside Royal Hospital, Produced for its Bicentenary, 1981; 44.

[36]Presly. A Sunnyside Chronicle 1781-1981...; 43.

[37]Pinel P. A Treatise on Insanity. Translated from the French by D. D. Davis. Sheffield: Printed by W Todd, for Messrs. Cadell and Davies, Strand, London, 1806; Footnote; 108-9.

[38]Pinel. A Treatise on Insanity...; 216.

[39]Pinel. A Treatise on Insanity...; Footnote, 216-18.

[40]Tuke S. Description of the Retreat: An Institution near York for Insane Persons of the Society of Friends Containing an Account of its Origin and Progress, the Modes of Treatment, and a Statement of Cases. York: Printed by W Alexander, and sold by him; also sold by M.M. and E. Webb, Bristol: and by Harvey, and Co; William Phillips; and W. Darton, London, 1813; 156.

[41]Tuke. Description of the Retreat...; 151.

[42]Poole R. Memoranda Regarding the Royal Lunatic Asylum of Montrose. Edinburgh: Black, and London: Longmans, 1841.

[43]Ellis Sir WC. A Treatise on the Nature, Symptoms, Causes and Treatment of Insanity, with Practical Observations on Lunatic Asylums and a Description of the Pauper Lunatic Asylum for the County of Middlesex, at Hanwell, with a Detailed Account of its Management. London: Samuel Holdsworth, 1838; 190.

[44]Ellis. A Treatise on the Nature, Symptoms, Causes and Treatment of Insanity...; 196-197.

[45]Unknown Author. The Philosophy of Insanity...; 70.

[46]Cheyne G. The English Malady: Or a Treatise of Nervous Diseases of all Kinds. London: Strahan and Leake, 1733; 177.

[47]Cheyne. The English Malady...; 180-181.

[48]Blundell JWF. The Muscles and their Story from the Earliest Times (an Adaptation of the 'Ars Gymnastica') including the Whole Text of Mercurialis, and the Opinions of other Writers Ancient and Modern on Mental and Bodily Development. London: Chapman & Hall, 1864; 34-36.

[49]Macdonald EM. World-Wide Conquests of Disabilities: The History, Development and Present Functions of the Remedial Services. London: Bailliere Tindall, 1981; 64.

[50]Southwood Smith T. The Philosophy of Health; Or an Exposition of the Physical and Mental Constitution of Man, With a View to the Promotion of Human Longevity and Happiness. Volume 1. London: Charles Knight. MDCCCXXXVI 1836-7; 73.

[51]Southwood Smith. The Philosophy of Health...; 75.

[52]Marr HC. Journal of Mental Science. July 1899.

[53]Watson F. Civilization and the Cripple. London: John Bale, Sons & Danielson, Ltd., 1930; 32.

[54]Groundes-Peace ZC. An outline of the development of occupational therapy in Scotland. The Scottish Journal of Occupational Therapy 1957, (30): 16-39.

[55]Philip R. Collected Papers on Tuberculosis. London: Humphrey Milford: Oxford University Press, 1937; 133-134. Originally published as: Rest and Movement in Tuberculosis. British Medical Journal, 24th December, 1910.

[56]Howard. J. An Account of the Principal Lazarettos in Europe; With Varios Papers Relative to the Plague: Together With further Observations on Some Foreign Prisons and Hospitals; And Additonal Remarks on the Present State of those in Great Britain and Ireland. Warrington: Printed by William Eyres MDCC LXXXIX. 1789; 140-142.

[57]Howard. An Account of the Principal Lazarettos in Europe...; 180.

[58]Unknown Author. The Philosophy of Insanity...; 70-72.

[59]Petrovic G. Praxis. In: Bottomore T, ed. A Dictionary of Marxist Thought...; 435-440.

[60]Morris. Useful work versus useless toil...; 604-605.

[61]Benedictine Rule. Cited in: Bettenson HS, ed. Documents of the Christian Church. New York: Springer, 1963.

[62]Smiles S. Self-Help: With Illustrations of Character and Conduct. London: John Murray, 1859.

[63]Bentham J. An introduction to the principle of morals and legislation. 1789. In: Burns JH, Hart HLA, eds. The Collected Works of Jeremy Bentham. Oxford: Clarendon, 1996.

[64]Southwood Smith. The Philosophy of Health...; 75.

[65]Ellis. A Treatise on the Nature, Symptoms, Causes and Treatment of Insanity...; Preface, v-vii.

[66]Locke. An Essay Concerning Humane Understanding...; 361-362.

[67]Pinel. A Treatise on Insanity... ; 25.

[68]Certificate of Incorporation of the National Society...; 4-5.

Legends of Frontispieces

The frontispieces provide a conceptual map of the material within the volume or chapter. They are encased in material illustrative of the social fabric of the times. Often that material is based on sections of art work of, or depicting the period.

Volume Frontispiece

The main frontispiece of each volume is based on the wonderful sepia frontispiece of Robert Burton's 17th century *Anatomy of Melancholy* which is pictured in chapter 5 of this volume: *The Renaissance, Humanism and Beyond: Occupational Regimes for Social and Mental Health* .

The collage for this volume illustrates, different aspects of occupation for health in different periods in history linked with the current British Association badge, and the early badges of English and Scottish Occupational Therapy Associations. The classical gods represent Asclepius, the god of medicine, and Hygiea, the goddess of health. Other representations include David playing the harp to sooth Saul with music; the occupations of the four seasons from early depictions of the Regimen Sanitatis, the six rules for health, which over the centuries maintained occupation, as action and rest as one of them; Chaucer riding his horse on a pilgrimage; disabled beggars earning their livelihood with drawings and lute playing; children dancing as part the social health initiatives at the industrial community of New Lanark; and a blind child in the nineteenth century being enabled to learn knitting.

Sketches after: G Hunt, Robert Owen's School at New Lanark, 1825, (New Lanark Conservation); Ellesmere Manuscript of the Canterbury Tales; Hieronymous Cock (1520-1570): Beggars; Dr Guillie, An Essay on Instructions and Amusments of the Blind, 1819; J. Curio's Regimen Sanitatis Salernitanum, (German edition of 1568. In: Croke 1830)

Chapter 2

The collage encapsulates the simple health giving occupations of a natural lifestyle. It includes an allusion to animal's and people's altruistic nature which was a necessary precursor to the evolution of any 'caring' profession. To the right, Eve suckles a child as Adam, with Death as his companion, tills the soil after being expelled from Eden and condemned to a life of occupational toil in order to survive. Within the conceptual map itself a sketch of an ancient Egyptian man with apparent disability and walking aid symbolises the religious based medical practice which was dominant for thousands of years.

Sketches after: John Richards, in: Burenhult G. The First Humans. The Illustrated History of Humankind. Hong Kong: University of Queensland, 1993; Frans De Waal photo in: De Waal F. Good Natured. The Origins of Right and Wrong in Humans and Other Animals. Cambridge: Harvard University Press, 1996; a Stele of XVIIIth Dynasty (Carlsberg Glyptothek at Copenhagen); Adam tills the Soil, a woodcut by Hans Holbein, 1530 (Wellcome Library).

Chapter 3

This collage depicts the ordered classical world of Greco-Roman citizens. An illustration of Socrates teaching pupils has been chosen to depict one of the occupations carried out in gymnasia, which multipurpose places of occupational health replaced many activities of daily living which were considered beneath humanness. Those were provided by slaves and conquered peoples, shown here as upholding the citizens way of life. Two giants of modern medicine, Hippocrates and Celsus, look down from the columns.

Sketches after: a relief of Socrates and his pupils (British Museum); reliefs: Banqueting Scene & Preparation in the Kitchen. 3rd century AD. (Tier Museum Neumahen); A Roman Farmer Milking a Goat. 4th century AD. (Museo della Civilta Romana, Rome); A Pharmacy, where Soap is Being Made (Uffizi Gallery, Florence); Harter J. Images of Medicine. NY: Bonzana Books, 1991.

Chapter 4

The border collage represents detailed and elaborate medieval manuscripts. They were, in the main, the work of monks and clerics, executed in monasteries who also provided the majority of health care. Within the conceptual map, monastic medicine is encased in a sketch of part of a Benedictine monastery. Pilgrimage was a frequent occupation for health of the period.

Sketches after: The Gospel of St. Luke. French 1000AD. (Pierpont Morgan Library, New York); The Annunciation. Bruges or Ghent, Late C15 and The Wedding Feast at Cana. Queen Mary's Psalter, Early C14, (British library); Walter Crane. in: Edmund Spenser's Fairie Queene (Victoria and Albert Museum); Ellesmere Manuscript of the Canterbury Tales; Monastery of Saint-Riquier, (Courtauld Institute of Art).

Frontispiece Chapter 5

Leonardo da Vinci is often considered a symbol of the renaissance. His simple

design of man set within a square and a circle, has been elongated for effect within this frontispiece. It was chosen and adapted to characterise the new spirit of individualism, creativity, and development which epitomised the time.

Illustration after Leonardo da Vinci.

Frontispiece Chapter 6

The collage of Tudor interior with 'renaissance man', fascinated by learning, and gesturing to the books in his library to indicate the new world that was opening up to scholars is set within splendid architecture of the Vatican Library.

Sketches after: J. Nash; G. M. Mitelli's Renaissance Man c.1700. (Wellcome Library); Melozzo da Forli's Foundation of the Vatican Library.

Frontispieces Chapter 7 and Chapter 8.

The Enlightenment collages are created with selected images of Hogarth. They provide contemporary scenes of business, exuberance, individuality, and creativity, as well as public and individual health horrors. Chapter 7 frontispiece features a few of the many people with physical disability that Hogarth depicted in his works. Chapter 8 frontispiece features a weaving and spinning factory to the right; one of his images of idleness and industry as a suspended business sign; and a group of young people enjoying what would be regarded as depraved occupation, possibly worthy of social rehabilitation in Bridewell.

Sketches after William Hogarth, 1697-1764.

Frontispiece Chapter 9

The collage for this chapter incorporates the mill at New Lanark set amongst the glorious countryside illustrating the suddenness of the lifestyle transformations from agriculture to industry for the majority of people. At the forefront are fragments of two images, the first relating to the Peterloo Massacre as a symbolic illustration of worker's powerlessness, and the second to the occupational deprivation of well-to-do women who were restricted to only a few genteel activities.

Sketches after New Lanark (New Lanark Trust); Mrs Henry McKarness, The Young Lady's Book. 1876, (Routledge); Cruikshank's Peterloo Massacre, (Mansell Collection).

Frontispiece Chapter 10

Set against a picture representing the transition from country to industry the inset collage represents the Victorian tradition of establishing large institutions, in this case, for the treatment of the sick. An outpatient's scene - receiving day at London Hospital, when patients wait quietly to see the surgeon, is combined with an engraving of the Hospital from the century before. The hospital is set between two symbols which appear appropriate to this history. One is the caduceus, the staff of Mercury, representing trade or the arts, and the other, the staff of Aesculepius, representing medicine.

The London Hospital, Whitechapel, receiving day for outpatients. Process Print after W.W. Russell. c. 1896. The London Hospital. Engraving. (Wellcome library).

Frontispiece Chapter 11

A collage of mental hospital buildings and patient's occupations, vocational, recreational and creative, are set on a background of a William Morris fabric design.

Bethlem Royal Hospital, Richard Dadd, artist and patient & ladies playing croquet, (The Bethlem Royal Hospital); Montrose Asylum 1840; A prize cow from the Montrose therapeutic farm. (Presly. A Sunnyside Chronicle' 1781-1981); The Farm of Crichton Royal Hospital,1894- behind Montrose's cow (Williams. History of Crichton Royal Hospital) Glasgow Lunatic Asylum (Andrews & Smith. Let There Be Light Again).

Frontispiece Chapter 12

The Victorian staircase used as a background to the last of the conceptual maps in this volume represents the gradual growth of knowledge throughout the centuries, and the window, a glimmering of understanding which was to lead to the development of a profession concerned with occupation for health. The collection of portraits on either side are of important figures in the development. Their stories have been told, or their work examined within previous chapters.

The central hallway, somewhat elongated: The Cedars, Derby School of Occupational Therapy; Portraits: (Wellcome Library & National Portrait Gallery).

Index

Indexer: Dr Laurence Errington

Abbreviations: OT, occupational therapy.

A

Aberdeen Royal Asylum, 507-8
Account of the Principal Lazarettos in Europe, 240
Ackroyd, Edward, 348
Acts (of British law)
    Act of 1349, 145
    Act of 1536, 146
    Act of 1563, 146
    Act of 1601 (Poor Law), 144-5, 145-8
    Factory Act (1833), 410, 411
    Lunacy (Scotland) Act (1857), 490
    Medical Act (1858), 401
    mining/colliery work (1842), 413
    public health acts (19th C), 406
    Vagrancy Act (1744), 301
    Workhouse Test Act (1723), 231
    see also Law
Acts, cooperative living, 34
Actuarius, 114
Adam and Eve, 30-1
    Cheyne's reference to, 267
Addams, Jane, 386, 388-90
Addison, Joseph, 236-7
Address to Persons of Quality and Estate, Ways and Methods of Doing Good, 226
Aegineta, Paulus, 102, 115
Aesculapius, 63-4, 75-6
Aetius of Almeda, 101-2
Africanus, Constantinus, 118-19
Age of Reason, *see* Enlightenment
Agricola, Georgius, 187-8
Agriculture/farming/gardening
    Gartnavel asylum, 491
    Perth asylum, 508
    the Retreat, 469
    see also Outdoor work
Aids and devices
    disabled (mobility aids etc.)
        Enlightenment, 271-4
        industrial era, 440-6, 551
        Renaissance, mobility, 211-14
    orthopaedic, Paré's, 204-5

    see also Prostheses; Splints
Aiken, John, 408
Airs, Waters and Places, 81
Alexander the Great and Aristotle, 74
Alienation, Marx on, 365-6
Alimentary (digestive) system, Galen's ideas, 87
Allen, Katherine, 317
Allen, William, 352, 354
Almshouses, 166
Alphanus, 118
Altruism, early humans, 24-5
America, moral treatment, 517-19
Amputee, prostheses, 90
Amsterdam, madhouse, 329
Anatomy, Renaissance studies, 181-2
Anatomy of Melancholy, 88, 532
Ancient civilisations, 40-7
    Greco-Roman times, *see* Classical times
    see also specific civilisations
Ancients, the, stories of, 22-3
Andre, Nicholas, 182, 201, 248
Anglicus, Gilbertus, 116
Animals
    behaviour of (ethology), 25, 26
    as therapy (mental illness), 457
Aphorisms
    Celsus, 84-5
    Hippocrates, 80, 81, 82
Apollo, 62
Apothecaries
    Enlightenment, 247
    Renaissance, 178
Arabic physicians, 101-2, 532
Archer, John, 265
Aristotle, 73-5, 129
Arm injuries, Tissot's recommendations, 275-6
Armstrong, George, 248
Armstrong, John, 270-1
Arnold, Thomas, 470-1
Art and Socialism, 373
Art of Preserving Health, 270-1
Arts and Crafts Movement, 368, 369, 371, 377, 533, 534, 539
Arts and Crafts Society, 389
Asclepiades, 82-3